NOBEL LECTURES

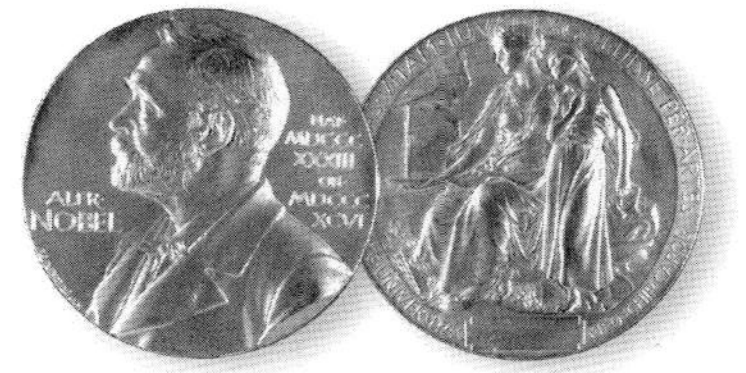

PHYSIOLOGY OR MEDICINE

2011–2015

Nobel Lectures

Including Presentation Speeches and Laureates' Biographies

Physics

Chemistry

Physiology or Medicine

Economic Sciences

NOBEL LECTURES

INCLUDING PRESENTATION SPEECHES
AND LAUREATES' BIOGRAPHIES

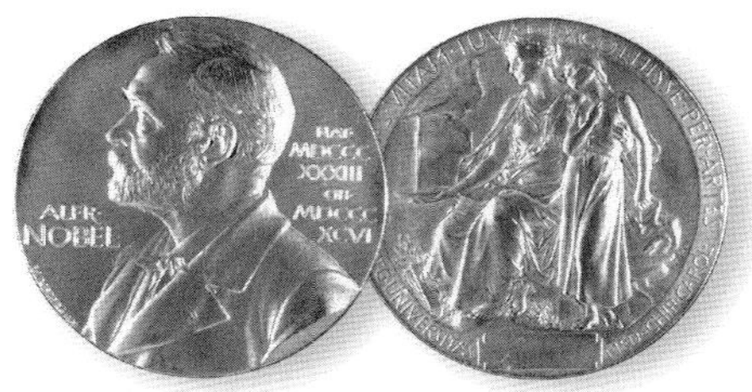

PHYSIOLOGY
OR
MEDICINE

2011–2015

EDITOR

Bo Angelin
Karolinska Institutet, Sweden

World Scientific

NEW JERSEY • LONDON • SINGAPORE • BEIJING • SHANGHAI • HONG KONG • TAIPEI • CHENNAI • TOKYO

Published by

World Scientific Publishing Co. Pte. Ltd.
5 Toh Tuck Link, Singapore 596224
USA office: 27 Warren Street, Suite 401-402, Hackensack, NJ 07601
UK office: 57 Shelton Street, Covent Garden, London WC2H 9HE

NOBEL LECTURES IN PHYSIOLOGY OR MEDICINE (2011–2015)

ISBN 978-981-124-558-9 (hardcover)
ISBN 978-981-124-682-1 (paperback)
ISBN 978-981-124-559-6 (ebook for institutions)
ISBN 978-981-124-560-2 (ebook for individuals)

For any available supplementary material, please visit
https://www.worldscientific.com/worldscibooks/10.1142/12510#t=suppl

Printed in Singapore

PREFACE

In this volume, great discoveries in Physiology or Medicine are presented based on the Nobel Prizes awarded in this field for the years 2011–2015. They represent the wide area of science related to the understanding of human biology in health and disease, and to the development of novel therapies. In addition to their lectures, the Laureates have also provided biographical sketches describing their life histories and their development as scientists. The introductory speeches given at the Prize ceremonies by representatives of the Prize-awarding Nobel Assembly at Karolinska Institutet summarize the ground-breaking discoveries which were:

- "the activation of innate immunity" to Bruce A. Beutler and Jules A. Hoffmann, who identified the gatekeepers of the immune system, and "the dendritic cell and its role in adaptive immunity" to Ralph M. Steinman, who described how the second line of immune defence is activated — in 2011. Their work resolved major questions regarding how the body is protected from infections, and has led to important advances by providing new tools to combat also other diseases such as cancer and inflammation.
- "that mature cells can be reprogrammed to become pluripotent" to Sir John B. Gurdon and Shinya Yamanaka — in 2012. Their work demonstrated that it is possible to unlock the differentiated state and allow mature cells to regain an immature state from which all types of cells can be derived. The possibility to engineer such stem cells has opened completely new avenues for development of diagnosis and therapy.
- "machinery regulating vesicle traffic, a major transport system in our cells" to James E. Rothman, Randy W. Schekman and Thomas C. Südhof — in 2013. Their work explained how molecules are positioned in cells with extraordinary precision, and how they can be packaged in vesicles for controlled transport both within and from the cells, knowledge that is of great importance both for diagnosis and therapy of many disease entities.

- "cells that constitute a positioning system in the brain" by John O'Keefe, May-Britt Moser and Edvard I. Moser — in 2014. Their work identified groups of cells in the brain which provide navigating systems making it possible for us to define orientation and movement (an internal "GPS"), a paramount basis also for the development of higher brain functions such as memory and cognition.
- "a novel therapy against infections caused by roundworm parasites" by William C. Campbell and Satoshi Ōmura, and "a novel therapy against Malaria" by Tu Youyou — in 2015. Their unique work was based on finding bioactive substances in extracts from bacteria in soil (Ivermectin) or from plants known from Chinese folk medicine (Artemisin) that could be shown to be effective in human diseases caused by parasite infections such as river blindness and malaria. The availability of these drugs has led to major improvements in global health.

According to the will of Alfred Nobel, all the Prizes to be awarded are to be given to "those who, during the preceding year, have conferred the greatest benefit to humankind". The Prize in Physiology or Medicine should be given to "the person who made the most important discovery within the domain". It is of relevance that the exact wording is different for Physics ("discovery or invention") and Chemistry ("discovery or improvement"). While these scientific prizes may be given for two separate discoveries, they cannot be shared by more than three persons each year; they are also not given posthumously. However, a unique situation occurred in the year 2011. While it was known that Ralph Steinman suffered from malignant disease since several years, the information that he had passed away 3 days before the decision-making meeting of the Nobel Assembly was not known at that time. After consultations with the Nobel Foundation, it was decided that he should receive the Prize as already announced. The lecture concerning his Prize was presented by his long-term collaborator Michel C. Nussenzweig; the Prize was received by his wife Claudia.

The wide range of scientific achievements in Physiology or Medicine is obvious from the varying discoveries awarded during these years. Even if the identification of the critical persons involved in making a "discovery" may sometimes be difficult, Nobel's vision to identify and award individuals making "paradigm-shifting" research remains a unique and challenging aspect of these Prizes, also considering the increasing role of large-scale collaborations in medical science. As always, it is also fascinating to take part of the personal histories of the Laureates. While each one is obviously unique, some themes seem to recur irrespective of background: an early interest in natural science, great curiosity, and some stubbornness together with sheer joy in finding solutions. The importance of being stimulated by teachers/mentors, both at an early stage and when choosing a more definite path for scientific work, also seems to be of high relevance for future success.

Bo Angelin
Senior Professor of Clinical Metabolic Research
Former Chairman of the Nobel Assembly and the Nobel Committee

CONTENTS

Physiology or Medicine 2011

Bruce A. Beutler and Jules A. Hoffmann

"for their discoveries concerning the activation of innate immunity"

Ralph M. Steinman

"for his discovery of the dendritic cell and its role in adaptive immunity"

The Nobel Prize in Physiology or Medicine

Speech by Professor Göran K. Hansson of the Nobel Assembly at Karolinska Institutet.

Your Majesties, Your Royal Highnesses, Honoured Nobel Laureates, Ladies and Gentlemen,

We live in a dangerous world. During the hour you spend here in the Concert Hall, you will be exchanging millions of bacteria and viruses with each other. Fortunately, you are equipped with a strong defence, and we do not expect that this hour will lead to any significant reduction of our guest list.

This defence constitutes our immunological protection against bacteria, viruses and other microorganisms. It consists of two lines of defence: the first one stops the invaders and the second one eliminates them.

Much research has been focused on the second line of defence with its antibodies and killer cells. But a major question remained unanswered: How can we survive an infection until antibodies have been formed? It can take several weeks before the antibody levels are sufficient, and by then we may already have recovered from our infected wound or our common cold. The first line of the immune defence, which is also called innate immunity, must have recognised and stopped the bacteria long before the antibodies had arrived on the scene.

Jules Hoffmann went on a quest to reveal the secrets of the first line of defence. He knew that insects lack the second line of defence, and therefore chose fruit flies as his research model. It turned out that flies with defects in a gene called Toll could not combat infections successfully. Hoffmann and his colleagues were able to unravel a detector system involving Toll that is activated by molecules derived from microorganisms, leading to mobilisation of the immune defence against the intruders. Thanks to Hoffmann's discovery, the sensors of the first line of host defence were finally identified.

Bruce Beutler was searching for the solution to another problem. He wanted to understand how bacteria such as Salmonella can elicit a life-threatening septic shock – what used to be called blood poisoning. By comparing the genome of different mouse strains, he could demonstrate that a single gene initiated the shock reaction. This gene turned out to be the mammalian counterpart of Toll, and it encodes a receptor that serves as a sensor on the cell surface. When bacterial components bind to this receptor, the immune system is activated, and antibacterial defence mechanisms are mobilised.

Thanks to Beutler's discovery, we understood how the sensors of the innate immune system operate to recognise infectious agents. Together, the two Nobel Laureates had clarified how the first line of defence is mobilised.

In parallel with these discoveries, Ralph Steinman was studying the activation of the second line of defence, which is also called adaptive immunity. More than 30 years ago, he isolated a new cell type called the dendritic cell. Through systematic research, he showed that dendritic cells patrol the organs searching for pathogens, and mobilise the second line of immune defence, with its antibodies and immunologic memory. The dendritic cells themselves are in fact activated by the Toll receptor that Beutler and Hoffmann had identified. This mechanism ties together the two lines of immune defence.

The three discoveries now awarded the Nobel Prize have identified the triggers for the innate and the adaptive immune system, and taught us how these two lines of defence are interconnected to protect us against infections. Today, knowledge about the sensors of innate immunity is exploited to improve vaccines and therapies, and dendritic cells are used to treat infections and cancer.

Dear Professor Beutler and Professor Hoffmann,

Your research has identified the gatekeepers of the immune system. Not only have your discoveries resolved a major enigma in immunology, they have offered new hope for mankind in its combat against infections, cancer, and inflammatory diseases. On behalf of the Nobel Assembly at Karolinska Institutet, I wish to convey to you our warmest congratulations.

Dear Mrs Steinman,

Your late husband's research has taught us how adaptive immunity is initiated and provided us with new tools in the struggle against disease. We deeply regret that Professor Steinman is no longer with us but we are happy that you are here to accept his Nobel Prize.

Professor Beutler, Professor Hoffmann and Mrs Steinman,

May I now ask you to step forward to receive the Nobel Prize from the hands of His Majesty the King.

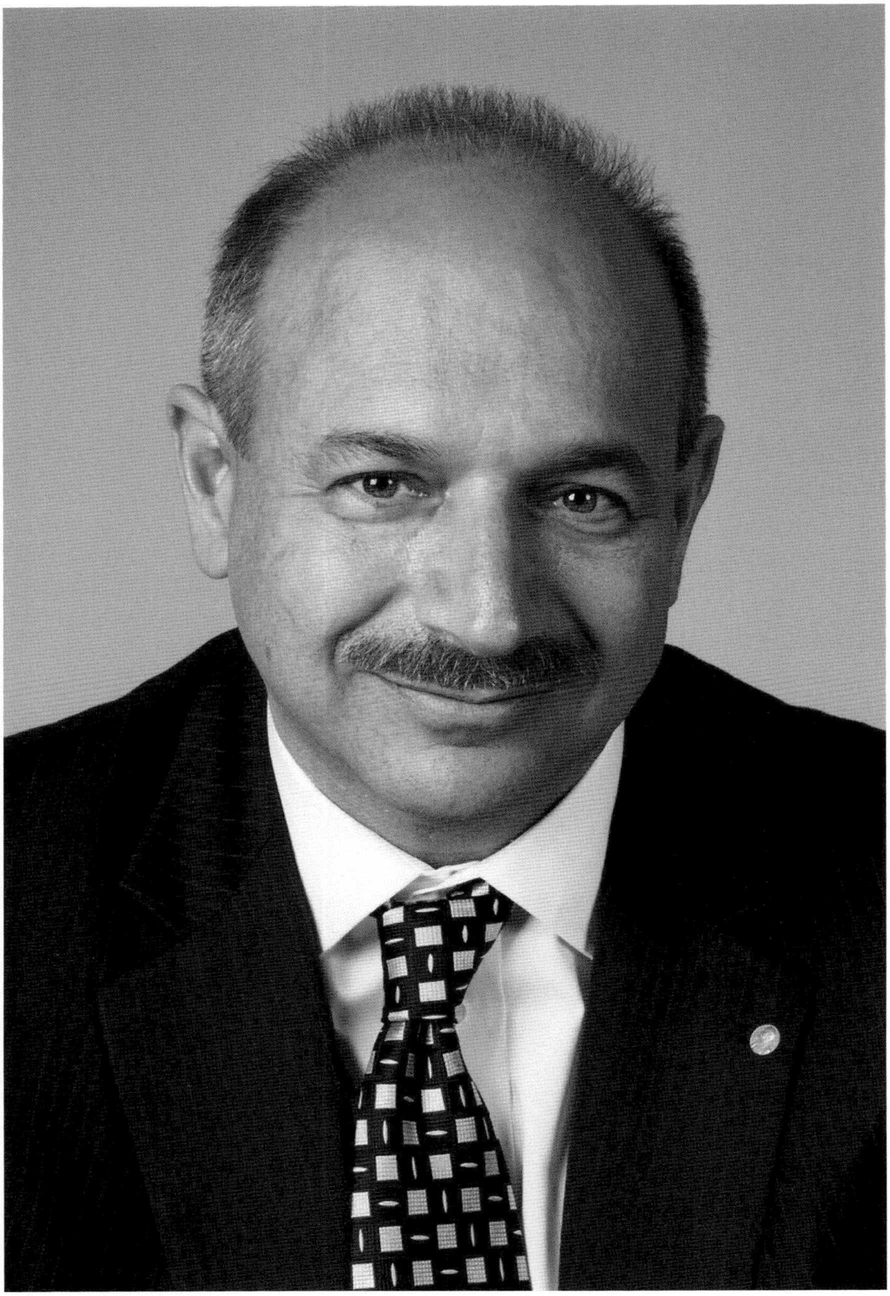

Bruce A. Beutler.

Bruce A. Beutler

ONE OF THE HAPPIEST DAYS OF MY LIFE

It was 2:30 a.m. on October 3, 2011, and I was at home, in my small condominium in San Diego, CA. I was sleepless, having recently returned from a trip to Hong Kong. There I had shared the Shaw Prize in Life Sciences: one of a series of prizes in recent years. The previous afternoon, as we visited our mother in La Jolla, my brother Earl had remarked that the Nobel Prize in Physiology or Medicine would be announced the next day. He also had asked if I was going to win it this year. This was on my mind as I lay awake.

Bleary-eyed, I looked at my cell phone to see if there was any email. There was a message: just one. The title line seemed to be "Nobel Prize." I reached for my glasses, looked again, and found I was correct. Nobel Prize. Perhaps this year the Committee had made a mass e-mailing of the announcement to members of various National Academies? I opened the message and read the first lines of a letter from Göran Hansson ...

"Dear Dr Beutler,
I have good news for you. The Nobel Assembly has today decided to award you the Nobel Prize in Physiology or Medicine for 2011. You will share the Prize with Drs Jules Hoffmann and Ralph Steinman. Congratulations!"

I was too excited to read more at that moment, and hurried downstairs. I called Betsy Layton, my longtime colleague and Administrative Manager. She was in Dallas, preparing the way for our relocation from the Scripps Research Institute to UT Southwestern, where we had earlier done some of our most important work. She had worked with me over the past 25 years, and had played an important part in finding the Lps mutation for which the Prize was awarded. I woke her from a sound sleep. "Bets," I said tentatively, "I think I won the Nobel

Prize!" She was ecstatic, but I cautioned her that I had to confirm it, and kept her on the line.

I tried to access the website Nobelprize.org, but found I couldn't; there was too much traffic. Then I went to news.google.com. I searched for my name, and within a minute or two, began to see it in reports emanating from all over the world. It was true. I told Betsy so, and she was so happy she began to cry! Yet still I was somehow disbelieving and only over the days and weeks that followed did the new reality settle in my mind.

Nadia Krochin, my dear friend and companion of many years, called me from the east coast before I could call her, and left a message on my voice mail that was almost incoherent with joy! I called my brother Earl; then my brother Steve; then my sons; then my friend Ari Theofilopoulos. I waited until about 4 a.m. to call my mother. Each person, though awakened abruptly, was nearly as happy as I had been.

By this time, my cell phone was ringing almost constantly, and it didn't stop ringing until late afternoon. Mostly reporters were calling, and I attempted to respond immediately to a few of them, hearing a constant beeping of incoming calls in the background as I did. Among those to whom I spoke during those first hours was a National Public Radio anchor, and it was on NPR, driving to work in various parts of the country, that many of my friends soon heard the news, along with my initial reaction. Emails were arriving every few seconds, and by the end of the day, I had more than a thousand of them. I realized it was hopeless to reply to them, and instead, via Betsy, I advanced my pre-existing plans to fly to Dallas. While waiting for my 10 a.m. flight, I went for a haircut earlier scheduled for 8 a.m. Hannah Andrusky, a charming lady who had cut my hair each month for several years, agreed to meet me an hour early that morning. I was her first client of the day, and she, too, knew of the Prize. She was as delighted and proud of me as everyone else had been. The haircut was free.

In Dallas I was greeted as a hero. A press conference was arranged for the next day, and after introductory speeches by the Dean, President, and Past President of UT Southwestern Medical Center, I stepped to the podium, met by a warm standing ovation. I spoke for several minutes from the heart, without slides, notes, or preparation of any kind. I felt a sense of self-confidence I hadn't known before. After all, I was a Nobel Laureate. Everyone present was elated and wished me well. I talked a bit about my life, about the steps that had brought me to the Nobel Prize, and also about some of the struggles and strains this entailed.

MY BACKGROUND

All of my grandparents immigrated to the United States to escape persecution as Jews, and I was reminded of this often from an early age. World War II had ended only 12 years before I was born, and recollections were fresh. My father was born in Germany, my mother in America to immigrant parents. My siblings, my cousins and I were always strongly conscious of our European origins, and of the extreme anti-Semitism that had recently prevailed in Europe. Probably we all felt a need to excel partly because of these facts; to show that we were as good as the other children in our schools.

My mother's parents, Aral ("Harry") Fleisher (1895–1953), and Miriam ("Mary") Fleisher, née Krasne (1893–1966), were both from Kiev, and moved separately to the USA near the turn of the century, settling in Chicago where they met and married in 1922. Harry initially worked in the insurance business. However, he was persuaded to join the company of Mary's father, Louis Krasne (L. Krasne and Sons). Mary and her brother Isador traveled to the west, ultimately settling in Tulsa, Oklahoma where they established a branch of L. Krasne and Sons that traded in "Leather and Findings." My mother, Brondelle May Fleisher, was born in Chicago but raised in Tulsa from the age of 11. She was the second of three children (Beverly was older and Lois younger), and she survives both her sisters today.

My mother's father died before I was born, but I knew my maternal grandmother well. Afflicted with a brittle form of diabetes (oddly at a mature age), she lived with us, was known as "Bubbie," and took care of me during my first few years of life. I remember her as a warm and kindly old woman with a strong Yiddish accent and extremely long hair, nearly touching the ground. Almost blind, she would spend much of her time in the garden, pulling weeds from the lawn, or otherwise trying to be useful. She was happy to talk to me, or walk with me or explore the yard. One of our routines was to "search for the Fountain of Youth" (which always turned out to be a drinking fountain in the back yard). She died within days of having a myocardial infarction at our California home in 1966.

My father's parents, Alfred Beutler (1891–1962) and Kaethe Beutler née Italiener (1896–1999) were both physicians: he an internist with a particular interest in cardiology, and she a pediatrician. They emigrated from Berlin, Germany in 1935 to escape Nazi persecution. I knew my father's father only slightly as he lived in Milwaukee, WI, visited only occasionally, and died when I was only four years old. My grandmother Kaethe, on the other hand, lived to be 102, residing near my parents' house for many of the last 40 years of her life. I had innumerable interesting conversations with her, beginning at a young age and continuing into my 40s. She was, on the one hand, kind to all her grandchildren, generally patient, and attentive to us. But occasionally she would lose her temper and shout at us with a strong German accent, which could be quite intimidating. She had an extraordinary vocabulary in English, was highly informed of current events, especially national and local politics, and spent much of her time reading books and political magazines. She was a lover of classical music and a competent pianist, who in her 60s and 70s, gave lessons to children in her neighborhood. She remained intellectually sharp, trading on the stock market and even learning to program a computer in her late 80s and early 90s. She had high standards, was quite strict about punctuality (once excoriating my sister when she showed up to an appointment at 3:17 pm rather than the designated 3:15 pm), and was hard to impress. She was not one to "ooh" and "ahh" over a child's drawing or any other minor accomplishment. On the other hand, she did encourage all of us, often through unstinting praise of great achievements in the world at large. It may well have been from her that I first heard the phrase "Nobel Prize" when I was still a small child, and on rare occasions, when I talked to her about science, I recall her saying "maybe someday you will win the Nobel Prize."

My grandmother was never comfortable as a Jew in German society at any time she lived there, although she was the physician to children of prominent gentile families in Berlin. Among her patients was the son of Magda Goebbels (from her marriage to Günther Quandt), about whom she spoke to me a few times. She described Magda as an "elegant, beautiful woman" who was quite pleasant prior to her marriage to Josef Goebbels, whereafter she visited no more. My grandmother did not foresee the Holocaust, even two years after Hitler's rise to power, but did foresee that her three children (my father, Ernst, his older brother Frederick, and his younger sister Ruth) would be denied an education and would have no future in Germany. She was the prime mover in the family's decision to leave. For a time, it was undecided whether they should emigrate to Palestine or to the United States. My grandfather actually visited Palestine, but found opportunities for physicians to be limited, and decided in favor of moving to America. This was reportedly contrary to my grandmother's wishes. "He asked me where I thought we should go. I said 'Palestine,' so of course we moved to America," she sometimes recounted. In the years that followed, she regretted that she could not take part in building the modern state of Israel. At the same time, she was relieved that her children did not need to fight in the wars that beset Israel from its founding.

Both of my parents were born in 1928, my father in Berlin, Germany, and my mother in Chicago, IL, USA. My father was said to have been a somewhat difficult child, often in conflict with his mother. However, he performed extraordinarily well at school, and at the age of 15 was enrolled in a special program developed by Robert Maynard Hutchins, then President of the University of Chicago, which permitted him to finish high school and college within two years and then go on to medical school. This he did, graduating as the valedictorian of his class, with a doctorate in medicine at the age of 21. He specialized in hematology, and in time became the pre-eminent academic hematologist of the 20th century. His scientific contributions extended to many areas of biomedical science, and he received numerous awards and distinctions in recognition of his work, including the Gairdner Prize in 1975, and election to the National Academy of Sciences and the Institute of Medicine in 1976. His most celebrated achievement was the 1962 discovery of random X chromosome inactivation in humans, made independently of Mary Lyon, who discovered it in mice. He made many other advances as well, in diverse fields of study, and he was to influence my own career dramatically.

My parents met at the University of Chicago, when my father was in his junior year of medical school. My mother was an undergraduate there, majoring in mathematics. They married June 15, 1950, and remained together until my father's death in October of 2008. In addition to me, they had three other children: Steven in 1952; Earl in 1954; and Deborah in 1962 (Figure 1). Like me, Steve and Debbie became physicians; Earl became a successful businessman. Our early years were mostly spent in southern California, because my father moved there in 1959 to accept a position as Chairman of the Department of Medicine at the City of Hope Medical Center in Duarte. My mother worked as a homemaker for about 18 years, spanning most of my childhood. She then began a late career as a technical writer, retiring in her mid-60s.

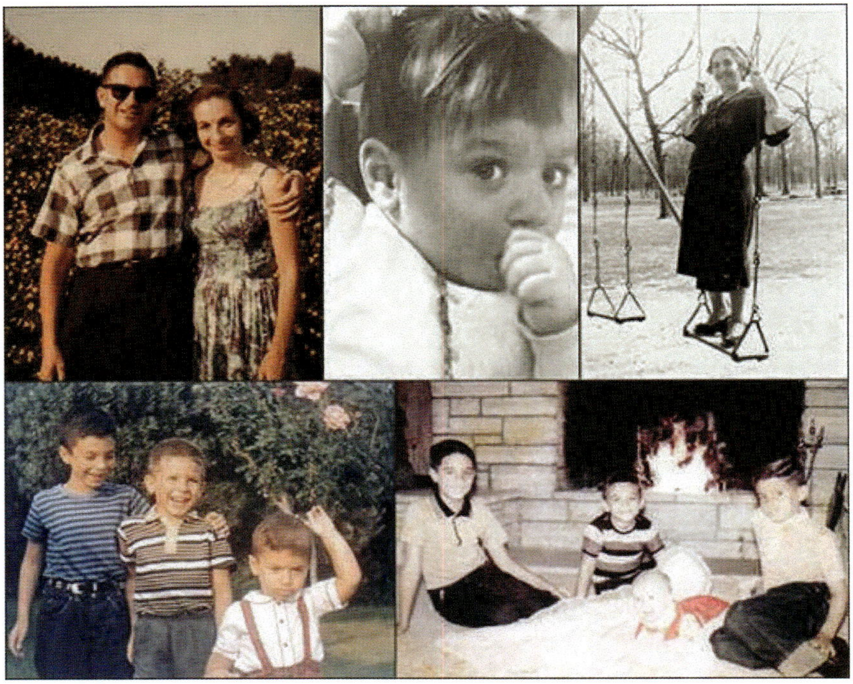

FIGURE 1. My early life and family. Clockwise from top left: My parents, standing in the front yard of our house in Arcadia, early 1960s (backdrop: a lantana bush often covered with skipper butterflies). Photograph taken of me at about 2 years of age, either before or after departure from Chicago for California. My maternal grandmother, Mary Fleisher ("Bubbie" to my sibs and me). My brothers and infant sister posing in front of the living room fireplace in 1962. From left: Steve, Bruce, Debbie, and Earl. My brothers and me, in the front yard of our home, ca. 1960. From left: Steve, Earl, and Bruce.

CA CHILDHOOD AND FRIENDS

I was born in Chicago, IL, on December 29, 1957. But I have only fleeting memories of my first years there. My earliest memory is of newly fallen snow in the autumn of 1959. Seeing that the world outside had changed overnight, I asked "Who did that?" I also remember crying when movers came to take everything out of my room, as the family was relocating to California, where, from the age of two, I grew up in Arcadia, a northeastern suburb of Los Angeles. I have warm recollections of my childhood in California, and often have dreams in the setting of the adobe brick house where I grew up, with its orange terra cotta tile roof, one-acre yard, orchard crammed with fruit trees, guest house (which served as my room from the ages of 12–16), large front lawn (which we called "the field,") and swimming pool (Figure 2). Generally speaking, I recall sunshine year round; heavy smog and hot weather during summer months; snow on the surrounding peaks and frost on the lawn in the mornings during winter; family vacations to national parks; and the fact that I had a strong interest in nature (particularly in animals). Over the years, I raised many animals (dogs, ducks, rabbits, mice, chameleons, tropical fish, turtles, and zebra finches), watching them and generally marveling at their behavior. As I grew up, I did lots of hiking (chiefly in the San Gabriel Mountains), birding, and bicycling. There were stresses to be sure: quarrels with my sibs and worries about deadlines in school, but nothing serious. On the whole I was very happy, even if I didn't always realize it.

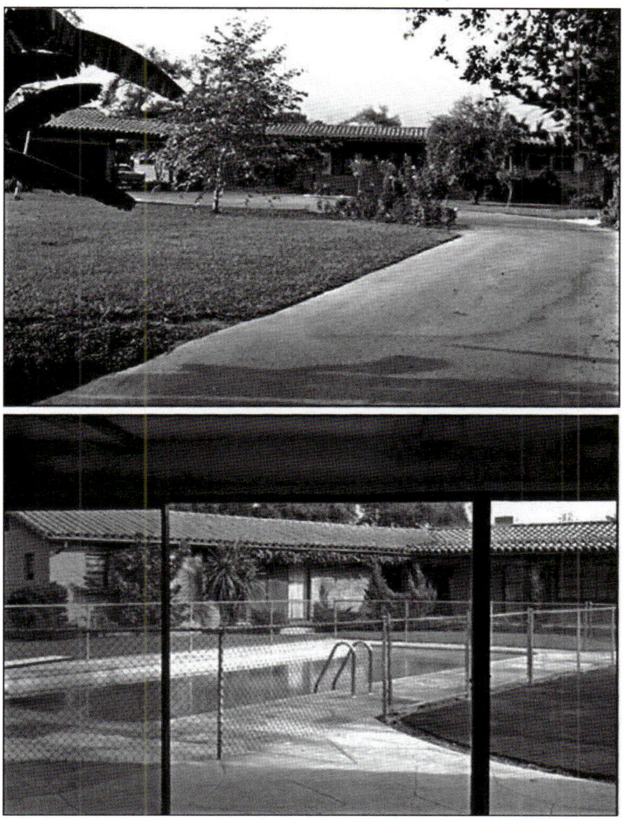

FIGURE 2. The house where I grew up (Arcadia, CA, early 1960s). A. Partial view of the front yard from the front gate, showing banana tree (bottom left) rose bushes and rose trees, a young sycamore tree and eucalyptus tree, olive tree, and adobe brick house with terra cotta tile roof. B. Partial view of the back yard and swimming pool, taken from inside the "guest house" (ultimately an annex to my room).

I began first grade early (at age 5), attending public school until I was 13 years old. I was then admitted to Polytechnic School, a college preparatory school in Pasadena, CA. The content of the curriculum at Polytechnic, and the pace at which we were taught, was quite different from what I had experienced in public school. It was something of a renaissance for me, and I regretted having wasted so much time beforehand. Not only was I taught more, and taught better at Polytechnic than at public school, but I also had exceptionally smart friends, and have remained close to some of them to this day. David Brittan, Paul Spiegel, Bob Kleinberg, John Taylor, and David Horowitz were among those friends, and with them, I could discuss almost any topic of the day, as they had a wide range of interests, spanning music, politics, literature, and science.

During three years at Polytechnic, I learned a lot about many things, and certainly changed a great deal, with some mental transformations literally occurring from one day to the next. For example, when I was 15 years old, I attended a performance of Bach's St. Matthew Passion. My father had intended to go, but could not, as he needed to rescue my brother Earl, who had been bicycling from San Francisco to Arcadia, and had become exhausted on the way; hence I went in his place. I had been exposed to classical music in my home as a child, but it didn't make any special impression on me. Yet I was completely electrified by this live performance of Bach's great choral masterpiece, the first I had heard, and at once began listening to other choral music and collecting it on vinyl records, especially pieces by Bach, Handel, Vivaldi, Mozart, and Haydn. I remember arranging my curriculum in such a way that I could bicycle to school early in the morning (a distance of eight miles), complete my classes by late morning, and then bicycle home to listen to a radio concert of Renaissance music in my father's study. Later I would do my homework (generally until quite late at night, and usually accompanied by Bach). I have remained a music lover ever since, ultimately settling on Bach as the center of my musical world. But although music became a deep and enduring interest of mine, I never learned to play any musical instrument proficiently.

EARLY INTEREST IN SCIENCE

From childhood, living things appealed to me aesthetically. I could relate to them, and I was amazed by their similarity to humans. I was aware that life forms had changed continuously on earth over many millions of years, and concepts of genetic variation, natural selection, and inheritance were second nature to me, even from the time I was in elementary school. In hiking and birding, and in looking at microbes through a microscope (one of my favorite diversions at some point), I enjoyed the observational side of science, which is where scientific inquiry normally begins. It was during high school, in the rich intellectual environment I have briefly described, that I first began to wonder about unanswered questions in science. The ability of inanimate molecules to assemble themselves into living matter was something that I found immeasurably interesting. My oldest brother, Steve, once introduced me to a quotation he attributed to Camus: "Life is the disease of matter." Probably it was actually from Goethe, who as I later learned, wrote "Viewed from the summit of reason, all life looks like a malignant disease." The idea resonated with me, not in a morbid sense, but because life was a process that compelled matter to do its bidding, co-opting it more or less automatically, and endowing it with special properties not seen in the inanimate world. In the early 1970s, I read the second edition of James Watson's "Molecular Biology of the Gene" (also a gift from my brother Steve, then in college at the University of California at San Diego) from cover to cover, and understood for the first time how DNA specifies the synthesis of proteins with specific functions, which in turn permit DNA replication, the development of a complex organism, meiosis, and the propagation of species. I became even more eager to participate in the study of living things, and to be an experimentalist rather than merely an admiring witness.

In high school and in college, I began to work in my father's laboratory, and it was at this stage that I began to do authentic research. I was guided by my father and his interests, and learned to assay erythrocyte enzymes, and to characterize their electrophoretic mobility. One of the enzymes I studied most was glutathione peroxidase, unusual because it was a seleno-enzyme. At one point, striking out on my own a bit, I decided to see whether bacteria might have glutathione peroxidase, and whether it might be subject to biosynthetic control based on the availability of selenium, like the genes of operons, which had been described not too long before by Jacob and Monod. Lysing E. coli, I first found that there was no glutathione peroxidase activity. My father suggested I should add sodium selenite to the culture. I did so, and found considerable activity, which I interpreted as a success: I believed the selenite had induced synthesis of the enzyme. "Boil it," said my father. The activity remained and was even slightly increased. Moreover, inorganic sodium selenite (and even more so, seleno-cysteine) exhibited catalytic activity. When seleno-cysteine was incorporated into the protein, this activity was enhanced many thousand fold. We proposed a reaction mechanism based on the catalytic properties of selenium in distinct oxidation states. We also found a polymorphism of erythrocyte glutathione peroxidase activity in members of my own family, and an electrophoretic polymorphism in others. I began to think as a biochemist, and to some extent, also as a geneticist, but only in a rather elementary way at that stage.

MY FATHER AS A ROLE MODEL

The foregoing vignette tells something of how my father influenced me. I was thrilled when he received the Gairdner Award, and when he was elected to the National Academy of Sciences, both of which occurred during my teenage years. Indeed, I sought to emulate him and took his advice seriously. When he suggested I read "Arrowsmith" by Sinclair Lewis, and "The Microbe Hunters" by Paul de Kruif, I did so, and just as they had earlier affected him, they also affected me. Among the most important pieces of advice he gave me was to go to medical school. The explanation he gave was that disease often reveals new and important biological principles; also, as a physician in training, one acquires broad knowledge of anatomy, physiology, histology, pathology, and pharmacology: sciences that come into play in understanding many biological phenomena. Throughout his life, my father was an advocate of working on "something important," rather than what he saw as esoteric topics. Generally speaking, he preferred authentic clinical research (with patients) to research with mice, and research with mice to research with flies or other distant model organisms. Notwithstanding his strong genetic and evolutionary orientation (which we shared), he tended more toward applied research than I myself did. And his judgment as to what was important rested chiefly on his medical experience, which was quite extensive.

With a strong focus and a sense of mission, I completed high school early (at the age of 16) and enrolled at the University of California at San Diego (UCSD), in Revelle College. I had taken certain examinations that gave me "advanced placement" credit, and I pursued an ambitious schedule in college. I worked through two summers, and graduated at the age of 18. I was a good student, but not an outstanding one. As a teenager and even for some years beyond, I was a bit emotionally volatile, often distracted by love interests, and generally speaking, in too much of a hurry. I took on an enormous course load, wishing to get through college quickly, go on to medical school, and become a scientist. It was an exciting time in biology, after all, with extraordinary advances in molecular cloning beginning to dawn. I was aware of what was going on, and impatient to be part of it. To my friend high school friend David Brittan (also my roommate for a time in college), I remember saying with frustration "The train of science is leaving without me."

But despite the hurry, I did learn a lot, and only realized how much later on. I had a truly stellar introduction to genetics in the laboratory of Dan Lindsley (Figure 3a), a distinguished Drosophila geneticist interested in spermatogenesis and spermiogenesis in the fly, among other topics. In his lab, I attempted to map the gene for hexosaminidase (a project inspired by my father, who had studied this enzyme in humans, where hexosaminidase deficiency causes Tay-Sachs disease). When I was 18, I spent the summer working in the lab of Abraham Braude, most immediately with his postdoctoral fellow Arthur Friedlander (who later became well known for his studies of anthrax lethal factor). In Braude's lab, I first heard the word "endotoxin," also known as lipopolysaccharide, or LPS. I understood it was pyrogenic, capable of activating leukocytes, and also heat stable (which made it a particular problem in our studies of chemotaxis). All glassware had to be heated to 180°C to destroy contaminating LPS. I also knew that Braude had tried to passively immunize humans against LPS to protect them against Gram-negative septic shock. But my interest in LPS was casual and tangential at that stage, probably because its biomedical importance was still an abstraction to me. I had never seen a patient with sepsis, and didn't grasp what a serious clinical problem it might be. The question of an LPS receptor did not occur to me at that time. I did not remotely imagine that searching for it would form the core of my Nobel Prize-winning work two decades later.

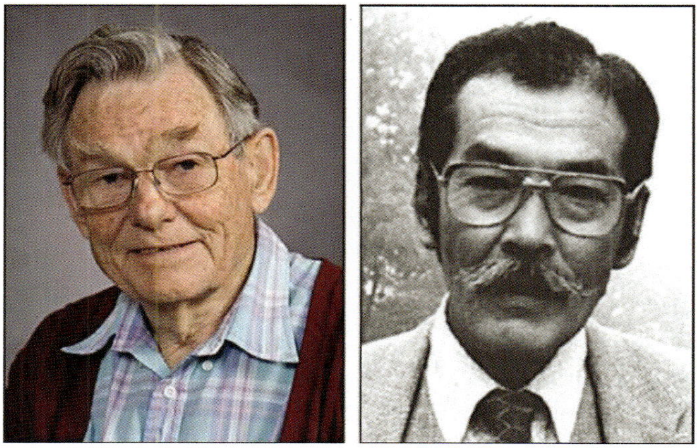

FIGURE 3. Teachers who influenced me. Left: Daniel Lindsley, photographed in the early 1990s. Right: Susumu Ohno (from a biographical memoir by Ernest Beutler, National Academy of Sciences, USA).

After completing college, I had still more exposure to genetics in the lab of Susumu Ohno (Figure 3b), a friend and colleague of my father at City of Hope Medical Center. I worked with Ohno for about nine months, and spent still another summer with him during medical school. A famous mammalian geneticist, Ohno had demonstrated that the Barr body observed in cells of female mammals was a condensed X chromosome. He had also developed the thesis that evolution depends upon gene duplication. He had written extensively on the phylogeny and origin of sex chromosomes. And he had observed that the genetic content of the X chromosome tends to be strongly conserved in all mammalian species. In short, he was a remarkable theoretical biologist at a time when experimental tools were not nearly what they are today.

Ohno inclined toward immunology after spending a sabbatical at the Basel Institute for Immunology. He hypothesized that major histocompatibility antigens act to anchor organogenesis-directing proteins. He adduced considerable experimental evidence supporting this hypothesis ... which we know today was entirely incorrect! The time I spent in Ohno's lab, working on this very subject, was quite enlightening for me from many points of view. In hindsight, perhaps the most important – if brutal – lesson was that even extremely intelligent scientists can deceive themselves if they embrace hypotheses too passionately. But I also learned much about immunology as it was understood in the mid-1970s.

I applied to several medical schools, confident that I would be admitted to most of them. I had good grades, extensive experience in laboratory research, several publications (including one first-author paper in Cell), and MCAT scores in the top percentile. But in the end, I was admitted to only one medical school: the University of Chicago. All others declined my application, perhaps because I was so young, and perhaps because I was unreservedly interested in science rather than clinical medicine. So I must be grateful to the University of Chicago for the chance it gave me. Luckily, it was (and remains) an outstanding institution. In the fall of 1977, I moved to Chicago and began my studies there at the age of 19, the youngest member of a class with more than 100 students.

MEDICAL SCHOOL

My first impression of Chicago was that it was a "real" city compared to the southern California suburbs I had known. But it was also somewhat dangerous (where I lived, at least), and comparatively unwelcoming. The Chicago winter was something for which I was not prepared. I arrived dressed as a Californian, and nearly froze when I tried to walk the mile from the University to my apartment during the first winter storm, in high winds and sub-zero temperatures. As I remember, my ears were insensate for about an hour, and I initially feared they would become gangrenous and fall off! I recall the first years as quite challenging. Anatomy and neuroanatomy were especially tough, requiring spatial memorization of a type that was unfamiliar to me, but in the end, both classes were rewarding. My classmates were for the most part smart and competitive, and I had to struggle to do well. I particularly enjoyed histology, physiology, and microbiology classes.

When it came to my introduction to clinical medicine, the work was more demanding than any I had ever known. Ultimately this was beneficial, because I came to expect equivalent discipline of myself and others when I worked in the laboratory. But I did not get the same joy out of clinical work that I did from laboratory work. I was often uncertain as to whether particular therapies and practices had a sound rational basis, and when patients got better, I did not always feel I could claim credit for it. After all, there was no control group. And very rightly, there was no leeway for experimentation on the wards. I did manage to work for some months in the laboratories of Patricia Spear, an outstanding young herpes virologist, and Barry Arnason, a neurologist with a strong interest in multiple sclerosis. But overall, there was little time for research, and I began to miss the lab.

In 1980, when I was 22, I married Barbara (Barbie) Lanzl, then a dental student at nearby University of Illinois. She was three years older than I, and had previously been married to my friend and medical school classmate Jiri Sonek. The marriage lasted 8 years, with phases in Chicago, Dallas, New York, and Dallas again, before ending in divorce. We had three bright, healthy sons, two born in Dallas and one in New York.

INTERNSHIP AND RESIDENCY

I graduated from the University of Chicago in 1981, and again acting according to my father's advice, decided to spend at least a year or two in residency, learning more about clinical medicine. I was matched with the internal medicine internship program and the neurology residency program at UT Southwestern Medical Center in Dallas. Dallas was my top choice, and arguably offered the finest clinical training in the country. It was known for giving interns and residents considerable responsibility and autonomy. During the year of my internship, for example, two interns and one resident would run the internal medicine emergency room alone through the night, with no attending physician present. And when necessary, medicine interns were expected to perform fairly invasive procedures, including intubation, placement of subclavian lines, cardiocentesis, insertion of chest tubes: in short, whatever was required, particularly during emergencies (which were not uncommon).

My father's twofold rationale in suggesting an internship and residency rather than a laboratory fellowship had been that I would become "a finished doctor;" also that I would have something to fall back on in the event that research did not pan out for me.

As to the first point, I believe he was correct. At least the year I spent in internal medicine internship taught me many things I hadn't known as a senior medical student. By the time I had finished, I feared no medical emergency; I felt secure in doing whatever needed to be done. But I also knew that medicine was not for me. I badly missed research and longed to return to it. I felt obligated to finish at least one year of neurology residency and did so. I learned quite a bit about neurology, which sometimes helps me to the present day in assessing mutations in mice. But perhaps the residency year gave me a bit more clinical training than I ever wanted.

As to the second point, my father was certainly being prudent. But to my recollection, I was supremely confident of success in science. I felt that no matter which lab I joined, and no matter what project I undertook, I would prevail, given the interconnectedness of biological processes, and my overall knowledge about how they worked. I was dead certain of my skills. I had a "feeling" for proteins and how to isolate them. I had a solid grounding in genetics and in immunology. And, true to my father's earlier advice, medicine had taught me much about how an organism functions: far more than I would have learned had I gone to graduate school. Perhaps I was brash, but in recalling my mental state at the time, I would say I was imbued with the enthusiasm of youth, and felt invincible.

ROCKEFELLER UNIVERSITY AND AN EARLY SUCCESS

I was 25 years old when, on the evening of July 4, 1983, Barbie and I arrived in New York City together with our infant son Danny, who had been born in Dallas. I remained in New York for three years, and during the second year, our second son Elliot was born. Most of the time, the four of us lived on the 11th floor of a high-rise apartment building across the street from the Rockefeller University campus, with a nice view of the East River.

I had joined the Cerami laboratory at Rockefeller. There I began to work on cachectin, an unidentified factor expressed by macrophages in response to activation by LPS, and defined by its ability to suppress lipoprotein lipase synthesis in adipocytes. The prevailing hypothesis in the laboratory at that time was that cachectin was responsible for wasting in chronic diseases such as tuberculosis, trypanosomiasis, and cancer. From the start, I was skeptical about the idea that a single factor could explain all cachexia, given the diversity of inciting causes. At least, there was no strong reason to think so. But I did see early on that a single factor responsible for suppression of lipoprotein lipase in fat cells was secreted by LPS-activated macrophages. Moreover, I saw that this factor was a protein, and I felt it could be purified.

At the time I started work in the lab, no progress at all had been made in isolating cachectin. Cachectin activity had been ascribed by my predecessors to a protein with a molecular weight of 70 kilodaltons (almost surely contaminating serum albumin). Moreover, they had purportedly excluded tumor necrosis factor (TNF) as a candidate mediator by exchanging material with the laboratory of Lloyd Old, who had discovered TNF and was then still trying to isolate it. They had erred in reaching this conclusion.

Within a year, I purified cachectin to homogeneity, raised an antibody against it, and affinity purified the antibody. I hypothesized that whatever role cachectin might have in cachexia, it was likely involved in endotoxic shock, as it was produced in large amounts when macrophages were activated by LPS, constituting about 2% of their secretory product. Moreover, I found that purified cachectin was capable of killing mice when as little as 20 micrograms was administered by an intravenous route. One evening, I passively immunized 5 mice against cachectin, and gave pre-immune globulin to 5 control animals. I had formally randomized the mice to the two treatment groups, and I waited for several hours to give the antibody time to distribute through all extracellular fluid compartments. I then challenged the animals with a carefully chosen dose of LPS: a low LD100. To my delight, I found the next morning that passive immunization protected all 5 recipients against LPS-induced death, while all 5 control mice had succumbed! I repeated the experiment many times and with many permutations, using hundreds of mice, and found the result to be robust and reproducible. I was thrilled because I knew I had isolated one of the key endogenous factors mediating the lethal effect of LPS. The inflammatory properties of cachectin, rather than an ability to induce wasting, proved to be immensely important.

Several months passed before I could determine the N-terminal sequence of cachectin, as my initial purification strategy left the protein N-terminally blocked. I needed to repurify it using an entirely different procedure. Eventually, 17 residues were called by Edman degradation. Initially, I believed cachectin was a novel protein. Its sequence did not appear in the rudimentary protein databases that existed at that time. However, I was soon alerted by the Ulevitch group at Scripps that my purified cachectin, sent to them for separate purposes, had high tumor necrosis factor activity. I directly compared the sequence of human TNF, only recently isolated and cloned at Genentech, to the sequence of mouse cachectin. I saw strong homology. Cachectin was the mouse orthologue of human TNF.

This worked to my advantage, perhaps, in that there was already great interest in TNF as an anti-neoplastic protein. Yet I had then shown that the protein also had toxic, inflammatory properties. In time, TNF became one of the most studied proteins in biomedicine, and attempts to block its activity with antibodies (or with recombinant proteins such as my group later developed) bore more fruit than attempts to administer it.

During my three years at Rockefeller, I published many papers, including several in high-ranking journals, and made a substantial name for myself in the rapidly developing cytokine field. Soon, many thousands of other publications cited my work. I obtained my own funding and was promoted to the rank of Assistant Professor at Rockefeller in 1985, but this post did not carry true autonomy. I wanted a lab of my own. When I was invited by Joe Sambrook to join the Howard Hughes Medical Institute (HHMI) at UT Southwestern Medical Center, I eagerly left New York to forge my own future.

DALLAS AND THE LPS LOCUS

Returning to Dallas in 1986, one of my first and best decisions was to hire Betsy Layton as my secretary. She was 19 years old at the time, and had just moved to Dallas from her native Pennsylvania, attracted by the image of Texas and by opportunities for work. When I interviewed her, she struck me first of all as nice, cheerful, smart, and friendly; also as someone who had a strong will to work and to do a good job. I was right on all of these calls. Meeting Betsy was one of the luckiest things that ever happened to me, because she was truly devoted to me over the many years that followed. She helped me to set up my lab, offered advice with appropriate tact and candor, and became a true partner in my professional life. In time, she became an administrative assistant; then an administrative manager. She accompanied me from Dallas to Scripps, and then back to Dallas, where she still works with me today. I hope this will always be the case. In the end, choosing outstanding people and guiding their work well becomes far more important than the work a biologist does with his own hands.

When I first settled in Dallas, I began to pursue several topics related to TNF. The most practical of these was to develop a means of blocking TNF activity in vivo. I engaged with this challenge partly because I knew that it would be useful to do so both in chronic inflammation and in septic shock, and partly because I wished, in the "pre-knockout" era, to see what a chronically TNF-deficient animal would be like. David Crawford, an MD/PhD student, and Karsten Peppel, a postdoc in my lab, developed a chimeric molecule in which the ectodomain of one of the TNF receptors was fused to part of an IgG heavy chain, including the hinge and Fc region. As we had hoped, this yielded a non-antigenic, stable, and extremely potent neutralizing reagent that could be administered to mice (or humans) to block TNF activity in vivo for long periods of time. We patented this protein, and eventually sold the patent to Immunex, which in turn was acquired by Amgen. Today, the molecule we invented is marketed as the drug Enbrel, and is used as an effective treatment for rheumatoid arthritis and several other inflammatory diseases.

On a more basic level, I focused my laboratory on the question of how TNF biosynthesis might be regulated. I viewed this as tantamount to the question of how the inflammatory response might be regulated as a whole, in that it was already apparent to me that TNF was an excellent marker of the inflammatory response. I had earlier shown, for example, that anti-inflammatory drugs such as glucocorticosteroids could entirely abolish TNF biosynthesis in response to LPS, and felt that this explained a large part of their inflammatory effect. I deduced that TNF biosynthesis was regulated both at transcriptional and translational levels. TNF gene transcription was dependent upon NF-κB, a factor soon seen to induce many cytokine genes. Translational repression depended upon a sequence my colleague Daniel Caput and I had discovered in the 3′-untranslated region of the TNF mRNA, consisting of overlapping and interleaved octamers with the sequence UUAUUUAU. A similar sequence, I had noted, was found in many cytokine encoding mRNAs. Activation of the macrophage by LPS overcame translational repression. Both Véronique Kruys and Jiahuai Han in my lab closely studied these phenomena, but we did not succeed in elucidating the biochemical details of translational regulation during those years.

The more central question as to how macrophages became activated by LPS remained elusive. At the core of the question was the issue of the LPS receptor. TNF was made in large amounts in response to LPS. Hence, I was inquiring into LPS signaling when I attempted to measure responses of the TNF gene and mRNA. Yet there was no understanding as to how LPS was perceived by cells in the first place. And long before most others in the innate immunity field, I regarded the question as one of the most fundamental and important in all of immunology.

After all, since microbes had been identified as the causative agents of infectious diseases in the mid-1800s by Pasteur and Koch, nobody had determined which receptors recognize their presence during infection. This was the first level of self/non-self discrimination by the immune system. LPS mimicked infection in all its complexity quite closely, and potentially, the LPS receptor might be responsible for all events that transpired during a real infection. In finding the LPS receptor, we could hope to know at least one key sensor used by the innate immune system to recognize microbes. Perhaps it might be a member of a receptor family; perhaps we would gain insight into how all microbes were detected within the first minutes following inoculation.

I was aware of two strains of mice that were specifically refractory to LPS, because of mutations affecting the so-called Lps locus. These were the C3H/HeJ and C57BL/10ScCr strains. For each, a closely related strain (C3H/HeN and C57BL/10ScSn, respectively) served as a control with normal LPS responses. And mice of both strains were known to be susceptible to Gramnegative infections. In my mind, these mutations abrogating LPS responses grew constantly in stature. What protein did they affect? Was it indeed the LPS receptor?

Positionally cloning the LPS locus was beyond my capabilities during the 1980s. I had isolated TNF in a lab in which molecular cloning had never been practiced, and I had to teach myself almost everything in the way of basic molecular biology methods. I understood what needed to be done, but did not at that time feel secure in tackling such an immense problem. I tried instead to look for a difference between control mice and mutants at the protein level. And I attempted to raise an antibody against the proteins of a WT mouse in a resistant animal (or vice versa) to discover a "missing" or altered protein in mutants. I also tried to use expression cDNA cloning to find a gene product that could rescue the LPS-resistant phenotype. We tried, too, to use insertional mutagenesis (with a retrovirus) to inactivate the LPS locus in heterozygous mice made by crossing C3H/HeN animals to C3H/HeJ animals. But as all of these approaches to finding the LPS receptor were unsuccessful, I began to think positional cloning might be the only way to go.

I began to pursue this strategy actively in 1993, when Christophe Van Huffel came to my laboratory from Belgium to work as a postdoctoral associate. He had a background in yeast genetics, which made me think he would be a good person to isolate the YA C clones we would need to build a contig across the critical region. We began mapping the mutation in C3H/HeJ mice to high resolution, ultimately including a total of 2093 mice in our meiotic analyses. We became stronger in our molecular skills, and gradually, more people were incorporated into the effort, until the entire lab had a single focus. Among these were Alexander Poltorak and Irina Smirnova, who worked devotedly and tirelessly to find the mutation, year after year. They were exceptionally able colleagues. Betsy too joined the effort, and helped to read sequence, organize data, pick colonies for sequencing. Alexander, Irina, and Betsy were as zealous as I was; they simply refused to give up.

I have not directly mentioned it to this point, but I tend to be an obsessive person in many ways. I am even somewhat proud of this, although in some circumstances it has brought me considerable suffering without tangible rewards. Finding the mutations that abolished LPS responses became one of the most gripping obsessions of my life. For years, it occupied much of my waking consciousness and sometimes my dreams as well. Once, in 1997, while staying in a hotel in the San Bernardino Mountains, I awoke from a dream in which I was sure I had come to understand what gene was affected by the mutation. I hastily wrote the name of the affected protein on a scrap of paper and happily returned to sleep. In the morning, I saw that the protein was complete nonsense; it did not exist (though from the suffix "ase," I could tell it must have been an enzyme)!

Positional cloning of the LPS locus was the toughest challenge I had ever faced for three reasons. First, the critical region was gigantic: by far the largest ever tackled in the mouse. 24 BAC clones and one YA C clone were needed to span it, and even then there was a small gap we never closed. We know today that the genomic interval was at least 5.6 million base pairs in size. To have such a region within which crossover was apparently forbidden was simply bad luck, and at that, we needed to explore about 90% of it before we found the mutation. Second, we had limited sequencing power. We began sequencing with radionuclides (mostly ^{35}S), loading gels by hand, drying them, and reading sequence ladders on X-ray film. Later we used slab gels with semi-automated fluorescence-based reading of sequence. But we never had capillary sequencers at our disposal. This made it difficult for us to examine the region for genes. Third, the methods used at the time to find genes were primitive. We began with exon trapping and hybridization selection. Only by the mid-1990s were complex expressed sequence tag (EST) databases available. Matches between genomic DNA in our interval of interest were sought in the EST databases using an algorithm called BLAST. And BLAST searching became a major chore, because we had insufficient local computing power. I taught myself to program in Perl in order to manage the many thousands of sequence files, and the output BLAST data in a semi-automated way. For years, no meaningful hits emerged. There were only hits derived from pseudogenes, which nonetheless had to be cloned, sequenced in full, and run to ground, so that we might be sure we could find no mutation distinguishing C3H/HeJ from the control strain C3H/HeN.

PRESSURES, CRITICISM, AND ANXIETY

Both personal and professional pressures weighed heavily on me during the years of the LPS cloning project. My youngest son, Jonathan, was born in 1987, and Barbara and I separated in 1988. The divorce proceedings were contentious, and went on for years, involving innumerable depositions, preliminary hearings, and a jury trial, ultimately leading to a joint custody order. Of course, life did not immediately normalize thereafter. Particularly during their teenage years, my sons were each difficult to manage. I am happy to say that all three are extremely close to me today. It was a special joy to bring Danny and Elliot to Stockholm for the Nobel Prize ceremony (unfortunately, Jonathan was unable to attend). But in the mid-1990s, there was a lot of stress, and tough times at home coincided with the toughest phase of the cloning work.

While the importance of finding the LPS mutations was obvious to me, it was less obvious to other people. Years elapsed with no publications to show, and some of my colleagues thought that we did not entirely know what we were doing; some believed that the gene might, in the end, not be particularly illuminating; all believed that we were taking a terrible risk. Among these was my father, who urged me to diversify my portfolio and not to "put all your eggs in one basket." I ignored his advice on this occasion; I simply couldn't abandon or in any way diminish the intense focus on the LPS locus, because I knew we wouldn't find the mutations if I did. In hindsight, I am sure I was correct about this.

At least two other groups were attempting to find the same gene. One was the group of Danielle Malo, in Montreal; another was the group of David Schwartz in Iowa. I worried in particular about Malo's effort, because she and her close colleagues had an impressive record in positional cloning. At one point, I offered to collaborate with her, but the offer was declined, which meant we were formally in a state of competition.

HHMI was increasingly impatient with me. Over the 14 years I worked as an HHMI investigator, my program was reviewed by the Medical Advisory Board five times. After our final review, in April of 1998, I was told I would be funded through August of 2000, but not beyond. This was disappointing, since we had indeed made progress, and I felt that success was imminent. But their indulgence was at an end.

I felt we must continue come what might, and we did so, though some of the postdoctoral fellows in my group, Christophe Van Huffel, Mu-Ya Liu, and Xiaolong He, left to find other laboratories, as did some of the technicians, who also sensed impending defeat. Hence, it was an anxious time. Most of the critical region had been explored in depth. Surely we would find the gene soon. Or else, perhaps, we had made a mapping error and were looking at the wrong part of the chromosome. Were we on the cusp of success? Or had I been a fool to reject wise counsel, and would our efforts end with nothing to show for them?

SUCCESS

The gene we had struggled with for five years was discovered very suddenly one night: on the 5th of September, 1998. I was reviewing the day's BLAST results as they returned from NCBI and from our own server where we had begun to run BLAST locally. I was shocked by what I saw, as there had been a long dry spell, and here was one ... then two ... matches with a real gene: Tlr4. Almost certainly it was not a pseudogene based on the quality of the hit. That in itself encouraged me to think that this was the "holy grail" we had been seeking: here was an authentic gene, and only a small amount of genetic material that remained unexplored. Moreover, a good story could immediately be made about the candidate. It appeared to be a cell surface receptor with a single membrane spanning domain. The ectodomain was rich in leucine, which might be expected to bind hydrophobic molecules like the acyl chains of LPS, and was similar in overall structure to CD14, earlier shown to be required for sensing LPS molecules. It was a member of a family of proteins related to Toll, which in Drosophila was known to have both an immune and a developmental function. And on the cytoplasmic side, it was similar to the IL-1 receptor, well known to deliver an inflammatory signal.

I related these facts breathlessly to my father (who was somewhat nonplussed, I must say), and to Alexander and Ira, who were very much more excited, sensing as I did that our battle might be nearing an end. But we would not be on firm ground until we were able to find a mutation distinguishing the

C3H/HeJ strain Tlr4 from the C3H/HeN strain Tlr4, and the C57BL/10ScCr strain Tlr4 from the C57BL/10ScSn strain Tlr4.

The very next day, we attempted to amplify the cDNA in all these strains by long-range PCR. Alexander succeeded in so doing using cDNA from the C3H/HeJ, C3H/HeN, and C57BL/10ScSn strains, but failed to do so using cDNA from the C57BL/10ScCr strain. We therefore concentrated first on the C3H/HeJ and C3H/HeN sequences, which Alexander established by shotgun sequencing. Within days, we saw the mutation for the first time: it was a single base pair change predicting the substitution of a conserved proline for a histidine in the cytoplasmic domain of the molecule. We later established that the gene was deleted in the C57BL/10ScCr strain. And this eliminated any remaining doubt that TLR4 was essential for LPS signaling.

I called James Gavin, my HHMI liaison, to tell him what we had done. In reply, he made no comment on our findings, but emphasized that the decision of HHMI was irrevocable. For my own part, I was so elated that we had made a truly great discovery that the blow was much softened. We submitted our work to Science, where it was promptly accepted for publication, and meanwhile, presented it at four international meetings, where it was received with acclaim (Figure 4). By now it has been cited over 4,000 times: more than any other paper in the innate immunity field.

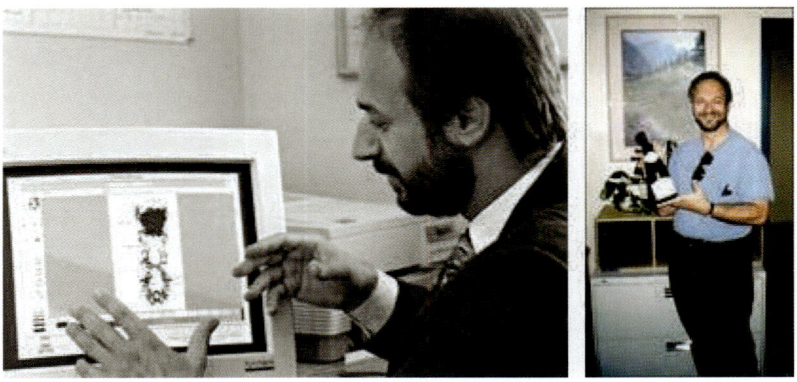

FIGURE 4. Left: Examining the predicted interaction of a TNF inhibitor molecule with TNF in a mock-up made by Dr. Steven Sprang, a colleague at UT Southwestern Medical Center. Photographed in 1995, courtesy David Gresham, UT Southwestern. Right: Holding a bottle of champagne in mid-September, 1998. Robert Munford, a colleague with a longstanding interest in LPS, brought it to our lab for a brief, impromptu celebration on hearing that the mutation had been identified. The bottle has been kept in my office to the present day as a memento.

Most exciting of all, perhaps, was the fact that the LPS receptor was indeed part of a protein family, and it could easily be imagined that other TLRs detected other molecules of microbial origin. In time, this proved to be the case. And in due course, we were able to show that TLR4 did in fact engage LPS in order to detect it. That is, TLR4 did not act as a signaling intermediate as its Drosophila homologue did, but as the receptor per se. We had opened a window into how mammals perceive microbes, and a great many laboratories began to study the question of how TLRs signal to initiate the inflammatory response, and how they might be involved in the pathogenesis of sterile inflammatory diseases.

LA JOLLA (2000–2011) AND ENU MUTAGENESIS

In 2000, I relocated my laboratory from UT Southwestern to The Scripps Research Institute (TSRI). Eager to dissect innate immunity in mammals, I invested heavily in ENU mutagenesis as a means of creating new and interesting phenotypes in the mouse. The plan was to create many exceptions to the norm using a random process, thus acquiring fresh paradigms of importance equal to the C3H/HeJ and C57BL/10ScCr mice (which bore spontaneous mutations, and taught us so much about microbe sensing). In this way, I felt, we could take innate immunity apart gene by gene, finding all the parts of an enormous puzzle, and do so without hypotheses and their attendant biases.

I chose the classical genetic route because I knew the mouse genome would soon be sequenced and annotated; hence positional cloning would become much easier. All candidates would be known within all critical regions, and only mapping would be required to exclude most genes from consideration. Never again would it be necessary to build a contig and explore it for genes: the two toughest parts of positional cloning. Moreover, sequencing candidate genes was becoming progressively easier. Capillary sequencing was replacing the slab gels, and there was great potential for automation. In time, I foresaw, entire genomes might be sequenced all at once. The main burden would be to generate phenotype for study: in our case, immunological phenotype.

But until sequencing technology had advanced further, the crucial point was to cover critical regions quickly and efficiently. Toward this goal, Yu Xia, an exceptionally skillful programmer in my group, wrote software that would analyze genes within a specific genomic interval, mask the sequence to hide common repeats, and design optimized primers for amplification and sequencing. He also wrote code that would permit mutation identification: a human observer no longer needed to search through trace files to find them.

This was a system that no other laboratory possessed, and using it, we were able to positionally clone as many as 50 mutations per year (as compared to one mutation in five years only a decade earlier).

As "next generation" sequencing became a reality, we modified Yu's system to validate mutations identified within the whole mouse genome. At last, only the most cursory mapping was required to define the location of a mutation, whereon it could then be found by machines that sequenced DNA a million times faster than we were able to sequence it in former times. This brings us to the present state of the art. My colleagues and I have found hundreds of mutations responsible for phenotype, many of them affecting immune function. Like all mechanists and reductionists, we regard the innate immune system as a highly complex machine. Surely we have far to go to understand its workings as we might understand those of a pocket watch. But just as surely, the innate immune system is a machine, and one day it will universally be seen as such.

Over the 13 years that elapsed between our discovery of the LPS receptor and the announcement of the Nobel Prize, I made a number of close friends in the innate immunity field. Shizuo Akira made enormous contributions, as he and his colleagues used reverse genetics to dissect the signaling pathways incorporating the receptors, adaptor proteins, kinases, and transcription factors that lead to activation of the inflammatory response. Jules Hoffmann, who with his colleagues had discovered the immunological role of Toll in the fruit fly, went forward to analyze the Drosophila imd pathway (evocative of the mammalian TNF signaling pathway, and used by the fly to detect Gramnegative bacteria) and the upstream proteins that activate Toll and imd signaling. Jules' group, Shizuo's group, and my own began to study antiviral defense in insects and mammals, collaborating in an open and congenial manner. I developed the highest respect for their scientific acumen and integrity. Jules and I, in particular, spent pleasant days together over the past decade hiking, discussing politics, and talking about history, science, and people.

I also developed strong friendships at Scripps, none stronger than with Argyrios (Ari) Theofilopoulos. Ari had worked for many years to understand autoimmunity, especially as represented in systemic lupus erythematosus (SLE). A part of the premise for searching for the LPS receptor was the likelihood that it might ultimately explain sterile inflammation. In fact, TLR7 (and conceivably other TLRs as well) turned out to have an essential facilitating role in SLE, at least as modeled in the mouse. Ari and I had numerous discussions about this, and collaborated quite extensively on studies of autoimmunity using TLR mutants and other mutants generated using ENU mutagenesis.

In time, our work in the innate immunity field was recognized by some major prizes: first the Robert Koch Prize (2004), then the Gran Prix Charles Leopold Mayer (2006), the William B. Coley Award (2006), the Balzan Prize (2007), the Albany Prize (2009), the Will Rogers Institute Prize (2009), the Shaw Prize (2011), and others in between. In 2008, I was elected both to the National Academy of Sciences and to the Institute of Medicine. Each of these distinctions was an occasion to celebrate, often with family, friends and colleagues in attendance (Figure 5). I was happy that my father was alive to mark most of these milestones with me. But to the sorrow of all my family, he passed away in October of 2008, after a year-long battle with mantle cell lymphoma.

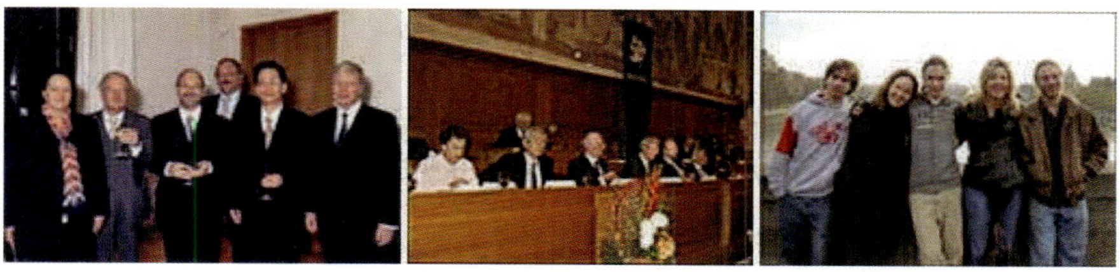

FIGURE 5. Top: Receiving the Robert Koch Prize with Shizuo Akira and Jules Hoffmann, 2004. Middle: Receiving the Balzan Prize in Berne, Switzerland, 2007. Left to right: Dame Rosalyn Higgins, Sumio Iijima, Michel Zink, Jules Hoffmann, Bruce Beutler, and Karlheinz Böhm. Lower: In Paris to receive the Charles-Leopold-Mayer Prize of the French Academy of Sciences, 2006. Left to right: Elliot Beutler, Nadia Krochin, Jonathan Beutler, Betsy Layton, and Daniel Beutler. (Photographed by Bruce Beutler).

THE PRESENT, THE FUTURE, AND ADVICE TO OTHERS WHO MAY FOLLOW ME

By March of 2011, I had decided to return to Dallas, and I had a dual appointment at Scripps and at UT Southwestern on October 3 of that year. By the time the Prize was awarded in December, I had completed my relocation. I have begun to build a Center for the Genetics of Host Defense, in which faculty with a forward genetic orientation, working with diverse model organisms, can join together to study the protective mechanisms that have developed to combat infection. They may also study autoimmune and autoinflammatory diseases: the destructive legacies of immunity, which was itself imposed on us by the enormous selective pressure that infections represent.

I must admit that many questions in biology appeal to me, and at times, it is difficult to maintain an intense focus on the immune system, important though immunity is. The great epiphany for me in solving a single, critical question

– the conundrum of LPS sensing – was the embrace of genetics. This is a golden age of genetics, in which one may find the cause of monogenic phenotype almost immediately. The destruction of all genes in the mouse by chemical and/or insertional mutagenesis and gene targeting will soon be a reality. At this writing, the ability to clone mice from somatic cells, and the availability of haploid embryonic stem cells for genetic experimentation, also promise to accelerate progress in biology. When I first began working in my father's laboratory, none of these technologies were foreseen by anyone then alive. It is fair to say that mankind's understanding of living things has advanced more during the past 50 years than it did during all of history before. I have been a direct witness to most of this progress. So have many others who are older than I, and have been practicing scientists for a longer time. This is to say that we live in an exciting era, and should feel lucky about it.

The Nobel Prize gives an opportunity for introspection, and to conclude this brief autobiography, I offer some thoughts that arose in my mind during the last few months, mostly prompted by specific questions from students, journalists, family and colleagues. "To what do you attribute your success?" they want to know. "How does one win a Nobel Prize?"

In my case, the path to the Nobel Prize began with a love of nature and an earnest curiosity about the phenomenon of life. I was lucky to have an understanding father, who was himself a distinguished scientist. He gave me excellent advice during my formative years. But this might have helped little had I not been industrious, enthusiastic, and optimistic in pursuing a career in biology. I did not worry or make contingency plans to be used in the event of failure; I ran blithely ahead with confidence that success would come to me.

I chose an undervalued question, viewing the mystery of the LPS response as the key to understanding inflammation and the recognition of microbes – and I based this assumption on a strong and well-studied phenotype. While the LPS receptor did not turn out to explain everything about how inflammation works, it did give major insights. The choice of a question is a matter of scientific taste; a matter of recognizing what is interesting and important. Such taste is partly innate and partly learned. To the extent that I learned scientific taste, I did so by studying medicine.

Much later than I might have, I embraced genetics, preferring its unbiased character to hypotheses, which often lead scientists astray, mainly because they don't like to be wrong. I do not eschew hypotheses. But not all scientists have the integrity to test them as they should be tested. Only the very best scientists do. The others try to "prove" their hypotheses. And this unfortunate fact is the cause of much error, wasted time, and wasted resources.

I have also learned that it is important to choose outstanding colleagues. Not only those who will frankly criticize one's work or provide fresh insight, but also those with whom one works directly, as a mentor or supervisor. Recognizing talent, acquiring it, nurturing it, and retaining it is among the hardest things a scientist must do. It is a skill quite separate from scientific ability per se. It will usually determine whether the scientist succeeds, because none of us can accomplish much in isolation.

Finally, and maybe most important of all, my principal achievements resulted from addressing a single problem with relentless obsession. Once convinced that something could be achieved, I was not deterred by discouraging advice from others. I would suggest the same course to anyone. In the event of failure, one may always select another problem and begin anew. That is what I would have done had I failed. As it happened, it was unnecessary.

HOW MAMMALS SENSE INFECTION: FROM ENDOTOXIN TO THE TOLL-LIKE RECEPTORS

Nobel Lecture, December 7, 2011

by

BRUCE BEUTLER

Center for Genetics of Host Defense, the University of Texas Southwestern Medical Center, Dallas, TX, USA.

HOW I CAME TO WORK ON THE QUESTION OF INNATE IMMUNE SENSING

About 30 years after the fact, I remembered a walk my father (Figure 1) and I took through a grove of redwoods in Sequoia National Park. I was perhaps 10 or 12 years of age. "Why is it that trees don't simply rot?" I asked him, aware that plants had none of the lymphoid or myeloid cells that confer immunity to vertebrates. He explained there were tannins and perhaps other molecules in trees that made them resistant to decay. "But they rot after they die, and the tannins are still there," I countered. The discussion went on, venturing into infections of live plants such as potatoes and wheat, and I tentatively concluded that plants must have some form of immunity that was actively maintained in the sense that it depended on their vitality. But at least to the two of us, not much seemed to be known about it. Of course, I didn't know then that I would discover a mechanism of disease resistance in mammals that had its counterpart in most multicellular life forms, including insects and plants. But our conversation in Sequoia was to return to my mind almost immediately when I did.

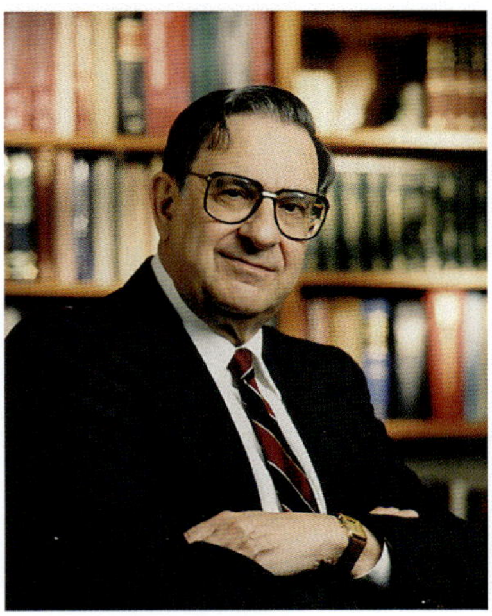

Figure 1. Ernest Beutler, M.D. (1928–2008).

This was one of many thousands of discussions about science I had with my father, who always challenged me, counseled me, and helped to prepare me for whatever I wanted to do. He encouraged my love of science from the time I was a small child. From him, I learned to work in the lab, to isolate and analyze proteins, to think in evolutionary terms, and to evaluate experimental results. It was he who suggested I should go to medical school, to gain broad familiarity with the special processes that make living things what they are. Among the most important pieces of advice I recall was to "know what problems are important." The message is one I try to pass on to students today. By the time my own interest in the field of innate immunity had become highly resolved, I felt secure in the knowledge that I was working on something of great importance. This inspired me to see a tough project through to its completion, despite all the difficulties my team and I encountered.

AMONG THINGS THAT ARE IMPORTANT, INFECTION IS A COMPLEX PROBLEM

In the depths of prehistory, infection probably killed most of our forebears. In historic times, there is no doubt that it did. Neither famine nor warfare nor cancer nor cardiovascular diseases have caused as many deaths as infection, for as long as humans have kept records of mortality and its causes. Even in the present century, with all our resources, infection claims nearly a quarter of all human lives[1] (Figure 2). Smallpox alone is said to have been the most frequent single cause of death among *Homo sapiens* during the 20th century,[2] and great plagues of other kinds may have been close behind. Particularly because they strike down so many people before or during reproductive age, microbes constitute the strongest selective pressure with which our species must contend, and we may assume that microbes have shaped the human genome more than any other selective pressure in recent times. The autoimmune and autoinflammatory diseases we experience – by themselves major causes of morbidity and sometimes death – are the legacy of the intense selection our species has endured.

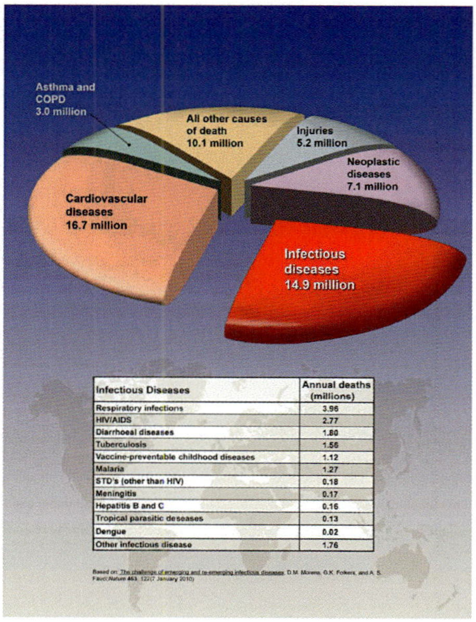

Figure 2. Leading causes of death worldwide. Approximately 15 million of the 57 (~25%) million annual deaths are the result of infectious diseases (listed in the table). Data were obtained from figures published by the World Health Organization (see http://www.who.int/whr/en). The figure above is adapted from Morens, Folkers, and Fauci.[3]

From almost any point of view, few phenomena are more complex than infections, which represent the clinical manifestations of the battle between host and microbe. Infection is a process in which thousands of biological processes go awry all at once as host and microbe compete with one another.

So many changes occur simultaneously during infection that it was once difficult to take a reductionist, mechanistic approach to the subject. The rhetorical question an investigator might ask was "where to begin?" But within this question was the seed of the right question, because there was reason to think that the host response might be initiated in a comparatively simple way: by a handful of receptors, recognizing the tell-tale molecular signatures of microbes and sounding an alarm. Our work was directed toward finding these receptors. Find them, we thought, and we would find the "eyes" of the immune system. Find them, and we might also understand how sterile inflammation is initiated. These were goals worth struggling for.

Genetics has provided the critical breakthrough in many biological problems, and it did so in the analysis of host responses to infection. By starting with distinguishable biological states (i.e., phenotypes) that are heritable, and identifying the genetic determinant of the difference, one may elucidate the molecules that play a key role in the phenomenon of interest. Using genetics, my colleagues and I determined one of the principal means by which mammals become aware of infection when it occurs, and deliver a response.

FRAMING THE QUESTION: INFECTIONS AND HOW THEY HARM US

Some of the most basic questions about how we fight infection remain unanswered to this day. The question as to how we sense infection was once in this category. To address it, we asked a more focused question: *how do we sense endotoxin, a structurally conserved component of Gram negative bacteria?* We did so in the hope that the answer would shed light on the more global picture of microbe sensing. We wanted to identify the first molecular events that initiate the immune response and all that goes with it.

The question about endotoxin was one that had endured for more than 100 years. Microbes had been discovered in the 17th century. But only in the late 19th century was their relationship to infection established, principally by Pasteur and Koch. It immediately occurred to many scientists of the time to ask how microbes actually do harm, and the possibility that toxins emanate from microbes was entertained.

Endotoxin was discovered by a German army surgeon, Richard Pfeiffer, who joined Koch and his team in 1887. Encouraged by Koch to study cholera, Pfeiffer noted that guinea pigs died when injected with a large inoculum of *V. cholerae,* even if passively or actively immunized against the microbe. Yet adaptive immunity had done its work: no living vibrio could be retrieved from the host. Pfeiffer's name became attached to this phenomenon, and he extended his observation, noting that heat-killed vibrio were also lethal to guinea pigs. He called the toxic principle "endotoxin,"[4] and endotoxin became a paradigmatic molecule in microbial pathogenesis (Figure 3).

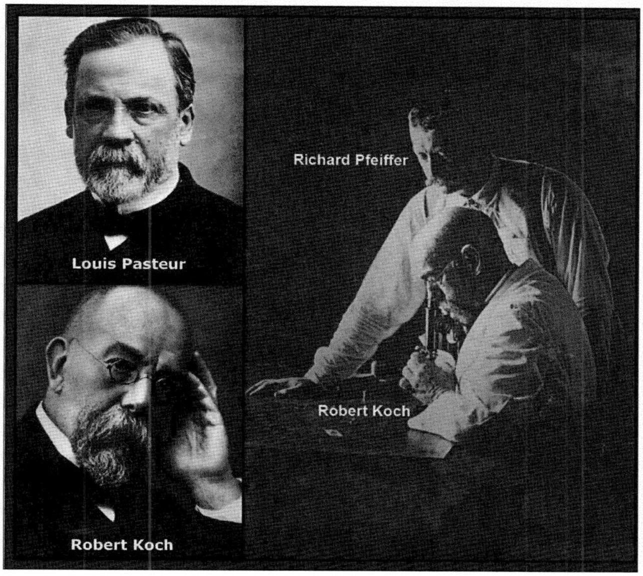

Figure 3. Louis Pasteur (1822–1895), Robert Koch (1843–1910), and Richard Pfeiffer (1858–1945), shown with Koch.

WHAT WAS ENDOTOXIN, AND HOW DID IT WORK?

With the passage of decades it was understood that endotoxin was, chemically speaking, a lipopolysaccharide (LPS). It was the major glycolipid of the outer leaflet of the outer membrane of nearly all Gram-negative bacteria.[5] Mesrobeanu and Boivin extracted LPS in fairly pure form in the 1930s;[6] Lüderitz and Westphal introduced a phenol extraction protocol for LPS isolation subsequently. Ultimately, LPS from diverse microbial sources was structurally characterized.[7] The lipid moiety of LPS, named "Lipid A," was seen to constitute the toxic center of LPS,[8] and by 1984, Lipid A had been synthesized artificially by Imoto et al., and shown to possess all of the activity of natural preparations.[9] The pathway by which LPS was naturally synthesized was also deciphered, principally by Christian Raetz and his colleagues.[10] LPS partial structures were isolated, and a number of structural rules for endotoxicity were established.[11] Of importance to our work later on, it was noted that some LPS partial structures are agonistic when applied to mouse cells, but antagonize LPS when applied to human cells. The best example of this was Lipid IVa, which lacked acyl-oxyacyl side chains, and had only four lipid chains.[12]

At nanomolar concentrations LPS was capable of activating leukocytes in vitro. If administered to living animals, it was strongly pyrogenic. It caused an immediate fall in the peripheral leukocyte count in animals as a result of the margination of circulating cells, and was also known to induce both the local and generalized Shwartzman reactions. If administered in sufficient quantities, just as Pfeiffer had observed, it could have a lethal effect. As a class, mammals are more sensitive to LPS than other vertebrates, and among mammals, humans, rabbits, ungulates, and certain other taxa were exquisitely sensitive to LPS. It was clear that LPS must contribute to the often dramatic shock and tissue injury observed in Gram-negative infections. For this reason more than any other, LPS became a central interest in biomedicine, and efforts were made to interdict and neutralize it, often with antibodies.

Intriguing "beneficial" effects of LPS were also noted. By the 1950s, Johnson et al. had shown that purified LPS was endowed with adjuvant activity,[13] greatly augmenting the antibody response to ovalbumin. Over the next decades, organized efforts to use LPS and LPS derivatives with diminished toxicity in vaccines were pursued by Ribi and others.[14] LPS could also induce non-specific resistance to infections for a period of time after its administration.[15] It was able to induce the necrosis of tumors in mice.[16] And it was known to have a protective effect against otherwise lethal doses of gamma irradiation.[17]

EVIDENCE FOR THE EXISTENCE OF AN LPS RECEPTOR, DEPENDENT UPON A SINGLE GENE.

There was no clear consensus as to *what* the LPS receptor might be. But as to the *existence* of an LPS receptor, there was a high degree of confidence from the 1960s onward. And much was known about the general characteristics of the receptor: that it could detect many structural variants of LPS, for example, but was not involved in the perception of other inflammatory molecules made by microbes. The evidence came from mouse genetics.

In 1965, Heppner and Weiss reported that mice of the C3H/HeJ strain were highly resistant to the toxic effects of LPS.[18] Sultzer later documented the absence of leukocyte responses to LPS in these mice, in that they failed to form a peritoneal exudate when injected with LPS.[19] The C3H/HeJ substrain had been separated from other C3H substrains only a few years earlier, and evidently, a recessive or semi-dominant mutation had become fixed in the population, forbidding responses to LPS. C3H/HeN mice, and C3H/OuJ mice stood as controls for LPS responsiveness, but were nearly identical to C3H/HeJ mice.

In 1977, Coutinho observed that mice of the strain C57BL/10ScCr mimicked mice of the C3H/HeJ strain, in that they had absent B cell responses to LPS.[20] Allelism testing showed that the mutation in C57BL/10ScCr mice affected the same locus that was affected in C3H/HeJ mice.[21]

Both C3H/HeJ and C57BL/10ScCr strains had highly specific defects. They responded normally to all microbial ligands tested, save LPS. This gave reason for confidence that the LPS receptor itself was affected by the mutations, rather than a broadly utilized transducing protein. And it suggested that the LPS receptor was quite specific. For example, certain lipopeptides from Borrelia burgdorferi seemed to utilize a distinct receptor to elicit TNF production.[22]

In 1974, Watson and Riblet determined that a single locus mutation abolished the response to LPS in C3H/HeJ mice.[23] In their study, they utilized B cell division and IgM production as indicators of the LPS response. Then, using classical phenotypic markers and a total of 14 recombinant inbred strains of mice derived from C57BL/6 and C3H/HeJ parents, they established linkage between the newly named *Lps* locus and the *Major Urinary Protein (Mup1)* locus on chromosome 4.[24] Using a backcross strategy, the *Lps* locus was further confined to the interval flanked by *Mup1* and *Polysyndactyly (Ps)* loci.[25] This critical region was of unknown size, but immense (occupying about 1/8 of the chromosome), and could not be narrowed until much later.

LPS-resistant mice revealed profound facts about endotoxicity. The lethal effect of LPS was shown to be conferred by cells of hematopoietic origin (although LPS undoubtedly triggers responses in other cells as well).[26] Mice that could not sense LPS were markedly compromised in their ability to survive infection by Gram-negative bacteria.[27] Therefore, whatever the harmful effects of LPS, detecting it operates to the benefit of the host under conditions in which a small inoculum of bacteria has been introduced. Moreover, all effects of LPS were apparently mediated by the *Lps* locus; hence adjuvant effects, B cell mitogenesis, IgM production, and lethality all depended on a single gene.

One of the most important conclusions of work with LPS-resistant mice concerned the affirmative link between LPS sensing and host resistance. If mice were unable to sense LPS, they were vulnerable to infection by Gram-negative microbes, despite the fact that they were spared damage caused by LPS itself. This was first observed in animals infected with *Salmonella typhimurium*,[28] then in *E. coli*,[29] and later *F. tularensis*[30] and *Rickettsia akari*.[31] One plausible interpretation of these results is that LPS sensing contributes to detection of microbes during the earliest stages of an infection, permitting the host to mount a response that contains or eliminates them. If the host remains ignorant of the infection, containment does not occur; hence the burden of microbes becomes much greater. By the time the microbes are detected because of other molecules they produce (for example, flagellin, lipopeptides, nucleic acids), it is too late to contain the infection, and the host is overwhelmed. The existence of inducers of an inflammatory response other than LPS, and specific receptors for their detection, is implicit in this interpretation. So, too, is the primacy of the LPS detection system where these particular Gram negative microbes are concerned.

MY OWN INTEREST IN LPS AND HOW IT DEVELOPED

Some of the discoveries described above took place before I was interested in LPS, and indeed before I was born. But I began to think about LPS at a young age. In 1975, during a summer term at UCSD where I was a student, I approached Abraham Braude (Figure 4) to ask whether I might work in his laboratory. Braude had been a pioneer in the use of passive immunization against LPS as a means of countering sepsis: an approach that never gained general broad acceptance by the medical community. He referred me to Arthur Friedlander, a postdoctoral associate in his group who was then studying the capsular polysaccharide of Cryptococcus, and its ability to induce chemotaxis. Friedlander, who later made impressive advances in the study of the lethal toxin of *Bacillus anthracis,* put me to work studying the responses of rabbit leukocytes to purified polysaccharide. In this environment, I first learned of LPS and its ability to activate leukocytes, induce fever, and cause shock. At that stage, my consciousness of LPS mainly concerned its potential to cause experimental artifacts, and the need to destroy it by baking glassware at 180°C (LPS is resistant to autoclaving).

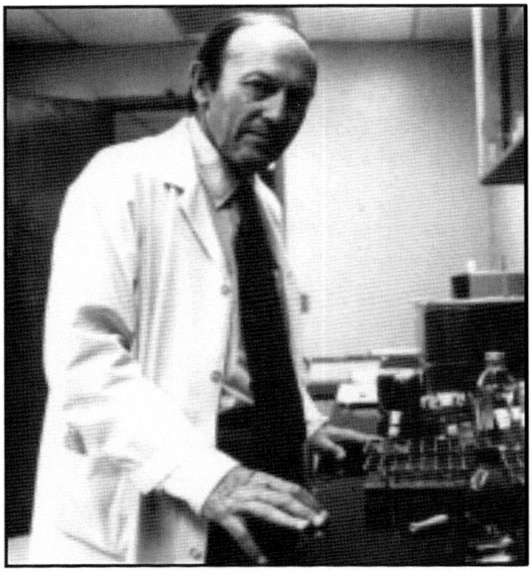

Figure 4. Abraham I. Braude, M.D, Ph.D. (1917–1984). Photograph provided by Josh Fierer.

As a medical student at the University of Chicago (1977–1981), and as a house officer at the University of Texas Southwestern Medical Center at Dallas (1981–1983), I treated patients suffering from Gram negative sepsis, and began to see the clinical effects of LPS firsthand. This certainly impressed me as to the importance of LPS as a clinical problem, and as to the magnitude of the disturbances LPS could cause. But my formal entry into the field of LPS research began later. As a postdoctoral associate and then an assistant professor, I worked in the lab of Anthony Cerami at the Rockefeller University (1983–1986). There I isolated and characterized cachectin, an LPS-induced macrophage factor.

Cachectin was named before my arrival in the lab, for its postulated role as mediator of cachexia, the wasting process seen in many chronic diseases. At the time I arrived, it was a crude factor, defined by its ability to suppress expression of lipoprotein lipase (LPL) produced by fat cells (or in the usual case, cultured 3T3-L1 pre-adipocytes). LPL is an enzyme required for the hydrolysis of triglycerides to generate free fatty acids, permitting the entry of plasma lipids into energy storage tissues. Cachectin activity was secreted in abundance by LPS-activated macrophages or LPS-activated immortalized macrophage cell lines. But no headway had been made in isolating the factor. Certain candidate mediators had been obtained as crude preparations from other laboratories, and tested for cachectin activity. One of the candidate mediators was tumor necrosis factor, obtained from the laboratory of Lloyd Old. It was found to have no cachectin activity; hence there was considerable surprise when I purified cachectin and determined what it actually was.

In succession I developed two purification protocols to isolate mouse cachectin from the conditioned medium of LPS-activated macrophages (RAW 264.7 cells). The first of these consisted of pressure dialysis, liquid-phase isoelectric focusing, ConA sepharose chromatography, and non-denaturing polyacrylamide gel electrophoresis (PAGE). This strategy allowed me to measure the quantity of cachectin produced by macrophages (it was about 2% of their secretory product during the early hours following LPS activation), to determine its specific activity, and to visualize it (Figure 5) as a 17.5 kD protein species on a polyacrylamide gel.[32] I also raised a strong antiserum against cachectin in rabbits. But it was not possible to obtain the amino acid sequence of the protein, which evidently became N-terminally modified in the course of purification.

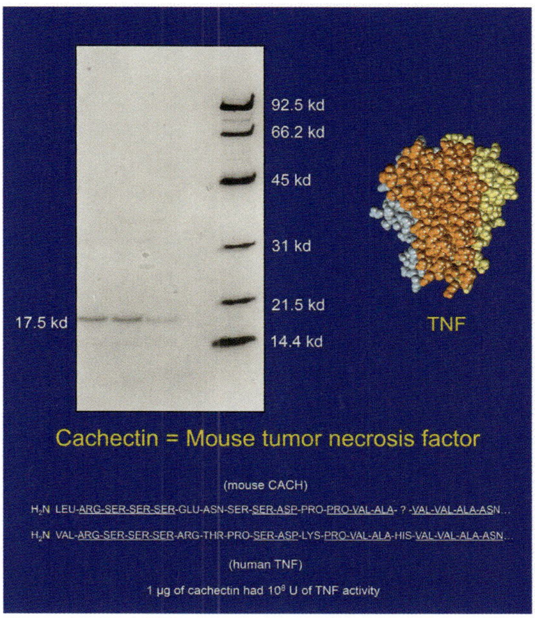

Figure 5. Cachectin purification from conditioned medium of LPS-activated macrophages (RAW 264.7 cells). Following pressure dialysis, ConA sepharose chromatography, liquid-phase isoelectric focusing, and non-denaturing polyacrylamide gel electrophoresis, cachectin was identified as a 17.5 kDa protein by polyacrylamide gel electrophoresis (SDS-PAGE). Cachectin was subsequently identified as the mouse orthologue of human tumor necrosis factor (TNF; space-filling representation shown on right).

I therefore devised a second purification method, involving the newly-developed FPLC system from Pharmacia, which included pressure dialysis, anion exchange (Mono Q) chromatography, and gel filtration (Superose 12). This yielded a product from which an N-terminal sequence could be obtained by Edman degradation.[33] Cachectin was strongly similar in sequence to human tumor necrosis factor (TNF), which had been isolated only a few months earlier by workers at Genentech.[34] Moreover, cachectin showed TNF bioactivity equivalent in terms of specific activity to that of purified recombinant human TNF: a fact first pointed out to us by John Mathison, a postdoctoral associate in the laboratory of Richard Ulevitch at The Scripps Research Institute, to whom we had sent some of our purified material.

It was thus suspected that cachectin was the mouse orthologue of human TNF: a conclusion verified by cDNA cloning a short time later.[35] However, its *de novo* purification from mouse cells, based on a different biological activity, opened a new window on what TNF actually did.

TNF, so-named by Lloyd Old, who worked at Sloan Kettering Cancer Research Institute across the street from Rockefeller University, had a history intertwined with the history of microbes and LPS. As described by Old,[36] the search for an endogenous mediator of tumor necrosis during sepsis was predicated on the observations of William Coley, who had used microbes and their products to induce remissions in patients with inoperable tumors during the early 20th century. Old had discovered TNF as the mediator of this effect, showing that LPS-injected mice produced a serum factor, apparently a protein, that could induce hemorrhagic necrosis of transplantable tumors grown in mice.[37] This factor was also capable of killing tumor cells, but not normal cells, in vitro.[38] It was viewed as a potentially nontoxic chemotherapeutic agent.

The fact that both TNF and cachectin activities emanated from a single molecule suggested to me that many of the effects of LPS might be TNF-dependent, and that TNF might mediate a strong inflammatory response. Indeed, I speculated that the lethal effect of LPS might depend upon TNF. In order to test this hypothesis, I raised an antibody against mouse TNF in rabbits, affinity purified the immunoglobulin, and made Fab'2 fragments from it.[39] I used both intact antibody and Fab'2 fragments to passively immunize mice prior to LPS challenge. Mice that were blocked in their ability to respond to TNF were demonstrably though partially LPS resistant, indicating that TNF was one of the major factors responsible for endotoxicity, though not the sole factor (Figure 6a). Moreover, I observed that TNF was remarkably toxic in mice, causing death when as little as 20 ug of active protein was administered intravenously (Figure 6b). All in all, the animals resembled mice that had been injected with LPS, developing diarrhea, prostration, and organ injury. Later, more detailed toxicological studies were performed in rats and primates, with more or less the same outcome.[40] In humans toxicity was observed also. While isolated limb perfusion with TNF did lead to remission of tumors such as melanoma,[41] systemic toxicity barred its routine use in chemotherapy.

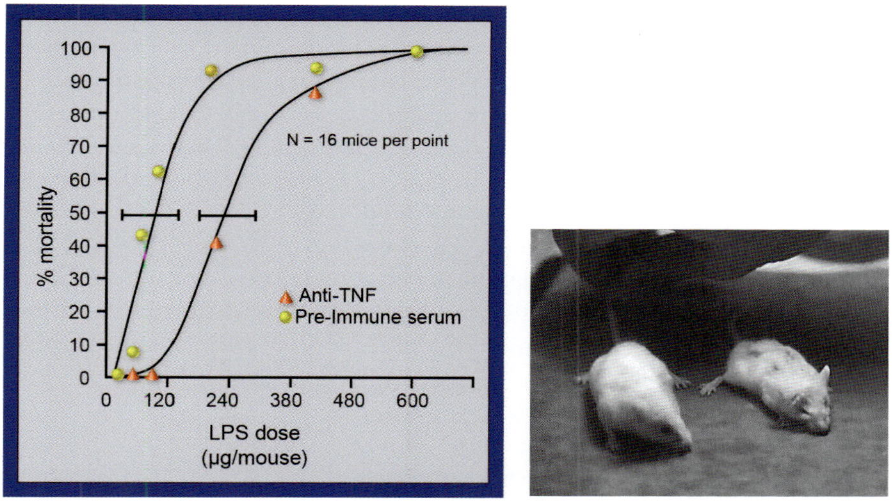

Figure 6. TNF is a major factor responsible for LPS-induced endotoxicity. (A) TNF blockade attenuates the lethal effect of LPS. Mice were treated with immune ("anti-TNF", triangles) and pre-immune serum, circles. Figure adapted from Beutler, Milsark, and Cerami.[42] (B) Mice injected with TNF (20 μg, purified from macrophages), became severely ill and often died. Animals injected with heat- inactivated material showed no untoward effects. These studies demonstrated that TNF was a major mediator of LPS toxicity.

The discovery that TNF could mediate the lethal effect of LPS led directly to experiments in many laboratories, in which the inflammatory potential of this cytokine was probed. It was found to be produced and influential in diverse model systems, and in particular, to affect both leukocytes and vascular endothelial cells so as to foster inflammatory responses (Figure 7). TNF blockade did not only prevent inflammation, but rendered animals highly susceptible to certain infections: especially infections with intracellular microbes such as *Listeria monocytogenes*[43] and *Mycobacterium bovis.*[44] TNF thus behaved as a clear executor of innate immunity.

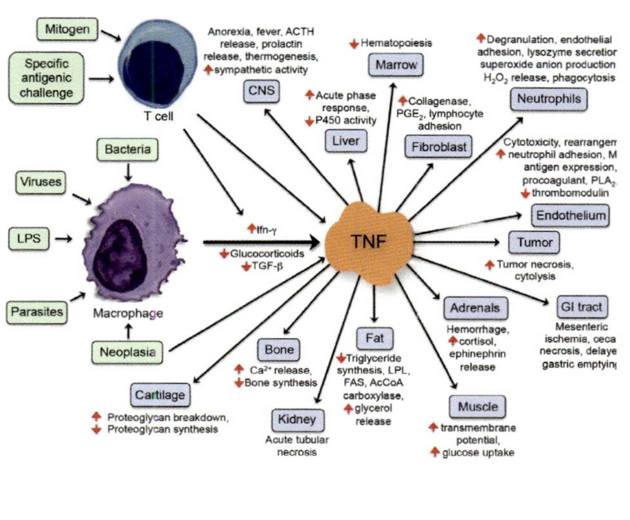

Figure 7. The many biological activities of TNF. Ligand binding to T cells (either T cell receptor specific or non-specific) and macrophages (e.g., by LPS or other microbial ligands) cause intracellular signaling that causes the secretion of TNF. Modulatory influences on signaling can be exerted by IFNγ, glucocorticoids, or TGF-β. Secreted TNF had measurable (usually inflammatory) effects on virtually all receptor-expressing cells.

TNF receptors, first isolated and cloned by David Wallach[45] and by David Goeddel[46] and their colleagues, were found to exist on many cells throughout the body, and to trigger inflammatory responses when exposed to the ligand. A practical consequence of our work was the use of anti-TNF antibodies and soluble versions of the TNF receptors as inhibitors of TNF activity in human inflammatory diseases. One of the inhibitors, a fusion protein in which the ectodomain of the TNF receptor was linked to the hinge and Fc fragment of an IgG heavy chain, was invented in my laboratory in Dallas,[47] patented, and sold to Immunex, which later manufactured an equivalent molecule, Enbrel. In time, TNF blockade was used to effectively treat several diseases, including rheumatoid arthritis, Crohn's disease, ankylosing spondylitis, and psoriasis (Figure 8).

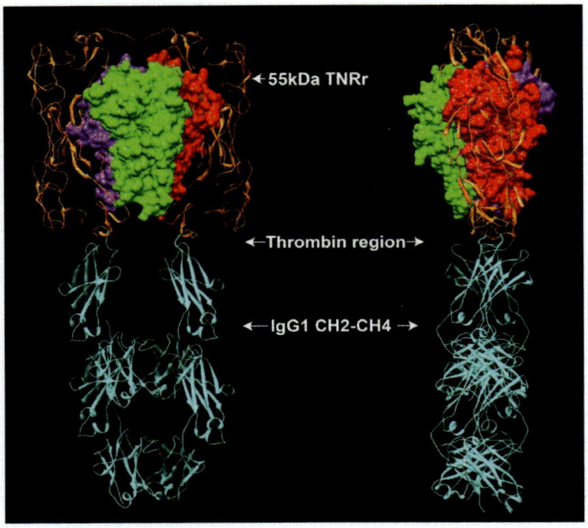

Figure 8. TNF blockade enforced by a recombinant TNF inhibitor. Two views of the inhibitor are presented. Shown is the interaction of the TNF trimer (red, green and purple subunits; space filling model) with the ectodomain of the 55 kDa TNF receptor (TNFr; gold ribbons). The ectodomain of TNFr was linked to the hinge and Fc fragment of an IgG heavy chain (cyan). Figures generated with USCF Chimera.

But a great question remained, relevant to all of these diseases. In sterile inflammation, what elicited production of TNF and other cytokines in the first place? And where Gram-negative infection was concerned, how did LPS trigger a biological response? In short, the cytokine response was clearly what orchestrated inflammation. But there was no understanding as to how the cytokine response began.

TNF was clearly a biologically relevant endpoint to follow in understanding responses to LPS. It was an "apex" cytokine, produced earlier than most other cytokines and capable of inducing many of them. Hence, I began to use TNF as a measurable marker of LPS-induced macrophage activation. And I did so with the conviction that a single molecule – the LPS receptor – must be found if we were to understand the very first events in the response to infection.

GROWING OBSESSION WITH THE C3H/HEJ MOUSE

It was during the course of my work with TNF that I first became aware of the existence of LPS resistant strains of mice: probably in 1983. Masanobu Kawakami, a postdoctoral associate who preceded me in the Cerami lab, had used macrophages from these animals as a control, to show that LPS induced cachectin activity and did not itself possess this activity when applied to adipocytes.[48] Despite all that had been learned from these mice, already discussed above, nothing was yet known about the LPS receptor, or how it signaled. Gradually, the genetic lesion of the C3H/HeJ mouse began to occupy center stage in my mind, particularly after I left the Rockefeller University and set up my own laboratory at UT Southwestern Medical Center at Dallas. There I was jointly appointed as a member of the Howard Hughes Medical Institute, and was encouraged to pursue a focused "high-risk, high-impact" project.

I began to reflect on the fact that aside from the N-formyl-methionyl-leucyl-phenylalanine (fMLP) receptor, known to be a plasma membrane GTP binding protein, almost no avenues for the perception of microbes had been established. While it was obvious that host cells perceived molecular signatures indicative of broad microbial taxa (fMLP and LPS being only two examples among many), little was known about how this was accomplished. And the fMLP receptor could not really compare with the LPS receptor in terms of its biological relevance: it had not been shown to be crucial for the events of sepsis or for resistance to infection. Finding the LPS receptor seemed the critical question in innate immunity, inasmuch as LPS itself was the archetypal microbial elicitor molecule. Finding the LPS receptor might tell how most infections sound an alarm.

How might one identify the protein affected by mutations of the *Lps* locus? Several "easy" methods were potentially at hand. For example, one might simply look for a distinction between C3H/HeJ mice and C3H/HeN mice at the protein level. Or one might attempt to raise an antibody against cells from C3H/HeN proteins in C3H/HeJ recipient. Such an antibody might pinpoint the protein defective in the C3H/HeJ strain. One might try insertional mutagenesis: make an F1 heterozygote by crossing C3H/HeJ to C3H/HeN; make an immortalized macrophage line (expected to be LPS responsive), and then attempt to destroy the one "good" copy of the *Lps* locus with a retrovirus and isolate an unresponsive clone. A standard cDNA rescue approach might also have worked. We went so far as to make an immortalized C3H/HeJ cell line in collaboration with Paola Ricciardi Castagnoli, hoping to use it in this way. Later, it was put to a different use, as described below.

Each of these approaches was diligently pursued, but each was unsuccessful. We understood that in other laboratories, affinity purification methods were used in an attempt to isolate the LPS receptor. But no substantial publications resulted. The nature of the LPS receptor remained entirely mysterious. There were, however, numerous papers hinting at what the receptor and/or the product of the *Lps* locus "might" be. Some referred to the putative involvement of the cell surface molecule CD18 in LPS signaling.[49] Through differential display studies, SLPI, a serine protease inhibitor, was indirectly implicated.[50] A small GTP binding protein called Ran/TC4 was suggested as well.[51] Studies with inhibitors suggested the involvement of a tyrosine kinase.[52] Or perhaps a histidine kinase was encoded by *Lps*, based on the upstream activator of the p38 equivalent in yeast, HOG1.[53] Or perhaps the *Lps* locus encoded a member of the protein kinase C family.[54] During the course of our positional cloning work, we needed to ignore such hints, because hypothesis-driven targeted searches would have distracted us from our primary mission: to find all candidate genes within the *Lps* critical region, and ultimately find the causative mutation responsible for LPS resistance.

One suggestion as to the nature of the LPS receptor could not be ignored, because it was so clearly true and compelling. In the year 1990, Sam Wright, working in Richard Ulevitch's group, showed that antibodies against the monocyte surface marker CD14 were able to inhibit responses to LPS.[55] The Ulevitch lab subsequently showed that overexpression of CD14 in 70Z/3 pre-B cells would greatly enhance LPS responsiveness in these cells, which were otherwise minimally responsive to LPS.[56] CD14, a leucine-rich repeat protein anchored to the surface of cells, had no obvious means of inducing a transmembrane signal, in that it had no cytoplasmic domain. Moreover, it was encoded by a gene unlinked to the *Lps* locus (it is now known to be on chromosome 18). It was considered, therefore, that CD14 might be part of the LPS receptor complex. But at least one missing part of the complex, crucial for signaling, would necessarily be encoded by the *Lps* locus (Figure 9).

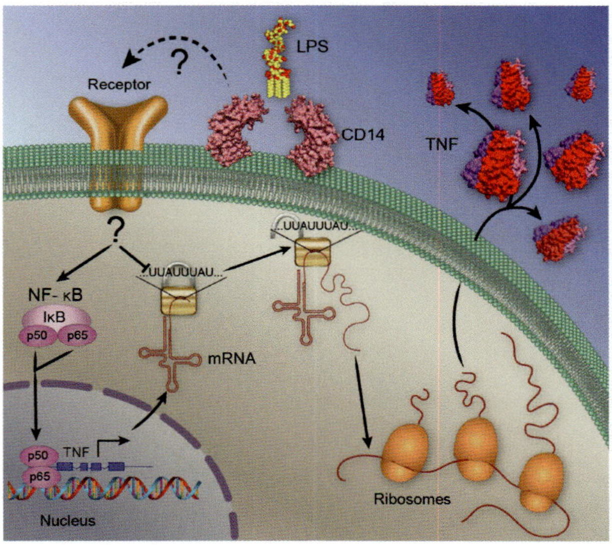

Figure 9. An unknown receptor in LPS-mediated TNF secretion. The figure reflects the state of knowledge that existed in the early 1990s. Overexpression of CD14 was observed to enhance LPS responses of 70Z/3 cells, although it had no means of inducing a transmembrane signal. Therefore CD14 was considered to be an essential part of the receptor complex, which must include an unknown membrane-spanning protein, likely defective in C3H/HeJ and C57BL/10ScCr mice. In unstimulated macrophages, TNF mRNA is repressed translationally through its AU-rich elements (AREs). In LPS- stimulated cells, the unidentified receptor relays a signal for the NF-κB subunits p50/p65 translocate to the nucleus and transcribe the TNF gene. The blockade of translation (via the AREs) is also alleviated upon LPS-mediated activation. The mRNA is subsequently translated and the TNF protein is processed and secreted.

During the late 1980s and early 1990s, my colleagues and I analyzed control points that governed biosynthesis of TNF in LPS-activated macrophages, with the general thought that we might work backward toward the receptor if we understood specific molecular events that transpired in the cell. We showed that both transcriptional and translational activation steps occurred in macrophages in response to LPS, and noted that acting in concert with one another, these regulatory mechanisms permitted a several thousand-fold increase in TNF secretion by activated cells as compared to quiescent cells.[57] From the work of Jongeneel and his colleagues, it was known that transcriptional activation depended minimally upon NF-κB translocation to the nucleus.[58] But the translational activation step remained quite enigmatic, and to a large extent still does. Consistent with earlier work of Kruys and Huez,[59] we concluded that translational repression of the TNF mRNA was maintained in quiescent cells by a cis-acting UA-rich sequence[60] which we had identified in the 3'-untranslated region of the molecule.[61] The same sequence motif, independently identified by others, was shown to cause instability of many mRNA molecules.[62]

We studied the effects of various inhibitory drugs (particularly glucocorticoids and pentoxifylline) on the TNF response to LPS,[63] and created reporter mice bearing a transgene in which a chloramphenicol acetyltransferase (CAT) coding sequence was substituted for the TNF coding sequence.[64] These animals permitted us to determine where TNF was produced during in vivo LPS challenge.[65] While useful, these analyses were tangential to the key question of what the receptor might be. Increasingly, I felt we were dancing around the problem rather than attacking it, and in 1993, I resolved to focus exclusively on the *Lps* locus.

POSITIONAL CLONING OF THE LPS LOCUS.

An unbiased genetic approach to finding the *Lps* locus became feasible when the density of markers in the mouse genome increased enough to permit at least some narrowing of the critical region established much earlier by Watson et al.[66] At the time we began our positional cloning work in 1993, only 317 microsatellite markers had been published,[67] and only a fraction of these were informative between any two selected strains. We set about to map the *Lps* locus to high-resolution, hopeful that we could confine the mutation to a relatively small part of mouse chromosome 4.

Christophe Van Huffel took the lead in this work, and was soon joined by Alexander Poltorak, Irina (Ira) Smirnova, Xiaolong He, and Mu-Ya Liu, all postdoctoral associates in my lab. Not all of them would see the work through to completion. Alexander and Ira were the exceptions, and deserve most of the credit for our success. They were truly devoted, smart, and innovative in their work, and passionate in their desire to find the mutation. I must also mention the contribution of Ms. Betsy Layton, my administrative assistant then and to the present day. She not only organized our work when it came to determining the position of markers and constructing accurate maps, but also participated in some of the laboratory effort, picking colonies, inoculating broth, and reading and searching DNA sequences. To these people, I owe a great debt of gratitude (Figure 10).

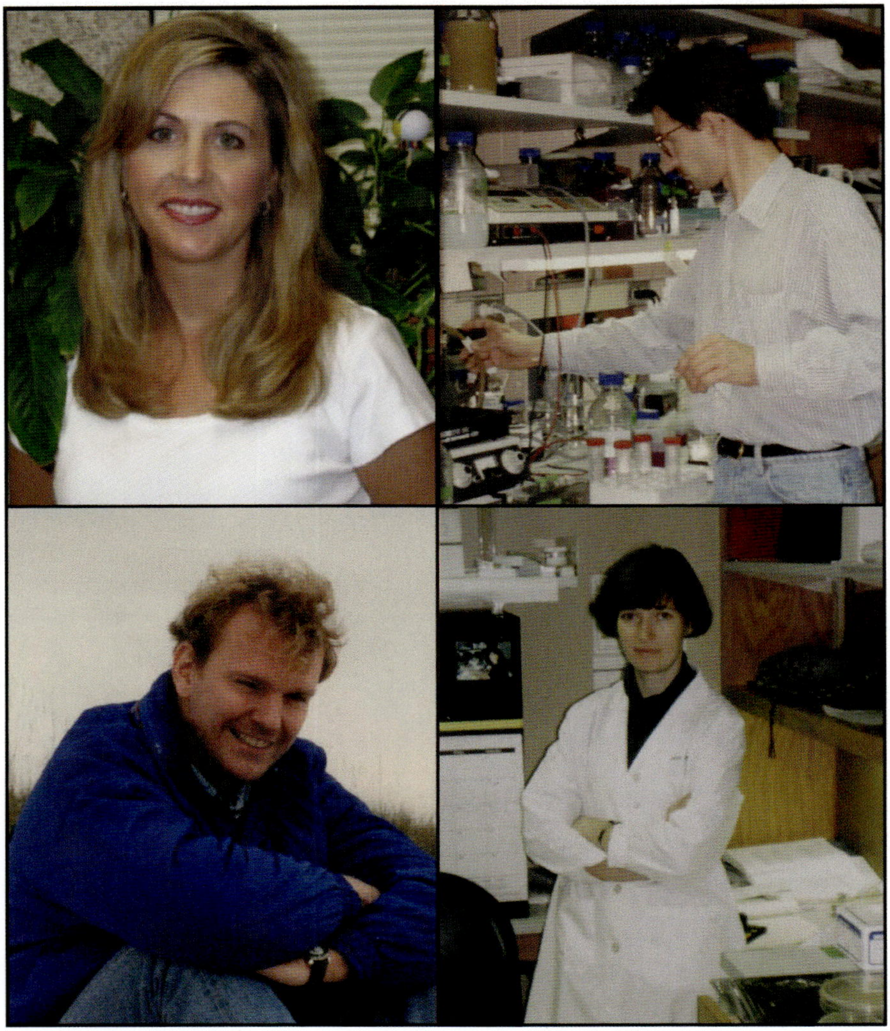

Figure 10. (clockwise, from top left) Ms. Betsy Layton, Dr. Alexander Poltorak, Dr. Irina (Ira) Smirnova and Dr. Christophe Van Huffel. Photos taken in early to middle 1990s.

The *Lps* cloning project grew to enormous proportions, although we never imagined it would in the beginning. It was accomplished in three phases. First came the *genetic mapping* phase. To narrow the critical region, we used a total 2,093 meioses, derived from crosses of C3H/HeJ to either SWR/J or C57BL/6J mice, with backcrosses of F1 hybrid animals to the C3H/HeJ parent. The F2 mice were examined for LPS responsiveness, measuring the ability of their peritoneal macrophages to secrete TNF when challenged with LPS, by means of a biological assay. The effort was not entirely straightforward, because the mutation was semi-dominant, and some phenotypic assignments were ambiguous. Mindful that a single mistake could put us out of the critical region, we tested and re-tested animals until we were absolutely sure of their *Lps* genotypes.

In the final analysis, we were able to confine the mutation to an interval 2.6 million base pairs (Mb) in length – or so we thought. This estimate was based on fluorescence *in situ* hybridization (FISH) studies using labeled bacterial artificial chromosomes (BACs) isolated from the region, on measurements of BAC sizes established through pulsed-field gel electrophoresis, and on probabilistic estimates of BAC overlap. In reality, all of these methods are rather imprecise, and the minimum size of the region, ultimately revealed by whole genome DNA sequencing, was approximately 5.8 Mb. No other critical region of such size had ever been successfully explored for a point mutation, at least in the mouse, and had we known the authentic size, we might have thought twice about continuing our work.

Try as we might, we could not reduce the critical region by genetic mapping. A large interval of the chromosome, incorporating approximately 5 Mb of DNA, was refractory to meiotic recombination, at least with the strain combinations we had selected.

The next phase, *physical mapping*, was actually initiated in parallel with the mapping work (which continued almost until the end of the project). The objective was to clone all of the genomic DNA of the critical region. Our purpose was both to estimate the physical size of the region and to explore it for genes, each of which would stand as a candidate until exonerated by DNA sequencing in C3H/HeN and C3H/HeJ strains. In the final *gene identification* phase, these candidates would be cloned and sequenced at the cDNA level, one by one.

It must be recalled that the draft sequence of the mouse genome was not published until the year 2002,[68] and the gene content of the *Lps* critical region was completely unknown. Moreover, exact details of its syntenic relationship with the human genome were also unknown: owing to an ancestral translocation event, the human *LPS* locus, if such existed, could either be on chromosome 9p or chromosome 9q (the likelihood was about equal for either possibility). And basic assumptions about the number of genes in the mouse genome were dramatically incorrect: it was typically bantered about that there must be "100,000 genes." If correct, there could easily have been 100 genes or more in the critical region we finally established. We now know that the total gene number was overestimated four-fold, and that the *Lps* critical region is rather poor in genes, though rich in pseudogenes.

Using D4Mit microsatellites as markers (they were listed at genetic intervals of 1 cM), we built a contiguous overlapping collection of yeast artificial chromosomes (YACs) and later BACs that covered the critical region. In common parlance, this is called a "contig." Ultimately a total of 66 BAC clones and 2 YAC clones were isolated to cover the region in depth. From close analysis of these clones, a minimum tiling path was established that contained a total of 24 overlapping BAC clones and one YAC clone (Figure 11).

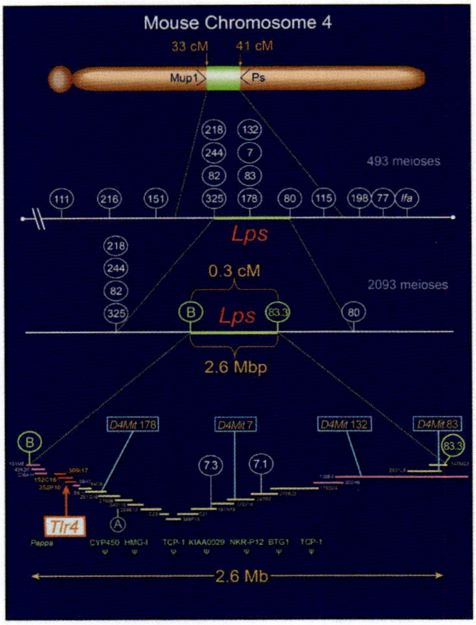

Figure 11. Physical map of the chromosomal region surrounding *Tlr4*. Mapping by Watson et al. confined Lps to an interval between *Mup1* and *Ps* loci (top). Mapping was repeated using microsatellite markers extending over approximately 1⁄4 of the chromosome (D4Mit111 through D4Mit77). On 493 meioses Lps was first confined to an interval bounded by D4Mit218 and D4Mit80), and physical mapping was initiated. On 1600 additional meiosis Lps was confined to an interval bounded by new markers B and 83.3 (isolated from the growing BAC and YAC contig). A contig was assembled to span the interval, which could not be genetically reduced although new polymorphic markers (circles) were identified within it. Each bar is a BAC, except the largest, which is a YAC. Yellow bars indicate sequencing to near-completion. Pink bars indicate heavy, but incomplete sequencing. Red bars indicate BACs that contained Tlr4. Genes are shown in green. Including a small gap near the 5' end of the contig, the entire critical region is known today to be approximately 5.8 Mb in size, rather than the 2.6 Mb that it was formerly believed to be, and the distance from Tlr4 to 83.3 is 4.2 Mb.

I will dispense with most of the details of the physical mapping and fine-mapping in this text. The map was published elsewhere as a prelude to publishing the identity of the *Lps* receptor.[69] But I would like it to be clear that physical mapping was a daunting task. The contig had, at first, "islands" of BACs separated from each other until they could be joined by chromosome walking. These islands would often flip in orientation, as we came to understand that one marker must be proximal to another; then the conjoined islands might flip again as they were extended to join with other islands. In the process of chromosome walking, we established new markers: unique sequences based on the ends of BAC clones, and also new microsatellites not seen by others. All microsatellites would be checked for polymorphism in the hope that we might use them in mapping, and a number of them could indeed be used. The final contig was the largest ever built in a mouse positional cloning foray, and no contig of equal size is likely to be built again.

It became unnecessary to build contigs once the genome of the mouse was sequenced and annotated.

One by one, the BAC and YAC clones were fragmented using ultrasound, and the fragments were polished, sub-cloned, and sequenced bidirectionally. When we began our work, there was no such assembly program as Phrap, which we later used extensively to generate long contiguous sequences (sometimes approaching 100 KB in length). In the beginning, we used much simpler programs such as Wordsearch and FastA to align sequences and reconstruct the landscape of each BAC, and to join BAC clones together.

HUNTING FOR GENES

The final phase of the project, as mentioned above, was the concerted search for genes, and for the mutation responsible for the defect in C3H/HeJ mice. In searching for genes within the trackless wilderness of our contig, we progressed from the most primitive methods (exon trapping and hybridization selection), to the most sophisticated (searching genomic sequences against expressed sequence tag [EST] databases using the matching algorithm BLAST [Basic Local Alignment Search Tool]) over the course of our search. We also used a computational method, the program GRAIL, developed by Richard Mural at ORNL,[70] to search for gene candidates in silico based on the base hexamer composition of genomic DNA. It proved remarkably sensitive and specific, although at first we had to use it essentially on faith.

Exon trapping, which soon went out of fashion, depended on cloning BAC DNA into special vectors with donor and acceptor splice sites. If a piece of DNA happened to have an exon in it, the exon would be spliced when the vector was transfected into mammalian cells, yielding a colony color difference based on the expression of beta-galactosidase activity. The cDNA would then be amplified from these cells, and the nature of the "trapped exon" would be determined by DNA sequencing. A total of 169 exons were trapped by Christophe Van Huffel, but many were from degenerate pseudogenes or from a fragment of the gene *Pappa* (encoding pregnancy associated plasma protein A), which we eventually eliminated as a candidate.

Hybridization selection depended upon the hybridization of cDNA from macrophages, which we knew to express the *Lps* locus, to BAC DNA of the contig (after appropriate blocking with Cot-1 DNA). The cDNA was then eluted and cloned, and a total of 568 cDNAs were isolated and identified in this manner. Among these were some validated candidate genes, but also a large number of false positive identifications, including conserved pseudogenes within the contig that were similar in sequence to mRNAs expressed from authentic genes elsewhere in the genome.

While we struggled with these difficult gene finding methods, EST databases were being developed, and these excited our interest. Some were proprietary (for example the TIGR database) and inaccessible to us without special subscription fees and institutional agreements; one (dbEST) was public. But there was a sense that one had to have access to all the data, lest the all-important gene go undetected. And for that matter, it might be important to continue exon trapping and hybridization selection because we couldn't be absolutely sure that these methods wouldn't lead to the identification of the gene we were seeking. Gradually, we gained confidence that EST searching was the best approach.

EST databases were simply databases of cDNA sequence, derived from processed mRNA expressed in many different tissues at many different embryonic stages. If one found a strong match between a genomic DNA sequence from the contig and an EST, one could be reasonably confident that this particular piece of genomic DNA must be expressed as mRNA. There were some caveats. EST databases were often contaminated with genomic DNA to some degree. Even foreign sequences (from other species, including microbes) had a way of creeping into the record. One could not therefore be totally confident about a particular match. But EST searching was certainly something we couldn't dispense with, and it became our preferred approach. Alexander and Ira became consummate artists at fragmenting BAC clones, producing complex libraries, and feeding the sequencing operation.

From the start, we were badly constrained by a shortage of sequencing power. When we began our work we were sequencing by hand. One of us would read the sequencing ladder on an X-ray film to another who would type it into a computer for later BLAST searching. There was a certain pathos to this, because we knew this was not the best way to proceed, but could not afford to purchase an automated sequencer with our existing funds, and HHMI declined to supplement our budget despite plaintive appeals on my part. Semi-automated slab sequencers, which could actually call bases, came into fairly wide use by the mid-1990s. We began to decentralize our operation, sending samples to three separate core sequencing labs. We also appealed to the UT Southwestern Sequencing Center (GESTEK) run by Glen Evans, hoping he might help us. We additionally turned to Bruce Roe, who ran a sequencing center at the University of Oklahoma. In this way we did manage to acquire hundreds and sometimes thousands of reads per week. Some of the sequencing was done by Dale Birdwell, a technician whom I paid out of pocket to work weekends. Still frustrated, I bought a somewhat antiquated ABI 373 sequencer at personal expense. Because it was under my exclusive control, we could run it around the clock to capture sequence. With this machine, as it happened, we made the critical breakthrough that allowed us to find the mutation. Later, when it was totally outmoded, I donated it to the San Diego Zoo. I don't know where it is today, but must confess I feel rather nostalgic about it.

Sequencing produced data that had to be analyzed in an efficient manner. It wasn't sufficient to BLAST a sequence once and then forget about it, because the EST databases were always being updated, and again, there was the feeling that one might miss the critical sequence. After a time, Betsy and I began to find that all our time was taken up with the manual submission of flat sequence files for blasting. At the advice of David Gordon, the author of consed (a program we had begun to use extensively to view sequences), I taught myself to program in Perl in order to automate the file manipulations needed for recursive sequence analysis. I wrote a script called Central_Command, which sent sequences for analysis and flagged those with likely matches for further analysis by a human observer. But every sequence was studied individually by a human observer at some point, because I feared we might otherwise miss a critical match. One day I received a telephone call from the National Center for Biotechnology Information. They complained that I was using an excess of computational resources by BLASTing on their servers and told me I must BLAST less or they would cut me off. Somehow I complied, decreasing the frequency of recursive searches and doing some of the BLAST searches on a Linux computer of our own.

FIRST GLIMPSE OF THE GENE

Psychologically, genetic work is addictive in the same way that gambling is addictive. We felt as gamblers at the slot machines probably do when we waited for crossovers that might help us narrow the critical region, and when reading through BLAST results to see whether we had found a new candidate gene. Most gamblers know how a losing streak feels, and in our own case, many months had elapsed with little progress either in genetic confinement of the mutation or in gene identification to show for the investment of time and money. But like a gambler who has committed a great deal of money without seeing a big payoff, we could hardly bear to give up having invested so much. At the same, we quietly begin to worry: are we in the correct area at all? Have we made a mistake in mapping, or in our contig construction?

These worries were compounded by external pressure. In April of 1998, I learned that my funding at HHMI would be terminated in September of 2000. I rued the decision, because we had indeed worked on an important problem with focus and industry. But we had not succeeded quickly enough. Like a gambler who sees he is down to his last few dollars, I decided to stay the course, whatever perils it might hold.

By our best estimates, approximately 90% of the critical region had been thoroughly explored by late summer of 1998, and only a modest collection of pseudogenes and a single authentic gene had been identified. Seemingly there were far fewer genes in the region than in most parts of the genome. One can invent a story about almost any gene – and even some pseudogenes – convincing oneself that at last the gene has been found. But a disciplined approach was necessary: the presence of a mutation distinguishing the gene in LPS sensitive mice from the gene in LPS resistant mice had to be found, or failing that, at least there needed to be a dramatic difference in expression. Time and again, the candidates failed these tests.

One of the candidates, known at the time as KIAA0029, was particularly fiendish, because it was large and complex, and expressed in an enormous number of variant splice forms. We began to wonder whether the innate immune system might depend upon splicing to generate receptor diversity, and whether one and only one splice variant might serve the recognition of LPS: a plausible idea at the time. We had, therefore, to look at hundreds of cDNA clones from this gene, to see whether a particular splice variant might be missing in C3H/HeJ. In the end, we decided this wasn't the case; moreover it became clear that the chromosome 4 version of KIAA0029 was a pseudogene. Irritatingly, it had absorbed much of our sequencing power while the intrigue lasted.

On the evening of September 5, 1998, I got my first look at the last gene we were to find in the contig. I was working at home, and it was about 9:30 pm. I was electrified by what I saw, but not entirely convinced we had reached the end of our search, given past experience.

Having endured a period of months during which I had seen absolutely nothing in terms of credible BLAST results, I was strongly confident that this was a genuine gene rather than a pseudogene. Two clones derived from BAC I17 scored as hits with the EST database, and both ESTs were derived from the same gene. Both matches were virtually flawless, and either end of the transcript was struck. By the next day, sequences from an overlapping BAC, C16, provided a third hit (and later a third overlapping BAC showed fragments of the gene). But as always, the proof would depend upon finding a distinguishing mutation.

The gene we had identified was *Tlr4*, and it was interesting to be sure. I saw immediately that it had cytoplasmic domain homology to the IL-1 receptor. I knew that Drosophila Toll had cytoplasmic domain homology to the IL-1 receptor as well: a fact that had surprised me since I learned of it in a lecture given by Steven Wasserman at UT Southwestern several years earlier. This had originally been noticed by Nick Gay in 1991. Why should a developmental protein in the fly resemble an immunological protein in the mouse? A quirk of evolution, I had thought, that common signals could be co-opted for very different purposes. The IL-1 receptor, of course, mediated inflammatory responses, and that was a good sign where the candidate LPS receptor was concerned. Moreover, the leucine-rich repeats of the TLR4 ectodomain were structurally reminiscent of CD14, which we knew on strong experimental grounds to be involved in LPS sensing.

I had a dim recollection that Toll was necessary for the response to fungal infection in Drosophila, which depended upon NF-κB mediated induction of Drosomycin, an antimicrobial peptide: the work of Jules Hoffmann, published in *Cell* two years earlier. Confirming this recollection within a few minutes, I realized that this situation was highly analogous to the LPS paradigm, since mutations affecting the LPS receptor had long been known to confer susceptibility to Gram-negative infection. There were differences as well: the fact that Toll engaged a protein ligand rather than a molecule of microbial origin. Nonetheless, I thought perhaps the host resistance mechanisms of the mouse and the fly were more similar than anyone had realized before.

That evening I also became aware for the first time of a paper from 1997 by Medzhitov, Preston-Hurlburt, and Janeway in which one member of the human TLR family had been cloned at the cDNA level and dubbed "hToll".[71] Unlike our work, theirs was derived from the discoveries of the Hoffmann group in Drosophila. They had demonstrated that human TLR4 could activate NF-κB if expressed as a fusion protein with extracellular CD4 sequences, designed to cause constitutive activation. It had been well established that both Toll and the IL-1 receptor could activate NF-κB; hence it was no surprise that TLR4 could do so. Transfected into myeloid cells, the modified TLR4 construct would cause upregulation of costimulatory molecules. It was suggested that this, too, might result from NF-κB activation.

The link to NF-κB was, by itself, no proof that TLR4 had an immunological function, since NF-κB has both developmental and immunological roles to play, in both mammals and in insects. In the fly, in fact, among nine members of the Toll family, only Toll itself has anything to do with immunity. Nonetheless, the paper advanced the hypothesis that TLR4 was a "pattern recognition receptor" using the name Janeway had earlier coined to designate innate immune receptors recognizing broadly conserved molecules such as LPS.[72] But it presented no evidence in support of this hypothesis, nor did it name the ligand that TLR4 was supposed to recognize.

All of the afore-mentioned considerations gave grounds for speculation, but only a mutational difference between *Tlr4* in LPS sensitive and resistant strains would provide strong evidence that TLR4 was involved in LPS signaling. Speculations notwithstanding, our positional data – and our positional data alone – pointed to TLR4 as the LPS receptor. In a telephone conversation that night, Alexander, Ira, and I all took note of the structural similarity between TLR4 and the IL-1 receptor and CD14, but mostly, we were swayed by the fact that the bulk of the contig had been explored. With only a few hundred thousand nucleotides (and presumably only a few thousand coding nucleotides) left to sequence in what seemed to be a gene desert, this was the only viable candidate in hand.

That night I designed primers to amplify the entire TLR4 cDNA by long-range PCR, and they were ready by the following afternoon. Alexander amplified both C3H/HeN and C3H/HeJ mRNA samples, extracted the bands, fragmented them with ultrasound, and shotgun cloned them into a sequencing vector. Within a week, we had sequenced both libraries, covering the cDNAs with 100 or more reads each: perhaps to a mean depth of ten reads or so. We first saw the mutation using the consed viewer on September 15th: a C→A transversion in the third exon of the gene. The mutation caused the substitution of a histidine for a conserved proline in the cytoplasmic domain of the protein (P712H). It was quickly verified at the genomic level. For some weeks, we kept returning to the computer screen to gaze at the trace file.

This discovery, while exciting, did not formally prove that *Tlr4* was the relevant gene in the *Lps* critical region, required for LPS responses. The mutation might have been an irrelevant and functionally neutral substitution that had occurred independently of the causative mutation, and like it, had become fixed in the C3H/HeJ strain. However, data developed from our analysis of the C57BL/10ScCr and C57BL/10ScSn strain combination were definitive. These strains, maintained for many years by our collaborators Chris Galanos and Marina Freudenberg, who provided us with much valuable insight into LPS biology both before and during the *Lps* cloning work, had been reserved for a final confirmatory experiment. Alexander was, in the case of LPS-unresponsive C57BL/10ScCr strain, unable to amplify the TLR4 cDNA. But he succeeded with amplification of the TLR4 cDNA in the case of the LPS-responsive C57BL/10ScSn strain. Northern and Southern blots suggested complete deletion of the Tlr4 locus had occurred in C57BL/10ScCr: a conclusion substantiated by DNA sequencing soon thereafter. A 74 kb interval of genomic DNA was cleanly excised, removing *Tlr4* but sparing all other genes (Figure 12).[73]

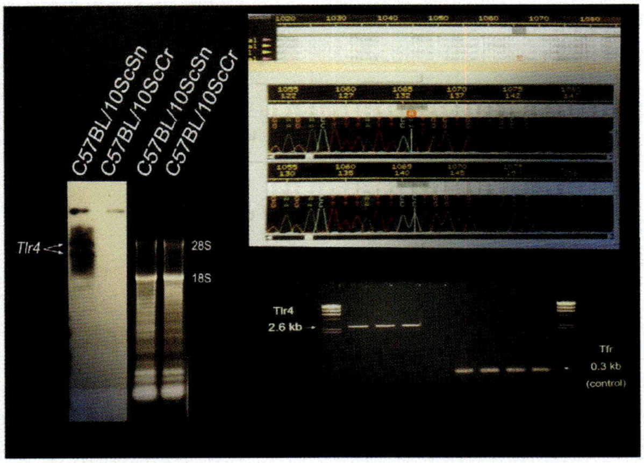

Figure 12. The mutations in C3H/HeJ and C57BL/10ScCr strains, as detected for the very first time. Right, top: photograph of computer screen, consed display, showing a C to A transversion in exon 3 at position 2342 of the C3H/HeJ *Tlr4* cDNA, causing the substitution P712H in the polypeptide chain. Left: Northern blot and ethidium stain of mRNA from C57BL/10ScSn (LPS responsive) and C57BL/10ScCr (LPS unresponsive) macrophages. Right, bottom: RT-PCR of *Tlr4* shows absence of detectable Tlr4 mRNA in C57BL/10ScCr strain mice, but not in closely related C57BL/10ScSn mice, nor in C3H/HeJ or C3H/HeN mice. Transferrin mRNA is expressed by all strains.

We thus knew of two allelic variants of *Tlr4*, one of them overtly destructive and the other likely to be. These variants were observed in the C3H/HeJ and C57BL/10ScCr strains, but not in closely related control strains that had normal LPS responses. Having published the mapping data on September 14,[74] we submitted our major paper establishing the identity of *Lps* and *Tlr4* to *Science* on September 30. It was accepted with minimal revisions and published on December 11, 1998.[75] It soon became the most highly cited publication in the innate immunity field because it had revealed the key sensors used by the mammalian innate immune system to detect infection, and had also revealed the conservation of this system for innate immune activation from mammals to insects (Figure 13). As I write this lecture, it has been cited 3,970 times.

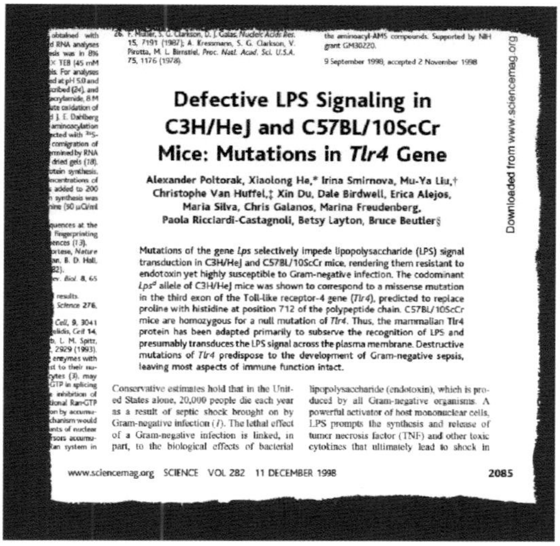

26. F. Müller, S. G. Clarkson, D. J. Galas, *Nucleic Acids Res.* 15, 7191 (1987); A. Kressmann, S. G. Clarkson, V. Pirotta, M. L. Birnstiel, *Proc. Natl. Acad. Sci. U.S.A.* 75, 1176 (1978).

the aminoacyl-AMS compounds. Supported by NIH grant GM30220.

9 September 1998; accepted 2 November 1998

Defective LPS Signaling in C3H/HeJ and C57BL/10ScCr Mice: Mutations in *Tlr4* Gene

Alexander Poltorak, Xiaolong He,* Irina Smirnova, Mu-Ya Liu,† Christophe Van Huffel,‡ Xin Du, Dale Birdwell, Erica Alejos, Maria Silva, Chris Galanos, Marina Freudenberg, Paola Ricciardi-Castagnoli, Betsy Layton, Bruce Beutler§

Mutations of the gene *Lps* selectively impede lipopolysaccharide (LPS) signal transduction in C3H/HeJ and C57BL/10ScCr mice, rendering them resistant to endotoxin yet highly susceptible to Gram-negative infection. The codominant *Lps*^{d} allele of C3H/HeJ mice was shown to correspond to a missense mutation in the third exon of the Toll-like receptor-4 gene (*Tlr4*), predicted to replace proline with histidine at position 712 of the polypeptide chain. C57BL/10ScCr mice are homozygous for a null mutation of *Tlr4*. Thus, the mammalian Tlr4 protein has been adapted primarily to subserve the recognition of LPS and presumably transduces the LPS signal across the plasma membrane. Destructive mutations of *Tlr4* predispose to the development of Gram-negative sepsis, leaving most aspects of immune function intact.

Conservative estimates hold that in the United States alone, 20,000 people die each year as a result of septic shock brought on by Gram-negative infection (*1*). The lethal effect of a Gram-negative infection is linked, in part, to the biological effects of bacterial lipopolysaccharide (endotoxin), which is produced by all Gram-negative organisms. A powerful activator of host mononuclear cells, LPS prompts the synthesis and release of tumor necrosis factor (TNF) and other toxic cytokines that ultimately lead to shock in

www.sciencemag.org SCIENCE VOL 282 11 DECEMBER 1998 2085

Downloaded from www.sciencemag.org

Figure 13. "Defective LPS Signaling in C3H/HeJ and C57BL/10ScCr Mice: Mutations in *Tlr4* gene," Poltorak, A. et al (1998) *Science 282,* 2085–2088.

Not long after our discovery, two published reports asserted that TLR2 was the LPS receptor. Workers at Genentech and Tularik, unaware of our work, each transfected mammalian cells to overexpress TLR2, and had found that high concentrations of LPS could drive NF-κB activation in these cells. Their papers, published in September and in December of 1998,[76] were not quantitative in the sense that there was no way to compare the magnitude of the LPS response to that in a positive control cell with truly normal LPS signaling potential (for example, a macrophage cell line). Moreover, no genetic test of the TLR2 hypothesis was made. To this day, it is not entirely clear why the observed results were obtained, but it has been suggested that the LPS preparations used were contaminated with lipopeptides that may have triggered a TLR2 response.

We knew immediately that the core conclusions of both studies were erroneous, and that the error occurred as a result of weak methodology: the use of transfection, rather than a true genetic approach, as the basis for inference. Lack of TLR4 signaling, as observed in C3H/HeJ or C57BL/10ScCr mice, completely abolished LPS sensing. This excluded the existence of an alternative pathway in which TLR2 might act as an autonomous LPS receptor. The notion that TLR2 could make any contribution to LPS signaling lost all credibility when Osamu Takeuchi and colleagues from the group of Shizuo Akira targeted *Tlr2,* and showed that TLR2 deficient mice respond normally to LPS.[77] Nonetheless, for the next few years, numerous publications referred to "two LPS receptors," until the idea faded away.

BUT IS TLR4 REALLY A RECEPTOR FOR LPS?

The discovery that TLR4 is necessary for LPS responses did not address the question as to whether it was indeed a physical receptor for LPS: a difficult question to answer given the hydrophobic character of the putative ligand, and the resultant difficulty of performing classical binding studies. In Drosophila, the homologous sensor Toll had no contact with any product of microbes, and genetic evidence indicated that the protein Spaetzle, cleaved by upstream proteases that were activated in response to infection, was the proximal ligand for Toll. Considerable doubt remained as to whether direct interaction between LPS and TLR4 actually occurred.

To address this question, we made use of a fact mentioned earlier: certain LPS partial structures, notably Lipid IVa, antagonize LPS when it is applied to human mononuclear cells, but act as agonists in the mouse. Lipid IVa differed from Lipid A only by the absence of two acyl side chains in the former and their presence in the latter. We hypothesized that TLR4 itself would "decide" whether those chains were present or absent, and if indeed it could do so, it must be in very close contact with lipid A or lipid IVa. A C3H/HeJ cell line had been created for us by Paola Ricciardi Castagnoli, and this cell line formed the perfect vehicle within which to test whether TLR4 actually made the decision. Lacking an active TLR4 molecule itself, but endowed with all of the other machinery needed to respond to LPS, this line was transfected to express either human or mouse TLR4 proteins, or neither. A clear outcome was obtained. In cells expressing mouse TLR4, both Lipid A and Lipid IVa could induce TNF production. In cells expressing human TLR4, only Lipid A, but not Lipid IVa, could induce TNF production.[78] We concluded that TLR4 must indeed directly "see" LPS: a conclusion also reached by Lien, et al., who used a conceptually similar approach (Figure 14).[79]

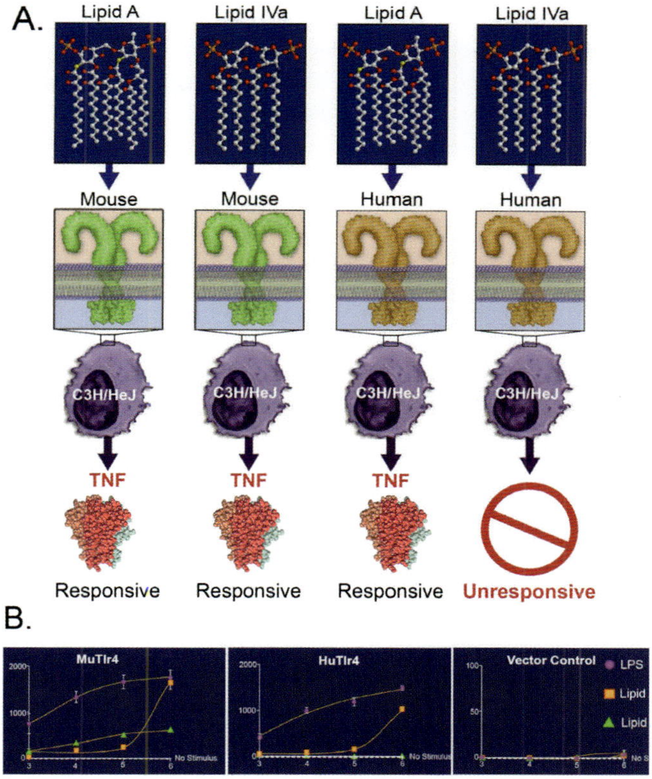

Figure 14. TLR4 and LPS interactions, established by genetic complementation. A. Experimental design and outcome. C3H/HeJ macrophages were transfected to express either human or mouse TLR4, and then challenged with either lipid A or lipid IVa. The species origin of the TLR predicted the response to lipid IVa (known to be agonistic in mice but antagonistic in humans). B. The data upon which the conclusions were based, adapted from (93). [80]

A little known paper published by our group inquired into the copy number of TLR4 on the surface of LPS-responsive macrophages. In the RAW 264.7 cell line, we estimated that only a few hundred receptors exist per cell.[81] Yet these cells respond vigorously to LPS, consistent with strong signal amplification. Knowing that the lethal effect of LPS is delivered by myeloid cells in the mouse, and knowing the approximate number of TLR4 molecules per cell, I calculated that the dramatic shock syndrome and lethal effect of LPS are delivered by only a few nanograms of TLR4 protein in the mouse. It was truly a tiny spark that lit the fire of endotoxic shock.

But not all of the receptor complex had been discovered in 1998. The following year, Miyake and colleagues reported that a small protein, MD-2, was tightly associated with TLR4 and was also important for LPS perception.[82] This report was soon verified by gene targeting. A study analyzing the ability of MD-2 to discriminate between agonistic and non-agonistic LPS partial structures soon indicated that this molecule, too, must have direct contact with the ligand.[83]

Several years elapsed before X-ray crystallography illustrated the exact mode of interaction between LPS and the receptor complex.[84] The acyl chains of Lipid A are mostly contained within a hydrophobic pocket formed by MD-2, but parts of the molecule also have direct contact with TLR4. A reaction mechanism favoring rotational rearrangement of the TLR4/MD-2 homodimer to produce a signal has been proposed, based on the different interactions of LPS as compared with an LPS antagonist (Figure 15).

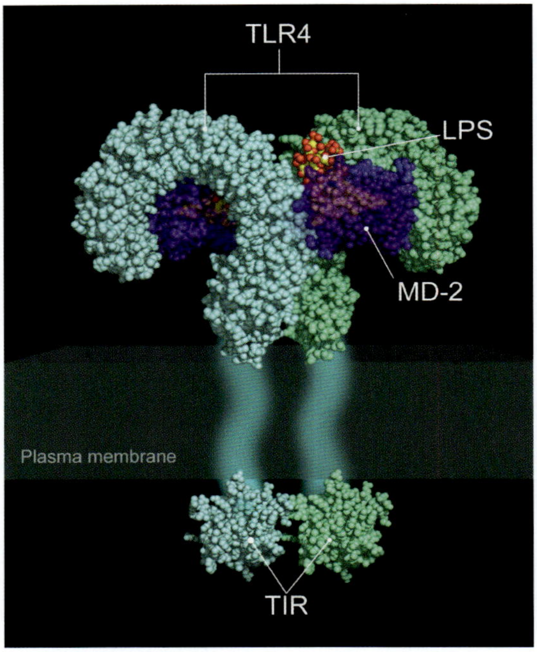

Figure 15. 3D crystallographic model of the interaction between LPS with the TLR4/MD-2 receptor complex. The acyl chains of the Lipid A component of LPS (yellow [carbons] and red [oxygens]) are mostly contained within a hydrophobic pocket formed by MD-2 (purple), but parts of the molecule also have direct contact with TLR4 (light blue/green). The TIR domain of TLR4 mediates homo- and heterotypic protein interactions during signal transduction. Reproduced from the work of Park, B.S. et al. (96).[85]

OTHER TLRS RECOGNIZE OTHER MICROBIAL LIGANDS

By the time TLR4 was identified as the LPS receptor, four other TLRs were already known to exist, and we and others were soon to identify and clone several others, until a total of 12 TLRs were identified in mice and 10 in humans. But the specificities of the other TLRs remained unknown. The fact that TLR4 is a specific receptor for LPS suggested the possibility that each of the other TLRs recognize other microbial ligands. Shizuo Akira led the way in testing this hypothesis, targeting all of the TLR-encoding genes in the mouse. In due course, it was clear that each TLR did recognize specific molecules of microbial origin. Hence, the qualitative similarity in responses to many different microbial ligands was explained by the similarity of their receptors.

X-ray crystallography has now shown that different ligands bind their respective TLRs in strikingly different ways (Figure 16). Some do so in conjunction with helper proteins, or co-receptors, as discussed below. In all instances, signaling is mediated by the recruitment of adaptor proteins, with structural similarity to the cytoplasmic domains of the TLRs themselves. In turn, protein kinases are recruited to the activation complex; then ubiquitin ligases modify and recruit still other proteins, some with other kinase activities. These events lead to the transcriptional and translational activation events seen in TLR signaling, and ultimately, to cytokine release and still more events downstream.

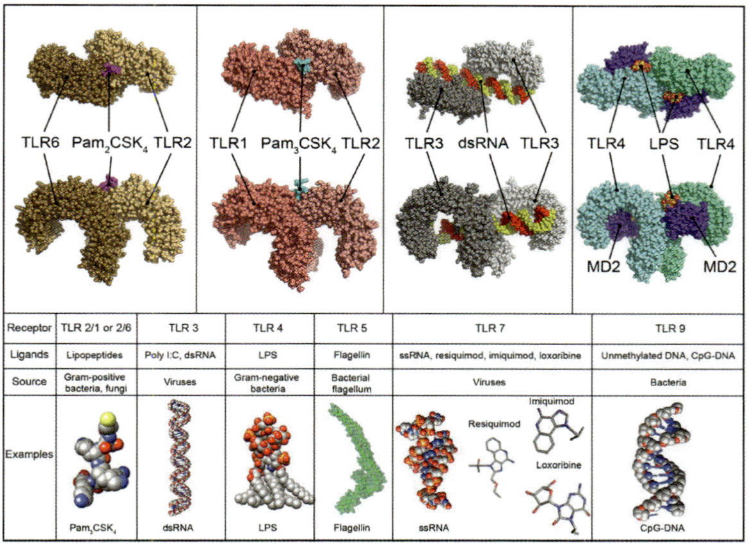

Figure 16. TLR ligands and interactions with receptors. (A) Three-dimensional structures of the lipopeptide Pam2CSK4 (from 3A79), double-stranded RNA (from 3CIY), LPS (from 3FXI), flagellin (3K8V), a tRNA as a model of single-stranded RNA (2L9E), and unmethylated CpG-DNA (from 3QMB). Gray, blue, red, orange, and yellow spheres represent carbon, nitrogen, oxygen, phosphorus, and sulfur atoms, respectively. The chemical structures of resiquimod, imiquimod, and loxoribine are also shown. Possible microbial sources of ligands are indicated. (B) Structures of TLR2–TLR6–Pam2CSK4 lipopeptide (3A79), TLR2–TLR1–Pam3CSK4 lipopeptide (2Z7X), TLR3-dsRNA (3CIY), and TLR4–MD-2–LPS (3FXI). Side view (upper panels) and top view (lower panels) are shown. Protein Databank ID numbers are indicated in parentheses. (All figures were generated with Schroedinger PyMol).

EVOLUTIONARY IMPLICATIONS: MAMMALS, INSECTS, AND PLANTS

As noted above, even before the immunological function of Toll was known in Drosophila, it had been noticed that the TIR domain of Toll and the IL-1 receptor were similar,[86] and furthermore, that both shared homology to certain plant pathogen resistance proteins;[87] hence the designation TIR (for <u>T</u>oll/<u>I</u>L-1 receptor/<u>R</u>esistance motif). It was soon noticed that leucine rich repeat motifs were commonly associated with resistance factors in plants, but for a time, the only examples were represented in cytoplasmic proteins, rather similar in overall domain structure to the NOD-like receptors (NLRs) of mammals. Pamela Ronald's discovery in 1995 of a cell surface LRR known as XA21, responsible for resistance to *Xanthomonas oryzae pv. Oryzae* in domestic rice (*Oryza sativa*), was exceptionally important, and receives far less attention than it should.[88] This protein does not signal by way of a TIR motif, but way of a non-RD kinase motif. Like TLRs in mammals (but not in flies), it recognizes a conserved molecule of microbial origin: as Ronald later showed, a sulfated peptide, AXYS22, produced by the microbe.[89] These discoveries cement the relationship between cell surface LRR proteins in mammals, insects, and plants as sensors of infection, and reveal how truly ancient and strongly conserved innate immune sensing mechanisms are (Figure 17). A related and strictly personal note: Pamela Ronald and I, whose interests in innate immunity developed entirely independently and then converged, are third cousins, both descendants of Fanny Frank (b. 1834) and Julius Rothstein (b. 1834) (Figure 18). Perhaps our mutual interest in innate immunity was itself innate!

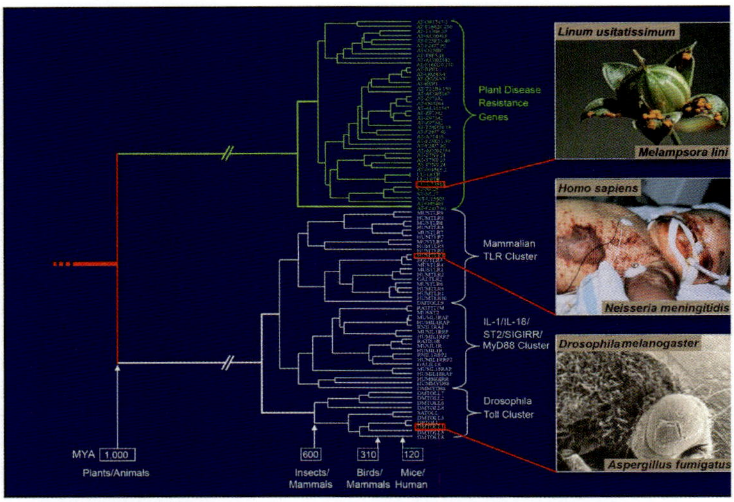

Figure 17. TIR domains in immunity across the tree of life. Plant disease resistance genes, Drosophila Toll, and mammalian Toll-like receptors all bear the TIR domain, which contributes to immunity. Some plant resistance proteins, such as XA21, have leucine-rich repeats (but no TIR domain) and directly engage microbial activators at the cell surface as Toll-like receptors do.

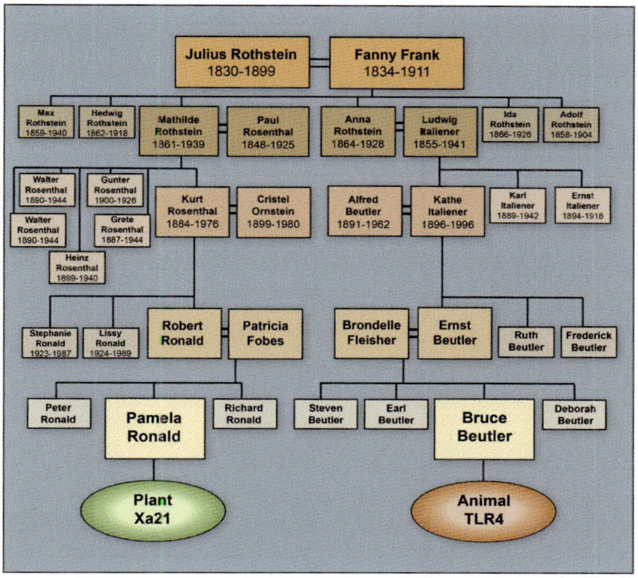

Figure 18. The Beutler and Ronald families, related by descent. XA21 and TLR4 may be as well, and have obvious functional similarity.

In insects, Jules Hoffmann and his colleagues identified a Toll-independent sensory system that recognizes Gram-negative bacteria. Termed the Imd pathway, it mimics at several points the mammalian TNF signaling pathway. One may therefore think of the mammalian TLR signaling pathways, inexorably linked to the production of TNF and then to TNF signaling, as equivalent to both the Toll and Imd pathways in the fruit fly (Figure 19). The "connecting" role of TNF, which joins the two pathways, gives some insight as to why TNF blockade is particularly effective as a therapy. TNF signaling is obviously one of the major mechanisms by which innate immunity and inflammation are implemented, and has been conserved across the evolutionary divide between vertebrates and invertebrates.

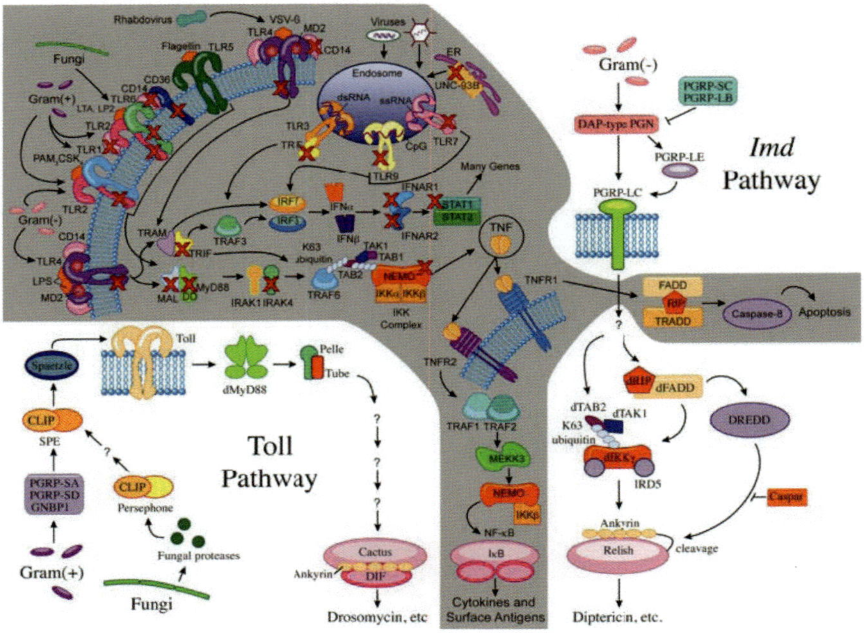

Figure 19. Comparison of the Toll and Imd signaling pathways with mammalian TLR and TNF signaling pathways. Each red X in the TLR signaling pathways corresponds to one or more mutations produced using ENU and isolated by its phenotypic effect. Homologues in the mammal and insect are given similar shapes and colors.

PUTTING PHENOTYPE FIRST: ENU MUTAGENESIS IN THE ANALYSIS OF INNATE IMMUNITY

When the positional cloning of Lps lay behind us, we sought to use forward genetics to further dissect innate immunity in mammals. We and others anticipated sweeping advances in mouse genetics, brought about by two developments. First, the sequencing and annotation of the mouse genome, soon to be completed, would make it unnecessary to build contigs or search for genes within critical regions. The complete gene content of the mouse would be known. Second, new sequencing technologies, a bit further off, would make it possible to find mutations with unprecedented speed. To exploit these advances, I foresaw the need to create new immunologically relevant phenotypes, and to do so using a random process.

In the year 2000, I relocated my laboratory to The Scripps Research Institute, where I began to mutagenize mice using the germline mutagen N-ethyl-N-nitrosourea (ENU) (Figure 20). In due course, we created hundreds of phenovariant mice, many with altered immune function. Over the years, we screened more than 150,000 animals for recessive defects of immunity, and identified many new and informative genetic diseases. We developed computational and robotic methods to target our search for mutations to the coding region and splice junctions of the mouse genome. This allowed us to tackle critical regions vastly larger than we could have in the past, which of course meant much less genetic mapping. In some instances, we were able to build quite elaborate models that shed light on immune reactions, based on the identification of dozens of mutations affecting defined immune phenomena.

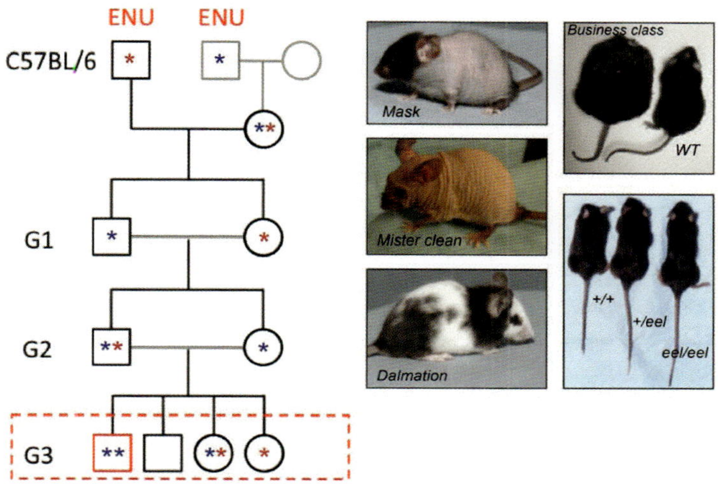

Figure 20. Making new phenotypes in mice. The germline N-ethyl-N-nitrosourea (ENU) mutagen was used to generate mutations in C57BL/6J mice. Left, the mating strategy used to generate G3 mice homozygous for a fraction of the ENU induced mutations (red box) from mutagenized (G0) progenitors. G3 mice were subjected to screening. Right, examples of appearance-altering mutations in G3 mice (clockwise, from top left): mutations in *Tmprss6* (mask), *Lepr* (business class), *npr3* (eel), *Sox10* (Dalmatian), and *Hr* (mister *clean).* Just as mutations cause visible and/or behavior phenotypes, they may also disrupt immune function. Mutations of this type can be detected by phenotypic screens that test immune competence. For more information on these mutations visit http://mutagenetix.utsouthwestern.edu/home.cfm.

For example, we asked: "what genes are essential for survival during infection with mouse cytomegalovirus?" Many mutations were found to affect survival, and a reasonable picture of the events that must occur to allow the host to survive could be assembled. In this particular case, TLR sensing (especially via TLRs 3 and 9) are crucial; so is activation and effector function in the NK cell compartment; and so is the ability to produce NK cells, conventional dendritic cells, and inflammatory monocytes,[90] along with the capacity for cardiovascular adaptation to the cytokine response.[91] Several postdoctoral associates, including Karine Crozat, Ben Croker, Micha Berger, Celine Eidenschenk, Nengming Xiao, and Carrie Arnold participated in finding these mutations and analyzing them (Figure 21).

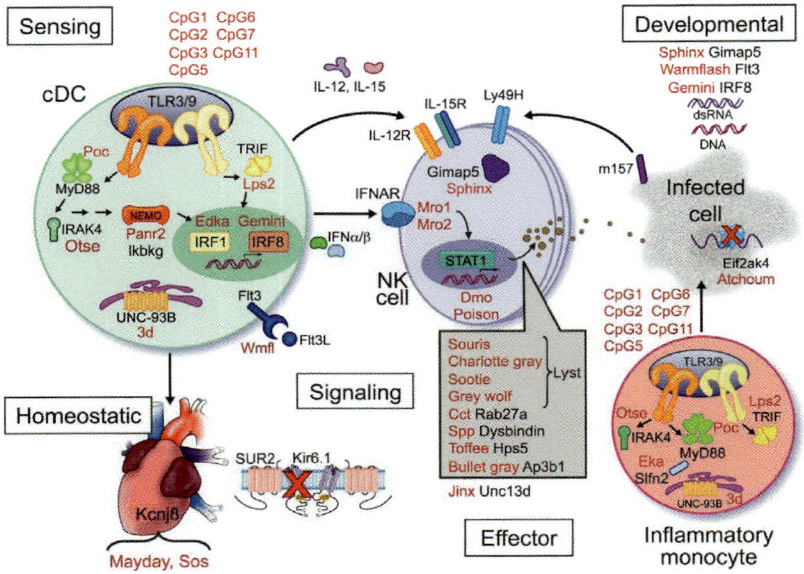

Figure 21. Genes essential for survival during mouse cytomegalovirus infection. Mutations causing MCMV susceptibility are denoted in red near their respective gene names (black) and/or protein structures. For more information on these mutations visit http://mutagenetix.utsouthwestern.edu/home.cfm. TLR signaling (specifically via TLRs 3 and 9) in conventional dendritic cells (cDCs) and inflammatory monocytes is crucial for survival; so is activation and effector function in the NK cell compartment; the ability to produce NK cells, cDCs, and inflammatory monocytes, and the capacity for cardiovascular adaptation to the cytokine response.

We also asked, "What genes maintain intestinal homeostasis when mice are challenged with oral dextran sodium sulfate (DSS)?" DSS, administered at a low dose, causes mild, reparable damage to the mucosa of the gastrointestinal tract. But exceptional mice develop severe inflammatory bowel disease as a result of mutations that interfere with mucosal proliferation, or with the immune function of hematopoietically derived cells adjacent to the epithelial layer. Again, TLRs were found to be involved in the repair process, and appear to act in mucosal cells, triggering the release of growth factors needed to close the wounds that DSS causes. Other essential events include the secretion of granules from Paneth cells and goblet cells; the degranulation of immune cells; the uptake of water within rapidly dividing cells of the epithelium; and the ability to manage ER stress. Katharina Brandl and Wataru Tomisato have taken the lead with this screen, which implies, overall, that there may be many monogenic causes of IBD, presumably in humans as in mice (Figure 22).

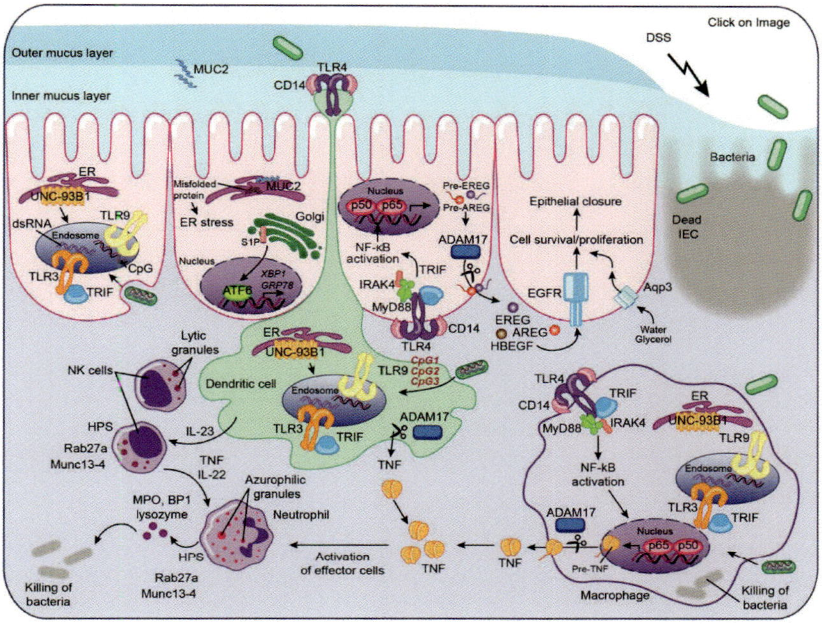

Figure 22. Maintenance of intestinal homeostasis after dextran sodium sulfate (DSS) challenge, as deduced from ENU mutagenesis. Microbe sensing after initial disruption of the epithelial barrier is accomplished by TLRs, which stimulate the release of growth factors needed to close epithelial defects. Other essential events include the secretion of granules from Paneth cells and goblet cells; the degranulation of immune cells; the uptake of water within rapidly dividing cells of the epithelium; and the ability to manage ER stress. For more information on these mutations visit http://mutagenetix.utsouthwestern.edu/home.cfm.

In more focused screens, we looked closely at the signaling pathways utilized by TLRs themselves, and found a number of surprises (Figure 23). TLRs 3, 7, and 9, which sense nucleic acids, must be escorted to endosomal compartments within which they signal. A protein called UNC93B1 is essential for this process, and a mutation identified in our laboratory, called 3d to connote a triple defect of nucleic acid sensing, could abrogate signaling via TLRs 3, 7, and 9.[92] Another mutation, called *Lps2* because it closely mimicked the phenotype imparted by the classical *Lps* mutation, was seen to inhibit TLR4 signaling and to completely abolish TLR3 signaling, suggesting a common adaptor protein. It was tracked to the gene encoding a new adaptor, independently identified and called TRIF by the Akira group,[93] and TICAM1 by the Seya group.[94] The *Lps2* allele, created prior to the knockout, first revealed the basis of MyD88-independent signaling by the TLRs.[95] A mutation called *Oblivious* revealed the importance of CD36, a class B scavenger receptor, in signaling via TLR2 heterodimers.[96] And a mutation called *Feeble* showed that a solute channel, SLC15A4, is essential for plasmacytoid dendritic cells to detect nucleic acids via TLRs 7 and 9.[97]

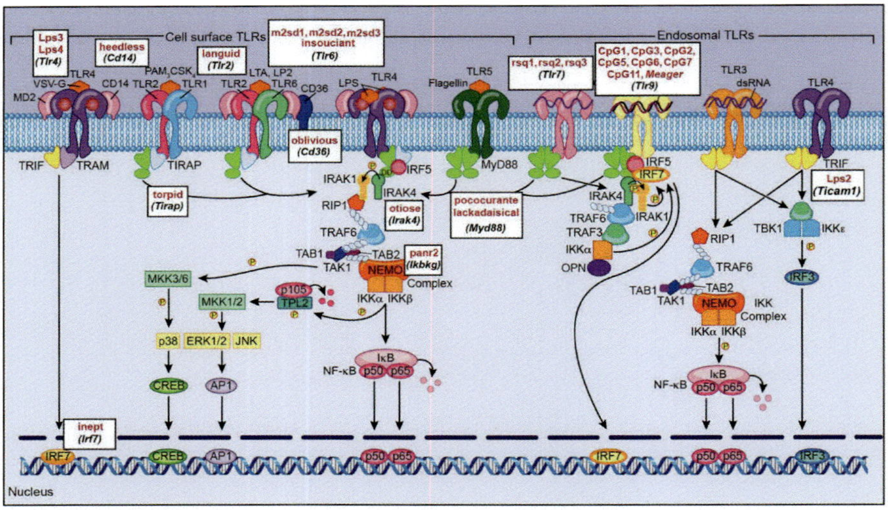

Figure 23. Overview of Toll-like receptor (TLR) signaling pathways. Shown are the signaling events downstream of TLR activation that ultimately lead to the induction of thousands of genes including TNF and type I IFN, which are critical in activating innate and adaptive immune responses. TLR1,2,4,5 and 6 are located at least largely at the cell surface, while TLR3,7, and 9 are located in endosomes. Once TLR complexes recognize their ligands, they recruit combinations of adaptor proteins (MyD88, TICAM, TRAM, TIRAP) via homotypic TIR domain interactions. Death domains (DD); osteopontin (OPN), vesicular stomatitis virus glycoprotein G (VSV-G); lipoteichoic acid (LTA); diacyl- lipopeptide (LP2). Phosphorylation events are represented by small yellow circles labeled with a "P". Other proteins are indicated with standard nomenclature. In boxes, ENU mutations, often representing multiple alleles of individual genes, that helped to elucidate pathways are listed (red text) with indication as to which genes they affect (black text). For more information on mutations in the TLRs or TLR-associated pathways visit http://mutagenetix.utsouthwestern.edu/home.cfm.

Another screen pursued by Carrie N. Arnold from my group in collaboration with Gunilla Karlsson Hedestam, Gerry McInerny, and Pia Dosenovic at the Karolinska Institute, has asked simply, "What is needed for an antibody response to an administered antigen?" This screen probes both T-dependent and T-independent immunization. One interesting observation is that while many mutations abolish the antibody response to an administered antigen, none of those identified to date seem to do so solely by virtue of an effect on the innate immune response.

The beauty of forward genetics is that one renounces hypothesis as much as possible. This is an act of humility; an admission that the system one is studying is too mysterious for guesses. Without hypotheses, the search for fundamental causes is far less susceptible to bias, and therefore, mistakes. At the same time, one may hope to discover the unexpected, because one *has* no strongly held expectations. And once a phenotype exists where none did before, it may spawn new views of how the system operates.

AFTERMATH AND FUTURE PROSPECTS

When a fundamental discovery has been made, there is a tendency to overreach. TLRs explain much of what happens during infection, and that is why they are so important. But not *everything* that happens during infection begins with TLRs. There are other systems for sensing infection, which emerged in the wake of the TLR4 discovery: the NOD-like receptors (NLRs), the RIG-I like helicases (RLHs), and the C-type lections (CTLs), for example. These must not be ignored in seeking to explain infection-related phenomena, and there may be still other sensors of which we are currently unaware.

As previously mentioned, LPS has an adjuvant effect, known since the 1950s.[98] It was well documented that this effect, like almost all effects of LPS, is dependent on the *Lps* locus.[99] Therefore, from the moment TLR4 was identified as the critically altered protein in C3H/HeJ mice, it was explicitly clear that TLR4 mediates the adjuvant effect of LPS.

However, blanket statements that the TLRs are "necessary" or "required" for adaptive immune responses are frankly incorrect. It is easy to demonstrate that TLRs are not necessary for adaptive immune responses to antigens administered with classical adjuvants, including those that employ microbes or their products.[100] And from what we know so far, few if any authentic infections depend upon TLR signaling to elicit an adaptive immune response. Nor are TLRs necessary for allograft rejection, although as discussed below, they do play an important part in the development of certain forms of autoimmunity, particularly systemic lupus erythematosus.[101] It may be inferred that the pathways leading to activation of an adaptive immune response are rather redundant.

What will our understanding of the TLRs do for us in the future? We have begun to realize, as with rheumatoid arthritis and Crohn's disease in the past, that the systems that evolved to limit infection are the same systems that malfunction to cause inflammatory diseases. Ann Marshak-Rothstein and her colleagues have shown that TLR signaling causes an important forward feedback loop that propels autoimmunity at the B cell level. It appears that a B cell with specificity for nucleic acids will engage DNA or RNA complexes upon encountering them. At that point, internalization of the nucleic acids may drive TLR-mediated expansion of the B cell clone. This general mechanism seems particularly important in systemic lupus erythematosus (SLE) pathogenesis, and may account for the prevalence of antibodies against nuclear components in that disease.

SLE is well modeled in mice of several strains; for example, the MRL^{Lpr} strain, with its critical Fas mutation, the NZW x NZB F1 hybrid, and the BXSB strain with its well-known Y-linked accelerator of autoimmunity (*Yaa*) locus. In the latter strain, the critical contribution of TLR signaling to development of autoimmunity was revealed by the observation that the *Tlr7* locus is duplicated within the pseudoautosomal region of the Y chromosome.[102] Homozygosity for *Tlr7* or *Myd88* knockout alleles, or for the *3d* allele of *Unc93b1*, will each suppress autoimmunity caused by the Fas^{Lpr} mutation.[103]

These observations give reason to think that highly specific therapies for amelioration of SLE may be based on antagonism of individual TLRs or proteins that support their action. Other autoimmune and autoinflammatory diseases may similarly be found to be TLR dependent.

We know, too, that death from infection sometimes results from mutational defects in the TLR signaling pathways. Innate immune deficiency is not a newly discovered phenomenon, but more and more mutations that cause it are being identified. The vulnerabilities these mutations impart may be relatively selective, and one wonders if each of us has his own Achilles' heel.

Finally, returning to infection, and to sepsis where our story began: might TLR blockade, instituted promptly and in conjunction with appropriate antibiotic therapy, spare some patients the severe injury that sepsis causes? One may hope so, and be reasonably optimistic.

REFERENCES

1. Morens, D. M., Folkers, G. K., and Fauci, A. S. (2004), "The Challenge of Emerging and Re-Emerging Infectious Diseases," *Nature 430, 242–249.*
2. Miller, J. S., Engelberg, S., and Broad, W. (2001), *Germs: The Ultimate Weapon,* Simon and Schuster, London; Oldstone, M. B. (1998), *Viruses, Plagues, and History,* Oxford University Press, New York.
3. Morens, D. M., Folkers, G. K., and Fauci, A. S. (2004), "The Challenge of Emerging and Re-Emerging Infectious Diseases," *Nature 430, 242–249.*
4. Rietschel, E. T., and Cavaillon, J. M. (2002), "Endotoxin and Anti-Endotoxin. The Contribution of the Schools of Koch and Pasteur: Life, Milestone-Experiments and Concepts of Richard Pfeiffer (Berlin) and Alexandre Besredka (Paris)," *J. Endotoxin Res. 8,* 3–16; Rietschel, E. T., and Cavaillon, J. M. (2002) Endotoxin and Anti-Endotoxin. the Contribution of the Schools of Koch and Pasteur: Life, Milestone-Experiments and Concepts of Richard Pfeiffer (Berlin) and Alexandre Besredka (Paris). *J. Endotoxin Res. 8,* 71–82.
5. Osborn, M. J., Rosen, S. M., Rothfield, L., Zeleznick, L. D., and Horecker, B. L. (1964), "Lipopolysaccharide of the Gram-Negative Cell Wall," Science 145, 783–789; Rietschel, E. T., and Westphal, O. (1999), "Endotoxin: Historical Perspectives," in Endotoxin in Health and Disease (H. Brade, S. M. Opal, S. N. Vogel, and D. C. Morrison, Eds.), pp 1–29, Marcel Dekker, New York.
6. Boivin, A., Mesrobeanu, I., and Mesrobeanu, L. (1933), "Extraction d'Un Complexe Toxique Et Antigenique a Partir Du Bacille d'Aertrycke," *Compt. rend. soc. biol. 114,* 307–310; Boivin, A., and Mesrobeanu, L. (1935), "Recherches Sur Les Antigènes Somatiques Et Sur Les Endotoxines Des Bactéries," *Rev. Immunol.* 1, 553–569.
7. Raetz, C. R., and Whitfield, C. (2002), "Lipopolysaccharide Endotoxins," *Annu. Rev. Biochem. 71,* 635–700.
8. Westphal, O., and Luderitz, O. (1954), "Chemische Erforshung Von Lipopolysacchariden Gramnegativer Bakterien," *Angew Chemie 66,* 407–417.
9. Imoto, M., Yoshimura, H., Kusumoto, S., and Shiba, T. (1984), "Total Synthesis of Lipid A, Active Principle of Bacterial Endotoxin," *Proc. Jpn. Acad. Sci.* 60, 285–288; Galanos, C., Luderitz, O., Rietschel, E. T., Westphal, O., Brade, H., Brade, L., Freudenberg, M., Schade, U., Imoto, M., Yoshimura, H., Kusumoto, S., and Shiba, T. (1985), "Synthetic and Natural Escherichia Coli Free Lipid A Express Identical Endotoxic Activities," *Eur. J. Biochem.* 148, 1–5.
10. Raetz, C. R., and Whitfield, C. (2002), "Lipopolysaccharide Endotoxins," *Annu. Rev. Biochem. 71,* 635–700; Raetz, C. R. H. (1990), "Biochemistry of Endotoxins," *Ann. Rev. Biochem.* 59, 129–170.
11. Galanos, C., Lehmann, V., Luderitz, O., Rietschel, E. T., Westphal, O., Brade, H., Brade, L., Freudenberg, M. A., Hansen-Hagge, T., and Luderitz, T. (1984), "Endotoxic Properties of Chemically Synthesized Lipid A Part Structures. Comparison of Synthetic Lipid A Precursor and Synthetic Analogues with Biosynthetic Lipid A Precursor and Free Lipid A," *Eur. J. Biochem. 140,* 221–227.
12. Kovach, N. L., Yee, E., Munford, R. S., Raetz, C. R., and Harlan, J. M. (1990), "Lipid IVA Inhibits Synthesis and Release of Tumor Necrosis Factor Induced by Lipopolysaccharide in Human Whole Blood Ex Vivo," *J. Exp. Med. 172,* 77–84.
13. Johnson, A. G., Gaines, S., and Landy, M. (1956), "Studies on the O Antigen of Salmonella Typhosa. V. Enhancement of Antibody Response to Protein Antigens by the Purified Lipopolysaccharide," *J. Exp. Med. 103,* 225–246.
14. Tomai, M. A., Solem, L. E., Johnson, A. G., and Ribi, E. (1987), "The Adjuvant Properties of a Nontoxic Monophosphoryl Lipid A in Hyporesponsive and Aging Mice," *J. Biol. Response Mod. 6,* 99–107; Johnson, A. G., Tomai, M., Solem, L., Beck, L., and Ribi, E. (1987), "Characterization of a Nontoxic Monophosphoryl Lipid A," *Rev. Infect. Dis. 9 Suppl 5,* S512–6.

15. Landy, M., and Pillemer, L. (1956), "Increased Resistance to Infection and Accompanying Alteration in Properidin Levels Following Administration of Bacterial Lipopolysaccharides," *J. Exp. Med. 104,* 383–409.
16. O'Malley, W. E., Achinstein, B., and Shear, M. J. (1962), "Action of Bacterial Polysaccharide on Tumors. I. Reduced Growth of S37, and Induced Refractoriness, by S. Marcescens Polysaccharide," *J. Natl. Cancer Inst. 29,* 1161–1168.
17. Ainsworth, E. J., and Chase, H. B. (1959), "Effect of Microbial Antigens on Irradiation Mortality in Mice," *Proc. Soc. Exp. Biol. Med. 102,* 483–485; Smith, W. W., Alderman, I. M., and Gillespie, R. E. (1957), "Increased Survival in Irradiated Animals Treated with Bacterial Endotoxins," *Am. J. Physiol. 191,* 124–130.
18. Heppner, G., and Weiss, D. W. (1965), "High Susceptibility of Strain A Mice to Endotoxin and Endotoxin-Red Blood Cell Mixtures," *J. Bacteriol. 90,* 696–703.
19. Sultzer, B. M. (1968), "Genetic Control of Leucocyte Responses to Endotoxin," *Nature 219,* 1253–1254.
20. Coutinho, A., Forni, L., Melchers, F., and Watanabe, T. (1977), "Genetic Defect in Responsiveness to the B Cell Mitogen Lipopolysaccharide," *Eur. J. Immunol. 7,* 325–328.
21. Coutinho, A., and Meo, T. (1978), "Genetic Basis for Unresponsiveness to Lipopolysaccharide in C57BL/10Cr Mice," *Immunogenetics 7,* 17–24.
22. Radolf, J. D., Norgard, M. V., Brandt, M. E., Isaacs, R. D., Thompson, P. A., and Beutler, B. (1991), "Lipoproteins of Borrelia Burgdorferi and Treponema Pallidum Activate cachectin/TNF Synthesis: Analysis using a CAT Reporter Construct," *J. Immunol. 147,* 1968–1974.
23. Watson, J., and Riblet, R. (1974), "Genetic Control of Responses to Bacterial Lipopolysaccharides in Mice. I. Evidence for a Single Gene that Influences Mitogenic and Immunogenic Responses to Lipopolysaccharides," *J. Exp. Med. 140,* 1147–1161.
24. Watson, J., Riblet, R., and Taylor, B. A. (1977), "The Response of Recombinant Inbred Strains of Mice to Bacterial Lipopolysaccharides," *J. Immunol. 118,* 2088–2093.
25. Watson, J., Kelly, K., Largen, M., and Taylor, B. A. (1978), "The Genetic Mapping of a Defective LPS Response Gene in C3H/HeJ Mice," *J. Immunol. 120,* 422–424.
26. Michalek, S. M., Moore, R. N., McGhee, J. R., Rosenstreich, D. L., and Mergenhagen, S. E. (1980), "The Primary Role of Lymphoreticular Cells in the Mediation of Host Responses to Bacterial Endotoxin," *J. Infec. Dis. 141,* 55–63.
27. O'Brien, A. D., Rosenstreich, D. L., Scher, I., Campbell, G. H., MacDermott, R. P., and Formal, S. B. (1980), "Genetic Control of Susceptibility to Salmonella Typhimurium in Mice: Role of the LPS Gene," *J. Immunol. 124,* 20–24; O'Brien, A. D., Rosenstreich, D. L., and Taylor, B. A. (1980), "Control of Natural Resistance to Salmonella Typhimurium and Leishmania Donovani in Mice by Closely Linked but Distinct Genetic Loci," Nature 287, 440–442; Hagberg, L., Hull, R., Hull, S., McGhee, J. R., Michalek, S. M., and Svanborg Eden, C. (1984), "Difference in Susceptibility to Gram-Negative Urinary Tract Infection between C3H/HeJ and C3H/HeN Mice," *Infect. Immun. 46,* 839–844.
28. O'Brien, A. D., Rosenstreich, D. L., Scher, I., Campbell, G. H., MacDermott, R. P., and Formal, S. B. (1980), "Genetic Control of Susceptibility to Salmonella Typhimurium in Mice: Role of the LPS Gene," *J. Immunol. 124,* 20–24.
29. Hagberg, L., Hull, R., Hull, S., McGhee, J. R., Michalek, S. M., and Svanborg Eden, C. (1984), "Difference in Susceptibility to Gram-Negative Urinary Tract Infection between C3H/HeJ and C3H/HeN Mice," *Infect. Immun.* 46, 839–844.
30. Macela, A., Stulik, J., Hernychova, L., Kroca, M., Krocova, Z., and Kovarova, H. (1996), "The Immune Response Against Francisella Tularensis Live Vaccine Strain in Lps(n) and Lps(d) Mice," *FEMS Immunol.* Med. Microbiol. 13, 235–238.
31. Anderson, G. W., Jr, and Osterman, J. V. (1980), "Host Defenses in Experimental Rickettsialpox: Genetics of Natural Resistance to Infection," *Infect. Immun. 28,* 132–136.

32. Beutler, B., Mahoney, J., Le Trang, N., Pekala, P., and Cerami, A. (1985), "Purification of Cachectin, a Lipoprotein Lipase-Suppressing Hormone Secreted by Endotoxin-Induced RAW 264.7 Cells, " *J. Exp. Med. 161,* 984–995.
33. Beutler, B., Greenwald, D., Hulmes, J. D., Chang, M., Pan, Y.-C.E., Mathison, J., Ulevitch, R., and Cerami, A. (1985), "Identity of Tumour Necrosis Factor and the Macrophage-Secreted Factor Cachectin," *Nature 316,* 552–554.
34. Aggarwal, B. B., Kohr, W. J., Hass, P. E., Moffat, B., Spencer, S. A., Henzel, W. J., Bringman, T. S., Nedwin, G. E., Goeddel, D. V., and Harkins, R. N. (1985), "Human Tumor Necrosis Factor. Production, Purification, and Characterization," *J. Biol. Chem. 260,* 2345–2354.
35. Caput, D., Beutler, B., Hartog, K., Brown-Shimer, S., and Cerami, A. (1986), "Identification of a Common Nucleotide Sequence in the 3'-Untranslated Region of mRNA Molecules Specifying Inflammatory Mediators," *Proc. Natl. Acad. Sci., USA 83,* 1670–1674; Fransen, L., Muller, R., Marmenout, A., Tavernier, J., Van der Heyden, J., Kawashima, E., Chollet, A., Tizard, R., Van Heuverswyn, H., Van Vliet, A., Ruysschaert, M.R., and Fiers, W. (1985), "Molecular Cloning of Mouse Tumour Necrosis Factor cDNA and its Eukaryotic Expression," *Nucleic Acids Res. 13,* 4417–4429.
36. Old, L. J. (1988), "Tumor Necrosis Factor. First Identified because of its Anticancer Activity, the Factor is Now Recognized to be One of a Family of Proteins that Orchestrate the Body's Remarkable Complex Response to Injury and Infection," *Sci. Am. 258,* 59–75.
37. Carswell, E. A., Old, L. J., Kassel, R. L., Green, S., Fiore, N., and Williamson, B. (1975), "An Endotoxin-Induced Serum Factor that Causes Necrosis of Tumors," *Proc. Natl. Acad. Sci. , USA 72,* 3666–3670.
38. Helson, L., Green, S., Carswell, E., and Old, L. J. (1975), "Effect of Tumour Necrosis Factor on Cultured Human Melanoma Cells," *Nature 258,* 731–732.
39. Beutler, B., Milsark, I. W., and Cerami, A. (1985), "Passive Immunization Against Cachectin/tumor Necrosis Factor (TNF) Protects Mice from the Lethal Effect of Endotoxin," *Science 229,* 869–871.
40. Tracey, K. J., Fong, Y., Hesse, D. G., Manogue, K. R., Lee, A. T., Kuo, G. C., Lowry, S. F., and Cerami, A. (1987), "Anti-cachectin/TNF Monoclonal Antibodies Prevent Septic Shock during Lethal Bacteraemia," *Nature 330,* 662–666; Tracey, K. J., Beutler, B., Lowry, S. F., Merryweather, J., Wolpe, S., Milsark, I. W., Hariri, R. J., Fahey, T. J. I., Zentella, A., Albert, J. D., Shires, G. T., and Cerami, A. (1986), "Shock and Tissue Injury Induced by Recombinant Human Cachectin," *Science 234,* 470–474.
41. Deroose, J. P., Eggermont, A. M., van Geel, A. N., de Wilt, J. H., Burger, J. W., and Verhoef, C. (2011), "20 Years Experience of TNF-Based Isolated Limb Perfusion for in-Transit Melanoma Metastases: TNF Dose Matters," *Ann. Surg. Oncol. 2012 Feb;19(2):627–35.*
42. Beutler, B., Milsark, I. W., and Cerami, A. (1985), "Passive Immunization Against Cachectin/tumor Necrosis Factor (TNF) Protects Mice from the Lethal Effect of Endotoxin," *Science 229,* 869–871.
43. Havell, E. A. (1989), "Evidence that Tumor Necrosis Factor has an Important Role in Antibacterial Resistance," *Journal of Immunology 143,* 2894–2899.
44. Kindler, V., Sappino, A., Grau, G. E., Piguet, P., and Vassalli, P. (1989), "The Inducing Role of Tumor Necrosis Factor in the Development of Bactericidal Granulomas during BCG Infection," *Cell 56,* 731–740.
45. Engelmann, H., Novick, D., and Wallach, D. (1990), "Two Tumor Necrosis Factor-Binding Proteins Purified from Human Urine. Evidence for Immunological Cross-Reactivity with Cell Surface Tumor Necrosis Factor Receptors," J. Biol. Chem. 265, 1531–1536; Engelmann, H., Aderka, D., Rubinstein, M., Rotman, D., and Wallach, D. (1989), "A Tumor Necrosis Factor-Binding Protein Purified to Homogeneity from Human Urine Protects Cells from Tumor Necrosis Factor Toxicity," *J. Biol. Chem. 264,* 11974–11980; Nophar, Y., Kemper, O., Brakebusch, C., Englemann, H., Zwang,

R., Aderka, D., Holtmann, H., and Wallach, D. (1990), "Soluble Forms of Tumor Necrosis Factor Receptors (TNF-Rs). the cDNA for the Type I TNF-R, Cloned using Amino Acid Sequence Data of its Soluble Form, Encodes both the Cell Surface and a Soluble Form of the Receptor," *EMBO J. 9,* 3269–3278; Novick, D., Engelmann, H., Wallach, D., Leitner, O., Revel, M., and Rubinstein, M. (1990), "Purification of Soluble Cytokine Receptors from Normal Human Urine by Ligand-Affinity and Immunoaffinity Chromatography," *J. Chromatogr. 510,* 331–337.

46. Lewis, M., Tartaglia, L. A., Lee, A., Bennett, G. L., Rice, G. C., Wang, G. H., Chen, E. Y., and Goeddel, D. V. (1991), "Cloning and Expression of cDNAs for Two Distinct Murine Tumor Necrosis Factor Receptors Demonstrate One Receptor is Species Specific," *Proc. Natl. Acad. Sci., USA 88,* 2830–2834; Tartaglia, L. A., Weber, R. F., Figari, I. S., Reynolds, C., Palladino, M. A., Jr, and Goeddel, D. V. (1991), "The Two Different Receptors for Tumor Necrosis Factor Mediate Distinct Cellular Responses," *Proc. Natl. Acad. Sci. U. S. A. 88,* 9292–9296.
47. Peppel, K., Crawford, D., and Beutler, B. (1991), "A Tumor Necrosis Factor (TNF) Receptor-IgG Heavy Chain Chimeric Protein as a Bivalent Antagonist of TNF Activity," *J. Exp. Med. 174,* 1483–1489.
48. Kawakami, M., and Cerami, A. (1981), "Studies of Endotoxin-Induced Decrease in Lipoprotein Lipase Activity," *J. Exp. Med. 154,* 631–639.
49. Flaherty, S. F., Golenbock, D. T., Milham, F. H., and Ingalls, R. R. (1997), "CD11/CD18 Leukocyte Integrins: New Signaling Receptors for Bacterial Endotoxin," *J. Surg. Res. 73,* 85–89; Ingalls, R. R., Arnaout, M. A., Delude, R. L., Flaherty, S., Savedra, R., Jr., and Golenbock, D. T. (1998), "The CD11/CD18 Integrins: Characterization of Three Novel LPS Signaling Receptors," *Prog. Clin. Biol. Res. 397,* 107–117; Ingalls, R. R., and Golenbock, D. T. (1995), "CD11c/CD18, a Transmembrane Signaling Receptor for Lipopolysaccharide," *J. Exp. Med. 181,* 1473–1479.
50. Jin, F. Y., Nathan, C., Radzioch, D., and Ding, A. (1997), "Secretory Leukocyte Protease Inhibitor: A Macrophage Product Induced by and Antagonistic to Bacterial Lipopolysaccharide," *Cell 88,* 417–426.
51. Kang, A. D., Wong, P. M., Chen, H., Castagna, R., Chung, S. W., and Sultzer, B. M. (1996), "Restoration of Lipopolysaccharide-Mediated B-Cell Response After Expression of a cDNA Encoding a GTP-Binding Protein," *Infect. Immun. 64,* 4612–4617.
52. Novogrodsky, A., Vanichkin, A., Patya, M., Gazit, A., Osherov, N., and Levitzki, A. (1994), "Prevention of Lipopolysaccharide-Induced Lethal Toxicity by Tyrosine Kinase Inhibitors," *Science 264,* 1319–1322.
53. Han, J., Lee, J. D., Bibbs, L., and Ulevitch, R. J. (1994), "A MAP Kinase Targeted by Endotoxin and Hyperosmolarity in Mammalian Cells," *Science 265,* 808–811; Han, J., Lee, J. D., Tobias, P. S., and Ulevitch, R. J. (1993), "Endotoxin Induces Rapid Protein Tyrosine Phosphorylation in 70Z/3 Cells Expressing CD14," *J. Biol. Chem. 268,* 25009–25014.
54. Shinji, H., Akagawa, K. S., and Yoshida, T. (1994), "LPS Induces Selective Translocation of Protein Kinase C-Beta in LPS-Responsive Mouse Macrophages, but Not in LPS-Nonresponsive Mouse Macrophages," *J. Immunol. 153,* 5760–5771.
55. Wright, S. D., Ramos, R. A., Tobias, P. S., Ulevitch, R. J., and Mathison, J. C. (1990), "CD14, a Receptor for Complexes of Lipopolysaccharide (LPS) and LPS Binding Protein," *Science 249,* 1431–1433.
56. Lee, J. D., Kato, K., Tobias, P. S., Kirkland, T. N., and Ulevitch, R. J. (1992), "Transfection of CD14 into 70Z/3 Cells Dramatically Enhances the Sensitivity to Complexes of Lipopolysaccharide (LPS) and LPS Binding Protein," *J. Exp. Med. 175,* 1697–1705.
57. Han, J., Brown, T., and Beutler, B. (1990), "Endotoxin-Responsive Sequences Control cachectin/TNF Biosynthesis at the Translational Level," *J. Exp. Med. 171,* 465–475.

58. Shakhov, A. N., Collart, M. A., Vassalli, P., Nedospasov, S. A., and Jongeneel, C. V. (1990), "KappaB-Type Enhancers are Involved in Lipopolysaccharide- Mediated Transcriptional Activation of the Tumor Necrosis Factor Alpha Gene in Primary Macrophages," *J. Exp. Med. 171,* 35–47.
59. Kruys, V., Marinx, O., Shaw, G., Deschamps, J., and Huez, G. (1989), "Translational Blockade Imposed by Cytokine-Derived UA-Rich Sequences," *Science 245,* 852–855; Kruys, V., Wathelet, M., Poupart, P., Contreras, R., Fiers, W., Content, J., and Huez, G. (1987), "The 3' Untranslated Region of the Human Interferon-Beta mRNA has an Inhibitory Effect on Translation," *Proc. Natl. Acad. Sci., USA 84,* 6030–6034; Kruys, V. I., Wathelet, M. G., and Huez, G. A. (1988), "Identification of a Translation Inhibitory Element (TIE) in the 3' Untranslated Region of the Human Interferon-Beta mRNA," Gene 72, 191–200.
60. Kruys, V., Kemmer, K., Shakhov, A., Jongeneel, V., and Beutler, B. (1992), "Constitutive Activity of the Tumor Necrosis Factor Promoter is Canceled by the 3' Untranslated Region in Nonmacrophage Cell Lines; a Trans-Dominant Factor Overcomes this Suppressive Effect," *Proc. Natl. Acad. Sci., USA 89,* 673–677.
61. Caput, D., Beutler, B., Hartog, K., Brown-Shimer, S., and Cerami, A. (1986), "Identification of a Common Nucleotide Sequence in the 3'-Untranslated Region of mRNA Molecules Specifying Inflammatory Mediators," *Proc. Natl. Acad. Sci., USA 83,* 1670–1674.
62. Shaw, G., and Kamen, R. (1986), "A Conserved AU Sequence from the 3' Untranslated Region of GM-CSF mRNA Mediates Selective mRNA Degradation," *Cell 46,* 659–667.
63. Han, J., Thompson, P., and Beutler, B. (1990), "Dexamethasone and Pentoxifylline Inhibit Endotoxin-Induced cachectin/TNF Synthesis at Separate Points in the Signalling Pathway," *J. Exp. Med. 172,* 391–394.
64. Beutler, B., and Brown, T. (1991), "A CAT Reporter Construct Allows Ultrasensitive Estimation of TNF Synthesis, and Suggests that the TNF Gene has been Silenced in Non-Macrophage Cell Lines," *J. Clin. Invest. 87,* 1336–1344.
65. Giroir, B. P., Johnson, J. H., Brown, T., Allen, G. L., and Beutler, B. (1992), "The Tissue Distribution of Tumor Necrosis Factor Biosynthesis during Endotoxemia," *J. Clin. Invest. 90,* 693–698.
66. Watson, J., Kelly, K., Largen, M., and Taylor, B. A. (1978), "The Genetic Mapping of a Defective LPS Response Gene in C3H/HeJ Mice," *J. Immunol. 120,* 422–424.
67. Dietrich, W., Katz, H., Lincoln, S. E., Shin, H. S., Friedman, J., Dracopoli, N. C., and Lander, E. S. (1992), "A Genetic Map of the Mouse Suitable for Typing Intraspecific Crosses," *Genetics 131,* 423–447.
68. Mouse Genome Sequencing Consortium, Waterston, R. H., Lindblad-Toh, K., Birney, E., Rogers, J., Abril, J. F., Agarwal, P., Agarwala, R., Ainscough, R., Alexandersson, M., An, P., Antonarakis, S. E., Attwood, J., Baertsch, R., Bailey, J., Barlow, K., Beck, S., Berry, E., Birren, B., Bloom, T., Bork, P., Botcherby, M., Bray, N., Brent, M. R., Brown, D. G., Brown, S. D., Bult, C., Burton, J., Butler, J., Campbell, R. D., Carninci, P., Cawley, S., Chiaromonte, F., Chinwalla, A. T., Church, D. M., Clamp, M., Clee, C., Collins, F. S., Cook, L. L., Copley, R. R., Coulson, A., Couronne, O., Cuff, J., Curwen, V., Cutts, T., Daly, M., David, R., Davies, J., Delehaunty, K. D., Deri, J., Dermitzakis, E. T., Dewey, C., Dickens, N. J., Diekhans, M., Dodge, S., Dubchak, I., Dunn, D. M., Eddy, S. R., Elnitski, L., Emes, R. D., Eswara, P., Eyras, E., Felsenfeld, A., Fewell, G. A., Flicek, P., Foley, K., Frankel, W. N., Fulton, L. A., Fulton, R. S., Furey, T. S., Gage, D., Gibbs, R. A., Glusman, G., Gnerre, S., Goldman, N., Goodstadt, L., Grafham, D., Graves, T. A., Green, E. D., Gregory, S., Guigo, R., Guyer, M., Hardison, R. C., Haussler, D., Hayashizaki, Y., Hillier, L. W., Hinrichs, A., Hlavina, W., Holzer, T., Hsu, F., Hua, A., Hubbard, T., Hunt, A., Jackson, I., Jaffe, D. B., Johnson, L. S., Jones, M., Jones, T. A., Joy, A., Kamal, M., Karlsson, E. K., Karolchik, D., Kasprzyk, A., Kawai, J., Keibler, E., Kells, C., Kent, W. J., Kirby, A., Kolbe, D. L., Korf, I., Kucherlapati,

R. S., Kulbokas, E. J., Kulp, D., Landers, T., Leger, J. P., Leonard, S., Letunic, I., Levine, R., Li, J., Li, M., Lloyd, C., Lucas, S., Ma, B., Maglott, D. R., Mardis, E. R., Matthews, L., Mauceli, E., Mayer, J. H., McCarthy, M., McCombie, W. R., McLaren, S., McLay, K., McPherson, J. D., Meldrim, J., Meredith, B., Mesirov, J. P., Miller, W., Miner, T. L., Mongin, E., Montgomery, K. T., Morgan, M., Mott, R., Mullikin, J. C., Muzny, D. M., Nash, W. E., Nelson, J. O., Nhan, M. N., Nicol, R., Ning, Z., Nusbaum, C., O'Connor, M. J., Okazaki, Y., Oliver, K., Overton-Larty, E., Pachter, L., Parra, G., Pepin, K. H., Peterson, J., Pevzner, P., Plumb, R., Pohl, C. S., Poliakov, A., Ponce, T. C., Ponting, C. P., Potter, S., Quail, M., Reymond, A., Roe, B. A., Roskin, K. M., Rubin, E. M., Rust, A. G., Santos, R., Sapojnikov, V., Schultz, B., Schultz, J., Schwartz, M. S., Schwartz, S., Scott, C., Seaman, S., Searle, S., Sharpe, T., Sheridan, A., Shownkeen, R., Sims, S., Singer, J. B., Slater, G., Smit, A., Smith, D. R., Spencer, B., Stabenau, A., Stange-Thomann, N., Sugnet, C., Suyama, M., Tesler, G., Thompson, J., Torrents, D., Trevaskis, E., Tromp, J., Ucla, C., Ureta-Vidal, A., Vinson, J. P., Von Niederhausern, A. C., Wade, C. M., Wall, M., Weber, R. J., Weiss, R. B., Wendl, M. C., West, A. P., Wetterstrand, K., Wheeler, R., Whelan, S., Wierzbowski, J., Willey, D., Williams, S., Wilson, R. K., Winter, E., Worley, K. C., Wyman, D., Yang, S., Yang, S. P., Zdobnov, E. M., Zody, M. C., and Lander, E. S. (2002), "Initial Sequencing and Comparative Analysis of the Mouse Genome," *Nature 420,* 520–562.

69. Poltorak, A., Smirnova, I., He, X. L., Liu, M. Y., Van Huffel, C., McNally, O., Birdwell, D., Alejos, E., Silva, M., Du, X., Thompson, P., Chan, E. K. L., Ledesma, J., Roe, B., Clifton, S., Vogel, S. N., and Beutler, B. (1998), "Genetic and Physical Mapping of the Lps locus- Identification of the Toll-4 Receptor as a Candidate Gene in the Critical Region," B*lood Cells Mol. Dis. 24,* 340–355.
70. Xu, Y., Mural, R. J., and Uberbacher, E. C. (1994), "Constructing Gene Models from Accurately Predicted Exons: An Application of Dynamic Programming," *Comput. Appl. Biosci. 10,* 613–623; Xu, Y., Mural, R., Shah, M., and Uberbacher, E. (1994), "Recognizing Exons in Genomic Sequence using GRAIL II," *Genet. Eng. (N.Y.) 16,* 241–253.
71. Medzhitov, R., Preston-Hurlburt, P., and Janeway, C. A.,Jr. (1997), "A Human Homologue of the Drosophila Toll Protein Signals Activation of Adaptive Immunity," *Nature 388,* 394–397.
72. Janeway, C. A., Jr. (1989), "Approaching the Asymptote? Evolution and Revolution in Immunology," *Cold Spring Harb. Symp. Quant. Biol. 54 Pt 1,* 1–13.
73. Poltorak, A., He, X., Smirnova, I., Liu, M. Y., Van Huffel, C., Du, X., Birdwell, D., Alejos, E., Silva, M., Galanos, C., Freudenberg, M. A., Ricciardi-Castagnoli, P., Layton, B., and Beutler, B. (1998), "Defective LPS Signaling in C3H/HeJ and C57BL/10ScCr Mice: Mutations in *Tlr4* Gene," *Science 282,* 2085–2088; Poltorak, A., Smirnova, I., Clisch, R., and Beutler, B. (2000), "Limits of a Deletion Spanning *Tlr4* in C57BL/10ScCr Mice," *J. Endotoxin Res. 6IS – 1,* 51–56.
74. Poltorak, A., Smirnova, I., He, X. L., Liu, M. Y., Van Huffel, C., McNally, O., Birdwell, D., Alejos, E., Silva, M., Du, X., Thompson, P., Chan, E. K. L., Ledesma, J., Roe, B., Clifton, S., Vogel, S. N., and Beutler, B. (1998), "Genetic and Physical Mapping of the *Lps* locus: Identification of the Toll-4 Receptor as a Candidate Gene in the Critical Region," *Blood Cells Mol. Dis. 24,* 340–355.
75. Poltorak, A., He, X., Smirnova, I., Liu, M. Y., Van Huffel, C., Du, X., Birdwell, D., Alejos, E., Silva, M., Galanos, C., Freudenberg, M. A., Ricciardi-Castagnoli, P., Layton, B., and Beutler, B. (1998), "Defective LPS Signaling in C3H/HeJ and C57BL/10ScCr Mice: Mutations in *Tlr4* Gene," *Science 282,* 2085–2088.
76. Yang, R.B., Mark, M. R., Gray, A., Huang, A., Xie, M. H., Zhang, M., Goddard, A., Wood, W. I., Gurney, A. L., and Godowski, P. J. (1998), "Toll-Like Receptor-2 Mediates Lipopolysaccharide-Induced Cellular Signalling," *Nature. 395,* 284–288; Kirschning, C. J., Wesche, H., Merrill, A. T., and Rothe, M. (1998), "Human Toll-Like Receptor

2 Confers Responsiveness to Bacterial Lipopolysaccharide," *J. Exp. Med. 188,* 2091–2097.

77. Takeuchi, O., Hoshino, K., Kawai, T., Sanjo, H., Takada, H., Ogawa, T., Takeda, K., and Akira, S. (1999), "Differential Roles of TLR2 and TLR4 in Recognition of Gram-Negative and Gram-Positive Bacterial Cell Wall Components," *Immunity 11,* 443–451.
78. Poltorak, A., Ricciardi-Castagnoli, P., Citterio, A., and Beutler, B. (2000), "Physical Contact between LPS and Tlr4 Revealed by Genetic Complementation," *Proc. Natl. Acad. Sci., USA 97,* 2163–2167.
79. Lien, E., Means, T. K., Heine, H., Yoshimura, A., Kusumoto, S., Fukase, K., Fenton, M. J., Oikawa, M., Qureshi, N., Monks, B., Finberg, R. W., Ingalls, R. R., and Golenbock, D. T. (2000), "Toll-Like Receptor 4 Imparts Ligand-Specific Recognition of Bacterial Lipopolysaccharide," *J. Clin. Invest. 105,* 497–504.
80. Poltorak, A., Ricciardi-Castagnoli, P., Citterio, A., and Beutler, B. (2000), "Physical Contact between LPS and Tlr4 Revealed by Genetic Complementation," *Proc. Natl. Acad. Sci., USA 97,* 2163–2167.
81. Du, X., Poltorak, A., Silva, M., and Beutler, B. (1999), "Analysis of Tlr4-Mediated LPS Signal Transduction in Macrophages by Mutational Modification of the Receptor," *Blood Cells Mol. Dis. 25,* 328–338.
82. Shimazu, R., Akashi, S., Ogata, H., Nagai, Y., Fukudome, K., Miyake, K., and Kimoto, M. (1999), "MD-2, a Molecule that Confers Lipopolysaccharide Responsiveness on Toll-Like Receptor 4," *J. Exp. Med. 189,* 1777–1782.
83. Muroi, M., Ohnishi, T., and Tanamoto, K. (2002), "MD-2, a Novel Accessory Molecule, is Involved in Species-Specific Actions of Salmonella Lipid A," *Infect. Immun. 70,* 3546–3550.
84. Park, B. S., Song, D. H., Kim, H. M., Choi, B. S., Lee, H., and Lee, J. O. (2009), "The Structural Basis of Lipopolysaccharide Recognition by the TLR4-MD-2 Complex," *Nature 458,* 1191–1195.
85. Shimazu, R., Akashi, S., Ogata, H., Nagai, Y., Fukudome, K., Miyake, K., and Kimoto, M. (1999), "MD-2, a Molecule that Confers Lipopolysaccharide Responsiveness on Toll-Like Receptor 4," *J. Exp. Med. 189,* 1777–1782.
86. Gay, N. J., and Keith, F. J. (1991), "Drosophila Toll and IL-1 Receptor," *Nature 351,* 355–356.
87. Whitham, S., Dinesh-Kumar, S. P., Choi, D., Hehl, R., Corr, C., and Baker, B. (1994), "The Product of the Tobacco Mosaic Virus Resistance Gene N: Similarity to Toll and the Interleukin-1 Receptor," *Cell 78,* 1101–1115.
88. Song, W. Y., Wang, G. L., Chen, L. L., Kim, H. S., Pi, L. Y., Holsten, T., Gardner, J., Wang, B., Zhai, W. X., Zhu, L. H., Fauquet, C., and Ronald, P. (1995), "A Receptor Kinase-Like Protein Encoded by the Rice Disease Resistance Gene, Xa21," *Science 270,* 1804–1806.
89. Lee, S. W., Han, S. W., Sririyanum, M., Park, C. J., Seo, Y. S., and Ronald, P. C. (2009), "A Type I-Secreted, Sulfated Peptide Triggers XA21-Mediated Innate Immunity," *Science 326,* 850–853.
90. Barnes, M. J., Aksoylar, H., Krebs, P., Bourdeau, T., Arnold, C. N., Xia, Y., Khovananth, K., Engel, I., Sovath, S., Lampe, K., Laws, E., Kronenberg, M., Steinbrecher, K., Hildeman, D., Grimes, H. L., Beutler, B., and Hoebe, K. (2010), "Loss of T and B Cell Quiescence and Development of Flora-Dependent Wasting Disease and Intestinal Inflammation in Gimap5-Deficient Mice," *J. Immunol. 184,* 3743–3754; Eidenschenk, C., Crozat, K., Krebs, P., Arens, R., Popkin, D., Arnold, C. N., Blasius, A. L., Benedict, C. A., Moresco, E. M., Xia, Y., and Beutler, B. (2010), "Flt3 Permits Survival during Infection by Rendering Dendritic Cells Competent to Activate NK Cells," *Proc. Natl. Acad. Sci. U. S. A. 107,* 9759–9764; Berger, M., Krebs, P., Crozat, K., Li, X., Croker, B. A., Siggs, O. M., Popkin, D., Du, X., Lawson, B. R., Theofilopoulos, A. N., Xia, Y., Khovananth, K., Moresco, E. M. Y., Satoh, T., Takeuchi, O., Akira, S., and Beutler, B. (2010), "An Slfn2 Mutation Causes Lymphoid and Myeloid Immunodeficiency due to Loss of Immune Cell Quiescence," *Nat. Immunol. 11,* 335–343.

91. Croker, B., Crozat, K., Berger, M., Xia, Y., Sovath, S., Schaffer, L., Eleftherianos, I., Imler, J. L., and Beutler, B. (2007), "ATP-Sensitive Potassium Channels Mediate Survival during Infection in Mammals and Insects," *Nat. Genet. 39,* 1453–1460.
92. Tabeta, K., Hoebe, K., Janssen, E. M., Du, X., Georgel, P., Crozat, K., Mudd, S., Mann, N., Sovath, S., Goode, J., Shamel, L., Herskovits, A. A., Portnoy, D. A., Cooke, M., Tarantino, L. M., Wiltshire, T., Steinberg, B. E., Grinstein, S., and Beutler, B. (2006), "The Unc93b1 Mutation 3d Disrupts Exogenous Antigen Presentation and Signaling Via Toll-Like Receptors 3, 7 and 9," *Nat. Immunol. 7,* 156–164.
93. Yamamoto, M., Sato, S., Hemmi, H., Hoshino, K., Kaisho, T., Sanjo, H., Takeuchi, O., Sugiyama, M., Okabe, M., Takeda, K., and Akira, S. (2003), "Role of Adaptor TRIF in the MyD88-Independent Toll-Like Receptor Signaling Pathway," *Science 301,* 640–643.
94. Oshiumi, H., Matsumoto, M., Funami, K., Akazawa, T., and Seya, T. (2003), "TICAM-1, an Adaptor Molecule that Participates in Toll-Like Receptor 3-Mediated Interferon-Beta Induction," *Nat. Immunol. 4,* 161–171.
95. Hoebe, K., Du, X., Georgel, P., Janssen, E., Tabeta, K., Kim, S. O., Goode, J., Lin, P., Mann, N., Mudd, S., Crozat, K., Sovath, S., Han, J., and Beutler, B. (2003), "Identification of Lps2 as a Key Transducer of MyD88-Independent TIR Signaling," *Nature 424,* 743–748.
96. Hoebe, K., Georgel, P., Rutschmann, S., Du, X., Mudd, S., Crozat, K., Sovath, S., Shamel, L., Hartung, T., Zahringer, U., and Beutler, B. (2005), "CD36 is a Sensor of Diacylglycerides," *Nature 433,* 523–527.
97. Blasius, A. L., Arnold, C. N., Georgel, P., Rutschmann, S., Xia, Y., Lin, P., Ross, C., Li, X., Smart, N. G., and Beutler, B. (2010), "Slc15a4, AP-3, and Hermansky-Pudlak Syndrome Proteins are Required for Toll-Like Receptor Signaling in Plasmacytoid Dendritic Cells," *Proc. Natl. Acad. Sci. U. S. A. 107,* 19973–19978.
98. Johnson, A. G., Gaines, S., and Landy, M. (1956), "Studies on the O Antigen of Salmonella Typhosa. V. Enhancement of Antibody Response to Protein Antigens by the Purified Lipopolysaccharide," *J. Exp. Med. 103,* 225–246.
99. Skidmore, B. J., Chiller, J. M., Morrison, D. C., and Weigle, W. O. (1975), "Immunologic Properties of Bacterial Lipopolysaccharide (LPS): Correlation between the Mitogenic, Adjuvant, and Immunogenic Activities. *J. Immunol. 114,* 770–775; Skidmore, B. J., Chiller, J. M., Weigle, W. O., Riblet, R., and Watson, J. (1976) Immunologic Properties of Bacterial Lipopolysaccharide (LPS). III. Genetic Linkage between the in Vitro Mitogenic and in Vivo Adjuvant Properties of LPS," *J. Exp. Med. 143,* 143–150.
100. Gavin, A. L., Hoebe, K., Duong, B., Ota, T., Martin, C., Beutler, B., and Nemazee, D. (2006), "Adjuvant-Enhanced Antibody Responses in the Absence of Toll-Like Receptor Signaling," *Science 314,* 1936–1938.
101. Baccala, R., Hoebe, K., Kono, D. H., Beutler, B., and Theofilopoulos, A. N. (2007), "TLR-Dependent and TLR-Independent Pathways of Type I Interferon Induction in Systemic Autoimmunity," *Nat. Med. 13,* 543–551; Kono, D. H., Haraldsson, M. K., Lawson, B. R., Pollard, K. M., Koh, Y. T., Du, X., Arnold, C. N., Baccala, R., Silverman, G. J., Beutler, B. A., and Theofilopoulos, A. N. (2009), "Endosomal TLR Signaling is Required for Anti-Nucleic Acid and Rheumatoid Factor Autoantibodies in Lupus," *Proc. Natl. Acad. Sci. U. S. A. 106,* 12061–12066.
102. Pisitkun, P., Deane, J. A., Difilippantonio, M. J., Tarasenko, T., Satterthwaite, A. B., and Bolland, S. (2006), "Autoreactive B Cell Responses to RNA-Related Antigens due to TLR7 Gene Duplication," *Science 312,* 1669–1672.
103. Kono, D. H., Haraldsson, M. K., Lawson, B. R., Pollard, K. M., Koh, Y. T., Du, X., Arnold, C. N., Baccala, R., Silverman, G. J., Beutler, B. A., and Theofilopoulos, A. N. (2009), "Endosomal TLR Signaling is Required for Anti-Nucleic Acid and Rheumatoid Factor Autoantibodies in Lupus," *Proc. Natl. Acad. Sci. U. S. A. 106,* 12061–12066.

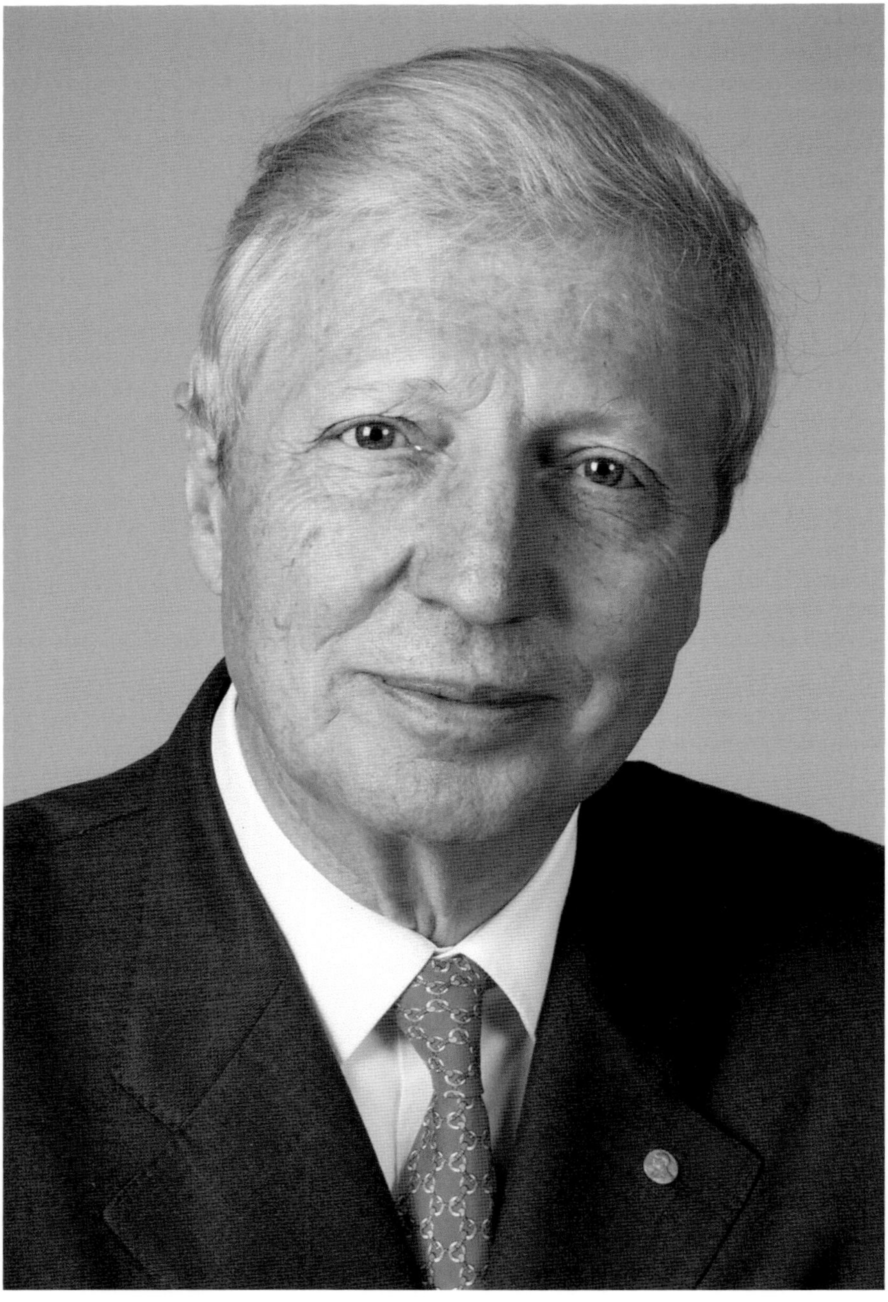

Jules A. Hoffmann. © The Nobel Foundation. Photo: U. Montan

Jules A. Hoffmann did not submit an autobiography. See https://www.nobelprize.org/prizes/medicine/2011/hoffmann/facts/

THE HOST DEFENSE OF INSECTS: A PARADIGM FOR INNATE IMMUNITY

Nobel Lecture, December 7, 2011

by

JULES HOFFMANN

Strasbourg, France.

I grew up in Luxembourg after the Second World War. My father (Figure 1) was a high school teacher, who spent his spare time collecting and describing insects in various settings, particularly around brooks and ponds in the countryside. From early age on, I accompanied him, and by and by participated in the identification of various insect species. This led me, with his obvious help, to publish at the age of 17 my first paper on the waterbug (Heteroptera) in Luxembourg. This period, which I dearly remember to this day, generated in me a fascination for insects, which represent the most important group of the present day fauna. It is believed that they make up some 80% of all extant animal species. They play a considerable role in human health by transmitting microbial pathogens that put close to one third of the human population at risk and yearly kill tens of thousands. They also have a strong impact on the economy: on the positive side through pollination, for instance, and on the negative side through the destruction of crops. It is estimated that one third of human crops are destroyed annually by insect pests world-wide.

After completing high school in Luxembourg, I left for Strasbourg University where I studied Life Sciences, in particular Zoology and Physiology. After graduation, I was fortunate to be accepted for Ph.D. studies by Professor Pierre Joly, the Chair of the Laboratory of General Biology at the Institute of Zoology (Figure 1). The Joly laboratory was the only group doing experimental research on insect models in Strasbourg. Their studies focused on the endocrine and neuroendocrine control of insect development and reproduction. The laboratory also had a particular interest in phase differentiation in grasshoppers *(Locusta migratoria)*, which represented a major plague in Northern and Western Africa at that time. Professor Joly proposed to me the study of antimicrobial defences in grasshoppers. In fact, as he explained, his laboratory had over decades transplanted endocrine organs and even whole brains from one insect to another without ever taking antiseptic precautions, but they had never observed the appearance of opportunistic infections. To Professor Joly, this could only be explained if efficient antimicrobial defences existed in these insects.

I was very excited by this project. A survey of the existing literature rapidly indicated that very little information was available on antimicrobial reactions in insects. At the end of the 19th century, Eli Metchnikoff had discovered phagocytosis in starfish larvae and established its role in water-flea antimicrobial defences ("cellular immunity") (Metchnikoff, 1884). Further, interesting studies by André Paillot and Rudolf Glaser in the early 20th century had pointed to the appearance of inducible antimicrobial activities in caterpillars following a microbial challenge ("humoral immunity") (Glaser, 1918; Paillot, 1919, 1933). Episodic investigations in a variety of insect species had analysed melanisation, tissue repair and other defence aspects (reviewed in Jehle, 2009), but in essence no clear-cut picture of these defences had emerged when I started my thesis work.

In the mid-sixties, the Joly laboratory was not equipped for biochemical studies and we relied on experimental biology, classical histology and electron microscopy to address this research topic. My initial investigations confirmed that phagocytosis was an essential arm of grasshopper antimicrobial defences. Injections of low doses of microbes (we used *Bacillus thuringiensis* during the first years of the project) induced a significant protection against subsequent administrations of higher and even lethal doses. I could correlate this induced protection with a strongly upregulated production of blood cells, namely of phagocytes. At that time, I was not able to detect any specificity in this mechanism of induction. The sometimes massive changes in the hemograms (blood cell counts) following experimental infections raised the question of the post-embryonic origin of blood cells in these insects. Hemopoiesis was not well understood in insects at that time, but through the combination of experimental biology (namely severe bleeding) and histology/ultrastructural studies, I eventually identified a well-organised hemopoietic tissue in the vicinity of the dorsal blood vessel in the abdomens of both larval and adult grasshoppers. Dr Aimé Porte (Figure 1), an exceptional cell biologist with a strong medical background, was my direct supervisor during this period and our thorough ultrastructural analysis of the grasshopper hemopoietic tissue revealed some unexpected similarities with hemopoiesis in mammals (Hoffmann et al., 1968, Hoffmann et al., 1970; Hoffmann 1973).

To establish the functional significance of this newly identified juxtacardiac hemopoietic tissue, I went on to submit it to selective X-ray treatment. The results were spectacular and were to orient the studies of the laboratory for many years to come. For one, grasshoppers which had their hemopoietic tissue selectively subjected to X-ray treatment rapidly succumbed to septicemia by opportunistic microbes; sham irradiated grasshoppers did not show a similar phenotype. This result underlined the crucial role of hemopoiesis in antimicrobial defences, namely through the massive production of phagocytes. A second, totally unexpected result was the observation that the endocrine control of moulting was upset. In short, grasshopper larvae undergo five cycles of moulting: it was understood that these cycles were dependent on a gland, referred to as prothoracic gland, and that this gland released the moulting hormone ecdysone (*ecdysis* meaning moult in Greek) at a precise moment within each larval instar (referred to as a "critical period"). When the X-ray treatment of the hemopoietic tissue was performed before this

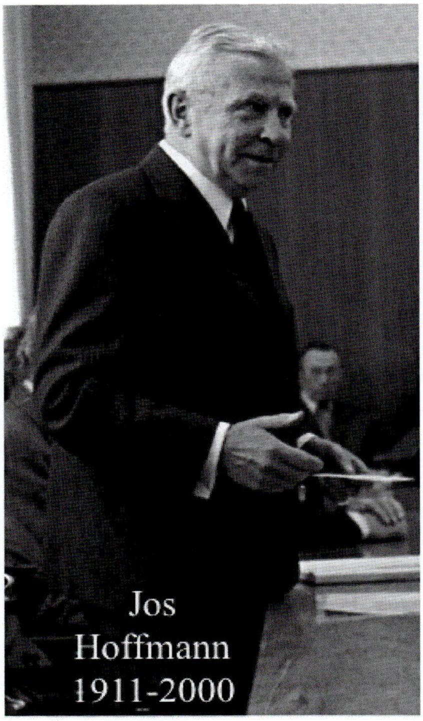

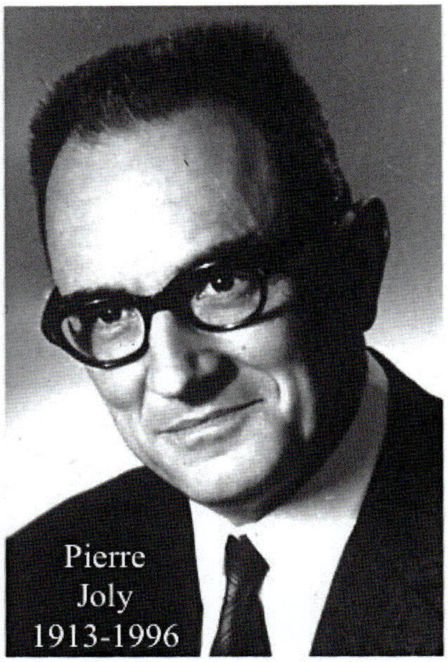

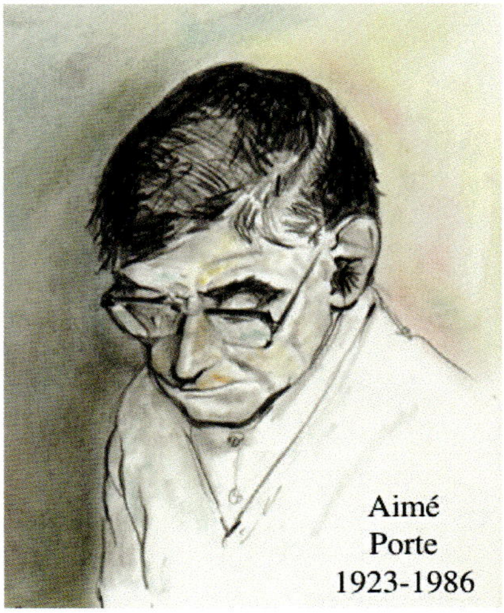

critical period within any instar, the following moults were blocked; if the treatment was performed after the critical period, the next moults was not blocked but subsequent moults were still suppressed. The moulting hormone ecdysone, a 27-carbon polar steroid, had been isolated and characterized by Professor Peter Karlson in Germany from the butterfly *Bombyx* (Butenandt and Karlson, 1954; Karlson et al., 1965). Professor Joly was particularly interested in the results of the X-ray treatment. He arranged for me to spend some time in the Karlson laboratory to relate our observations with the studies on the synthesis, blood transport and metabolism of ecdysone which were being undertaken by Professor Karlson and Dr Jan Koolman at the Institute of Chemical Physiology of the University of Marburg – a 4 hour drive from Strasbourg. Meanwhile, he suggested, the antimicrobial defence studies in grasshoppers should be continued in Strasbourg by my first doctoral student (who actually was my wife Danièle whom I had met in the Joly laboratory some time before). For years, our laboratory carried the official CNRS denomination “Endocrinology and Immunology of Insects” and was renamed only in 1994

"Immune Response and Development in Insects". I will not recount here the fruitful years that we spent with our colleagues from Marburg investigating the biosynthesis, metabolism, and mode of action of the steroid hormone ecdysone in grasshoppers. These studies became a hallmark of our laboratory for many years, during which we collaborated with the Department of Organic Chemistry in Strasbourg, and specifically with Professor Guy Ourisson and Dr Luu Bang. Thanks mainly to the enthusiastic involvement of Marie Lagueux and Charles Hetru, the "Ecdysone years" allowed our group to mature in the fields of biochemistry and analytical chemistry, to invest in appropriate equipment and to recruit talented scientists. Eventually, we were in excellent condition when we concentrated on the immune studies in flies from the mid-80s on.

In spite of strenuous efforts we were not able in the 70s and 80s to get hold of any significant inducible antimicrobial substances in challenged grasshoppers, beyond that of lysozyme. Professor Hans Boman, from Stockholm, was a member of the Ph.D. defence committee of Danièle Hoffmann (1978) and he proposed that she join his laboratory for a postdoctoral period. Right at that time, Boman and his associates were about to identify the inducible antimicrobial peptide cecropin from challenged pupae of the moth *Hyalophora cecropia* (Steiner et al, 1981). Danièle joined the Boman laboratory in 1979 to work with Dan Hultmark on another lepidopteran insect, *Galleria mellonella* (D. Hoffmann et al, 1981). Once Danièle was back from Stockholm, she developed a severe allergy to the dust present on the wings (elytra) of grasshoppers. There were no real perspectives that we could use *Locusta* for genetic studies and we decided that we would shift our studies on insect antimicrobial defences to dipteran species and abandon grasshoppers. Our objectives were to eventually turn to the genetically tractable *Drosophila melanogaster* model. In the early 80s the methodologies available to us still prevented the direct characterisation of inducible antimicrobial substances from small organisms, like fruit flies. We therefore chose the large fly *Phormia terranovae*, which could be mass-raised in our laboratory and which provided ample amounts of blood for biochemical analysis. The project was to subsequently characterise inducible antimicrobial substances in the fruit fly through homology cloning based on the peptide sequences from the molecules identified in large flies. In retrospect, this was an excellent decision as we now know that grasshoppers do not rely for their antimicrobial defences on the massive secretion of antibacterial peptides into their blood, in contrast to flies, as we shall see below. By that time, the number of persons in our laboratory working on antimicrobial defences had significantly increased. In addition to Danièle, we now had Jean-Luc Dimarcq, Daniel Zachary and Jean-Marc Reichhart working on this topic. The members working on the endocrine aspects (steroids, neurohormones) included Marie Lagueux, Christine Kappler, Charles Hetru, Marie Meister and Maurice Charlet.

Our efforts directed at identifying inducible antimicrobial peptides in *Phormia* eventually led in the late 80s to the characterisation of a glycine-rich 82-residue polypeptide which we named Diptericin (from Diptera, two-winged insects) (Dimarcq et al, 1988). It had taken 100 ml of blood from challenged larvae to generate this sequence, indeed a formidable task, which the spectacular progress of physico-chemical methods in the following years has fortunately made obsolete. We cloned the corresponding gene and followed its expression pattern in flies challenged by an injection of a mix of bacteria (Reichhart et al, 1989). Activity spectra of purified Diptericin showed that it was particularly active against Gram-negative bacteria. Importantly for our future studies, we were able to clone a *Diptericin* homologue in *Drosophila* in 1990 (Wicker et al, 1990). From 1990 on, we felt confident that we were able to directly identify inducible antimicrobial substances from challenged fruit flies (Figure 2), in spite of their small size. Through the intense work of Charles Hetru, Jean-Luc Dimarcq, Philippe Bulet and others in the group,

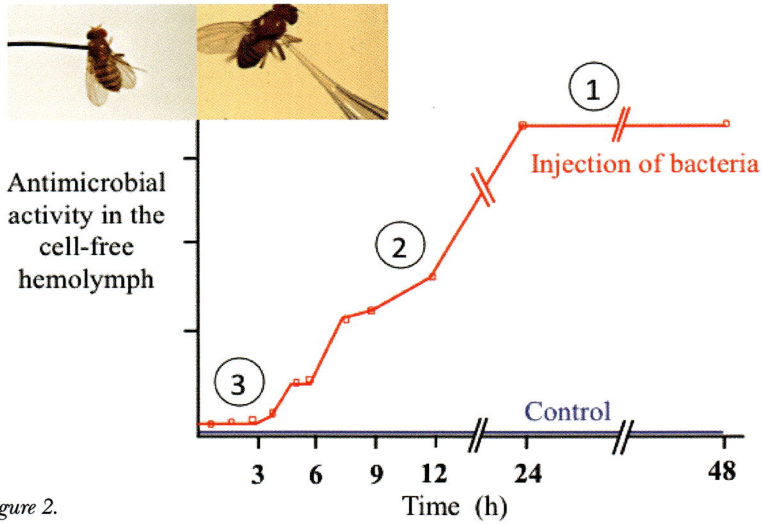

Figure 2.

we actually identified several antimicrobial peptides (Figure 3), namely the disulphide-bridged Defensin (Dimarcq et al. 1994), whereas our colleagues in the Boman laboratory cloned genes encoding *Drosophila* homologues of the linear polypeptides Cecropins and Attacins, which they had initially identified in the *Cecropia* moth (Kylsten et al. 1990, Åsling et al. 1995). Altogether, there was now evidence that the fruit fly fat body, an equivalent of the mammalian liver, produces several families of potent antibacterial peptides, with distinct and sometimes overlapping activity spectra against either Gram-positive or Gram-negative bacteria. The corresponding genes are transcribed rapidly after microbial challenge and after translation of the corresponding mRNAs, the prepropeptides are matured and the mature peptides are secreted into the blood of the fly at remarkably high concentrations, where they oppose invading microorganisms via membrane-disruptive mechanisms (the mode of action is reviewed in Shai, 2002).

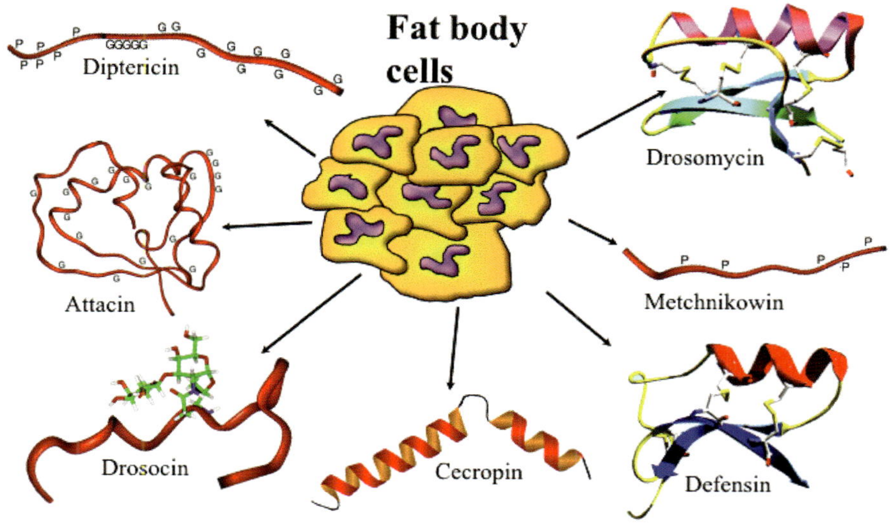

Figure 3.

As mentioned above (Figure 2), a paramount feature of the antimicrobial peptides of *Drosophila* is the rapid inducibility of their expression following challenge. This rapid induction of a potent antimicrobial activity illustrated immediately to us the potentials of this experimentally easily amenable system for a molecular genetic analysis of the immune induction of the antimicrobial defences in *Drosophila*. Further, as described below, once the genes encoding some of the antimicrobial peptides were cloned, it became apparent that their promoters contained sequences similar to mammalian NF-κB binding sites in immune response genes (Sen and Baltimore, 1986). I had read recently papers from Professor Charles Janeway at Yale University (Janeway, 1989) and from Professor Alan Ezekowitz (Sastry et al., 1991) at Harvard and, in June 1992, I visited their laboratories and presented our data on the inducibility of antimicrobial peptides during the host defence of *Drosophila* and the presence of NF-κB binding sites in the promoter of the *Diptericin* gene. At that time we knew that these sites were mandatory for the immune-inducibility of this gene (see below). Both Janeway and Ezekowitz felt attracted by the fly model, and we decided that we would embark on a collaboration, with the aim of understanding and comparing sensing and signalling in mice and flies during infections. In 1993, Charlie Janeway, Shunji Natori from Tokyo University (working on the fly model *Sarcophaga peregrina*) and I organised a conference at Versailles near Paris on the topic of innate immunity (Figure 4). In retrospect, this may have been the first international meeting on innate immunity, a term still not in universal use at that time. We decided with Charlie Janeway, Shunji Natori and Alan Ezekowitz, after the Versailles meeting to submit a formal grant application to the Human Frontiers in Science Programme (HFSP), whose General Office is based in Strasbourg. Fotis Kafatos, who had just been named Director General of the European Molecular Biology Laboratory at Heidelberg and had started

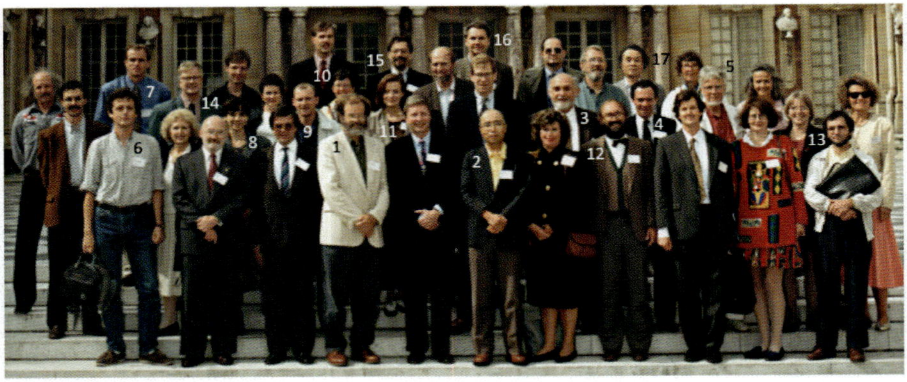

Figure 4.

working on antiparasitic reactions in mosquitoes, also joined our collaborative project. On behalf of our five laboratories, I submitted the project to HFSP. Much to our delight it was accepted in 1995 and generously funded. For four years, the five groups met regularly to exchange and discuss results and ideas. It is through these meetings that I became acutely aware of the problems raised by the interactions between innate immunity and adaptive immunity in mammals (*Drosophila* lacks adaptive immunity) and that our colleagues followed the developments of our studies on activation of immune defences in challenged flies. After termination of this grant in 1998, Alan Ezekowitz coordinated a follow-up project of our groups, which was funded by the NIH. A common article in *Science*, on the Phylogenetic Perspectives of Innate Immunity, published in 1999, is a testimony to our fruitful and happy interactions during these pioneering years (Hoffmann et al., 1999).

Let me turn back to the period of the Versailles meeting. We had by that time, as already mentioned, found the presence of NF-κB binding sites in the *Diptericin* promoter (Reichhart et al., 1992) and shown by site-directed mutagenesis that they were mandatory for inducibility of this gene by microbial challenge (Kappler et al., 1993; Meister et al., 1994). In parallel, Ylva Engström in Stockholm and her colleagues, had obtained similar results for the *Cecropin* gene in flies (Engström et al., 1993) (of note, the presence of NF-κB binding sites had been first reported in the *Attacin* gene of *Hyalophora cecropia* by Ingrid Faye (Sun et al., 1991). NF-κB was known to be a transcriptional activator responsible for the challenge-induced expression of many immune and stress proteins in mammals (Sen and Baltimore, 1986), and the *Drosophila* genome also contained at least one member of this family, namely the *Dorsal* gene (Steward, 1987) (Figure 5). In *Drosophila*, the groundbreaking work of Christiane Nüsslein-Volhard (Nüsslein-Volhard et al., 1980) had shown by unbiased mutagenesis experiments that the *Dorsal* gene was involved in dorso-ventral patterning in the early embryo (Figure 6). Further mutagenesis screens by her laboratory and that of Trudi Schupbach identified a cascade of genes that direct the nuclear translocation of the Dorsal protein, which subsequently controls the expression of developmental genes (reviewed in Belvin and Anderson, 1996). Kathryn Anderson worked out the

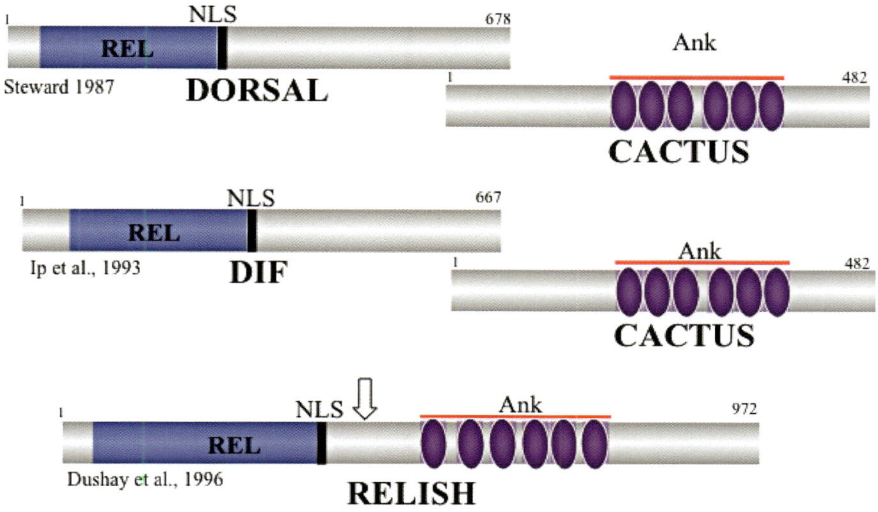

Figure 5.

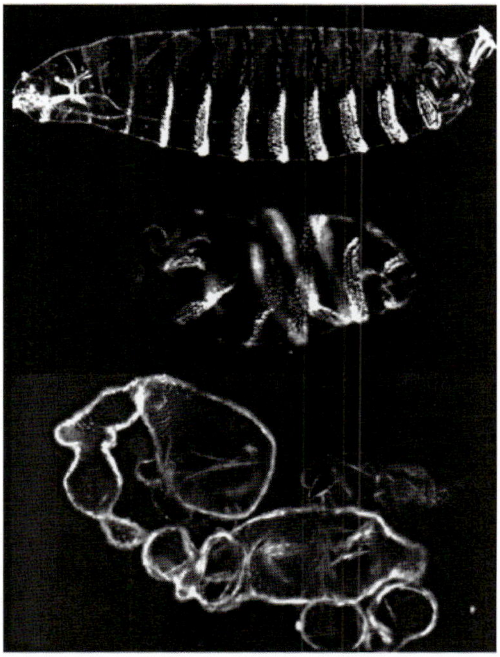

Figure 6.

role of a key gene in this signalling pathway, namely *Toll* (Anderson et al., 1985a, 1985b), which had originally been isolated in the zygotic screens that won the Nobel Prize for Christiane Nüsslein-Volhard and Eric Wieschaus. This cascade involves several extracellular serine proteases and culminates in the cleavage of the cysteine-knot polypeptide Spätzle. Cleaved Spätzle then activates the type I transmembrane receptor Toll and triggers an intracellular series of events which result in the phosphorylation of the inhibitor protein

Cactus, inducing its dissociation from Dorsal (also reviewed in Belvin and Anderson, 1996). Although these genes had initially been characterized by Nüsslein-Volhard and her colleagues because of their maternally expressed phenotypes, we confirmed that they were also expressed in larvae and adults, including males, and notably, that their expression was upregulated by microbial challenge (Reichhart et al., 1993). We also showed, using appropriate antibodies in collaboration with Ruth Steward, that an immune challenge induces the nuclear translocation of the Dorsal protein in fat body cells (Reichhart et al., 1993; Lemaitre et al., 1995a). Further, we found that a microbial challenge induced the appearance in these cells of a protein complex binding to the NF-κB sites of the *Diptericin* gene, that this complex was competed off by excess probe and supershifted by an antibody specific to Dorsal (Reichhart et al, 1993; Kappler et al., 1993; Georgel et al., 1993).

For a short moment, I believed that we were close to solving the problem of the control of antimicrobial gene expression. But then, to my utter dismay, we found that in loss-of-function mutants for *Dorsal*, the *Diptericin* gene was induced like in wild-type flies (Reichhart et al., 1993; see also Lemaitre et al., 1995b). We were of course aware at that time of the report by the Levine and Engström laboratories of the existence of a second NF-κB family member, namely DIF (for Dorsal related immunity factor) (Ip et al., 1993), but *Dif* mutants would only be generated years later (Meng et al., 1999; Rutschmann et al., 2000a). Several mutants with potentially abnormal defence reactions were available in the community at that time, namely *mbn-2* (Gateff, 1978) and *Black cells* (Rizki et al., 1980), which was considered to have a block in the phenol-oxidase cascade that normally leads to the formation of melanin and is activated by injury. Bruno Lemaitre, a *Drosophila* geneticist, who had joined our group in the fall of 1992, shortly after his Ph.D. defence, and who was to become a driving force in the *Toll* saga in the laboratory, analysed the expression of *Diptericin* in *Black cells* mutants and observed that the induction of this antibacterial peptide gene was blocked. The *Black cells* mutation had been created by ethyl methane sulphonate (EMS) mutagenesis by Grell in 1969. I had shared our preliminary and unpublished results on the effect of the *Black Cells* mutation with Professor Michael Levine when I visited his group in San Diego in 1993. Given that the role of proteolytic cascades in immune defences had been highlighted by the studies of Professor Sadaaki Iwanaga at Fukuoka University on immune defences in the horse-shoe crab (reviewed in Iwanaga, 2002), and that the *Black Cells* mutation was considered to affect such a cascade, it was tempting to speculate on the potential similarities in the induction of the immune responses in the two systems. The Levine laboratory had had access to a *Black Cells* mutant line, and they informed us that they could not reproduce our results on the lack of inducibility of the antibacterial peptide with that line. Given that both groups were certain of their data, the only valid explanation that came to our minds was that our EMS-mutated line carried a second-site recessive mutation. This mutation would be responsible for the failure of *Diptericin* induction and be unrelated to the phenol-oxidase cascade, which had led to the initial isolation of the mutant strain. Bruno Lemaitre, Elisabeth Kromer and Marie Meister set out to isolate the mutant gene and found that it mapped one centiMorgan away from the *Black Cells* locus (Lemaitre et al., 1995b). We called this mutation *immune deficiency* (imd). This first allele was a weak hypomorph. Null alleles of the *shadok* class of alleles that would be generated some years later by Dominique Ferrandon display a much stronger sensitivity to immune challenges (Gottar et al., 2002). The *imd* locus resides in a genetically poorly characterised region. Its identification entailed considerable mapping efforts, with the generation of an overlapping set of deletions. The region corresponding to the relevant deletions was sequenced in 1999 by our collaborators of Exelixis Inc (San Francisco), as the *Drosophila* genome sequence was not yet available. The identification of the correct gene in the 30 kilobases region was facilitated by the detection of three mutations in the most likely candidate gene in the three alleles of *imd* that were available at this time. With Silvia Naitza, Philippe Georgel and other colleagues from our laboratory and from Exelixis Inc. we found that *imd* encoded a death domain protein that shared significant similarities with that of mammalian RIP (TNF-receptor interacting protein) (Georgel et al., 2001).

In 1995, then, we understood that the immune induction of the antibacterial peptide Diptericin was dependent on the *imd* gene and independent of the Dorsal member of the NF-κB family. Given the biochemical competence of the laboratory, we considered the possibility of purifying the proteins of the complex bound to the NF-κB response elements of the *Diptericin* gene. For this, Christine Kappler and Emma Langley spent more than a year to produce massive quantities of spinner cultures of LPS-treated cells and to purify the nuclear protein extracts by affinity chromatography with multiple NF-κB binding nucleotide sequences. As a result of these efforts, a faint band of a size in the range of the Dorsal (or DIF) protein, and an additional one of higher molecular weight (with hindsight, this might have corresponded to the Relish NF-κB family member, see below) were detected by gel electrophoresis in the pooled protein extracts. These samples were further analysed by mass spectrometry after an "in-gel trypsic digestion" by Andrej Shevchenko from the group of Mathias Mann at the EMBL in Heidelberg. Unfortunately, the quantities of the purified proteins were below the resolution limits of mass spectrometry at that time and in the absence of the genome sequence of *Drosophila*, the small fragments of protein that were sequenced were of no help.

This was obviously a delicate moment in our efforts. Fortunately, a breakthrough then occurred in the laboratory with the discovery of the antifungal peptide Drosomycin. Let me briefly recount how this came about. The biochemists in the group had so far isolated antibacterial peptides on the basis of growth inhibition assays, a classical procedure used by the Boman laboratory to isolate cecropins and attacins in the early 80s. In 1992 we decided with Jean-Luc Dimarcq, Philippe Bulet and Charles Hetru to engage in a massive experiment of comparing chromatographic profiles from several thousands of individually challenged flies with those of as many naive flies, independently of their potential antimicrobial effects. One objective was to view the immune response in *Drosophila* beyond the simple induction of antimicrobial peptides, and to isolate other types of immune response polypeptides. In pooled extracts of these flies, we noted the appearance, following challenge, of a major absorption peak. Upon sequencing of the peptide contained within this peak, Jean-Luc Dimarcq, Philippe Bulet and Charles Hetru identified a 5-kDa molecule with four disulphide bridges. The inducible peptide was inactive, however, against all the bacterial strains available to us. It was not an inhibitor of circulating proteases either– an idea which we had favoured at a given moment, given the structure of the peptide. At a session on antimicrobial peptides at the 1993 meeting of the Federation of European Biochemical Societies in Stockholm, to which Hans Boman had invited me, I heard the presentation by Professor Willem Broeckaert from Leuwen University in Belgium on plant antimicrobial peptides and was struck by the similarity between one of the peptides from *Raphanus sativus* (Rs-Antifungal Peptide 1) and our novel 5-kDa inducible peptide from challenged fruit flies. We rapidly started collaboration between our two laboratories and in 1994 we showed that the fly peptide was potently antifungal against some filamentous fungi, hence the name "Drosomycin" proposed in our joint paper (Fehlbaum et al., 1994).

At this point, things began to come together. The *Drosomycin* gene was rapidly cloned by Jean-Marc Reichhart and Lydia Michaut. Bruno Lemaitre then added *Drosomycin* to the set of probes for RNA blots to study the expression of this and the other inducible antimicrobial peptide genes in wild-type and mutant fly lines. The data which he generated were compelling: the *Drosomycin* gene was perfectly inducible by immune challenge (bacterial mix) in *imd* mutants, but was clearly NOT induced in Toll pathway mutants by the same challenge. Particularly striking were the results obtained with *Cactus*-deficient flies, in which the *Drosomycin* gene was strongly expressed in the absence of infection, but not the *Dipterincin* gene (Figure 7). Bruno Lemaitre went on to probe the immune induction of the characterised antimicrobial

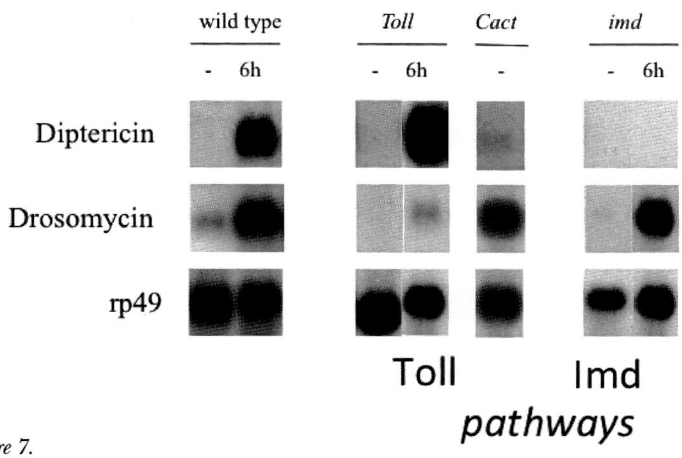

Figure 7.

peptide genes in all the available mutants affecting the dorsoventral regulatory cascade. These studies were published in *Cell* in 1996 (Lemaitre et al., 1996). They demonstrated that: (1) essential components of the dorsoventral pathway, namely the *Spätzle/Toll/Cactus* gene cassette, control expression of the gene encoding the antifungal peptide Drosomycin; (2) two distinct pathways control the expression of the antimicrobial peptide genes (Toll controlling *Drosomycin,* IMD driving *Diptericin* and *Drosocin* – possibly a combined action of both pathways on *Cecropin, Attacin,* and *Defensin* expression); (3) the induction of all antimicrobial peptide genes is impaired in double mutant flies for the *Toll* and *imd* genes, which excludes the existence of additional pathways for this particular aspect of the immune defence; (4) mutations which affect the synthesis of antimicrobial peptide genes dramatically lower the resistance of flies to infection. More specifically to this point: the collaboration with the Broeckaert laboratory had led to the introduction of fungal strains into our laboratory (up to that stage, our studies had focused on antibacterial defences). Bruno Lemaitre developed comparative survival tests to bacterial and fungal infections in mutant backgrounds and showed that the Toll pathway essentially protects against fungal infections, (and, as later shown by Dominique Ferrandon and Julien Royet, also against some Gram-positive bacterial infections; Michel et al., 2001; Rutschmann et al., 2002), whereas the *imd* gene is mostly involved in fighting Gram-negative infections (Figure 8) (Lemaitre et al., 19956b; see also below, Lemaitre et al., 1997)

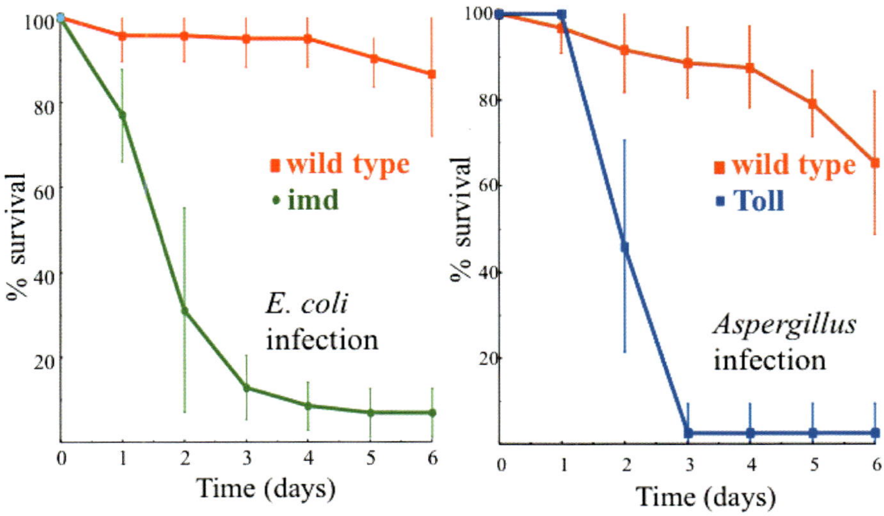

Figure 8.

Studies later performed with microarray analysis (De Gregorio et al., 2001; Irving et al., 2001; De Gregorio et al., 2002; Boutros et al., 2002) indicated that the Toll pathway and the IMD pathway (which had been largely characterised by that time, see below) each control the expression of hundreds of genes, with some overlap (De Gregorio et al., 2002).

The results summarised above were obtained in an ebullient context where several laboratories were searching for the receptors of innate immune cells that would be capable of recognising conserved microbial cell wall components ("Pattern Recognition Receptors", Janeway, 1989) and, in response, activate NF-κB to direct the synthesis of immune-response genes. In the case of mammals, it was proposed that this would not only lead to the expression of innate defence genes but would also stimulate adaptive immune responses (Janeway, 1989). It had been known for some time that in mammals, lectin-like molecules (Fraser et al., 1998) and scavenger receptors (Krieger, 1997) were able to recognise the molecular patterns that adorn bacteria, but the link between recognition and signalling had remained elusive. The Toll transmembrane receptor, initially cloned in the context of the dorsoventral patterning system (Hashimoto et al., 1988), contains an extracellular leucine-rich repeat domain, evocative of that of the LPS-binding protein CD14 (GPI-anchored and hence incapable of signalling to NF-κB) (Wright et al.,1990). Its intracytoplasmic domain is highly similar to the intracellular signalling domain of the IL-1 receptor (referred to as TIR domain, for Toll-Interleukin Receptor), an established activator of NF-κB (Gay and Keith, 1991; Schneider et al., 1991; Rosetto et al., 1995). I first presented our data on the immune function of the Toll pathway in flies at our regular HFSP meeting held in June 1996 in Annisquam and hosted by Charlie Janeway. I vividly remember the interest and receptiveness they generated with our colleagues. Although our laboratory in Strasbourg never worked directly on mammalian models, we were delighted to observe over the following years the relevance that our work on innate immunity in *Drosophila* took across the phylogenetic spectrum. To this day, we remain in close contact with the community working on mammalian models.

The sequencing of the *Drosophila* genome revealed in 2000 that this species has nine genes encoding Toll receptors (Adams et al., 2000). Jean-Luc Imler in our group investigated the potential roles of the eight other Toll receptors and of DmelMyD88 in the control of antimicrobial peptide gene expression (Tauszig et al., 2000; Tauszig-Delamasure et al., 2002). In spite of an in-depth analysis, we and others have been unable so far to demonstrate that, with the marked exception of Toll, any of the other Tolls is involved in an NF-κB driven expression of these peptides during systemic infections (Ooi et al., 2002; Yagi et al., 2010; Narbonne-Reveau et al., 2011; Akhouayri et al., 2011).

In spite of the progress described above, the question remained as to how Toll is activated during infection, all the more so when it became clear that the Toll pathway responds both to fungal and Gram-positive bacterial infection (see above). The spectacular results on the identities of the ligands activating the various mammalian Toll-like Receptors (reviewed in Kawai and Akira, 2011) continued to bring up the questions in meetings whether a similar situation might not prevail, or at least occur, in insects. In 1999, Elena Levashina, Emma Langley, Jean-Marc Reichhart and colleagues, when analysing loss-of-function mutants for a gene encoding an inhibitor of serine proteases, the serpin Necrotic, found that a proteolytic cascade leads to the cleavage of Spätzle in the blood of adult flies and can activate Toll (Levashina et al., 1999). This cascade is different from that which cleaves Spätzle during embryogenesis, as already noted by Bruno Lemaitre (Lemaitre et al., 1996). Biochemical analysis by Nick Gay (Cambridge) and Jean-Luc Imler in the laboratory further showed that proteolytic processing of Spätzle allows its binding with high affinity to the Toll extracellular domain, thus triggering the intracellular signalling cascade (Weber et al., 2003). It is of interest here to mention that Spätzle is a member of a family of neurotrophin-like proteins that play essential roles in the development of the nervous system (Parker et al., 2001; Zhu et al., 2008). Of the six members of this family (now referred to as DNT- *Drosophila* neurotrophins) only one member, *i.e.*, Spätzle, has conclusively been shown to date to activate an immune response – in addition to its developmental role. Why evolution has selected one Toll member out of a family of nine, and one Spätzle/DNT out of a family of six to play an immune function, is one of the intriguing questions in this field.

Experiments performed by Bruno Lemaitre in 1997 had indicated that the *Drosophila* innate immune system is able to discriminate between various classes of invading microbes (Lemaitre et al., 1997). Expression data of various antimicrobial peptide genes in response to various microbial challenges indeed showed that the IMD pathway is strongly induced by Gram-negative bacteria and Gram-positive bacilli (which contain a peptidoglycan in their envelope which is distinct from that of other Gram-positive bacteria, see below). In contrast, the Toll pathway is stimulated preferentially by fungi and Gram-positive bacteria, and to a lesser extent by Gram-negative bacteria. These findings suggested the existence of receptors able to discriminate between these various classes of microorganisms. When we finally addressed this question around 2000, the genome of *Drosophila* had been sequenced and many candidate genes attracted interest. However, the answers to the questions regarding the identities of the receptors for microbial ligands with potential to activate NF-κB, came from unbiased genetic approaches, which had been initiated in our laboratory by Dominique Ferrandon in 1995 on the second chromosome and by Louisa Wu and Kathryn Anderson (Wu et al., 2001) on the third chromosome. In essence, the Ferrandon screen in Strasbourg was initially based on large-scale EMS mutagenesis using transgenic flies expressing distinct reporter genes as read-outs for each pathway (Jung et al., 2001). These screens and later, additional ones performed by the Lemaitre (by then at Gif-sur-Yvette) (X chromosome) and Schneider (Stanford) (P-element insertions) laboratories identified several genes in the IMD pathway, as described below. The Ferrandon screen as based on the use of a dual reporter system, also allowed identifying genes involved in the Toll pathway, for instance the only known *Dif* point mutants (Rutschmann et al., 2000a). By applying the unbiased reporter screening approach on the first chromosome, Julien Royet isolated in 2001 the first mutant fly line in which the Toll pathway was not activated by Gram-positive bacteria, but was still responsive to fungal infection (Michel et al., 2001). Upon cloning, the mutated gene turned out to be Peptidoglycan Recognition Protein-SA, a member of a protein family previously characterised in Lepidoptera (Kang et al. 1998; Ochiai et al., 1999). Genomic data mining and expression profile studies by Dan Hultmark, Håkan Steiner and colleagues later established that *Drosophila* encodes 13 members of the PGRP family of proteins (Werner et al., 2000). They are either circulating, intracellular or transmembrane proteins (Figure 9) and have in common a domain (called PGRP homology domain) that is derived from an evolutionary ancient amidase enzyme, already present in some bacteriophages. Remarkably, the amidase function is conserved in 7 out of the 13 fly PGRPs whereas the others have lost their catalytic function and today serve as recognition PGRPs (reviewed in Royet and Dziarski, 2007). Shortly after the identification of PGRP-SA, Dominique Ferrandon and Julien Royet demonstrated that one of the transmembrane PGRP family members, that is PGRP-LC, is required for activation of the IMD pathway and resistance to Gram-negative bacteria (Gottar et al., 2002). The role of PGRP-LC was independently established, at the same time, in the laboratories of Kathryn Anderson (Choe et al., 2002) and Alan Ezekowitz (Rämet et al., 2002). Biochemical and structural studies performed by several groups subsequently established that the PGRP homology domain has a well-defined groove to which peptidoglycan binds for enzymatic cleavage, or for recognition (Chang et al., 2004; Chang et al., 2006; Lim et al., 2006). Importantly, depending on the PGRP member, the groove can selectively bind a Lysine-type peptidoglycan which is predominant in most Gram-positive bacteria or alternatively, a diaminopimelic acid form of peptidoglycan which is typical for Gram-negative bacteria (these amino acids are in position 3 of the stem peptides linking the two glycan chains of peptidoglycan (Leulier et al., 2003; Kaneko al., 2004; see also the reviews of Royet and Dziarski, 2007 and Royet et al., 2011 for PGRPs in general).

The detection of microorganisms is, however, not restricted to the PGRP

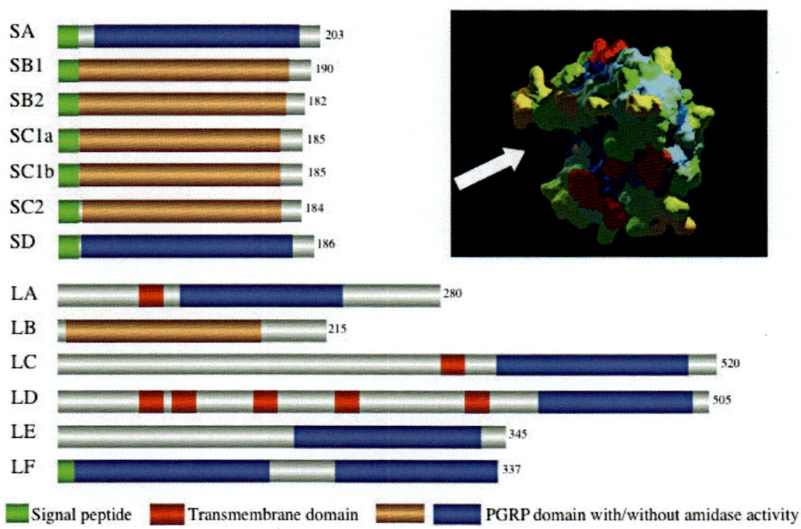

Figure 9.

family and involves a second family, the GNBP/ßGRP family. Dominique Ferrandon in the laboratory demonstrated that a circulating protein that interacts with fungal ß-(1,3)-glucan triggers the proteolytic cascade leading to the cleavage of Spätzle and the activation of the Toll pathway (Figure 10) (Gottar et al., 2006; Mishima et al., 2009). This protein, GNBP3, is a member of a small family of proteins initially characterised in the silkworm Bombyx mori. The first member was reported to bind Gram-negative bacteria, hence the name GNBP for Gram-negative binding protein (Lee et al., 1996). The GNBP3 orthologue of *B.mori* had originally been identified in the Ashida laboratory for its ability to bind to ß-(1,3)-glucans and trigger the phenol-oxidase cascade (Ochiai et al., 1988; see also Ochiai et al., 2000). Of note, another Drosophila member of the family, GNBP1, appears to function as a coreceptor of PGRP-SA for the detection of Lys-type peptidoglycan Gram-positive bacteria, both in Diptera and Coleoptera (Gobert et al., 2003; Filipe et al., 2005; Wang et al., 2006a; Park et al., 2007).

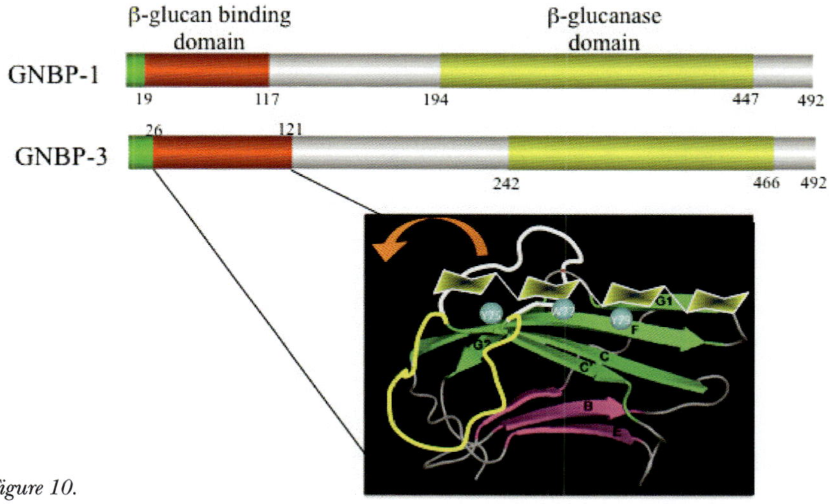

Figure 10.

Figure 11 summarizes our view as it had emerged in the early 2000s. Two essential microbial inducers, *i.e.* Lys-PGN and ß-Glucan trigger the Toll pathway by activating an upstream proteolytic cascade upon recognition by PGRPs or GNBPs respectively. In addition, as shown by Dominique Ferrandon and Jean-Marc Reichhart, proteases secreted by invading entomopathogenic fungi, or bacteria, interact with a dedicated circulating serine-protease (dubbed *Persephone* by Petros Ligoxygakis, see Ligoxygakis et al., 2002) which also feeds into the proteolytic cascade upstream of Spätzle and Toll (Gottar et al., 2006; El Chamy et al., 2008). Thus the systemic immune response of *Drosophila* is not only activated by "pattern recognitions receptors" (Janeway, 1989) but also by sensing the catalytic activity of microbial virulence factors. The IMD pathway, in turn, is activated via a direct interaction of DAP-PGN with the transmembrane PGRP-LC. In this case, no evidence exists for a circulating amplification cascade, as opposed to the interaction described above for Toll activation. Studies in several groups have identified most of the players of the proteolytic cascades upstream of Spätzle. The ultimate protease, termed Spätzle Processing Enzyme (SPE), was identified in 2006 by Won-Jae Lee and colleagues (Jang et al., 2006). The molecular mechanisms that lead from binding of ß-glucans to GNBP-3 or of Lys-peptidoglycan to PGRP-SA, to activation of the upstream serine proteases are still under investigation.

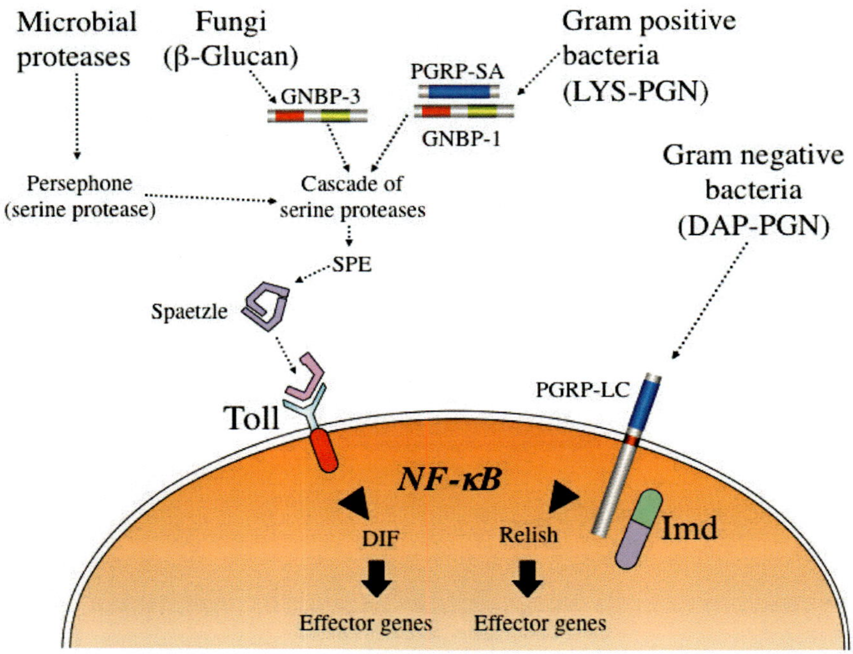

Figure 11.

We and others have devoted many efforts to decipher the intracellular pathways which lead to the expression of antimicrobial peptide genes downstream of either the Toll or the PGRP-LC transmembrane proteins. A simplified picture is presented for both pathways in Figures 12 and 13. Basically, both pathways direct activation of dormant cytoplasmic NF-κB family members. These are in the case of the Toll pathway the Dorsal or DIF proteins in larvae or the sole DIF protein in adults (Meng et al., 1999; Manfruelli et al. 1999; Rutschman et al., 2000a). Both proteins are retained in the cytoplasm by their interactions with the ankyrin-repeat inhibitor protein Cactus. Phosphorylation of Cactus leads to the dissociation from either Dorsal and/or DIF and to subsequent degradation of the inhibitor by the proteasome. Upon the ensuing nuclear translocation, Dorsal or DIF control the expression of hundreds of immune response genes, predominantly but not exclusively, in fat body cells. Prominent among these is the antifungal

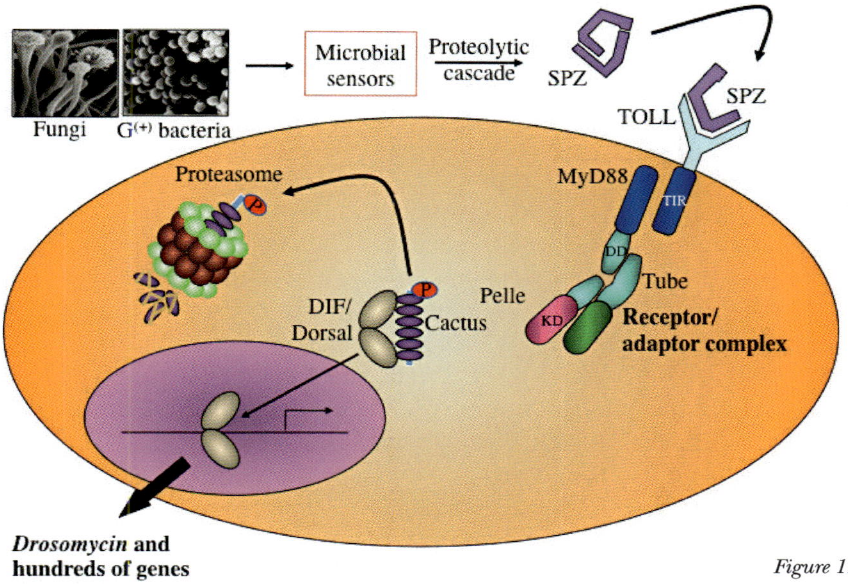

Figure 12.

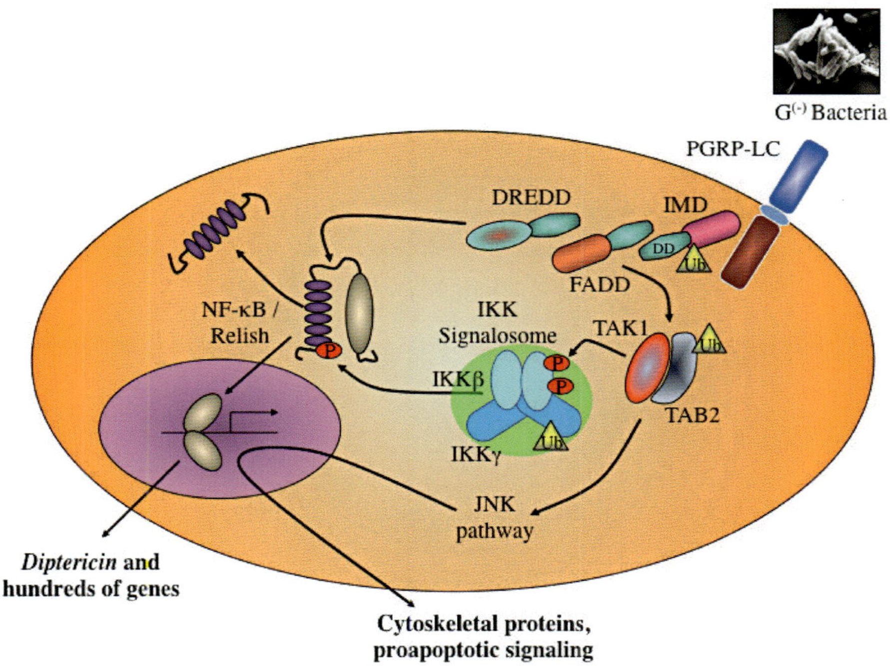

Figure 13.

peptide Drosomycin and a significant number of small (3-9kDa) peptides (Uttenweiler-Joseph et al., 1998), the functions of which have eluded analysis so far. The molecular mechanisms linking the binding of Spätzle to the phosphorylation of Cactus warrant further investigation. Recent studies have proposed that the Spätzle-Toll complex is internalised into endocytic vesicles (Huang et al., 2010; Lund et al., 2010). The kinase Pelle, which is present in the Toll-receptor-adaptor complex together with MyD88 and the death domain protein Tube, has similarities to mammalian IRAKs (Towb et al., 2009). Pelle does not appear to act as the Cactus-kinase (Grosshans et al., 1994), and this kinase still remains to be identified, in spite of many efforts in the recent past by several laboratories. In the case of the IMD pathway, the NF-κB family member controlling immune gene expression is called Relish. This large-sized protein, identified by Dan Hultmark in 1996, carries at its C-terminus, the inhibitory functions of Cactus (ankyrin repeats) (Dushay et al., 1996). Activation of Relish consequently occurs via a proteolytic cleavage roughly in the middle of the protein (Stöven et al., 2000; Leulier et al., 2000; Stöven et al., 2003; Ertürk-Hasdemir et al., 2009). Cleaved Relish translocates into the nucleus to control expression of antimicrobial peptides. As for the Toll intracellular signalling cascade, the IMD pathway is as yet not completely understood in mechanistic terms. Activation of the PGRP-LC receptor (which comes in three distinct splice isoforms, Werner et al., 2000) by binding to DAP-Peptidoglycan (Leulier et al., 2003) leads to the association of a protein complex involving the adaptor protein IMD (Choe et al., 2005; Kaneko et al., 2006), the caspase-8 homologue DREDD, the homologue of mammalian FADD (Naitza et al., 2002; Leulier et al., 2002) and the inhibitor of Apoptosis DIAP2 (Kleino et al., 2005, Gesellchen et al., 2005). This complex activates the MAP-3 kinase TAK1 (associated with the non catalytic protein TAB 2) via an as yet undefined mechanism (Vidal et al., 2001; Silverman et al., 2003) that in turn phosphorylates both IRD5 (Lu et al., 2001), a fly homologue of mammalian IKKβ (Silverman et al., 2000) and the JUN-kinase pathway (Silverman et al., 2003). The IKK beta homologue IRD5 in turn associates with a homologue of mammalian IKKγ (Kenny) (Rutschman et al., 2000b) leading to phosphorylation of Relish (Silverman et al., 2000). Relish is thought to be cleaved by the Caspase DREDD, followed by the nuclear translocation of the N-terminal, phosphorylated part, and participates in the control of gene expression, and namely of the genes encoding Diptericin and Drosocin (Leulier et al., 2000; Stöven et al., 2000; Stöven et al., 2003; Ertürk-Hasdemir et al., 2009). As is the case for the Toll pathway, the IMD cascade controls the expression not only of antimicrobial peptides, but of many hundreds of other immune genes the functions of which remain mostly poorly understood in the context of the antimicrobial defences. Some evidence suggests that DIAP2 (in conjunction with its associated proteins Ue1va and Ubc13) functions as an E3 ligase that K63-ubiquitinates IMD, the TAB2 protein (associated with TAK1) and the IKKγ homologue Kenny. It is plausible that polyubiquitin chains bring many of the members of this signalling cascade into close proximity, as suggested recently by Neal Silverman (Paquette et al., 2010 and references therein). With Hidehiro Fukuyama in the laboratory, we have recently engaged on a functional analysis of the interactome of the IMD pathway proteins and detected protein-protein interactions between the eleven canonical members of the pathway described so far and a total of more than 300 proteins. Functional characterisation of the newly-identified genes is currently under way, but RNAi knockdown of many of them affects IMD signalling. Significantly, half of the proteins yielding a phenotype under these conditions are conserved between flies and mammals (Fukuyama et al. in preparation).

CONCLUDING REMARKS AND PERSPECTIVES

Innate immunity was a relatively neglected field of research twenty years ago. Insects were considered by most immunologists at that time to be too primitive and distant from mammals to represent an interesting model. Indeed, the second half of the 20th century was a time of ground-breaking discoveries on the roles of lymphocytes, the generation of very large repertoires of antigen receptors, clonal expansion and memory cells. Nevertheless, invertebrates, including the extremely large class of insects, represent around 95% of all living species on earth today, and they apparently cope well with invading microbes by solely relying on innate immunity. A primary incentive to start our studies was to unravel the mechanisms of this remarkable resistance. It was the physico-chemical identification of the molecules responsible for the "humoral immunity" observed by Glaser and Paillot, which gave us an opening into the field, once these methods had been introduced into our laboratory. The initial identification of the linear antimicrobial peptide cecropin by Hans Boman in butterflies, and our subsequent characterisation of disulphide-bridged inducible peptides in fruit flies, were essential steps that provided us with an easily amenable system to analyse the upstream mechanisms of this defence. It is now understood that all multicellular organisms (animals as well as plants) produce antimicrobial peptides for their defences. Most of these molecules are small-sized, cationic, and membrane-active. Although they show a great diversity during evolution, some are remarkably similar between groups. To give just one example, Mihai Netea and colleagues (Simon et al., 2008) have recently identified an antimicrobial peptide in human skin, which is structurally so close to *Drosophila* Drosomycin that they named it Human Drosomycin Like peptide. Whether this similarity reflects convergent evolution or a common ancestry remains an open question. Antimicrobial peptides are mostly expressed in the various zoological groups on barrier epithelia and in blood cells. In recent insect groups (holometabolous orders) they are in addition secreted into the blood stream to oppose microbes that have succeeded in breaching epithelial barriers (Tzou et al., 2000). We do not yet know how widespread this "systemic response" is among the various zoological groups, in addition to the common "epithelial response".

Antimicrobial peptide genes are mostly expressed under the control of the transcriptional activator NF-κB, which has by now been found in nearly every animal group (an exception is C. *elegans*, which appears to have lost a number of pathways). Strikingly, the intracellular signalling cascades that lead to the activation of NF-κB during immune responses show marked similarities throughout evolution. These similarities are not only structural, but also functional, as illustrated by the comparison between *Drosophila* and mice. Obviously, much of our information on the gene products in these cascades still relies on data mining of recently sequenced genomes, but as more and more experimental data become available, they tend to confirm the assumption of a high degree of functional conservation in the NF-κB activating cascades during evolution (see for example recent studies on the sea anemone *Nematostella vectensis* (Wolenski et al., 2011) (Figure 14).

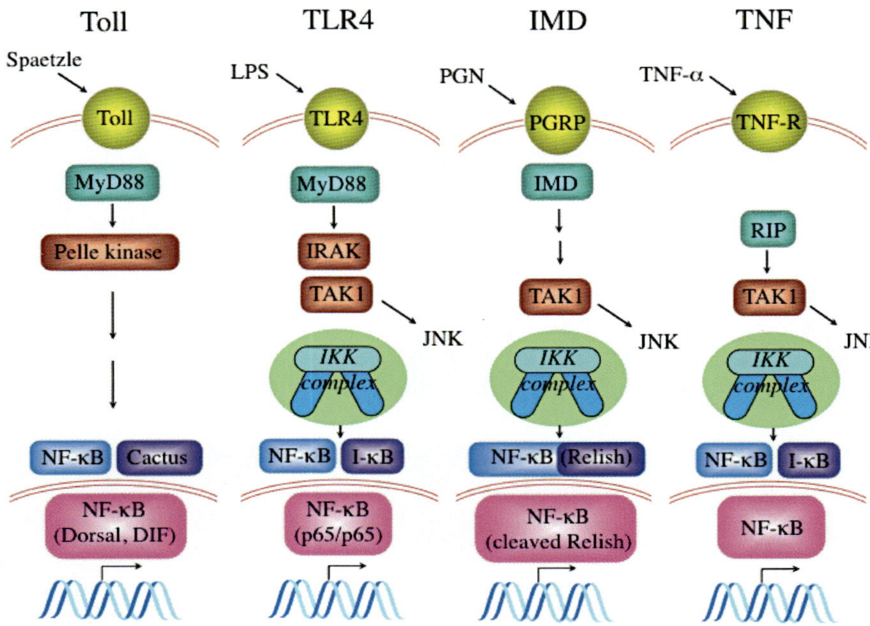

Figure 14.

Finally, we now know that Toll transmembrane receptors are present through evolution from Sponges to Mammals. Tolls are typically associations between extracellular leucine-rich recognition/interaction domains and intracellular TIR domains which often associate with adaptor proteins to signal to immune responsive transactivators (and namely to NF-κB). These domains of Toll show structural variabilities, in particular as regards the extracellular domains, which can have variable numbers and positions of cysteine clusters. Phylogenetic trees illustrate the high degree of complexity in the evolution of the Toll family (Roach et al., 2005). We also have to be aware that in invertebrates at least, Tolls can have developmental as well as defence roles. Whether this duality evolved very early in life history and when/why it was lost, is one of the challenging questions.

Drosophila is generally credited with having significantly contributed to a renewed interest in innate immunity and to our present view of a high conservation of its molecular and cellular mechanisms throughout evolution. Using a metaphor of which Hans Boman was fond, we may ask here as a final reflexion, which are today the Golden Apples of the Hesperides in the orchard of the studies on fruit fly immune defences?

A first obvious apple relates to the study of antiviral defences. *Drosophila* is under the continuous threat of viral infections and several defence mechanisms have been unravelled over the last decade. Paramount among these is RNA interference (Galiana-Arnoux et al., 2006; Wang et al., 2006b; van Rij et al. 2006), but viral infections also induce the expression of genes encoding polypeptides with poorly understood roles in opposing the development of viruses (see *e.g.*, Deddouche et al., 2008). Viral infections have also been shown to induce cytokine productions which lead to some gene reprogramming via the conserved JAK-STAT pathway (Dostert et al., 2005). A possible role in the fight against viruses of the Toll and IMD pathways discussed above in the context of antibacterial and antifungal defences, has been proposed. Further investigations are required to substantiate this involvement and to define the levels at which genes of these pathways could play a role in the control of the viral load (reviewed in Imler and Hoffmann, 2012; see also references therein).

A second apple in the orchard is the rapidly evolving field of epithelial immune defences in *Drosophila*, and namely of the gut and tracheal epithelia. Significant progress has been made recently in this field and it is now understood that the IMD, and not the Toll, pathway mediates the induction of antimicrobial peptide expression in epithelia (Ferrandon et al., 1998, Tzou et al., 2000; Liehl et al., 2006; Ryu et al., 2006, Nehme et al., 2007). However, its activation is finely regulated at multiple levels by negative feedback loops, especially in the intestinal epithelium so as to tolerate commensal microbiota (Ryu et al., 2008; Lhocine et al., 2008, Ragab et al., 2011). Of note, antimicrobial peptide-mediated responses are complemented in the gut by a potent reactive oxygen species response generated by the dual oxidase enzyme (Ha et al., 2005).

A third apple is the deciphering of *Drosophila* defence reactions in a non-infectious context. As already pointed out in this text, a series of instances have been reported in which the IMD pathway (and probably also the Toll pathway) are activated by endogenous ligands. Our information on the endogenous inducers and their receptors is almost non-existent. There are potential parallels here with mammalian responses to so-called "danger signals" (Gallucci and Matzinger, 2001) and this field of research is bound to attract much interest in the future. Possibly some, if not many, of the genes induced by the IMD and Toll pathways, and whose roles we fail to understand in the present "anti-infectious context", are functionally related to responses to endogenous ligands. It remains to be established whether some of these target genes might be involved in another facet of host defence that has been referred to initially as tolerance by phytopathologists (Schneider and Ayres, 2008) (endurance, homeostasis). Briefly, this relates to the ability of the organism to withstand and repair damage inflicted either by microbial virulence factors or by the host's own immune response. This concept is well illustrated by the proliferation of intestinal stem cells that compensates the loss of apoptotic enterocytes and thus maintains the homeostasis of the intestinal epithelium (Cronin et al., 2009; Jiang et al., 2009; Buchon et al., 2009).

Insects are the largest group of extant species, as outlined at the beginning of this presentation. Insect immunity can of course not be restricted to that of *Drosophila*. At the present time, studies on immune defences are performed on several species representative of various orders such as Hymenoptera, Coleoptera, and Lepidoptera. Of particular medical interest are investigations on disease transmitting insects such as mosquitoes. To give but one example, the antiparasitic reactions of the vector insect *Anopheles* towards *Plasmodium* species, have been the focus of intense research in a dozen of groups over the last 20 years. Cellular and molecular analyses of these reactions have shed significant insights into the mechanisms that the mosquito uses to oppose invading parasites, and have namely unravelled the roles of complement-like proteins (thioester containing proteins, TEPs) in parasite killing – a process not paralleled in *Drosophila* in which the role of TEPs is still not well understood (Levashina et al., 2001; Blandin et al., 2004; Blandin et al., 2009). Mosquitoes also transmit viruses of great impact on human health, and here the investigations show marked parallels with the antiviral reactions of fruit flies. In particular, RNA interference and inducible responses regulated by the JAK/STAT pathways appear to be shared assets of antiviral host defences in flies and mosquitoes (Fragkoudis et al. 2009).

In ending this presentation, I would simply like to remind the reader that it was not intended to be a classical review, but rather a narrative of our work on innate immunity put into a historical and societal context. Many aspects of *Drosophila* antimicrobial defences are therefore understandably not covered here (for detailed reviews, see e.g. Lemaitre and Hoffmann, 2007; Ferrandon et al., 2007; Aggarwal and Silverman, 2008).

My final message will be to young scientists who feel interested in the studies presented here and who ponder whether or not to engage in this field: our investigations so far have really only touched the tip of the iceberg of invertebrate immunity and many important discoveries lie ahead for the next generation. The methodologies for this type of research have evolved beyond what I could ever have dreamt of, and our current understanding of the evolution of the innate immune system warrants that the results that will be obtained with insect studies will be one way or another relevant throughout the whole phylogenetic spectrum, including humans (Figure 15).

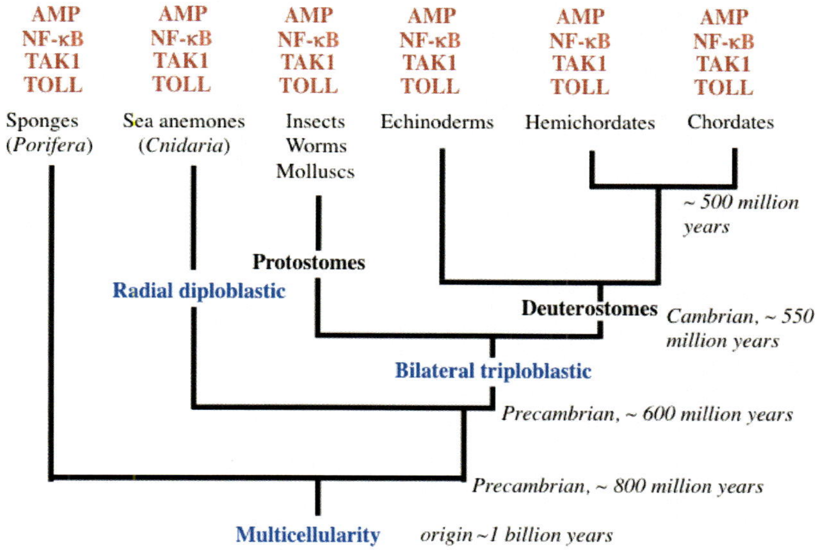

Figure 15.

ACKNOWLEDGMENTS

It goes without saying that the scientific achievements of our laboratory over the many years, as recounted above, are to be credited to a long list of collaborators of high intellectual and human calibre. Many in this list are now Distinguished Class Professors and Directors of Scientific Departments or heads of well-recognised groups in the field, in this and in other countries. I express my deep admiration and warm gratitude to all of them, and in particular to Marie Lagueux, Charles Hetru, Jean-Marc Reichhart, Jean-Luc Dimarcq (Institut Hospitalo-Universitaire, Strasbourg), Marie Meister (Zoological Museum, Strasbourg), Philippe Bulet (Grenoble), Bruno Lemaitre (EPFL, Lausanne), Elena Levashina (Strasbourg/MPI Berlin), Jean-Luc Imler, Dominique Ferrandon, Julien Royet (IBDM Marseille) and Christine Kappler, for their exceptional contributions to our common endeavour. I am further indebted to many colleagues from other institutions in various countries and would like to make a special mention here of Alan Ezekowitz, who has accepted to do a critical reading of the present text. I warmly remember very constructive discussions with Charlie Janeway, Fotis Kafatos and Shunji Natori. Since the early 2000s, we have had a close interaction with Bruce Beutler and Shizuo Akira on the phylogeny of antiviral defences. I would like to warmly thank Charles Hetru, Dominique Ferrandon, Jean-Luc Imler, Jean-Marc Reichhart, Elena Levashina, Jean-Luc Dimarcq and Christine Kappler for their dedicated and constructive help in the preparation of this text and its illustrations. I would also like to acknowledge the significant contributions of many colleagues from other laboratories worldwide to the field of insect immunity, and in particular that of the colleagues of the Boman group in Stockholm. Our studies were supported by the French National Research Agency CNRS, the University of Strasbourg, the Human Science Frontiers Program, the European Union, the US National Institutes of Health, the Fondation pour la Recherche Médicale and the companies Rhone-Poulenc, Exelixis and EntoMed.

REFERENCES

Adams, M.D., Celniker, S.E., Holt, R.A., Evans, C.A., Gocayne, J.D., Amanatides, P.G., Scherer, S.E., Li, P.W., Hoskins, R.A., Galle, R.F., et al. (2000), "The genome sequence of Drosophila melanogaster," *Science* **287,** 2185–2195.

Aggarwal, K., Silverman, N. (2008), "Positive and negative regulation of the Drosophila immune response," *BMB Rep.* **41**(4):267–77.

Akhouayri, I., Turc, C., Royet, J., Charroux, B. (2011), "Toll-8/Tollo negatively regulates antimicrobial response in the Drosophila respiratory epithelium," *PLoS Pathog.* **7**(10):e1002319.

Alder, M.N., Herrin, B.R., Sadlonova, A., Stockard, C.R., Grizzle, W.E., Gartland, L.A., Gartland, G.L., Boydston, J.A., Turnbough, C.L. Jr, Cooper, M.D. (2008), "Antibody responses of variable lymphocyte receptors in the lamprey," *Nat Immunol.* **9**(3):319–27.

Anderson, K.V., Bokla, L., Nüsslein-Volhard, C. (1985a), "Establishment of dorsal-ventral polarity in the Drosophila embryo: the induction of polarity by the Toll gene product," *Cell* **42**(3):791–8.

Anderson, K.V., Jürgens, G., Nüsslein-Volhard, C. (1985b), "Establishment of dorsal-ventral polarity in the Drosophila embryo: Genetic studies on the role of the Toll gene product," *Cell* **42**(3):779–89.

Åsling, B., Dushay, M.S., Hultmark, D. (1995), "Identification of early genes in the Drosophila immune response by PCR-based differential display: the Attacin A gene and the evolution of attacin-like proteins," *Insect Biochem Mol Biol.* **25**(4):511–8.

Belvin, M.P., Anderson, K.V. (1996), "A conserved signaling pathway: The Drosophila Toll-dorsal pathway," *Annu Rev Cell Dev Biol.* **12**:393–416.

Blandin, S., Shiao, S.H., Moita, L.F., Janse, C.J., Waters, A.P., Kafatos, F.C., Levashina, E.A. (2004), "Complement-like protein TEP1 is a determinant of vectorial capacity in the malaria vector Anopheles gambiae," *Cell* **116**(5):661–70.

Blandin, S.A., Wang-Sattler, R., Lamacchia, M., Gagneur, J., Lycett, G., Ning, Y., Levashina, E.A., Steinmetz, L.M. (2009), "Dissecting the genetic basis of resistance to malaria parasites in Anopheles gambiae," *Science* **326**(5949):147–50.

Boutros, M., Agaisse, H., Perrimon, N. (2002), "Sequential activation of signaling pathways during innate immune responses in Drosophila," *Dev Cell.* **3**(5):711–22.

Buchon, N., Broderick, N.A., Chakrabarti, S., Lemaitre, B. (2009), "Invasive and indigenous microbiota impact intestinal stem cell activity through multiple pathways in Drosophila," *Genes Dev.* **23**(19):2333–44.

Butenandt, A., and Karlson, P. (1954), "Über die Isolierung eines Metamorphose-Hormone der Insekten in kristallisierter Form," *Z. Naturforsch.* **9b**, 389–391.

Chang, C.I., Pili-Floury, S.S., Herve, M., Parquet, C., Chelliah, Y., Lemaitre, B., Mengin-Lecreulx, D., Deisenhofer, J. (2004), "A Drosophila pattern recognition receptor contains a peptidoglycan docking groove and unusual l,d-carboxypeptidase activity," *PLoS Biol* **2**, E277.

Chang, C.I., Chelliah, Y., Borek, D., Mengin-Lecreulx, D., Deisenhofer J., (2006), "Structure of tracheal cytotoxin in complex with a heterodimeric pattern-recognition receptor," *Science* **311**(5768):1761–4.

Choe, K.M., Werner, T., Stöven, S., Hultmark, D., Anderson, K.V. (2002), "Requirement for a peptidoglycan recognition protein (PGRP) in Relish activation and antibacterial immune responses in Drosophila," *Science* **296**(5566):359–62.

Choe, K.M., Lee, H., Anderson, K.V. (2005), "Drosophila peptidoglycan recognition protein LC (PGRP-LC) acts as a signal-transducing innate immune receptor," *Proc Natl Acad Sci USA*. **102**(4):1122–6.

Cronin, S.J., Nehme, N.T., Limmer, S., Liegeois, S., Pospisilik, J.A., Schramek, D., Leibbrandt, A., Simoes Rde, M., Gruber, S., Puc, U., Ebersberger, I., Zoranovic, T., Neely, G.G., von Haeseler, A., Ferrandon, D., Penninger, J.M. (2009), "Genome-wide RNAi screen identifies genes involved in intestinal pathogenic bacterial infection," *Science* **325**(5938):340–3.

De Gregorio, E., Spellman, P.T., Rubin, G.M., Lemaitre, B. (2001), "Genome-wide analysis of the Drosophila immune response by using oligonucleotide microarrays," *Proc Natl Acad Sci USA*. **98**(22):12590–5.

De Gregorio, E., Spellman, P.T., Tzou, P., Rubin, G.M., Lemaitre, B. (2002), "The Toll and Imd pathways are the major regulators of the immune response in Drosophila," *EMBO J.* **21**(11):2568–79.

Deddouche, S., Matt, N., Budd, A., Mueller, S., Kemp, C., Galiana-Arnoux, D., Dostert, C., Antoniewski, C., Hoffmann, J.A., Imler, J.L. (2008), "The DExD/H-box helicase Dicer-2 mediates the induction of antiviral activity in drosophila," *Nat Immunol.* **9**(12):1425–32.

Dimarcq, J.L., Keppi, E., Dunbar, B., Lambert, J., Reichhart, J.M., Hoffmann, D., Rankine, S.M., Fothergill, J.E., Hoffmann J.A. (1988), "Insect immunity. Purification and characterization of a family of novel inducible antibacterial proteins from immunized larvae of the dipteran Phormia terranovae and complete amino-acid sequence of the predominant member, diptericin A," *Eur J Biochem.* **171**(1-2):17–22.

Dimarcq, J.L., Hoffmann D., Meister, M., Bulet, P., Lanot, R., Reichhart, J.M., Hoffmann, J.A. (1994), "Characterization and transcriptional profiles of a Drosophila gene encoding an insect defensin. A study in insect immunity," *Eur J Biochem.* **221**(1):201–9.

Dostert, C., Jouanguy, E., Irving, P., Troxler, L., Galiana-Arnoux, D., Hetru, C., Hoffmann, J.A., Imler, J.L. (2005), "The Jak-STAT signaling pathway is required but not sufficient for the antiviral response of Drosophila," *Nat Immunol.* **6**(9):946–53.

Dushay, M.S., Asling, B., Hultmark, D. (1996), "Origins of immunity: Relish, a compound Rel-like gene in the antibacterial defense of Drosophila," *Proc Natl Acad Sci USA.* **93**(19):10343–7.

El Chamy, L., Leclerc, V., Caldelari, I., Reichhart, J.M. (2008), "Sensing of 'danger signals' and pathogen-associated molecular patterns defines binary signaling pathways 'upstream' of Toll," *Nat Immunol.* **9**(10):1165–70.

Engström, Y., Kadalayil, L., Sun, S.C., Samakovlis, C., Hultmark, D., Faye, I. (1993), "kappa B-like motifs regulate the induction of immune genes in Drosophila," *J Mol Biol.* **232**(2):327–33.

Ertürk-Hasdemir, D., Broemer, M., Leulier, F., Lane, W.S., Paquette, N., Hwang, D., Kim, C.H., Stöven, S., Meier, P., Silverman, N. (2009), "Two roles for the Drosophila IKK complex in the activation of Relish and the induction of antimicrobial peptide genes," *Proc Natl Acad Sci USA.* **106**(24):9779–84.

Fehlbaum, P., Bulet, P., Michaut, L., Lagueux, M., Broekaert, W.F., Hetru, C., Hoffmann, J.A. (1994), "Insect immunity. Septic injury of Drosophila induces the synthesis of a potent antifungal peptide with sequence homology to plant antifungal peptides," *J Biol Chem.* **269**(52):33159–63.

Ferrandon, D., Jung, A.C., Criqui, M., Lemaitre, B., Uttenweiler-Joseph, S., Michaut, L., Reichhart, J., Hoffmann, J.A. (1998), "A drosomycin-GFP reporter transgene reveals a local immune response in Drosophila that is not dependent on the Toll pathway," *EMBO J.* **17**(5):1217–27.

Ferrandon, D., Imler, J.L., Hetru, C., Hoffmann, J.A. (2007), "The Drosophila systemic immune response: sensing and signalling during bacterial and fungal infections," *Nat Rev Immunol.* **7**(11):862–74.

Filipe, S.R., Tomasz, A., Ligoxygakis, P. (2005), "Requirements of peptidoglycan structure that allow detection by the Drosophila Toll pathway," *EMBO Rep* **6**(4): 327–333

Fragkoudis, R., Attarzadeh-Yazdi, G., Nash, A.A., Fazakerley, J.K., Kohl, A. (2009), "Advances in dissecting mosquito innate immune responses to arbovirus infection," *J Gen Virol.* **90**(Pt 9):2061–72.

Fraser, I.P., Koziel, H., and Ezekowitz, R.A.B. (1998), "The serum mannose-binding protein and the macrophage mannose receptor are pattern recognition molecules that link innate and adaptive immunity," *Seminars Immunol* **10**:363–372.

Galiana-Arnoux, D., Dostert, C., Schneemann, A., Hoffmann, J.A., Imler, J.L. (2006), "Essential function in vivo for Dicer-2 in host defense against RNA viruses in drosophila," *Nat Immunol.* **7**(6):590–7.

Gallucci, S., Matzinger, P. (2001), "Danger signals: SOS to the immune system," *Curr Opin Immunol.* **13**(1):114–9.

Gateff, E. (1978), "Malignant neoplasms of genetic origin in Drosophila melanogaster," *Science* **200**(4349):1448–59.

Gay, N.J., Keith, F.J. (1991), "Drosophila Toll and IL-1 receptor," *Nature* **351**(6325):355–6.

Georgel, P., Meister, M., Kappler, C., Lemaitre, B., Reichhart, J.M., Hoffmann, J.A. (1993), "Insect immunity: The diptericin promoter contains multiple functional regulatory sequences homologous to mammalian acute-phase response elements," *Biochem Biophys Res Commun.* **197**(2):508–17.

Georgel, P., Naitza, S., Kappler, C., Ferrandon, D., Zachary, D., Swimmer, C., Kopczynski, C., Duyk, G., Reichhart, J.M., Hoffmann, J.A. (2001), "Drosophila immune deficiency (IMD) is a death domain protein that activates antibacterial defense and can promote apoptosis," *Dev Cell.* **1**(4):503–14.

Gesellchen, V., Kuttenkeuler, D., Steckel, M., Pelte, N., Boutros, M. (2005), "An RNA interference screen identifies Inhibitor of Apoptosis Protein 2 as a regulator of innate immune signalling in Drosophila," *EMBO Rep.* **6**(10):979–84.

Glaser, R.W. (1918), "On the existence of immunity principles in insects," *Psyche* **25**, 39–46.

Gobert, V., Gottar, M., Matskevich, A.A., Rutschmann, S., Royet, J., Belvin, M., Hoffmann, J.A., Ferrandon, D. (2003), "Dual activation of the Drosophila toll pathway by two pattern recognition receptors," *Science* 3**02**(5653):2126–30.

Gottar, M., Gobert, V., Michel, T., Belvin, M., Duyk, G., Hoffmann, J.A., Ferrandon, D., Royet, J. (2002), "The Drosophila immune response against Gram-negative bacteria is mediated by a peptidoglycan recognition protein," *Nature* **416**(6881):640–4.

Gottar, M., Gobert, V., Matskevich, A.A., Reichhart, J.M., Wang, C., Butt, T.M., Belvin, M., Hoffmann, J.A., Ferrandon, D. (2006), "Dual detection of fungal infections in Drosophila via recognition of glucans and sensing of virulence factors," *Cell.* **127**(7):1425–37.

Grell, R.F. (1969), "New Mutant Report," *D.I.S.*, **44**:46–47

Grosshans, J., Bergmann, A., Haffter, P., Nüsslein-Volhard, C. (1994) "Activation of the kinase Pelle by Tube in the dorsoventral signal transduction pathway of Drosophila embryo," *Nature* **372**(6506):563–6.

Ha, E.M., Oh, C.T., Bae, Y.S., Lee, W.J. (2005), "A direct role for dual oxidase in Drosophila gut immunity," *Science* **310**(5749):847–50.

Hashimoto, C., Hudson, K.L. and Anderson, K.V. (1988), "The Toll gene of Drosophila, required for dorsal-ventral embryonic polarity, appears to encode a transmembrane protein," *Cell* **52**, 269–279.

Hoffmann, D., Hultmark, D., Boman, H.G. (1981), "Insect immunity – Galleria mellonella and other Lepidoptera have cecropia P9 like factors active against Gram-negative bacteria," *Insect Biochem.* **11**, 537–548.

Hoffmann, J.A., Porte, A., Joly, P. (1968), "Sur la nature hématopoiétique de l'"organe phagocytaire" (Cuénot) de Gryllus bimaculatus (Orthoptère Ensifère)," *C.R. Acad. Sciences, Paris* **267**: 776–777.

Hoffmann, J.A. (1970), "Les organes hématopoiétiques de deux insectes Orthoptères Locusta migratoria et Gryllus bimaculatus," *Z. Zellforsch.* **106**:451–472

Hoffmann, J.A. (1973), "Blood-forming tissues in Orthopteran Insects: an analogue to Vertebrate hemopoietic organs," *Experientia* **29**:50–51

Hoffmann, J.A., Kafatos, F.C., Janeway, C.A., Ezekowitz, R.A. (1999), "Phylogenetic perspectives in innate immunity," *Science* **284**(5418):1313–8.

Huang, H.R., Chen, Z.J., Kunes, S., Chang, G.D., Maniatis, T. (2010), "Endocytic pathway is required for Drosophila Toll innate immune signalling," *Proc Natl Acad Sci USA* **107**(18):8322–7.

Imler, J.L., Hoffmann, J.A. (2012), "Antiviral responses in invertebrates," in *Nucleic acid sensors and antiviral immunity*, eds. T. Fujita & P. Sambhara, Landes Bioscience, Austin, 2012.

Ip, Y.T., Reach, M., Engström, Y., Kadalayil, L., Cai, H., González-Crespo, S., Tatei, K., Levine, M. (1993), "Dif, a dorsal-related gene that mediates an immune response in Drosophila," *Cell* **75**(4):753–63.

Irving, P., Troxler, L., Heuer, T.S., Belvin, M., Kopczynski, C., Reichhart, J.M., Hoffmann, J.A., Hetru, C. (2001), "A genome-wide analysis of immune responses in Drosophila," *Proc Natl Acad Sci USA* **98**(26):15119–24.

Iwanaga, S. (2002), "The molecular basis of innate immunity in the horseshoe crab," *Curr Opin Immunol.* **14**(1):87–95.

Janeway, C.A. Jr. (1989), "Approaching the asymptote? Evolution and revolution in immunology," *Cold Spring Harb Symp Quant Biol.* **54** Pt 1:1–13.

Jang, I.H., Chosa, N., Kim, S.H., Nam, H.J., Lemaitre, B., Ochiai, M., Kambris, Z., Brun, S., Hashimoto, C., Ashida, M., Brey, P.T., Lee, W.J. (2006), "A Spätzle-processing enzyme required for Toll signaling activation in Drosophila innate immunity," *Dev Cell* **10**, 45–55.

Jehle, J.A. (2009), "André Paillot (1885–1944): His work lives on," *J Invertebr Pathol.* **101**(3):162–8.

Jiang, H., Patel, P.H., Kohlmaier, A., Grenley, M.O., McEwen, D.G., Edgar, B.A. (2009) "Cytokine/Jak/Stat signaling mediates regeneration and homeostasis in the Drosophila midgut," *Cell* **137**(7):1343–55.

Jung, A.C., Criqui, M.C., Rutschmann, S., Hoffmann, J.A., Ferrandon, D. (2001), "Microfluorometer assay to measure the expression of beta-galactosidase and green fluorescent protein reporter genes in single Drosophila flies," *Biotechniques* **30**(3):594–8, 600–1.

Kaneko, T., Goldman, W.E., Mellroth, P., Steiner, H., Fukase, K., Kusumoto, S., Harley, W., Fox, A., Golenbock, D., Silverman, N. (2004), "Monomeric and polymeric gram-negative peptidoglycan but not purified LPS stimulate the Drosophila IMD pathway," *Immunity* **20**(5):637–49.

Kaneko, T., Yano, T., Aggarwal, K., Lim, J.H., Ueda, K., Oshima, Y., Peach, C., Ertürk-Hasdemir, D., Goldman, W.E., Oh, B.H., Kurata, S., Silverman, N. (2006), "PGRP-LC and PGRP-LE have essential yet distinct functions in the drosophila immune response to monomeric DAP-type peptidoglycan," *Nat Immunol.* **7**(7):715–23.

Kang, D., Liu, G., Lundstrom, A., Gelius, E., Steiner, H. (1998), "A peptidoglycan recognition protein in innate immunity conserved from insects to humans," *Proc Natl Acad Sci USA* **95**, 10078–10082.

Kappler, C., Meister, M., Lagueux, M., Gateff, E., Hoffmann, J.A., Reichhart, J.M. (1993) "Insect immunity. Two 17 bp repeats nesting a kappa B-related sequence confer inducibility to the diptericin gene and bind a polypeptide in bacteria-challenged Drosophila," *EMBO J.* **12**(4):1561–8.

Karlson, P., Hoffmeister, H., Hummel, H., Hocks, P., Spiteller, G. (1965), "Zur Chemie des Ecdysons, VI Reaktionen des Ecdysonmoleküls," *Chem. Ber.* **98**, 2394–2402.

Kawai, T., Akira, S. (2011), "Toll-like receptors and their crosstalk with other innate receptors in infection and immunity," *Immunity.* **34**(5):637–50.

Kleino, A., Valanne, S., Ulvila, J., Kallio, J., Myllymäki, H., Enwald, H., Stöven, S., Poidevin, M., Ueda, R., Hultmark, D., Lemaitre B., Rämet, M. (2005), "Inhibitor of apoptosis 2 and TAK1-binding protein are components of the Drosophila Imd pathway." *EMBO J.* **24**(19):3423–34.

Krieger, M. (1997), "The other side of scavenger receptors: Pattern recognition in host defense," *Curr Opin Lipidol.* **5**:275–280.

Kylsten, P., Samakovlis, C., Hultmark, D. (1990), "The cecropin locus in Drosophila; a compact gene cluster involved in the response to infection," *EMBO J.* **9**(1):217–24.

Lee, W.J., Lee, J.D., Kravchenko, V.V., Ulevitch, R.J., Brey, P.T. (1996), "Purification and molecular cloning of an inducible gram-negative bacteria-binding protein from the silkworm, Bombyx mori," *Proc Natl Acad Sci USA* **93**(15):7888–93.

Lemaitre, B., Meister, M., Govind, S., Georgel, P., Steward, R., Reichhart, J.M., Hoffmann, J.A. (1995a), "Functional analysis and regulation of nuclear import of dorsal during the immune response in Drosophila," *EMBO J. 14*(3):536–45.

Lemaitre, B., Kromer-Metzger, E., Michaut, L., Nicolas, E., Meister, M., Georgel, P., Reichhart, J.M., Hoffmann, J.A. (1995b), "A recessive mutation, immune deficiency (imd), defines two distinct control pathways in the Drosophila host defense," *Proc Natl Acad Sci USA* **92**(21):9465–9.

Lemaitre, B., Nicolas, E., Michaut, L., Reichhart, J.M., Hoffmann, J.A. (1996), "The dorsoventral regulatory gene cassette spätzle/Toll/cactus controls the potent antifungal response in Drosophila adults," *Cell* **86**(6):973–83.

Lemaitre, B., Reichhart, J.M., Hoffmann, J.A. (1997), "Drosophila host defense: differential induction of antimicrobial peptide genes after infection by various classes of microorganisms," *Proc Natl Acad Sci USA* **94**(26):14614–9.

Lemaitre, B., Hoffmann, J.A. (2007), "The host defense of Drosophila melanogaster," *Annu Rev Immunol.* **25**:697–743.

Leulier, F., Rodriguez, A., Khush, R.S., Abrams, J.M., Lemaitre, B. (2000), "The Drosophila caspase Dredd is required to resist Gram-negative bacterial infection," *EMBO Rep.* **1**(4):353–8.

Leulier, F., Vidal, S., Saigo, K., Ueda, R., Lemaitre, B. (2002), "Inducible expression of double-stranded RNA reveals a role for dFADD in the regulation of the antibacterial response in Drosophila adults," *Curr Biol.* **12**(12):996–1000.

Leulier, F., Parquet, C., Pili-Floury, S., Ryu, J.H., Caroff, M., Lee, W.J., Mengin-Lecreulx, D., Lemaitre, B. (2003), "The Drosophila immune system detects bacteria through specific peptidoglycan recognition," *Nat Immunol.* **4**(5):478–84.

Levashina, E.A., Langley, E., Green, C., Gubb, D., Ashburner, M., Hoffmann, J.A., Reichhart, J.M. (1999), "Constitutive activation of Toll-mediated antifungal defense in serpin-deficient Drosophila," *Science* **285**(5435):1917–9.

Levashina, E.A., Moita, L.F., Blandin, S., Vriend, G., Lagueux, M., Kafatos, F.C. (2001), "Conserved role of a complement-like protein in phagocytosis revealed by dsRNA knockout in cultured cells of the mosquito, Anopheles gambiae," *Cell* **104**(5):709–18.

Lhocine, N., Ribeiro, P.S., Buchon, N., Wepf, A., Wilson, R., Tenev, T., Lemaitre, B., Gstaiger, M., Meier, P., Leulier, F. (2008), "PIMS modulates immune tolerance by negatively regulating Drosophila innate immune signalling," *Cell Host Microbe* **4**(2):147–58.

Liehl, P., Blight, M., Vodovar, N., Boccard, F., Lemaitre, B. (2006), "Prevalence of local immune response against oral infection in a Drosophila/Pseudomonas infection model," *PLoS Pathog.* **2**(6):e56.

Ligoxygakis, P., Pelte, N., Hoffmann, J.A., Reichhart, J.M. (2002), "Activation of Drosophila Toll during fungal infection by a blood serine protease," *Science* **297**(5578):114–6.

Lim, J.H., Kim, M.S., Kim, H.E., Yano, T., Oshima, Y., Aggarwal, K., Goldman, W.E., Silverman, N., Kurata, S., Oh, B.H. (2006), "Structural basis for preferential recognition of diaminopimelic acid-type peptidoglycan by a subset of peptidoglycan recognition proteins," *J Biol Chem.* **281**(12):8286–95.

Lu, Y., Wu, L.P., Anderson, K.V. (2001), "The antibacterial arm of the drosophila innate immune response requires an IkappaB kinase," *Genes Dev.* **15**(1):104–10.

Lund, V.K., DeLotto, Y., DeLotto, R. (2010), "Endocytosis is required for Toll signaling and shaping of the Dorsal/NF-kappaB morphogen gradient during Drosophila embryogenesis," *Proc Natl Acad Sci USA* **107**(42):18028–33.

Manfruelli, P., Reichhart, J.M., Steward, R., Hoffmann, J.A., Lemaitre, B. (1999), "A mosaic analysis in Drosophila fat body cells of the control of antimicrobial peptide genes by the Rel proteins Dorsal and DIF," *EMBO J.* **18**(12):3380–91.

Medzhitov, R., Preston-Hurlburt, P., Janeway, C.A. Jr. (1997), "A human homologue of the Drosophila Toll protein signals activation of adaptive immunity," *Nature.* **388**(6640):394–7.

Meister, M., Braun, A., Kappler, C., Reichhart, J.M., Hoffmann, J.A. (1994), "Insect immunity: A transgenic analysis in Drosophila defines several functional domains in the diptericin promoter," *EMBO J.* **13**(24):5958–66.

Meng, X., Khanuja, B.S., Ip, Y.T. (1999), "Toll receptor-mediated Drosophila immune response requires Dif, an NF-kappaB factor," *Genes Dev.* **13**(7):792–7.

Metchnikoff, E. (1884). "Untersuchung über die intracellular Verdauung bei Wirbellosen Tieren," *Arbeiten aus dem zoologischen Institut der universität zu Wien* **2**, 241.

Michel, T., Reichhart, J.M., Hoffmann, J.A., Royet, J. (2001), "Drosophila Toll is activated by Gram-positive bacteria through a circulating peptidoglycan recognition protein," *Nature* **414**(6865):756–9.

Mishima, Y., Quintin, J., Aimanianda, V., Kellenberger, C., Coste, F., Clavaud, C., Hetru, C., Hoffmann, J.A., Latgé, J.P., Ferrandon, D., Roussel, A. (2009), "The N-terminal domain of Drosophila Gram-negative binding protein 3 (GNBP3) defines a novel family of fungal pattern recognition receptors," *J Biol Chem.* **284**(42):28687–97.

Naitza, S., Rossé, C., Kappler, C., Georgel, P., Belvin, M., Gubb, D., Camonis, J., Hoffmann, J.A., Reichhart, J.M. (2002), "The Drosophila immune defense against gram-negative infection requires the death protein dFADD," *Immunity* **17**(5):575–81.

Narbonne-Reveau, K., Charroux, B., Royet, J. (2011), "Lack of an antibacterial response defect in Drosophila Toll-9 mutant," *PLoS One.* **6**(2):e17470.

Nehme, N.T., Liégeois, S., Kele, B., Giammarinaro, P., Pradel, E., Hoffmann, J.A., Ewbank, J.J., Ferrandon, D. (2007), "A model of bacterial intestinal infections in Drosophila melanogaster," *PLoS Pathog.* **3**(11):e173.

Nusslein-Volhard, C., Lohs-Schardin, M., Sander, K., Cremer, C. (1980), " A dorso-ventral shift of embryonic primordia in a new maternal-effect mutant of Drosophila," *Nature* **283**, 474–476.

Ochiai, M., Ashida, M. (1988), "Purification of a beta-1,3-glucan recognition protein in the prophenoloxidase activating system from hemolymph of the silkworm, Bombyx mori," *J Biol Chem.* **263**, 12056–12062.

Ochiai, M., Ashida, M. (1999), "A pattern recognition protein for peptidoglycan : Cloning the cDNA and the gene of the silkworm, Bombyx mori," *J Biol Chem.* **274**, 11854–11858.

Ochiai, M., Ashida, M. (2000), "A pattern-recognition protein for beta-1,3-glucan: The binding domain and the cDNA cloning of beta-1,3-glucan recognition protein from the silkworm, Bombyx mori," *J Biol Chem.* **275**, 4995–5002.

Ooi J.Y., Yagi Y., Hu X., Ip Y.T. (2002) The Drosophila Toll-9 activates a constitutive antimicrobial defense," *EMBO Rep.* **3**(1):82–7.

Paillot, A. (1919), "Immunité naturelle chez les insects," *C. R. Acad Sci Paris.* **169**, 202–204.

Paillot, A. (1933), *L'infection chez les insects.* Imprimerie G. Patissier, Trévoux, 535p.

Paquette, N., Broemer, M., Aggarwal, K., Chen, L., Husson, M., Ertürk-Hasdemir, D., Reichhart, J.M., Meier, P., Silverman, N. (2010), "Caspase-mediated cleavage, IAP binding, and ubiquitination: Linking three mechanisms crucial for Drosophila NF-kappaB signalling," *Mol Cell* **37**(2):172–82.

Park, J.W., Kim, C.H., Kim, J.H., Je, B.R., Roh, K.B., Kim, S.J., Lee, H.H., Ryu, J.H., Lim, J.H., Oh, B.H., Lee, W.J., Ha, N.C., Lee, B.L. (2007), "Clustering of peptidoglycan recognition protein-SA is required for sensing lysine-type peptidoglycan in insects," *Proc Natl Acad Sci USA* **104**(16):6602–7.

Parker, J.S., Mizuguchi, K., Gay, N.J. (2001), "A family of proteins related to Spätzle, the Toll receptor ligand, are encoded in the Drosophila genome," *Proteins* **45**(1):71–80.

Poltorak, A., He, X., Smirnova, I., Liu, M.Y., van Huffel, C., Du, X., Birdwell, D., Alejos, E., Silva, M., Galanos, C., Freudenberg, M., Ricciardi-Castagnoli, P., Layton, B., Beutler, B. (1998), "Defective LPS signaling in C3H/HeJ and C57BL/10ScCr mice: mutations in Tlr4 gene," *Science* **282**(5396):2085–8.

Ragab, A., Buechling,,T., Gesellchen, V., Spirohn, K., Boettcher, A.L., Boutros, M. (2011), "Drosophila Ras/MAPK signalling regulates innate immune responses in immune and intestinal stem cells," *EMBO J.* **30**(6):1123–36.

Rämet, M., Manfruelli, P., Pearson, A., Mathey-Prevot, B., Ezekowitz, R.A. (2002), "Functional genomic analysis of phagocytosis and identification of a Drosophila receptor for E. coli," *Nature* **416**(6881):644–8.

Reichhart, J.M., Essrich, M., Dimarcq, J.L., Hoffmann, D., Hoffmann, J.A., Lagueux, M. (1989), "Insect immunity: Isolation of cDNA clones corresponding to diptericin, an inducible antibacterial peptide from Phormia terranovae (Diptera). Transcriptional profiles during immunization," *Eur J Biochem.* **182**(2):423–7.

Reichhart, J.M., Meister, M., Dimarcq, J.L., Zachary, D., Hoffmann, D., Ruiz, C., Richards, G., Hoffmann, J.A. (1992), "Insect immunity: Developmental and inducible activity of the Drosophila diptericin promoter," *EMBO J.* **11**(4):1469–77.

Reichhart, J.M., Georgel, P., Meister, M., Lemaitre, B., Kappler, C., Hoffmann, J.A. (1993), "Expression and nuclear translocation of the rel/NF-kappa B-related morphogen dorsal during the immune response of Drosophila," *C.R. Acad Sci III.* **316**(10):1218–24.

Rizki, T.M., Rizki, R.M., Grell, E.H. (1980), "A mutant affecting the crystal cells in Drosophila melanogaster," Rouxs Arch. Dev. Biol. 188(2): 91–99.

Roach, J.C., Glusman, G., Rowen, L., Kaur, A., Purcell, M.K., Smith, K.D., Hood, L.E., Aderem, A. (2005), "The evolution of vertebrate Toll-like receptors," *Proc Natl Acad Sci USA.* **102**(27):9577–82.

Rosetto, M., Engström, Y., Baldari, C.T., Telford, J.L., Hultmark, D. (1995), "Signals from the IL-1 receptor homolog, Toll, can activate an immune response in a Drosophila hemocyte cell line," *Biochem Biophys Res Commun.* **209**(1):111–6.

Roth, S., Schüpbach, T. (1994), "The relationship between ovarian and embryonic dorsoventral patterning in Drosophila," *Development* **120**(8):2245–57.

Royet, J., Dziarski, R. (2007), "Peptidoglycan recognition proteins: Pleiotropic sensors and effectors of antimicrobial defences," *Nat Rev Microbiol.* **5**(4):264–77.

Royet, J., Gupta, D., Dziarski, R. (2011), "Peptidoglycan recognition proteins: Modulators of the microbiome and inflammation," *Nat Rev Immunol.* **11**(12):837–51.

Rutschmann, S., Jung, A.C., Hetru, C., Reichhart, J.M., Hoffmann, J.A., Ferrandon, D. (2000a), "The Rel protein DIF mediates the antifungal but not the antibacterial host defense in Drosophila," *Immunity.* **12**(5):569–80.

Rutschmann, S., Jung, A.C., Zhou, R., Silverman, N., Hoffmann, J.A., Ferrandon, D. (2000b), "Role of Drosophila IKK gamma in a Toll-independent antibacterial immune response," *Nat Immunol.* **1**(4):342–7.

Rutschmann, S., Kilinc, A., Ferrandon, D. (2002), "Cutting edge: The Toll pathway is required for resistance to gram-positive bacterial infections in Drosophila," *J Immunol.* **168**(4):1542–6.

Ryu, J.H., Ha, E.M., Oh, C.T., Seol, J.H., Brey, P.T., Jin, I., Lee, D.G., Kim, J., Lee, D., Lee, W.J. (2006), "An essential complementary role of NF-kappaB pathway to microbicidal oxidants in Drosophila gut immunity," *EMBO J.* **25**(15):3693–701.

Ryu, J.H., Kim, S.H., Lee, H.Y., Bai, J.Y., Nam, Y.D., Bae, J.W., Lee, D.G., Shin, S.C., Ha, E.M., Lee, W.J. (2008), "Innate immune homeostasis by the homeobox gene caudal and commensal-gut mutualism in Drosophila," *Science* **319**(5864):777–82.

Sastry, K., Zahedi, K., Lelias, J.M., Whitehead, A.S., Ezekowitz, R.A. (1991), "Molecular characterization of the mouse mannose-binding proteins: The mannose-binding protein A but not C is an acute phase reactant," *J Immunol.* **147**(2):692–7.

Schneider, D.S., Hudson, K.L., Lin, T.Y., Anderson, K.V. (1991), "Dominant and recessive mutations define functional domains of Toll, a transmembrane protein required for dorsal-ventral polarity in the Drosophila embryo," *Genes Dev.* **5**(5):797–807.

Schneider, D.S., Ayres, J.S. (2008), "Two ways to survive infection: What resistance and tolerance can teach us about treating infectious diseases," *Nat Rev Immunol.* **8**(11):889–95.

Sen, R., Baltimore, D. (1986), "Inducibility of kappa immunoglobulin enhancer-binding protein NF-kappa B by a posttranslational mechanism," *Cell* **47**(6):921–8.

Shai, Y. (2002), "Mode of action of membrane active antimicrobial peptides," *Biopolymers.* **66**(4):236–48.

Silverman, N., Zhou, R., Stöven, S., Pandey, N., Hultmark, D., Maniatis, T. (2000), "A Drosophila IkappaB kinase complex required for Relish cleavage and antibacterial immunity," *Genes Dev.* **14**(19):2461–71.

Silverman, N., Zhou, R., Erlich, R.L., Hunter, M., Bernstein, E., Schneider, D., Maniatis, T. (2003), "Immune activation of NF-kappaB and JNK requires Drosophila TAK1," *J Biol Chem.* **278**(49):48928–34.

Simon, A., Kullberg, B.J., Tripet, B., Boerman, O.C., Zeeuwen, P., van der Ven-Jongekrijg, J., Verweij, P., Schalkwijk, J., Hodges, R., van der Meer, J.W., Netea, M.G. (2008), "Drosomycin-like defensin, a human homologue of Drosophila melanogaster drosomycin with antifungal activity," *Antimicrob Agents Chemother.* **52**(4):1407–12.

Steiner, H., Hultmark, D., Engström, A., Bennich, H., Boman, H.G. (1981), "Sequence and specificity of two antibacterial proteins involved in insect immunity," *Nature* **292**(5820):246–8.

Steward, R. (1987), "Dorsal, an embryonic polarity gene in Drosophila, is homologous to the vertebrate proto-oncogene, c-rel.," *Science* **238**(4827):692–4.

Stöven, S., Ando, I., Kadalayil, L., Engström, Y., Hultmark, D. (2000), "Activation of the Drosophila NF-kappaB factor Relish by rapid endoproteolytic cleavage," *EMBO Rep.* **1**(4):347–52.

Stöven, S., Silverman, N., Junell, A., Hedengren-Olcott, M., Ertürk, D., Engström, Y., Maniatis, T., Hultmark, D. (2003), "Caspase-mediated processing of the Drosophila NF-kappaB factor Relish," *Proc Natl Acad Sci USA* **100**(10):5991–6.

Sun, S.C., Lindström, I., Lee, J.Y., Faye, I. (1991), "Structure and expression of the attacin genes in Hyalophora cecropia," *Eur J Biochem.* **196**(1):247–54.

Tauszig, S., Jouanguy, E., Hoffmann, J.A., Imler, J.L. (2000), "Toll-related receptors and the control of antimicrobial peptide expression in Drosophila," *Proc Natl Acad Sci USA.* **97**(19):10520–5.

Tauszig-Delamasure, S., Bilak, H., Capovilla, M., Hoffmann, J.A., Imler, J.L. (2002), "Drosophila MyD88 is required for the response to fungal and Gram-positive bacterial infections," *Nat Immunol.* **3**(1):91–7.

Towb, P., Sun, H., Wasserman, S.A. (2009), "Tube Is an IRAK-4 homolog in a Toll pathway adapted for development and immunity," *J Innate Immun.* **1**(4):309–21.

Tzou, P., Ohresser, S., Ferrandon, D., Capovilla, M., Reichhart, J.M., Lemaitre, B., Hoffmann, J.A., Imler, J.L. (2000), "Tissue-specific inducible expression of antimicrobial peptide genes in Drosophila surface epithelia," *Immunity* **13**(5):737–48.

Uttenweiler-Joseph, S., Moniatte, M., Lagueux, M., van Dorsselaer, A., Hoffmann, J.A., Bulet, P. (1998), "Differential display of peptides induced during the immune response of Drosophila: A matrix-assisted laser desorption ionization time-of-flight mass spectrometry study," *Proc Natl Acad Sci USA* **95**(19):11342–7.

van Rij, R.P., Saleh, M.C., Berry, B., Foo, C., Houk, A., Antoniewski, C., Andino, R. (2006), "The RNA silencing endonuclease Argonaute 2 mediates specific antiviral immunity in Drosophila melanogaster," *Genes Dev.* **20**(21):2985–95.

Vidal, S., Khush, R.S., Leulier, F., Tzou, P., Nakamura, M., Lemaitre, B. (2001), "Mutations in the Drosophila dTAK1 gene reveal a conserved function for MAPKKKs in the control of rel/NF-kappaB-dependent innate immune responses," *Genes Dev.* **15**(15):1900–12.

Wang, L., Weber, A.N., Atilano, M.L., Filipe, S.R., Gay, N.J., Ligoxygakis, P. (2006a), "Sensing of Gram-positive bacteria in Drosophila: GNBP1 is needed to process and present peptidoglycan to PGRP-SA," *EMBO J.* **25**(20):5005–14.

Wang, X.H., Aliyari, R., Li, W.X., Li, H.W., Kim, K., Carthew, R., Atkinson, P., Ding, S.W. (2006b), "RNA interference directs innate immunity against viruses in adult Drosophila," *Science* **312**(5772):452–4.

Weber, A.N., Tauszig-Delamasure, S., Hoffmann, J.A., Lelièvre, E., Gascan, H., Ray, K.P., Morse, M.A., Imler, J.L., Gay, N.J. (2003), "Binding of the Drosophila cytokine Spätzle to Toll is direct and establishes signalling," *Nat Immunol.* **4**(8):794–800.

Werner, T., Liu, G., Kang, D., Ekengren, S., Steiner, H., Hultmark, D. (2000), "A family of peptidoglycan recognition proteins in the fruit fly Drosophila melanogaster," *Proc Natl Acad Sci USA* **97**(25):13772–7.

Wicker, C., Reichhart, J.M., Hoffmann, D., Hultmark, D., Samakovlis, C., Hoffmann, J.A. (1990), "Insect immunity: Characterization of a Drosophila cDNA encoding a novel member of the diptericin family of immune peptides," *J Biol Chem.* **265**(36):22493–8.

Wolenski, F.S., Garbati, M.R., Lubinski, T.J., Traylor-Knowles, N., Dresselhaus, E., Stefanik, D.J., Goucher, H., Finnerty, J.R., Gilmore, T.D. (2011), "Characterization of the core elements of the NF-κB signaling pathway of the sea anemone Nematostella vectensis," *Mol Cell Biol.* **31**(5):1076–87.

Wright, S.D., Ramos, R.A., Tobias, P.S., Ulevitch, R.J., Mathison, J.C. (1990), "CD14, a receptor for complexes of lipopolysaccharide (LPS) and LPS binding protein," *Science.* **249**(4975):1431–3.

Wu, L.P., Choe, K.M., Lu, Y., Anderson, K.V. (2001), "Drosophila immunity: Genes on the third chromosome required for the response to bacterial infection," *Genetics* **159**(1):189–99.

Yagi, Y., Nishida, Y., Ip, Y.T. (2010), "Functional analysis of Toll-related genes in Drosophila," *Dev Growth Differ.* **52**(9):771–83.

Zhu, B., Pennack, J.A., McQuilton, P., Forero, M.G., Mizuguchi, K., Sutcliffe, B., Gu, C.J., Fenton, J.C., Hidalgo, A. (2008), "Drosophila neurotrophins reveal a common mechanism for nervous system formation," *PLoS Biol.* **6**(11):e284.

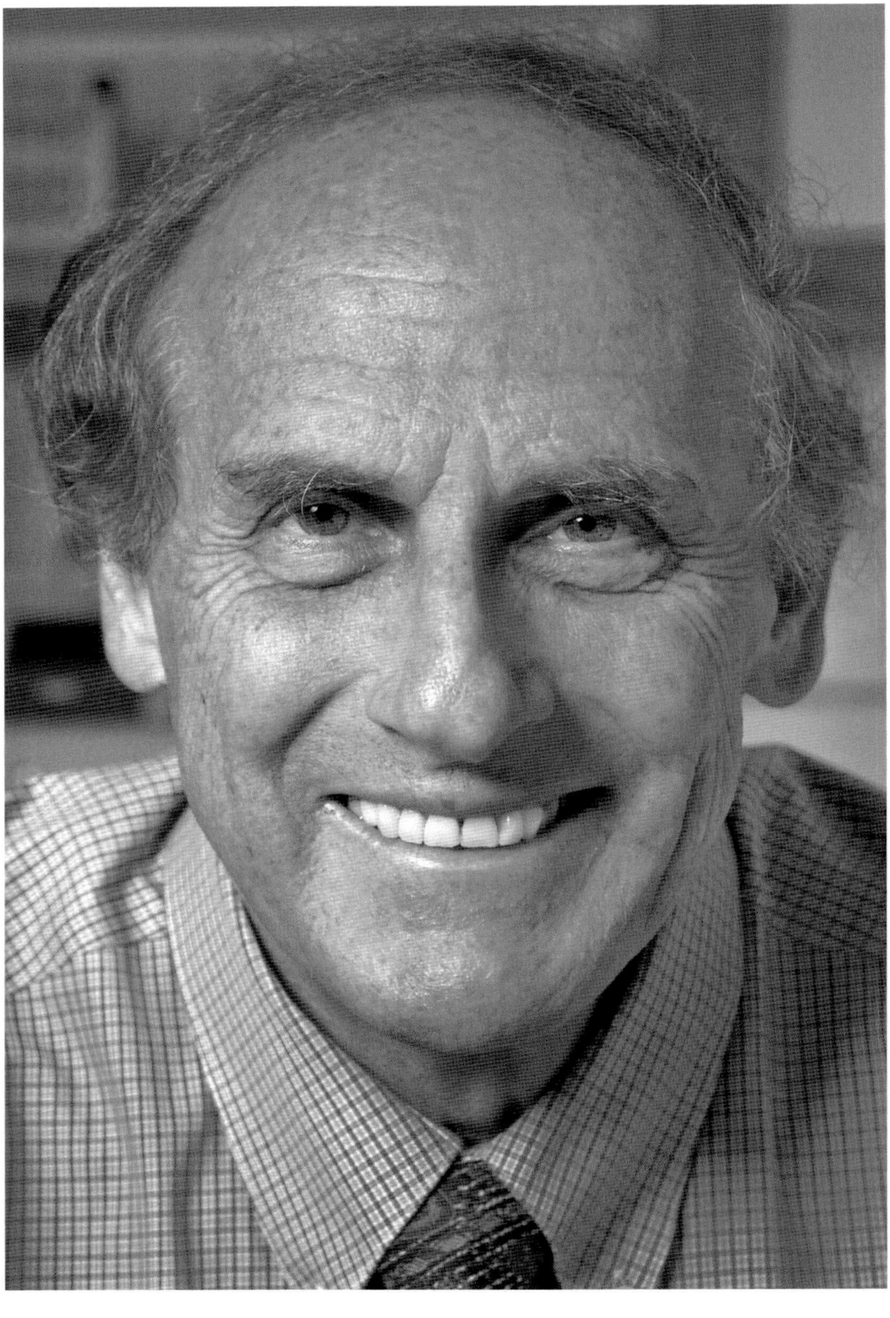

Ralph M. Steinman. Photo: The Rockefeller University

Ralph M. Steinman

Ralph M. Steinman was born in Montreal, Canada, on 14 January 1943, the second of four children. His father Irving, a Jewish immigrant from Eastern Europe, and his mother Nettie owned a department store in Sherbrooke near Montreal. His father wanted him to continue in the family business, but in high school Ralph became interested in science. He received a B.S. with honors from McGill University in 1963, and an M.D. magna cum laude from Harvard Medical School in 1968. While at Harvard, he spent a year as a research fellow in the laboratory of Elizabeth Hay, who introduced him to cell biology and the immune system. During his internship and residency at the Massachusetts General Hospital, Steinman met Claudia Hoeffel, who was a medical social worker in the hospital. They married in 1971.

After completing his medical training, he was drawn to biomedical research. He joined The Rockefeller University in 1970 as a postdoctoral fellow in the Laboratory of Cellular Physiology and Immunology headed by physician-scientists Zanvil A. Cohn and James G. Hirsch. This laboratory was founded by the premier microbiologist René Dubos, who recognized the need to study the host during infection. Dubos, Cohn, and Hirsch were Steinman's ideal mentors whose approach was not limited to immunology but embraced cell biology and biochemistry. He spent his entire career at Rockefeller, where he was appointed assistant professor in 1972, associate professor in 1976, and professor in 1988. He was named Henry G. Kunkel Professor in 1995 and director of the Christopher Browne Center for Immunology and Immune Diseases in 1998.

Steinman's early research in collaboration with Cohn was an attempt to understand the white cells of the immune system that operate in a variety of ways to spot, apprehend, and destroy infectious microorganisms and tumor cells. In 1973, Steinman and Cohn discovered dendritic cells, a previously unknown class of immune cells that constantly formed and retracted their processes. This discovery changed the field of immunology.

For the next four decades, until his death in 2011, Steinman's laboratory was at the forefront of dendritic cell research. He and his colleagues established that dendritic cells are critical sentinels of the immune system that control both its innate and adaptive responses – from silencing to actively resisting its challenges. He also showed that dendritic cells are the 2 main initiators of T cell-mediated immune responses. Steinman's deep insights into medicine led him to take his dendritic cell research into the treatment of human disease. His most recent studies were focused on the interface of several diseases with the immune system and included clinical studies using dendritic cell- and immune-based vaccines and therapies for such medical conditions as graft rejection, resistance to tumors, autoimmune diseases, and infections. In 2010, he initiated at The Rockefeller University Hospital a phase I clinical trial with the first dendritic cell-targeted vaccine against HIV.

Steinman's dynamic personality, boundless energy, and persistent leadership during these four decades allowed him to build international collaborations with many immunologists and scientists in other fields and to create an entire new field of dendritic cell biology. As part of his efforts in establishing this science, he personally trained and mentored more than a hundred postdoctoral fellows and graduate students in his laboratory. He published some 450 scientific papers. Beginning in 1978, he became editor of the *Journal of Experimental Medicine* and was one of its guiding forces. He also served as advisory editor of *Human Immunology*, the *Journal of Clinical Immunology*, the *Journal of Immunologic Methods* and the *Proceedings of the National Academy of Sciences*.

For the first two decades of Steinman's research, dendritic cells were underappreciated, but by the mid-1990s, the scientific community began to recognize his work on their critical role in the immune system. Steinman received numerous honors, including the Freidrich-Sasse (1996), Emil von Behring (1996), and Robert Koch (1999) Prizes, the Rudolf Virchow (1997) and Coley (1998) Medals. In 2004, he received the New York City Mayor's Award for Science and Technology. He was honored with the Gairdner Foundation International Award in 2003, the Albert Lasker Award for Basic Medical Research in 2007, the Albany Medical Prize in 2009, and the A.H. Heineken Prize for Medicine in 2010. He was awarded honorary degrees from the University of Innsbruck, Free University of Brussels, Erlangen University, and the Mount Sinai School of Medicine. He was elected a member of the National Academy of Sciences in 2001 and the Institute of Medicine in 2002. He was also a corresponding fellow of the Royal Society of Edinburgh. In 2012, the Ralph M. Steinman Center for Cancer Vaccines was established in his honor at the Baylor Institute for Immunology Research in Dallas, Texas.

Steinman was a trustee of the Trudeau Institute in Saranac Lake, New York. He also served as a scientific advisor to several organizations including the Charles A. Dana Foundation, the Campbell Family Institute of Breast Cancer Research in Toronto, Canada, the M. D. Anderson Cancer Center for Immunology Research in Houston, Texas, Baylor Institute for Immunology Research, RIKEN Center for Allergy and Immunology Research in Yokohama, Japan, and CHAVI Center for HIV-AIDS Vaccine Immunology, Durham, North Carolina. Steinman was a member of the American Society of Clinical Investigation, the American Society of Cell Biology, the American Association of Immunologists, the Harvey, the Kunkel, and the Practitioners' Societies, and the Society for Leukocyte Biology.

Diagnosed with pancreatic adenocarcinoma in March 2007, Steinman believed that dendritic cells had the potential to fight his aggressive tumor. With many collaborators and leading-edge technology, he designed dendritic cell-based immunotherapies for himself that he thought might also advance medical science. For four-and-a-half years after his diagnosis, he remained quite healthy and continued to travel, lecture, and pursue new laboratory studies. Steinman died on 30 September 2011, three days before his Nobel Prize was announced. Unaware of his death at the time of its announcement, the Nobel Committee made an unprecedented decision that his award would stand. In addition to his wife Claudia, Steinman was survived by his three children Adam, Alexis, and Lesley, three grandchildren Isadola, Syla, and Robert; his mother Nettie; his brothers Seymour and Mark; his sister Joni; his daughter-in-law Jenny and his son-in-law Joseph.

Claudia Steinman and her children have donated the entire proceeds of Dr. Steinman's Nobel Prize to charity, $500,000 of which they are giving to the Cohn-Steinman Professorship at the Rockefeller University and $250,000 to The Steinman Family Foundation to support the careers of young scientists and science education.

RALPH STEINMAN AND THE DISCOVERY OF DENDRITIC CELLS

Nobel Lecture, December 7, 2011

by

MICHEL C. NUSSENZWEIG

Laboratory of Molecular Immunology and Howard Hughes Medical Institute, The Rockefeller University, New York, NY 10065, USA.

In science, it is a rare event for one individual to make a discovery that opens a new scientific field, work at the forefront of its research for forty years, and live to see his endeavors transformed into novel medical interventions. Ralph Steinman was such an individual. His discovery of dendritic cells changed immunology.

HISTORICAL BACKGROUND

The dendritic cell discovery was a key breakthrough in immunology because it brought together the work of Paul Ehrlich and Ilya Metchnikov, who shared the Nobel Prize in Physiology or Medicine in 1908 for their work on immunity (Fig. 1).

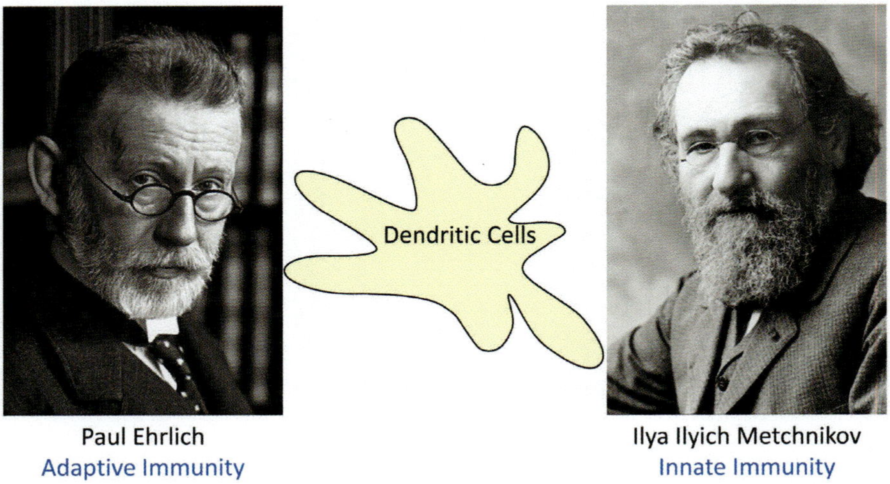

Figure 1. Dendritic cells connect the adaptive and innate immune systems featured in the work of Paul Ehrlich and Ilya Metchnikov, who were awarded the Nobel Prize in Physiology or Medicine in 1908.

Ehrlich focused on adaptive immunity and the exquisite specificity of the serologic response by the immune system to produce antitoxins, each of which was unique. He suggested a model whereby cells with receptors for the toxins would recognize the toxins and then release excess toxin receptors into circulation. Ehrlich was also the first to frame the problem of diversity: if the immune system can respond to any invading organism and destroy it, how does it know the difference between self and non-self antigens so that it prevents attacks on self, a condition he called *horror autotoxicus* known today as autoimmunity.

Metchnikov, on the other hand, focused on innate immunity. He discovered phagocytosis in starfish larvae and proposed there are innate cells, particularly macrophages, that internalize and kill microbes. There was nothing for cells to learn because the immune system provided an instinctive response for phagocytes to destroy pathogens.

How the adaptive and innate immunity are related was entirely not clear at the time, but we now know dendritic cells are the missing link that connects Ehrlich and Metchnikov. Dendritic cells are a part of the innate system and they orchestrate adaptive immunity.

Steinman learned about immunity at Harvard Medical School and especially during courses he took in cell biology during the 1960s (Fig. 2). Those were heady times for immunology. The immune system was being linked to a number of mysterious diseases like lupus and arthritis, which are due to *horror autotoxicus,* and there were successful new vaccines against infectious diseases that were making an enormous difference in public health.

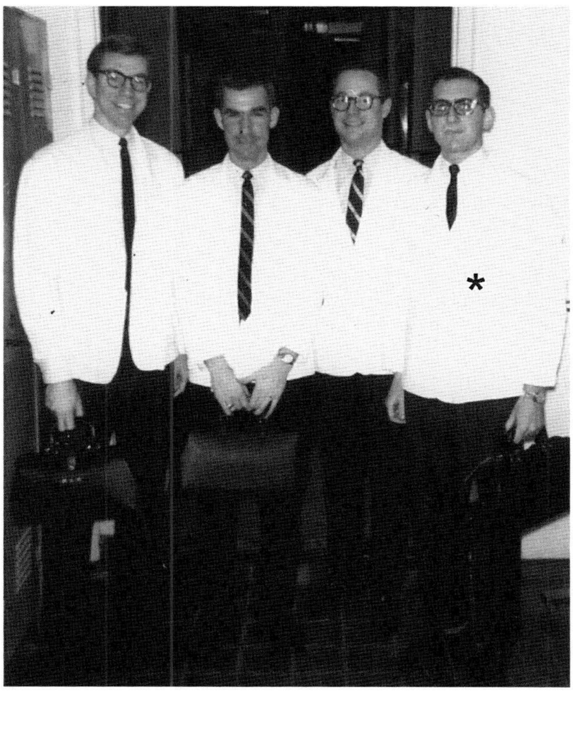

Figure 2. Ralph Steinman, far right, as a medical student at Harvard in the 1960s when he started to learn about the immune system.

Steinman was particularly interested in the work of Macfarlane Burnet and Peter Medawar, who were awarded the Nobel Prize in Medicine or Physiology in 1960 for their work on acquired immune tolerance (Fig. 3). Burnet, in particular, had published several lectures in which he tried to establish a theoretical framework to explain Ehrlich's dilemma about how the immune system distinguishes self from non-self. Burnet outlined the three cardinal features of immunity as Specificity, Diversity, and Memory. Specificity, going back to Ehrlich, meant immune responses that recognize one toxin do not cross-react with a different toxin. Diversity, a concept championed in the 1930s at The Rockefeller Institute by Nobel laureate Karl Landsteiner, referred to the finding that even substances that do not exist in nature can induce an immune response, thus leading to the conclusion that the immune system can recognize any invading organism, pathogen, or toxin. Memory, going back to Edward Jenner and smallpox in the 18th century, is a basic property of vaccines; once the immune system sees a toxin and it reappears, the system recognizes it and can respond faster and better.

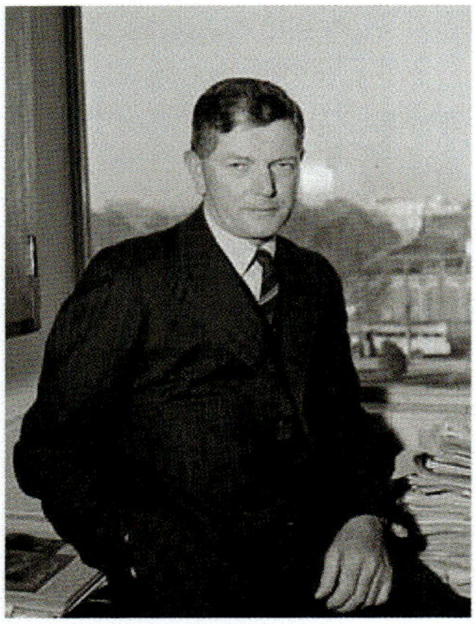

Macfarlane Burnet
Clonal Selection

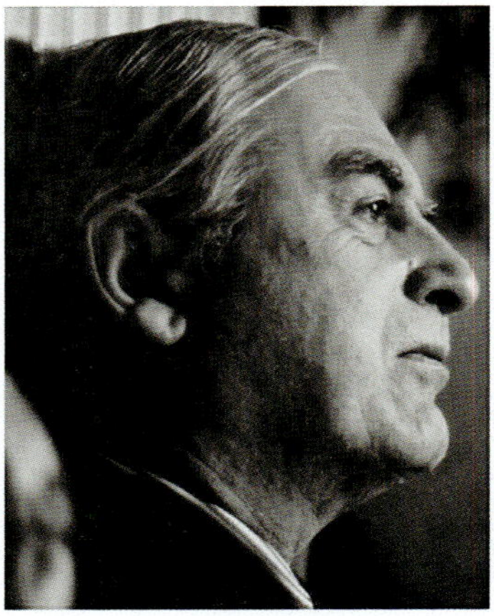

Peter Medawar
Immune Tolerance

Figure 3. Macfarlane Burnet and Peter Medawar, who were awarded the Nobel Prize in Physiology or Medicine in 1960 for their work on immunological tolerance.

To account for these properties, Burnet (Burnet, 1957; Burnet, 1958) contemporaneously with David Talmage (Talmage, 1957) suggested that the immune system is composed of clones of cells, each expressing a unique receptor (Fig. 4). Specificity would come from the receptor expressed on these cells (as hypothesized by Ehrlich) and would be unique for each cell. Diversity would be accounted for by the large number of individual clones emerging during development. According to Burnet's theory, when antigen comes into the system, it selects the right clone and that clone is expanded and memory is induced. Nobel laureate Joshua Lederberg added to this idea by suggesting that any self-reactive clones that arise during development would be deleted during encounters with self antigens (Lederberg, 1959). Finally, immune responses begin when a pathogen or antigen enters the system and causes expansion of the specific clone, whereas memory involves simply more cells that are specific for the pathogen so there is a faster and better response the second time around.

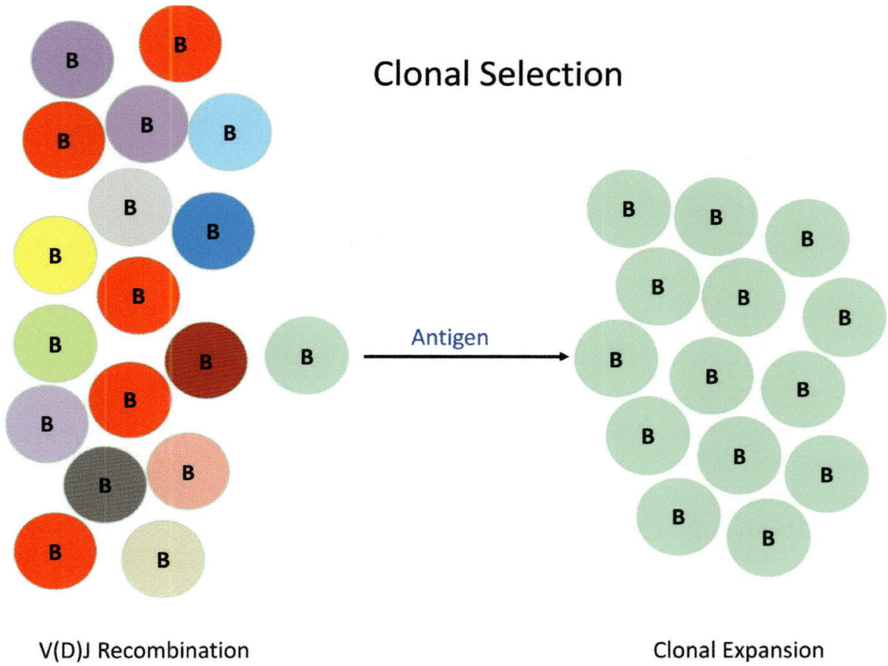

Figure 4. The clonal selection theory. Clones of lymphocytes, each with a different unique receptor (represented by a different color), are present before antigen is introduced into the system. The antigen selects the clone with the best cognate receptor for expansion.

The most intriguing problem in immunology during the 1960s was how to create sufficient diversity to account for adaptive immunity. But neither Burnet nor Steinman was interested in this problem. Steinman wanted to learn how an immune response begins, and he believed that understanding this feature of immunity would make it possible to regulate immune responses, both to prevent autoimmunity and to create vaccines.

DISCOVERY

In 1970, Steinman joined physician-scientists Zanvil A. Cohn and James G. Hirsch in The Rockefeller University laboratory of René Dubos, a microbiologist (Fig. 5) who was a disciple of Oswald T. Avery, in whose Rockefeller laboratory he discovered the natural antibiotic gramicidin in 1939 (Hirsch and Moberg, 1989; Moberg and Steinman, 2003, 2009). The Dubos laboratory had evolved from studying microbes to focus on interactions of the host with pathogens. Metchnikov became the hero for Cohn and Hirsch.

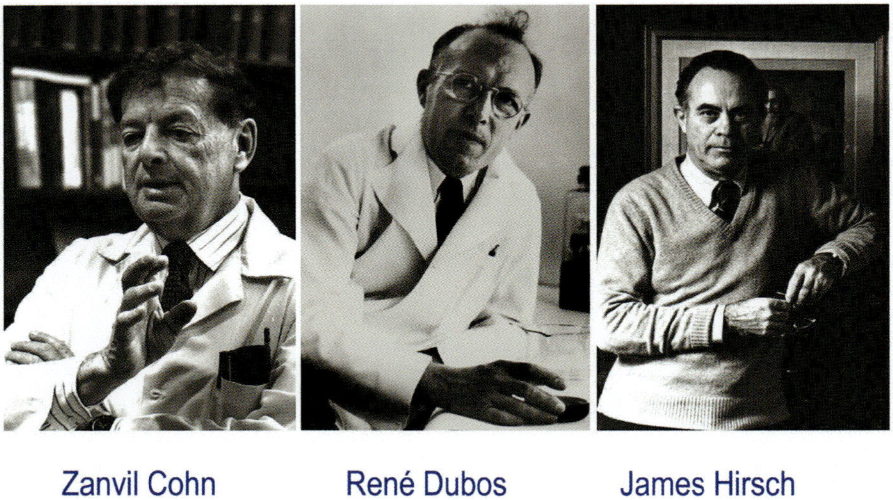

Figure 5. Ralph Steinman's mentors at The Rockefeller University.

An important breakthrough in immunology in 1967 was the development of a method to study specific immune responses in vitro. The system developed by Robert Mishell and Richard Dutton involved mixing antigens with lymphocytes and measuring antibody responses (Mishell and Dutton, 1967). An unexpected finding was that lymphocytes alone were not sufficient to produce immune responses and that accessory cells were required to initiate immunity (Fig. 6). Although the nature of the accessory cells was unknown, it was a cell that was adherent to glass and its role was to present antigen to lymphocytes.

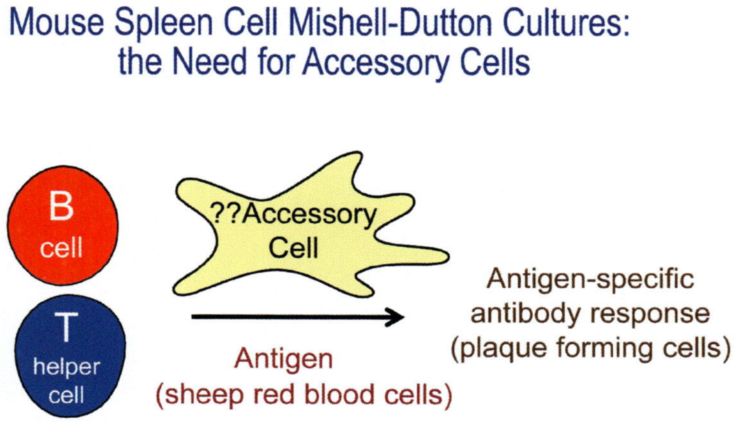

Figure 6. The diagram summarizes the observation that T and B cells are not sufficient to induce antibody immune responses in vitro and that reaction requires an accessory cell.

Following his interests in initiation of immunity, Steinman worked closely with Cohn to look for the accessory cells. Most workers in the field at the time believed the accessory cell was a macrophage. In vivo studies by other laboratories showed cells looking like macrophages were associated with antigens in lymph nodes (Nossal et al., 1968) , and when macrophages were loaded with antigens, they induced immune responses (Unanue and Cerottini, 1970).

However, Cohn had spent his career studying macrophages and had shown with Barbara Ehrenreich that when antigens such as albumin were captured by macrophages, they were degraded to amino acids (Ehrenreich and Cohn, 1967). Steinman's first assignment as a postdoctoral fellow in the Cohn laboratory was to explore that finding. He developed a method using horseradish peroxidase and horseradish peroxidase-immune complexes to see whether this protein could be detected on macrophage surfaces where it would be displayed to lymphocytes that would induce immunity. While this method allowed quantitative measurements and ultrastructural visualization of ingested antigens, Steinman failed to find antigen uptake or retention by macrophages. Instead, he made an important discovery in cell biology when he found that the uptake of horseradish peroxidase was so rapid that he and Cohn concluded that macrophages must be constantly recycling their membranes (Steinman and Cohn, 1972a, b).

To look for a different accessory cell, Steinman and Cohn decided to study adherent cells from mouse spleen instead of from the peritoneal cavity. They were fortunate to have help from their Rockefeller colleagues, two cell biologists who won the 1974 Nobel Prize in Physiology or Medicine for their discoveries of cell structure and function (Fig. 7). George Palade's laboratory pioneered fixation and electron microscopy of cells, tools that Steinman used to identify dendritic cells. Christian de Duve's laboratory was expert in centrifugation methods to separate subcellular components, a technique that Steinman adapted in devising a scheme to purify dendritic cells.

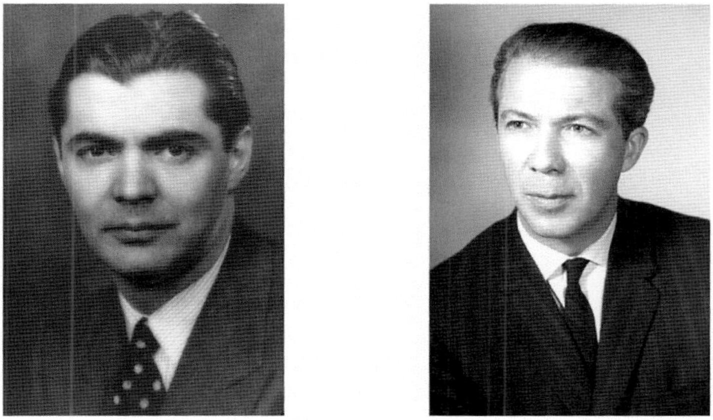

Figure 7. George Palade and Christian de Duve, who were awarded the Nobel Prize in Physiology or Medicine in 1974 for their work in cell biology, were instrumental in developing techniques used by Ralph Steinman to characterize and purify dendritic cells (DC). Courtesy of The Rockefeller Archive Center.

What Steinman and Cohn found in 1973 when they looked through a phase contrast microscope was a different cell (Steinman and Cohn, 1973). It had dendritic processes but no prominent phagocytic vacuoles (Fig. 8). This is the discovery that was honored with the 2011 Nobel Prize in Physiology or Medicine. Steinman and Cohn used electron microscopy to confirm their phase contrast observations and saw features that were distinct from typical macrophages and monocytes (Steinman and Cohn, 1973). The cells were elongated with tree-like processes that were constantly forming and retracting. Steinman named them dendritic cells, from the Greek word *dendreon* for tree. The dendritic cells also had a few, small lysosomes and lacked the typical membrane ruffling seen in phagocytes. With micro-cinematography they observed dendritic cell behavior that was dynamic and distinct from macrophages that were sedentary. Using the best microscopic and ultra-structural techniques available, they were confident they had found a novel cell.

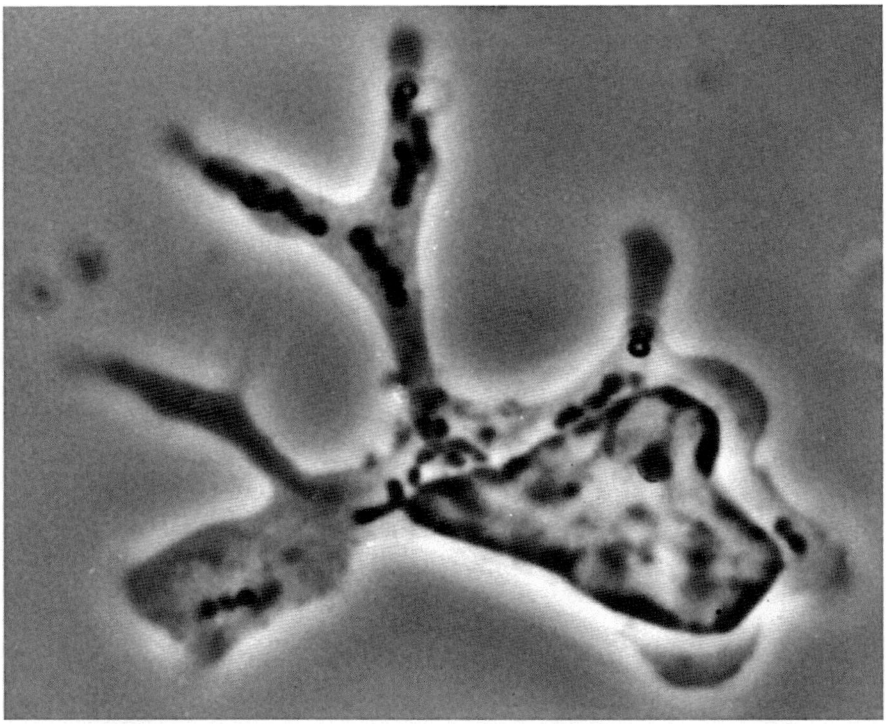

Figure 8. Phase contrast micrograph of a dendritic cell (Steinman and Cohn, 1973).

PURIFICATION

Steinman intuited that the newly discovered cell was the accessory cell, but he needed to devise a method to purify the cells before he could test this idea (Steinman and Cohn, 1974). At the time there were no easy procedures for cell purification and it took him a couple years to develop a technique based on physical properties of dendritic cells (Fig. 9). A suspension of spleen cells was subjected to de Duve's methods of density gradient centrifugation in a column of bovine serum albumin, on which semi-purified dendritic cells rose to the top and small lymphocytes went to the bottom. Steinman then placed this low-density fraction on glass for an hour and then delicately washed away all except the adherent dendritic cells and macrophages. Following an overnight culture, the dendritic cells detached from the glass. Steinman then devised a method for removing the lingering macrophages by adding antibody-coated sheep red blood cells that formed rosettes by virtue of their Fc receptor expression. The rosetted macrophages went to the bottom of a second gradient centrifugation and the dendritic cells were collected from the light interphase. Unfortunately, the yield of dendritic cells by this method was poor and there were never enough cells to do all the experiments that Steinman wanted to do. Moreover, it was difficult for others to replicate this tedious procedure. In addition, the techniques were familiar to cell biologists but not to immunologists. As a result, Steinman and his students had dendritic cell studies all to themselves for the next fifteen years.

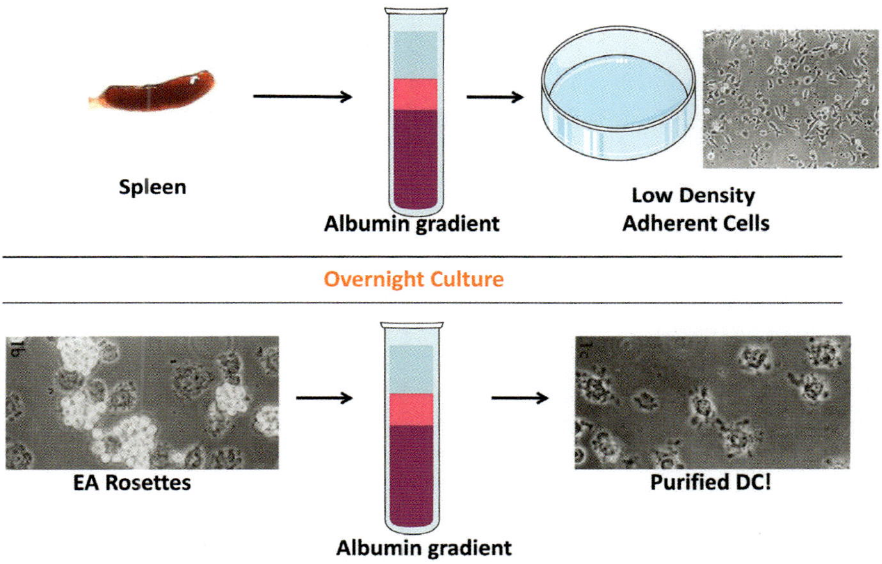

Figure 9. Original method for dendritic cell purification. Spleen cell suspensions are fractionated on albumin density gradients and low density cells placed on glass to capture adherent cells. Following overnight culture, cells that come off the glass are incubated with antibody coated erythrocytes (EA). The mixture is separated by a second round of albumin gradient centrifugation to obtain purified dendritic cells.

MIXED LEUKOCYTE REACTION

To demonstrate that dendritic cells were functionally unique, Steinman and Maggi Witmer-Pack used the mixed leukocyte reaction (MLR) (Fig. 10). This model had been used for tissue typing to predict whether a patient would accept or reject a transplanted graft. In this experiment, dendritic cells from one mouse strain were mixed with T cells from another mismatched strain and the T cell proliferative response to the mismatched dendritic cells was measured. Steinman found that dendritic cells were nearly 100 times more potent in inducing the MLR than non-fractionated mixtures of spleen cells. Since the dendritic cells account for only 1–2% of all cells in the spleen, he concluded that dendritic cells were the key stimulators of this reaction. He also made the leap to suggest that dendritic cells might be the accessory cells (Steinman and Witmer, 1978).

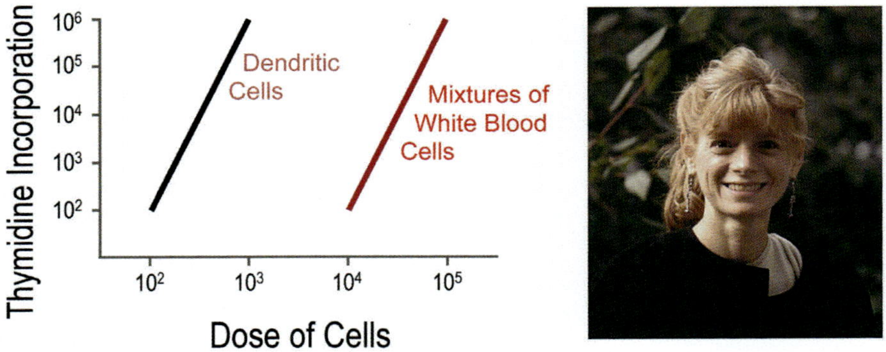

Figure 10. Dendritic cells are potent stimulators of the mixed leukocyte reaction (Steinman and Witmer, 1978). The graph shows a comparison of the stimulatory activity of dendritic cells and unfractionated spleen cells. The photograph shows Maggi Witmer-Pack, who worked with Ralph Steinman on these experiments.

Nevertheless, most immunologists did not accept this conclusion, as William Paul pointed out in his commentary in Cell on the 2011 Nobel Prize in Physiology and Medicine: "This report was initially received with some skepticism, based on the widely held view that the major antigen presenting cells were the far more numerous macrophages and on the uncertainty that many immunologists had about the assay that Steinman and Cohn used to establish the function of their dendritic cells (Paul, 2011)." In other words, the MLR was not thought to be a typical adaptive immune response but more like a spontaneous, innate response. Also, the precise nature of the antigen and the reacting cells were not well defined.

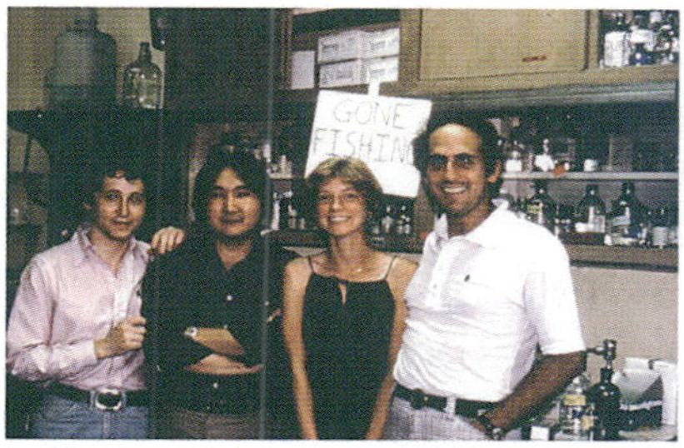

Michel Nussenzweig · Bodma Gutchinov · Maggi Pack · Ralph Steinman — 1980

DENDRITIC CELLS ARE ACCESSORY CELLS FOR THE DEVELOPMENT OF ANTI-TRINITROPHENYL CYTOTOXIC T LYMPHOCYTES*

BY MICHEL C. NUSSENZWEIG, RALPH M. STEINMAN,‡ BODMA GUTCHINOV, AND ZANVIL A. COHN

From The Rockefeller University, New York 10021

"DC are the critical accessory cells, whereas macrophages regardless of source or expression of Ia (MHC II) are without significant activity."

Figure 11. Investigators who demonstrated that dendritic cells are antigen presenting cells and the title of that 1980 paper (Nussenzweig et al., 1980).

ANTIGEN PRESENTATION

By 1978, an experimental system was needed to measure a more typical antigen-specific adaptive response and show that dendritic cells are antigen presenting cells. Steinman's first graduate student, Michel Nussenzweig, developed such an assay based on Karl Landsteiner's pioneering work that utilized haptens as the antigens to elicit responses (Fig. 11). The assay adapted to dendritic cells involved modifying cells with the nitrophenyl moiety and measuring the development of cytotoxic or killer T lymphocytes. Dendritic cell responses were compared to those of macrophages and other accessory cells (Nussenzweig et al., 1980). Results of these experiments showed that "dendritic cells are the critical accessory cells whereas macrophages regardless of source or Ia (MHCII) are without significant activity." With these experiments Steinman and Nussenzweig established the important principle that dendritic cells present antigen to T cells to initiate immunity.

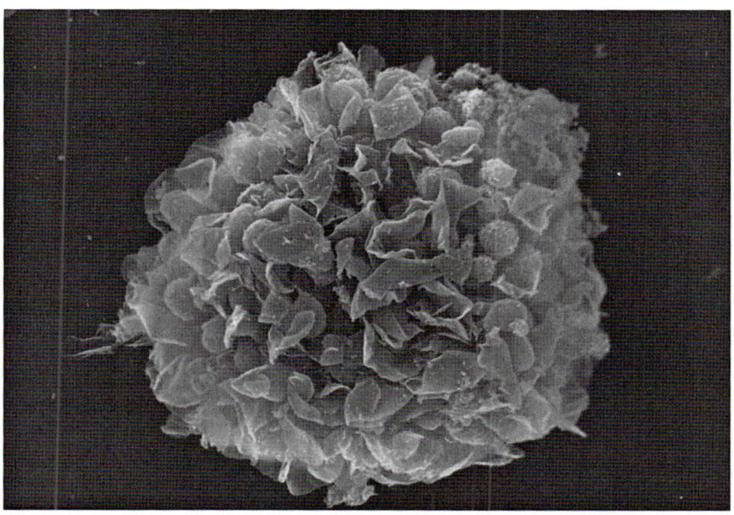

Figure 12. Scanning electron micrograph of a cluster of T cells and dendritic cells illustrates their large membrane projections. Courtesy of Dr. Gilla Kaplan.

By 1980, it was clear that dendritic cells had unique morphological features (Fig. 12), behaved differently, had specific physical properties that allowed their purification, and had remarkable T cell stimulatory activity *in vitro*. However, methods did not exist to eliminate dendritic cells from cell mixtures or to locate them in the organism. Moreover, since there were no molecular markers for dendritic cells, it was still difficult to convince anyone that they were really a distinct cell type. The first step in that direction was the development by Michel Nussenzweig of the monoclonal antibody 33D1 that is specific for the major dendritic cell subset in spleen (Nussenzweig et al., 1982). It was used to visualize dendritic cells in tissue sections and to deplete dendritic cells from complex mixtures of cells. T cell responses were decreased when dendritic cells were depleted from cell mixtures of cells (Fig. 13, (Steinman et al., 1983)). Although only 1% of the cells were killed, there was a very significant decrease in the ability of spleen cell mixtures to stimulate the mixed leukocyte reaction. Therefore, the 33D1 monoclonal antibody became a molecule that distinguished dendritic cells from other cells and a tool that could determine their role in cell mixtures.

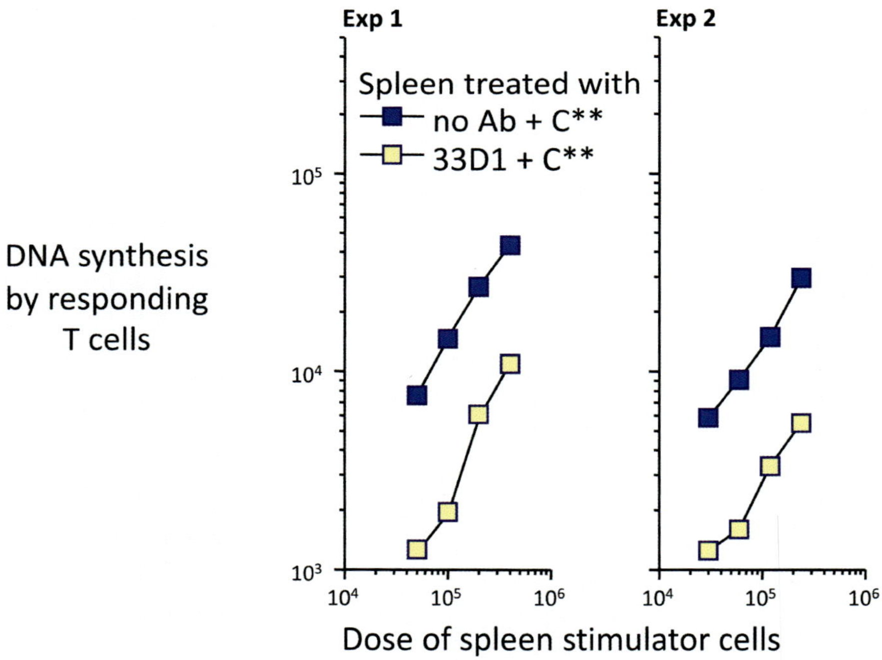

Figure 13. Graph shows results of mixed leukocyte reactions in which mixtures of spleen cells were treated with anti-33D1 monoclonal antibody to eliminate dendritic cells carrying this surface antigen and compared to untreated controls (Steinman et al., 1983). The Y axis displays DNA synthesis as measured by H3Thymidine incorporation and the X axis shows the dose of stimulator cells added to the culture. C** refers to Complement. Ab refers to antibody.

Steinman had two early collaborators who added important contributions to establishing the antigen presentation properties of dendritic cells (Fig. 14). Wes Van Voorhis, an MD-PhD student in the laboratory, was the first to study human dendritic cells; he showed they exist in blood, are distinct from blood monocytes, and are antigen presenting cells (Van Voorhis et al., 1982).

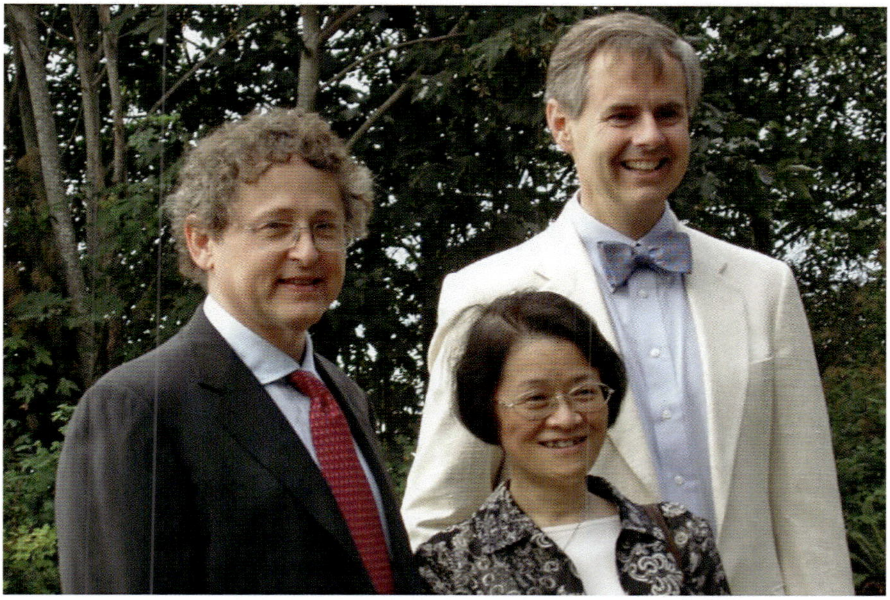

Figure 14. Ralph Steinman's early collaborators. From left to right: Michel C. Nussenzweig, Kayo Inaba, and Wesley Van Voorhis.

Kayo Inaba, who had shown independently in Japan that a non-macrophage in spleen could function as an accessory cell (Inaba et al., 1981), continued the work on antigen presentation in a variety of different systems, most notably the Mishell-Dutton system (Inaba et al., 1983a; Inaba and Steinman, 1985). When accessory functions of purified dendritic cells were compared to adherent cells or dendritic cell-depleted adherent cells, dendritic cells were found to be far superior antigen presenting cells compared to mixtures of adherent cells. Furthermore, depletion of dendritic cells from mixtures of cells using 33D1 led to a loss of accessory activity (Fig. 15) (Inaba et al., 1983a)

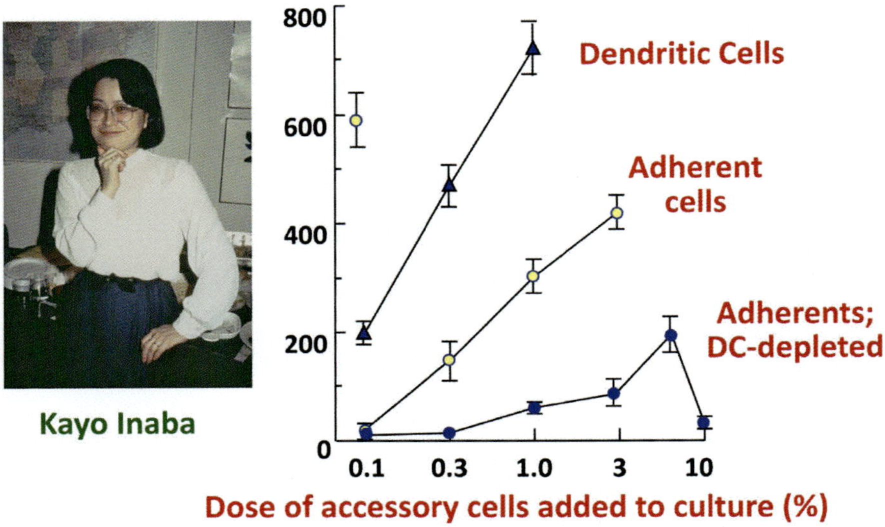

Figure 15. Kayo Inaba is shown on the left. On the right a plaque forming cell response in Mishell Dutton cultures where T and B cells are supplemented with increasing number of dendritic cells, mixtures of adherent cells or adherent cells depleted of dendritic cells that express the 33D1 antigen (Inaba and Steinman, 1985; Inaba et al., 1983b). Y axis shows the number of plaque forming cells and the X axis the number of accessory cells added to the cultures.

Based on their work at the The Rockefeller University, Nussenzweig, Inaba, and Steinman put forward a model to explain how dendritic cells capture and process the antigen and present it to T cells (Fig. 16). The interaction between T cells and dendritic cells is a cognate interaction in which T cells recognize the specific antigen being displayed by the dendritic cell. Most importantly, the interaction leads to T cell activation and allows them to perform their various effector functions. Under some conditions, the activated T cell stimulates cognate B cells to produce antibody (Fig. 16).

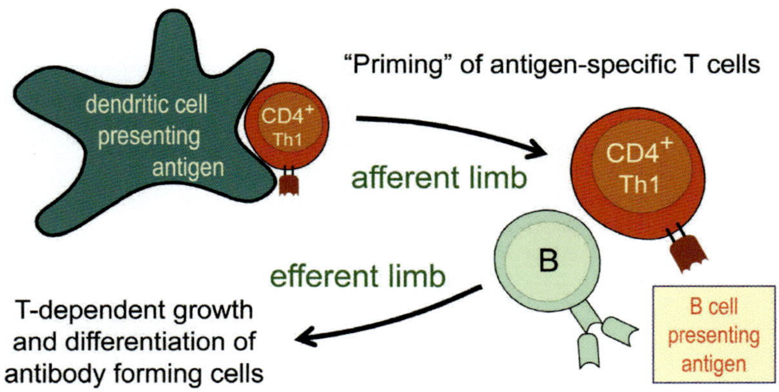

Figure 16. A model put forward by Ralph Steinman and his colleagues to explain the role of dendritic cells in inducing B cell antibody responses. Dendritic cells present antigen to and activate T cells which then interact with antigen specific B cells, by virtue of antigen presentation by the B cells.

Inaba and Steinman did an additional ground breaking experiment on anti-tumor and anti-viral activities of dendritic cells. When they removed dendritic cells from mice, loaded them with antigen, and re-infused them into mice, there was strong protective immunity (Fig. 17, (Inaba et al., 1990)). This finding established the significant principle that antigen presentation of dendritic cells in vivo could be the basis for immunotherapy experiments.

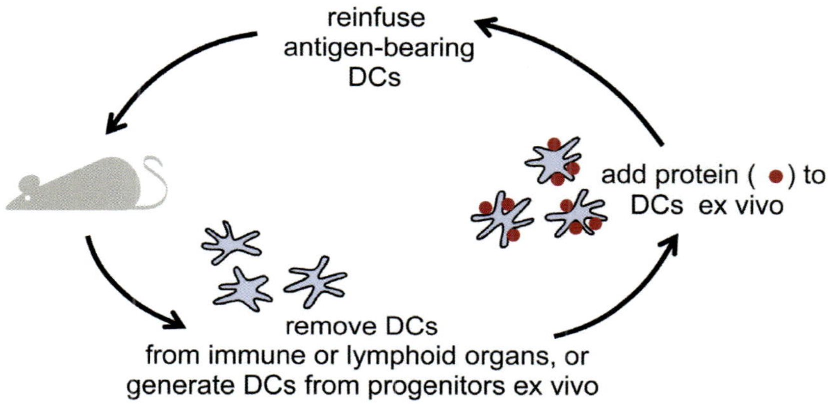

Figure 17. Diagram of the protocol for showing how antigen-loaded dendritic cells can be re-infused into mice to induce potent immune responses (Inaba et al., 1990).

Currently, immunotherapy is used in humans and is being tested by Steinman's clinical collaborators (Fig. 18). In this treatment dendritic cells are removed from the patient, expanded in culture, and loaded with the tumor antigen before being re-infused into the patient. This is the basis for the therapy of the first drug, Provenge, approved by the U.S. Food and Drug Administration to treat prostate cancer. This is also the basis for the therapy Steinman used to treat his own pancreatic cancer.

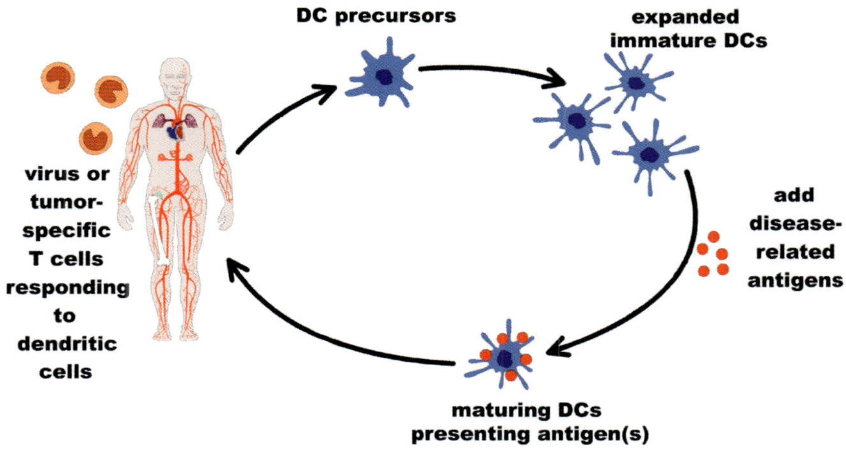

Figure 18. Diagram of the protocol for immunizing humans with antigen-loaded monocyte derived dendritic cells.

Together, these early experiments brought a new essential element to Burnet's theory concerning immune responses (Fig. 19). Burnett's idea remains that clones of lymphoid cells with specific receptors are selected to expand in response to the pathogen, but what is new is that the response depends on antigen capture and presentation by an innate cell. In this new model, the dendritic cell carries the antigen and selects the lymphocyte that is clonally expanded. This process, which was not anticipated by early immunologists, turns out to be an essential step in initiating immunity.

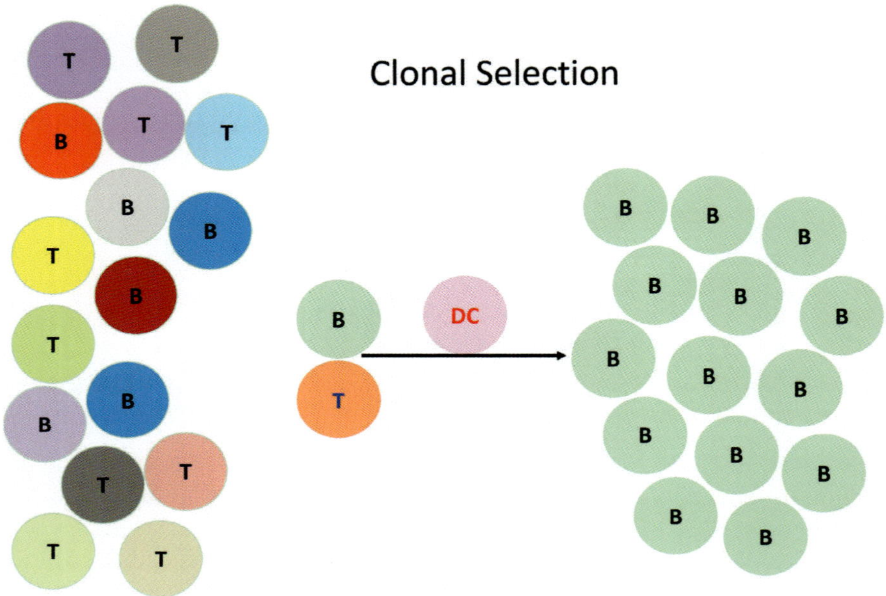

Figure 19. The role of dendritic cells in clonal selection. Antigen no longer activates the lymphocytes directly as originally proposed by Burnet and shown in Figure 4. Instead, antigen is presented to T lymphocytes or B cells by dendritic cells to initiate immunity.

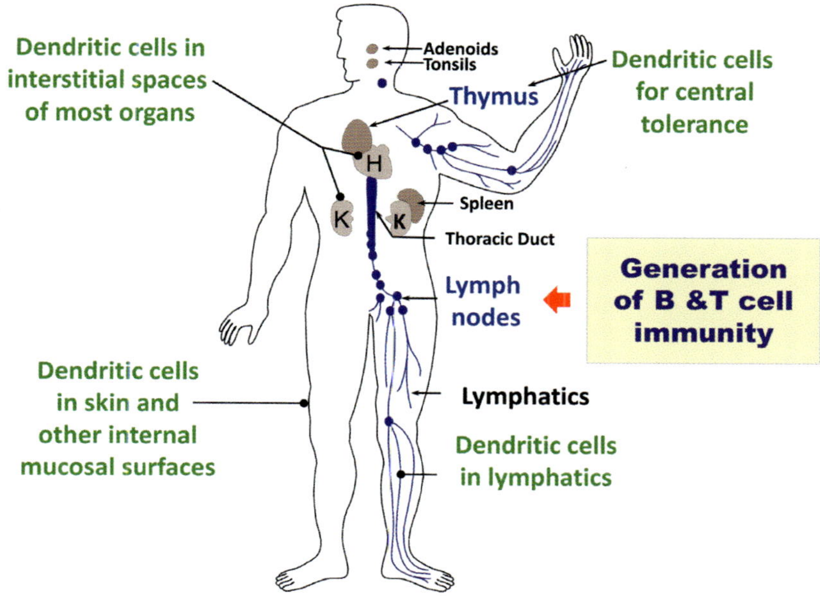

Figure 20. Diagram of the human body indicating the lymphoid organs and the location of dendritic cells in non-lymphoid organs. H referrers to heart, K referrers to kidneys.

Where are the dendritic cells located in the body (Fig. 20)? Soon after antibodies to dendritic cells became available, Steinman and his colleagues systematically investigated their location throughout the organism. The immune system, unlike the brain or the liver or heart, is a collection of cells that migrate through all the tissues in the organism. Dendritic cells are present at all the interfaces between the body and environment: airway epithelium (Fig. 21), skin, and mucosal surfaces. In other words, they are perfectly positioned to be sentinels and to capture antigens when and where they enter the organism.

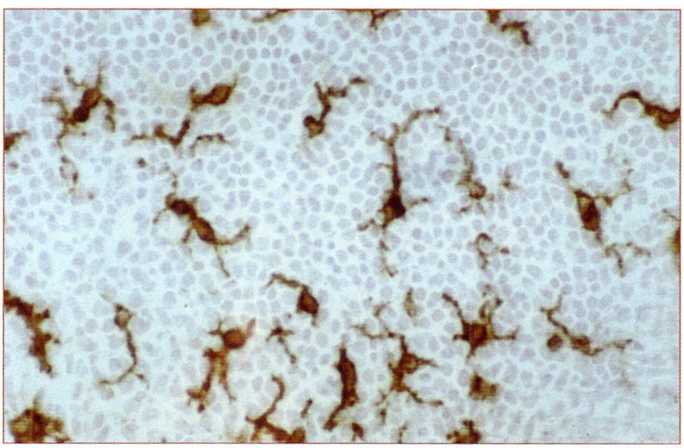

Figure 21. Micrograph showing dendritic cells in the airway epithelium. Courtesy of Dr. Patricia Holt.

Most importantly, collections of dendritic cells are found in lymphoid organs: lymph nodes (Fig. 22), spleen, tonsils, and thymus. In a movie made by 2-photon live imaging by Gabriel Victora, the dendritic cells in the T cell zone extend their processes throughout and create a dense network of cells (Movie #1). The T cells are migrating around and through this network in search of antigens on the dendritic cells (Movie #2). And when they meet an antigen on the dendritic cell, they stop, communicate, and receive the signal that activates their immune response (Movie #3). Again, the dendritic cells are in the right place where they interact with T cells in the adaptive immune system to initiate their immune response.

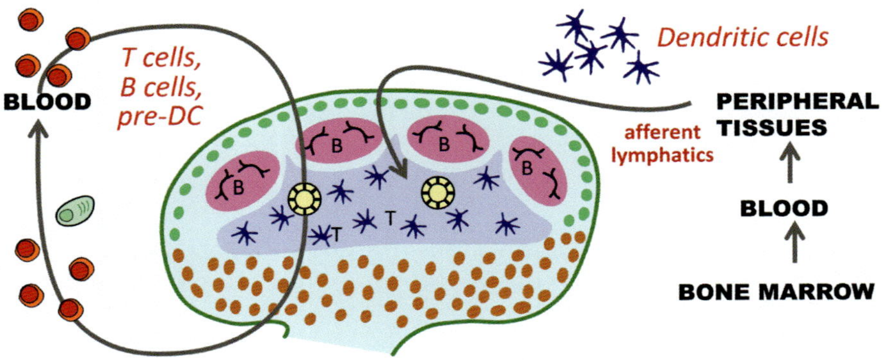

Figure 22. Diagram of a lymph node showing the position of dendritic cells in the T area. Dendritic cells arrive in the lymph node from the blood as pre-DC and from the tissues via the lymph. T and B cells circulate through the lymph nodes.

Thus, the histology showed that dendritic cells are positioned as sentinels in the innate immune system, as conceived by Metchnikov, and they are also positioned to connect with the adaptive immune system cells, as conceived by Ehrlich, to initiate the responses by effector cells.

Movie 1. Mouse lymph node with CD11c-YFP (Lindquist et al., 2004) labeled dendritic cells shown in yellow. Dendritic cells form a network in the T cell area of the node. Most cells remain in their position, and increase their surface area of antigen presentation with membrane extensions which are actively motile. Courtesy of Dr. Gabriel Victora.

Movie 2. Highlights the searching behavior displayed by the migrating blue fluorescent protein expressing T cells in a lymph node where dendritic cells are yellow labeled with CD11c-YFP.

Movie 3. Highlights T cell behavior upon meeting a dendritic cell presenting its cognate antigen. The T cell (fuchsia) remains in contact with the dendritic cell for a prolonged period of time.

DENDRITIC CELL MATURATION

Another important discovery made by Steinman and colleagues during the mid-1980s was that dendritic cells do not exist in just one state. In order to initiate immune responses, they need to be activated by signals from pathogens or other activated immune cells. Steinman called this step maturation. Working with Gerold Schuler, a dermatologist, and Nikolaus Romani (Fig. 23) (Schuler and Steinman, 1985), Steinman found that immature dendritic cells are either poor stimulators or unable to induce immunity. However, once dendritic cells received activation signals, such as innate signals from Toll receptors, they matured, expressed high levels of MHC antigens, and became excellent antigen presenting cells (Fig. 24). Ira Mellman at Yale University working closely with Steinman uncovered the cellular basis of this phenomenon (Pierre et al., 1997). They showed that the switch between inactive and active states could in part be explained by re-distribution of MHC Class II molecules from lysosomes in immature dendritic cells to their cell surface during maturation where they would be recognized by T cells (Fig. 24).

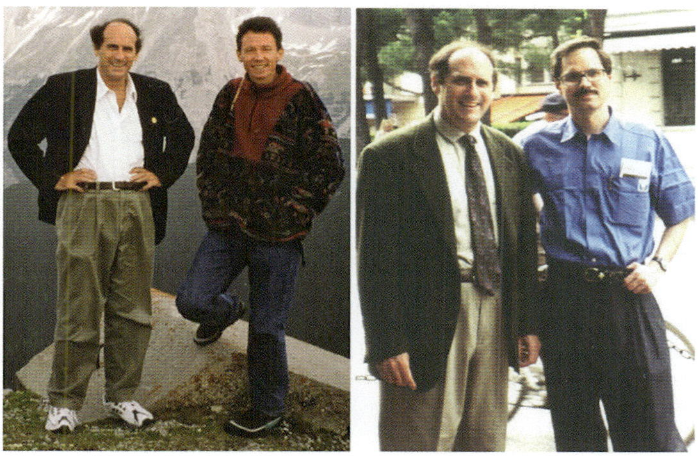

Figure 23. Ralph Steinman's collaborators Nikolaus Romani (left) and Gerold Schuler (right).

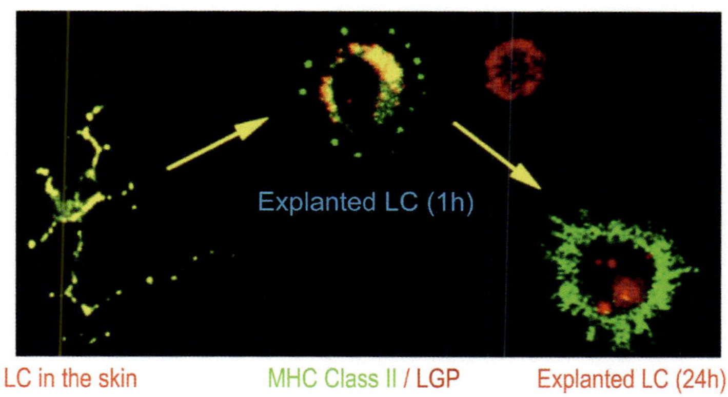

Figure 24. Cell biological basis for dendritic cell maturation. MHC Class II is found in vesicles inside the cell in the immature state and translocated to the cell surface in mature dendritic cells (Pierre et al., 1997). LGP is lysosomal membrane protein lgp-b/lamp-2. LC is Langerhans cell.

Based on these experiments, Steinman and his colleagues proposed the following model (Fig. 25). Dendritic cells can be found in two states of activation. In the immature state, they express antigen capture receptors and pattern recognition receptors that can induce activation. In the activated or mature state, they express high levels of co-stimulatory molecules for T cell activation and MHC surface antigens. The transition between these two states can be modulated by microbial products including Toll receptor ligands as well as by signals such as cytokines and ligation of the costimulatory protein CD40 (Fig. 25).

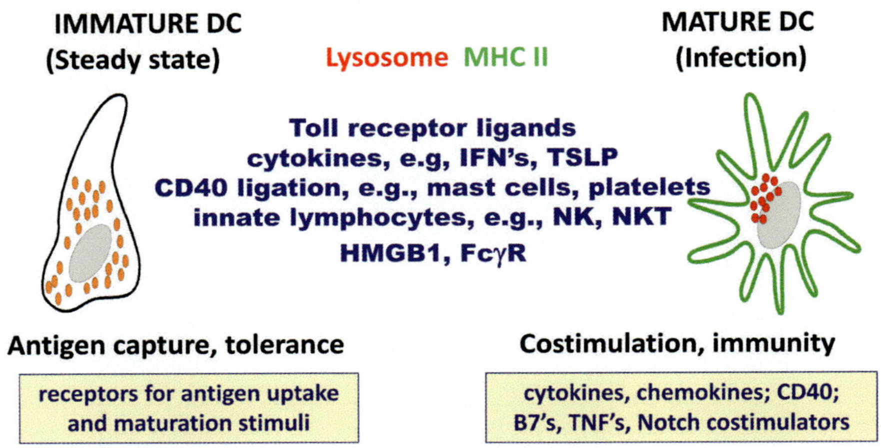

Figure 25. The diagram summarizes the idea that dendritic cells act as sensors which can be induced to undergo maturation as a result of Toll like receptor signaling or signaling by a number of other pathways. In the immature state dendritic cells are specialized for antigen capture, and in the mature state they up-regulate surface molecules required for T cell activation and polarization.

Steinman then suggested the following paradigm (Fig. 26). When a dendritic cell at a body surface receives an innate signal from the incoming pathogen by virtue of, for example, Toll receptor ligation, it becomes activated or mature. The mature dendritic cell then migrates to the local lymph node to join the networks of dendritic cells that contact migrating T and B cells. In addition to presenting antigen, the dendritic cell orchestrates the adaptive immune response by activating effector T cells. The activated T cells then leave the dendritic cell network in the lymphoid organ and patrol the body for invading pathogens.

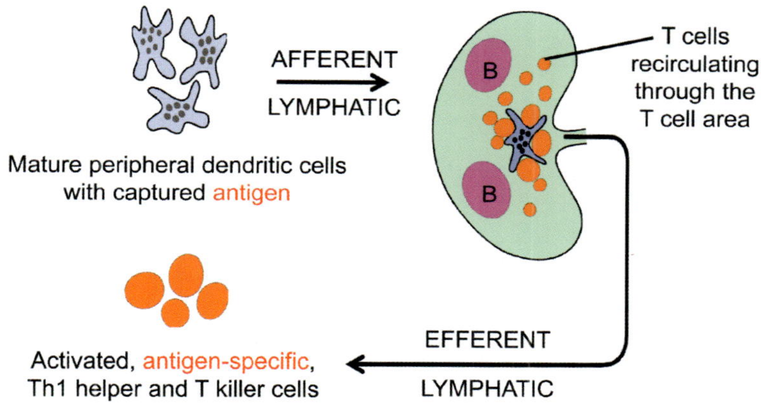

Figure 26. Proposed pathway for antigen capture and activation by peripheral dendritic cells and traffic to the lymph nodes where they present antigen to T cells. Activated T cells leave the lymph nodes and circulate in the organism.

IMMUNE TOLERANCE

An important test of the idea that dendritic cells initiate immunity was to deliver an antigen to dendritic cells in vivo. Until 2001 all experiments showing that dendritic cells activate immunity had been performed by removing dendritic cells from their natural environment and testing their function after in vitro manipulations. Daniel Hawiger, a graduate student in Nussenzweig's laboratory devised a system to test dendritic cell function in vivo by delivering antigen to these cells in situ (Hawiger et al., 2001). What he did was to engineer a monoclonal antibody specific to a molecule on dendritic cells, DEC-205 (Jiang et al., 1995) (Fig. 27), that would then serve as a specific delivery vehicle to carry the antigen to the dendritic cell (Fig. 28). When injected into a mouse, the chimeric antibody bound to dendritic cells and thereby delivered the antigen. Antigen delivered to dendritic cells in this manner was far more efficient than soluble antigen in inducing T cell responses (Fig. 29). Moreover, because antibodies have a long half-life (Fig. 30), their targeting of dendritic cells lasted for days, and there were prolonged T cell responses with immunity strong enough to reject tumors or handle a viral infection (Bonifaz et al., 2004)

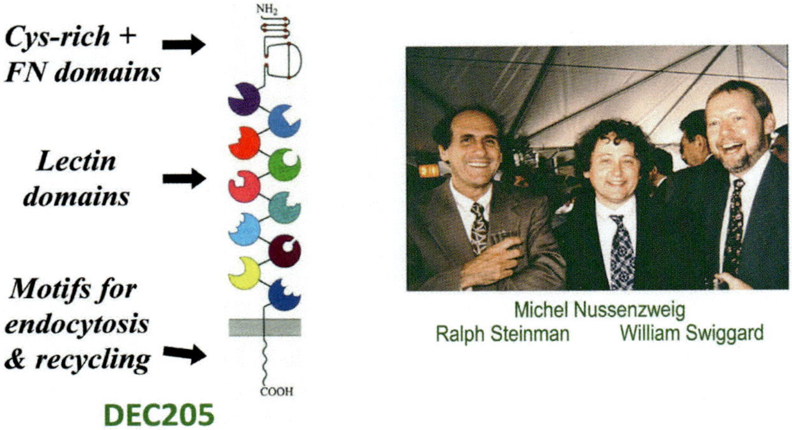

Figure 27. Diagram shows the domain structure of the DEC-205 molecule (left). Photograph of Ralph Steinman, Michel Nussenzweig and William Swiggard, who with Wanping Jiang cloned the molecule (Jiang et al., 1995).

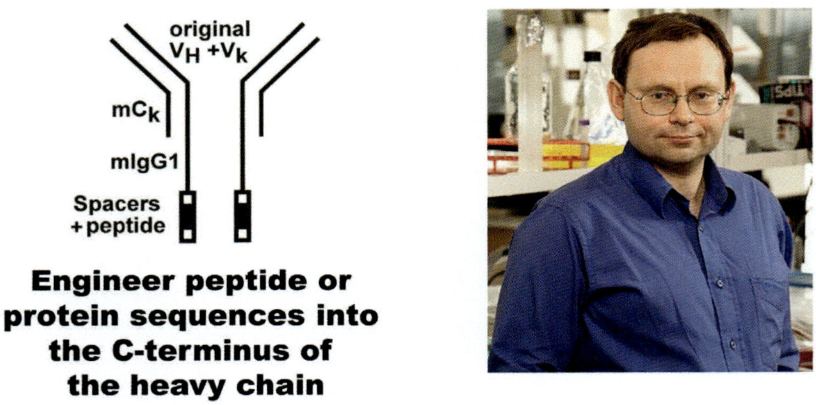

Figure 28. The diagram shows strategy for delivering antigens to dendritic cells in vivo using anti-DEC-205 fusion antibodies (left) developed by Daniel Hawiger (photograph right) (Hawiger et al., 2001).

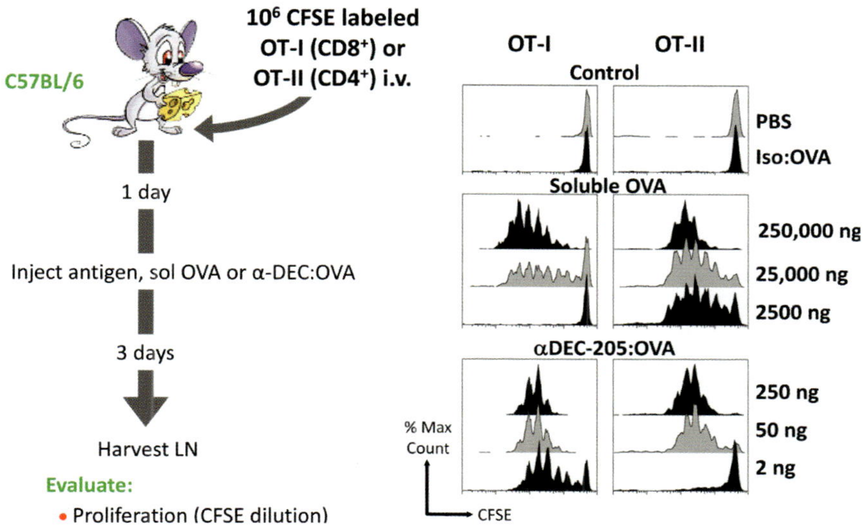

Figure 29. Dendritic cell targeted antigen is far more efficient than soluble antigen in inducing T cell responses. Experimental protocol (left) and OTI class I restricted, ovalbumin specific CD8+) or OTII (class II restricted, ovalbumin specific CD4+) T cell responses to injected soluble antigen, or antigen targeted to dendritic cells by DEC-205 (right) (Hawiger et al., 2001). OVA is ovalbumin.

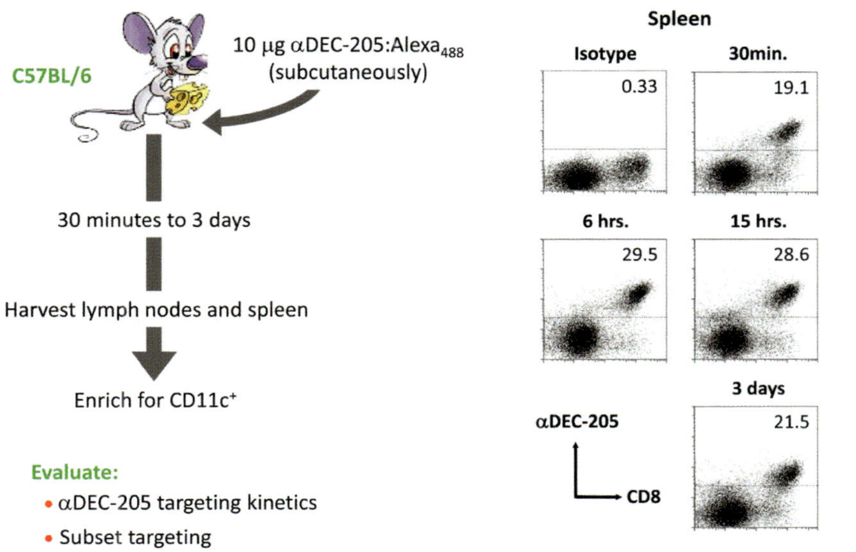

Figure 30. Dendritic cell targeting by DEC-205 fusion antibodies results in long lasting antigen targeting to dendritic cells. Experimental protocol (left) and time course showing long lasting dendritic cell associated DEC-205 in vivo (right) (Hawiger et al., 2001).

When dendritic cells were activated by Toll receptor ligation or some other stimulus by giving antigen along with a maturation stimulus, the result was robust immunity (Fig. 31, (Hawiger et al., 2001)). But when the antigen was administered alone, T cells, instead of becoming effector cells for immune responses, were stopped from responding by one of a number of different mechanisms. They were either deleted, silenced (anergized), or actively induced to become regulatory T cells (Fig. 32, (Hawiger et al., 2001; Hawiger et al., 2004; Kretschmer et al., 2005)).

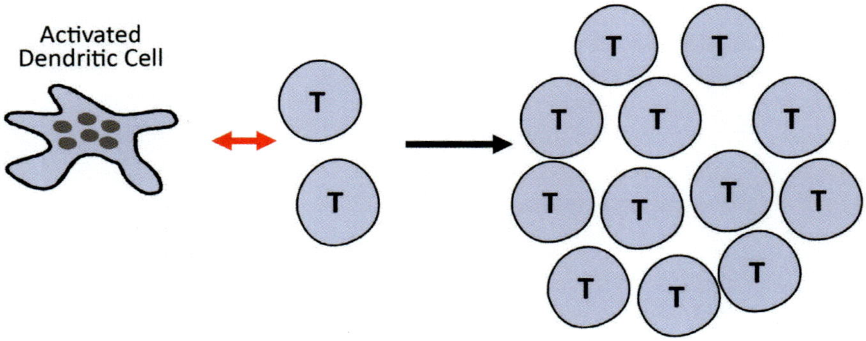

Figure 31. The diagram shows antigen specific T cell clonal expansion and activation by dendritic cells that present antigen after activation by CD40 or Toll receptor ligands (Hawiger et al., 2001).

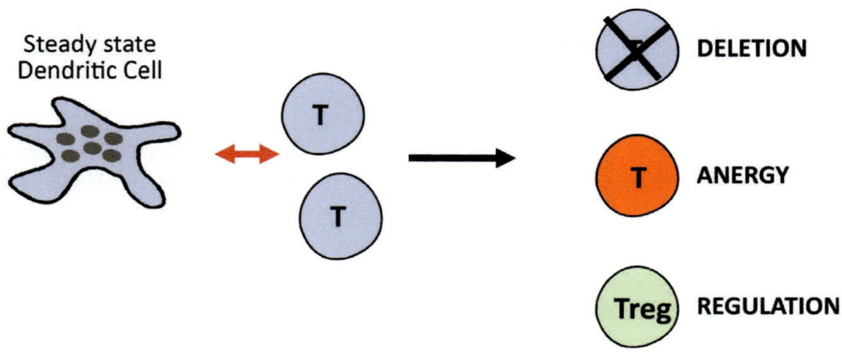

Figure 32. The diagram summarizes the observation that antigen presentation by steady state dendritic cells results in T cell tolerance by deletion, anergy or induction of T regulatory cells (Hawiger et al., 2001; Hawiger et al., 2004; Kretschmer et al., 2005).

This important experiment added an unanticipated role of dendritic cells to maintain tolerance. The model put forward by Nussenzweig and Steinman is that under resting conditions, dendritic cells are continually capturing self-antigens from serum or dying cells. These antigens are also continually being presented to T cells. In the absence of an activation signal, the self-reactive cells are silenced (Steinman and Nussenzweig, 2002). This is one of the mechanisms by which the immune system averts Ehrlich's horror autotoxicus. During viral infections, for example, the dendritic cells pick up a mixture of self and non-self antigens, all of which are presented to T cells. The previous silencing of the self-reactive cells allows the immune system to avoid attacking self and to focus on the invading viruses, bacteria, or toxins (Fig. 33).

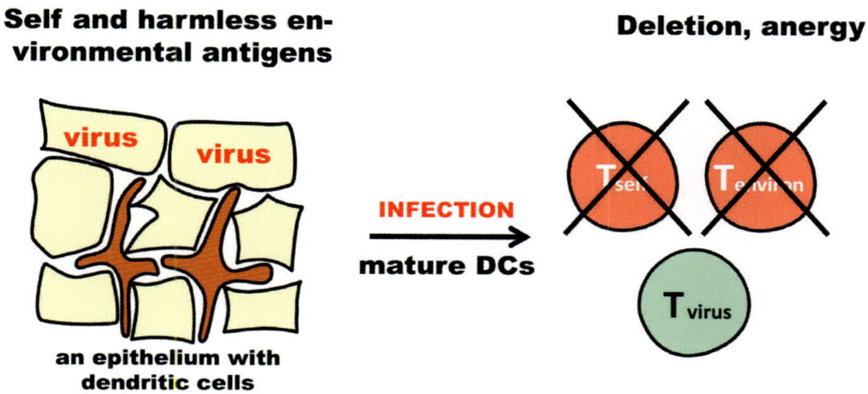

Figure 33. Induction of T cell tolerance by steady state DCs is required to prevent anti-self reactivity during immune responses to pathogens. Steady state dendritic cells capture, process and present self-antigen to T cells resulting in tolerance. The same self-antigens are also processed and presented by dendritic cells when they capture pathogen-infected cells, but the immune response is focused on the pathogen because the anti-self reactive T cells were previously silenced in the steady state (Steinman and Nussenzweig, 2002).

Thus, the dendritic cell discovery and its role in directing both tolerance and immunity not only connects innate and adaptive immune responses but also helps to explain how self-reactivity is removed from the adaptive repertoire to prevent autoimmunity, or Ehrlich's horror autotoxicus.

DENDRITIC CELL LINEAGE AND DEVELOPMENT

From the beginning, Steinman was interested in the relationship of dendritic cells to monocytes and macrophages. Many laboratories have contributed to solving this problem, but the first breakthrough came from Frederic Geissman (Fogg et al., 2006). He fractionated developing bone marrow cells looking for progenitors of dendritic cells and found that myeloid progenitors could give rise to dendritic cells whereas lymphoid progenitors did not. Most importantly, Geissman defined a bone marrow progenitor that was restricted to producing dendritic cells and monocytes, but not lymphoid cells or granulocytes (Fogg et al., 2006).

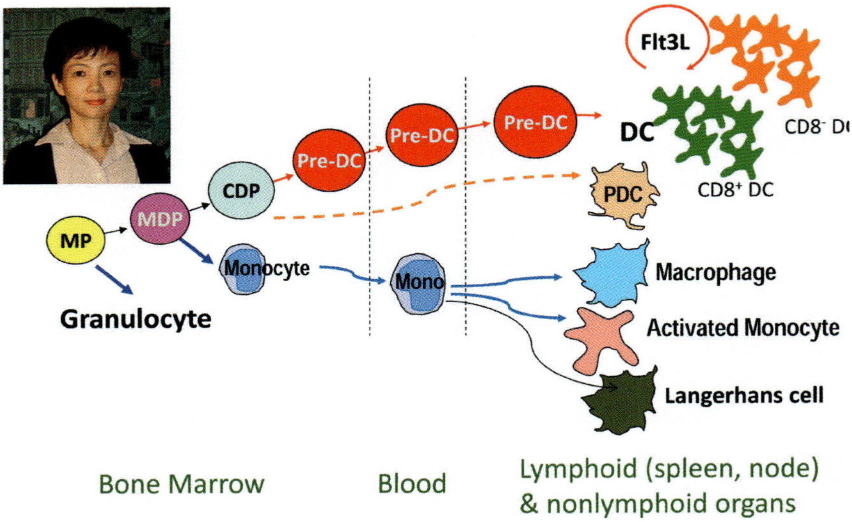

Figure 34. Dendritic cell development. Kang Liu (photograph left) and a diagram of the cellular intermediates in the dendritic cell development pathway in the bone marrow blood and tissues. The dendritic cell pathway splits from the monocyte pathway in the bone marrow after the common macrophage and dendritic cell precursor state. Pre-dendritic cells leave the bone marrow and enter the tissues (Liu et al., 2009). MP is myeloid progenitor, MDP is monocyte-dendritic cell progenitor, CDP is common dendritic cell progenitor, and PDC is plamacytoid dendritic cell.

Kang Liu and Claudia Waskow accomplished the next key experiments during their postdoctoral fellowships in Nussenzweig's laboratory (Fig. 34). (Liu et al., 2009; Waskow et al., 2008) They found that monocyte and dendritic cell lineages split from each other in the bone marrow. The monocyte-dendritic cell progenitor discovered by Geissman produces monocytes and also produces a more developed progenitor that is committed to the dendritic cell lineage and can no longer produce monocytes. Instead, this dendritic cell committed progenitor is limited to producing plasmacytoid dendritic cells and pre-dendritic cells that leave the bone marrow and enter tissues where they further divide in response to a hematopoietic growth factor called Flt3L to give rise to the two major subsets of dendritic cells in lymphoid and non-lymphoid tissues. Exactly how these differentiation steps are controlled is still not known.

DENDRITIC CELL-BASED VACCINES

Steinman liked to emphasize that vaccines by and large have not been created by immunologists. Instead microbiologists, like Pasteur, used attenuated microbes to stimulate the immune system. Steinman's frequently stated goal was to use immunology to create vaccines. He spent the last four years of his life investigating ways to harness dendritic cells to produce vaccines.

The features of dendritic cells that Steinman wanted to exploit to produce immunity were 1) specific receptors for antigen uptake and processing, such as DEC-205; 2) pattern recognition receptors that activate or mature dendritic cells, such as the Toll like receptor ligand; and 3) the various pathways of dendritic cell development into their different subsets (Fig. 35).

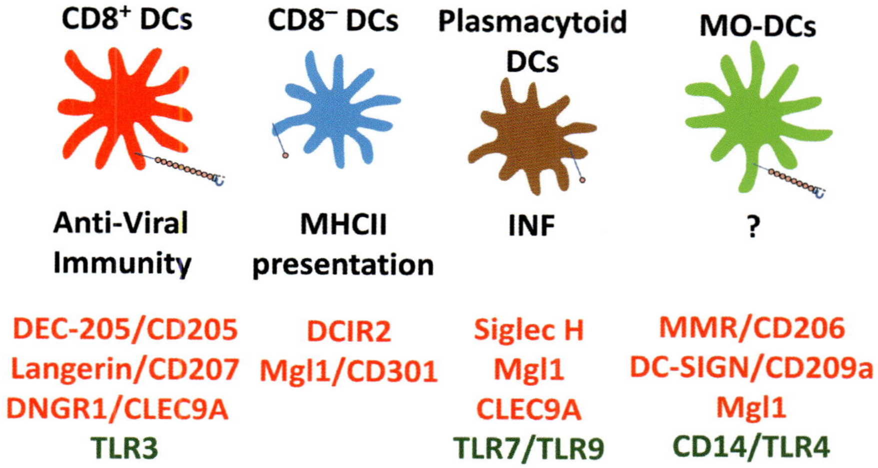

Figure 35. Subsets of dendritic cells, their functional specializations, and receptors that might be used to target or activate each one specifically.

The conceptual framework for Steinman's new vaccines was based on Daniel Hawiger's experiment (Hawiger et al., 2001), that is, using antigens specific for HIV, tuberculosis, allergy, diabetes, or cancer tied to a specific antibody serving as a delivery vehicle that would reach dendritic cells (Fig. 36). In addition, this type of immunization would require different adjuvants to activate dendritic cells. Unlike other vaccines, this one would be delivered to dendritic cells throughout the body because the antibody would carry the antigen to all dendritic cells. The idea was that by using different receptors to target different dendritic cells and different innate stimuli, these vaccines could activate different types of immunity. For example, Steinman ambitiously considered and planned vaccines to prevent or treat cancer and infection as mediated by Th1 and Th2 immunity as well as vaccines to regulate allergy and inflammation by inducing regulatory T cells.

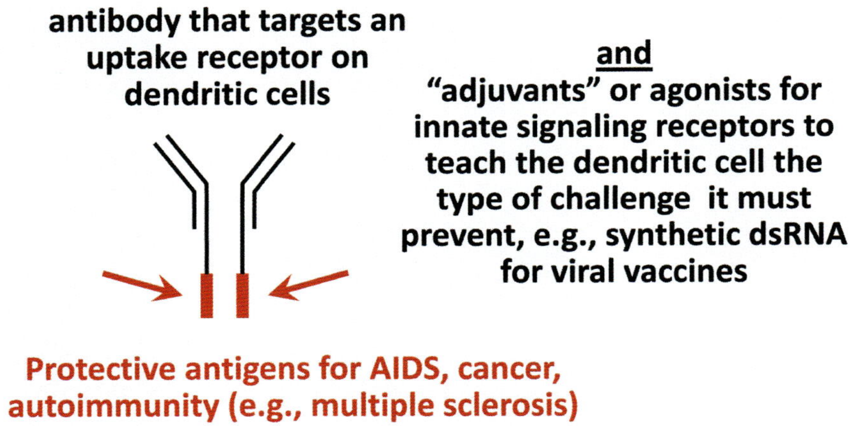

Figure 36. Suggested approach to dendritic cell-based vaccines for humans. Antibodies to endocytic receptors on dendritic cells are used as fusion proteins to target antigens to specific dendritic cells in vivo (left). Toll receptor ligands or other agents activate dendritic cells in specific ways (right).

Steinman's success in mouse models with anti-cancer (Fig. 37) and anti-viral immune responses encouraged him to use this approach in humans. His clinical group at The Rockefeller University Hospital is currently conducting the first proof-of-concept study in a phase one clinical trial (Fig. 38). The vaccine consists of a HIV gag p24 protein engineered into anti-DEC-205 antibody and is administered together with a Toll receptor 3 ligand (Poly ICLC) as the adjuvant to mature the dendritic cells.

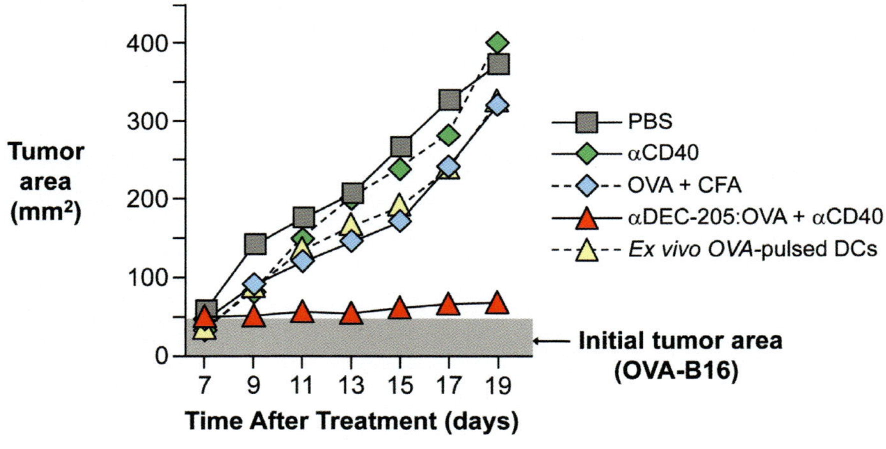

Figure 37. Strong protective immunity to B16-OVA melanoma after vaccination with anti-DEC-205-OVA and CD40 ligation. X axis is time after tumor challenge, Y axis is tumor size. OVA is ovalbumin. (Bonifaz et al., 2004).

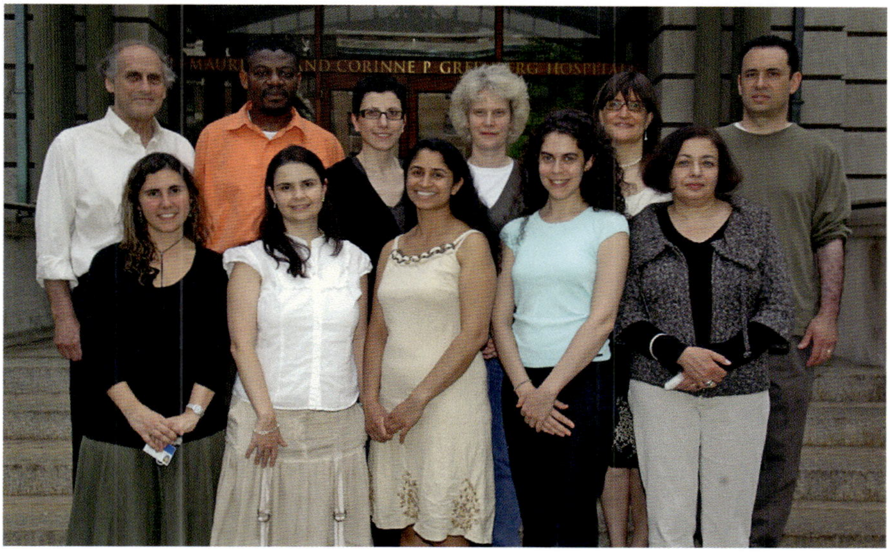

Figure 38. Ralph Steinman's clinical team standing in front of The Rockefeller University Hospital. Top left to right: Ralph Steinman, Godwin Nchinda, Leonia Bozzacco, Christine Trumpfheller, Sarah Schlesinger, Jules Hoffman. Bottom, left to right: Paula Longhi, Marina Caskey, Niroshana Anandasabapathy, Sarah Pollak, Irina Shimeliovich. 28 April 2009, courtesy of The Rockefeller University.

EPILOGUE

Ralph Steinman created a revolution in immunology when he discovered a beautiful cell by just looking through a microscope. During the following forty years at The Rockefeller University, he characterized this cell and elucidated its roles in immunity. He showed that dendritic cells are critical for initiating the most important immune responses. He described their three central features. Dendritic cells are "Sentinels" that capture pathogens, as Metchnikov suggested. They are "Sensors" for infection that use their cell surface pattern recognition receptors like Toll to become activated. And, once activated, they become "Conductors" of the immune orchestra whose individual cells play harmonious roles to protect and regulate the body's immune system. Dendritic cells link Metchnikov to Ehrlich (Fig. 39).

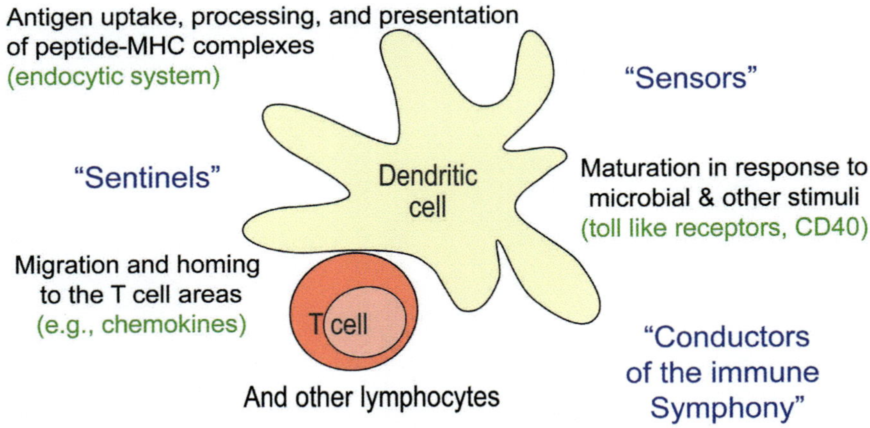

Figure 39. Dendritic cells are innate cells that activate adaptive responses. The diagram shows that dendritic cells are sentinels positioned in tissues to detect pathogens or inflammation; they act as sensors by virtue of expression of receptors that detect pathogens or other inflammatory signals; and they are conductors of the immune symphony as they process and present antigen to activate adaptive immune responses.

Ralph Steinman was excited in 1973 when he discovered dendritic cells. And in 2011, he was confident they would form the basis of still unknown medical advances.

ACKNOWLEDGMENTS

Dr. Svetlana Mojsov for discussions, Drs. Svetlana Mojsov and Carol Moberg for help with the manuscript, and Judy Adams for help with the figures.

BIBLIOGRAPHY

Bonifaz, L.C., Bonnyay, D.P., Charalambous, A., Darguste, D.I., Fujii, S., Soares, H., Brimnes, M.K., Moltedo, B., Moran, T.M., and Steinman, R.M. (2004), "In vivo targeting of antigens to maturing dendritic cells via the DEC-205 receptor improves T cell vaccination," *J Exp Med* **199**, 815–824.

Burnet, F.M. (1957), "A modification of Jerne's thory of antibody production using the concept of clonal selection," *Australian Journal of Science* **20**, 67–68.

Burnet, M. (1958), *The clonal selection theory of acquired immunity* (Nashville, Vanderbilt University Press).

Ehrenreich, B.A., and Cohn, Z.A. (1967), "The uptake and digestion of iodinated human serum albumin by macrophages in vitro," *J Exp Med* **126**, 941–958.

Fogg, D.K., Sibon, C., Miled, C., Jung, S., Aucouturier, P., Littman, D.R., Cumano, A., and Geissmann, F. (2006), "A clonogenic bone marrow progenitor specific for macrophages and dendritic cells," *Science* **311**, 83–87.

Hawiger, D., Inaba, K., Dorsett, Y., Guo, M., Mahnke, K., Rivera, M., Ravetch, J.V., Steinman, R.M., and Nussenzweig, M.C. (2001), "Dendritic cells induce peripheral T cell unresponsiveness under steady state conditions in vivo," *The Journal of experimental medicine* **194**, 769–779.

Hawiger, D., Masilamani, R.F., Bettelli, E., Kuchroo, V.K., and Nussenzweig, M.C. (2004), "Immunological unresponsiveness characterized by increased expression of CD5 on peripheral T cells induced by dendritic cells in vivo," *Immunity* **20**, 695–705.

Hirsch, J.G., and Moberg, C.L. (1989), "Rene Dubos," *Biographical Memoirs of the National Academy of Sciences* **58**, 132–161.

Inaba, K., Granelli-Piperno, A., and Steinman, R.M. (1983a), "Dendritic cells induce T lymphocytes to release B cell-stimulating factors by an interleukin 2-dependent mechanism," *J Exp Med* **158**, 2040–2057.

Inaba, K., Metlay, J.P., Crowley, M.T., and Steinman, R.M. (1990), "Dendritic cells pulsed with protein antigens in vitro can prime antigen-specific, MHC-restricted T cells in situ," *The Journal of experimental medicine* **172**, 631–640.

Inaba, K., Nakano, K., and Muramatsu, S. (1981), "Cellular synergy in the manifestation of accessory cell activity for in vitro antibody response," *J Immunol* **127**, 452–461.

Inaba, K., and Steinman, R.M. (1985), "Protein-specific helper T-lymphocyte formation initiated by dendritic cells," *Science* **229**, 475–479.

Inaba, K., Steinman, R.M., Van Voorhis, W.C., and Muramatsu, S. (1983b), "Dendritic cells are critical accessory cells for thymus-dependent antibody responses in mouse and in man," *Proc Natl Acad Sci USA* **80**, 6041–6045.

Jiang, W., Swiggard, W.J., Heufler, C., Peng, M., Mirza, A., Steinman, R.M., and Nussenzweig, M.C. (1995), "The receptor DEC-205 expressed by dendritic cells and thymic epithelial cells is involved in antigen processing," *Nature* **375**, 151–155.

Kretschmer, K., Apostolou, I., Hawiger, D., Khazaie, K., Nussenzweig, M.C., and von Boehmer, H. (2005), "Inducing and expanding regulatory T cell populations by foreign antigen," *Nat Immunol* **6**, 1219–1227.

Lederberg, J. (1959), "Genes and antibodies," *Science* **129**, 1649–1653.

Lindquist, R.L., Shakhar, G., Dudziak, D., Wardemann, H., Eisenreich, T., Dustin, M.L., and Nussenzweig, M.C. (2004), "Visualizing dendritic cell networks in vivo," *Nat Immunol* **5**, 1243–1250.

Liu, K., Victora, G.D., Schwickert, T.A., Guermonprez, P., Meredith, M.M., Yao, K., Chu, F.F., Randolph, G.J., Rudensky, A.Y., and Nussenzweig, M. (2009), "In vivo analysis of dendritic cell development and homeostasis," *Science* **324**, 392–397.

Mishell, R.I., and Dutton, R.W. (1967), "Immunization of dissociated spleen cell cultures from normal mice," *J Exp Med* **126**, 423–442.

Moberg, C.L., and Steinman, R. (2003), "James Gerald Hirsch, 1922–1987," *Biographical Memoirs of the National Academy of Sciences* **84**, 182–203.

Moberg, C.L., and Steinman, R. (2009), "Zanvil Cohn, 1926–1993," *Biographical Memoirs of the National Academy of Sciences.*

Nossal, G.J., Abbot, A., Mitchell, J., and Lummus, Z. (1968), "Antigens in immunity. XV. Ultrastructural features of antigen capture in primary and secondary lymphoid follicles," *J Exp Med* **127**, 277–290.

Nussenzweig, M.C., Steinman, R.M., Gutchinov, B., and Cohn, Z.A. (1980), "Dendritic cells are accessory cells for the development of anti-trinitrophenyl cytotoxic T lymphocytes," *J Exp Med* **152**, 1070–1084.

Nussenzweig, M.C., Steinman, R.M., Witmer, M.D., and Gutchinov, B. (1982), "A monoclonal antibody specific for mouse dendritic cells," *Proc Natl Acad Sci USA* **79**, 161–165.

Paul, W.E. (2011), "Bridging innate and adaptive immunity," *Cell* **147**, 1212–1215.

Pierre, P., Turley, S.J., Gatti, E., Hull, M., Meltzer, J., Mirza, A., Inaba, K., Steinman, R.M., and Mellman, I. (1997), "Developmental regulation of MHC class II transport in mouse dendritic cells," *Nature* **388**, 787–792.

Schuler, G., and Steinman, R.M. (1985), "Murine epidermal Langerhans cells mature into potent immunostimulatory dendritic cells in vitro," *The Journal of experimental medicine* **161**, 526–546.

Steinman, R.M., and Cohn, Z.A. (1972a), "The interaction of particulate horseradish peroxidase (HRP)-anti HRP immune complexes with mouse peritoneal macrophages in vitro," *J Cell Biol* **55,** 616–634.

Steinman, R.M., and Cohn, Z.A. (1972b), "The interaction of soluble horseradish peroxidase with mouse peritoneal macrophages in vitro," *J Cell Biol* **55**, 186–204.

Steinman, R.M., and Cohn, Z.A. (1973), "Identification of a novel cell type in peripheral lymphoid organs of mice. I. Morphology, quantitation, tissue distribution," *J Exp Med* **137**, 1142–1162.

Steinman, R.M., and Cohn, Z.A. (1974), "Identification of a novel cell type in peripheral lymphoid organs of mice. II. Functional properties in vitro," J Exp Med 139, 380–397.

Steinman, R.M., Gutchinov, B., Witmer, M.D., and Nussenzweig, M.C. (1983), "Dendritic cells are the principal stimulators of the primary mixed leukocyte reaction in mice," *J Exp Med* **157**, 613–627.

Steinman, R.M., and Nussenzweig, M.C. (2002), "Avoiding horror autotoxicus: the importance of dendritic cells in peripheral T cell tolerance," *Proc Natl Acad Sci USA* **99**, 351–358.

Steinman, R.M., and Witmer, M.D. (1978), "Lymphoid dendritic cells are potent stimulators of the primary mixed leukocyte reaction in mice," *Proc Natl Acad Sci USA* **75**, 5132–5136.

Talmage, D.W. (1957), "Allergy and immunology," *Annu Rev Med* **8**, 239–256.

Unanue, E.R., and Cerottini, J.C. (1970), "The immunogenicity of antigen bound to the plasma membrane of macrophages," *J Exp Med* **131**, 711–725.

Van Voorhis, W.C., Hair, L.S., Steinman, R.M., and Kaplan, G. (1982), "Human dendritic cells. Enrichment and characterization from peripheral blood," *J Exp Med* **155**, 1172–1187.

Waskow, C., Liu, K., Darrasse-Jeze, G., Guermonprez, P., Ginhoux, F., Merad, M., Shengelia, T., Yao, K., and Nussenzweig, M. (2008), "The receptor tyrosine kinase Flt3 is required for dendritic cell development in peripheral lymphoid tissues," *Nat Immunol* **9**, 676–683.

Physiology or Medicine 2012

Sir John B. Gurdon and Shinya Yamanaka

"for the discovery that mature cells can be reprogrammed to become pluripotent"

The Nobel Prize in Physiology or Medicine

Speech by Professor Thomas Perlmann of the Nobel Assembly at Karolinska Institutet.

Your Majesties, Your Royal Highnesses, Honoured Nobel Laureates, Ladies and Gentlemen,

We can assume that more than one of us here at the Stockholm Concert Hall has sometimes thought it might be desirable to once again be young, wild and maybe a little crazy – and perhaps be offered the opportunity to grow up another time and try a different path than the one we chose early in life. Now, if this person were not an adult human being but instead a mature cell, such a journey through time would actually be possible. This has been demonstrated through the discoveries that are being honoured with this year's Nobel Prize in Physiology or Medicine.

Each of us developed from a fertilised egg cell that – by means of cell divisions – gave rise to all the different types of cells that form a complete human being. During this controlled developmental process, immature cells successively form all the specialised cell types found in our organs, such as the liver, lungs and brain.

For a long time, it was believed that this could only be a one-way journey. After all, development always progresses from immature cells in the early embryo towards specialisation in adult humans. It was assumed that perhaps cells do not retain all the genetic information that is needed to produce all types of cells, so the return journey is no longer possible.

This picture fundamentally changed as a result of John Gurdon's cloning experiments, which were published in the 1960s. Gurdon destroyed the nucleus with its genetic material in a frog's egg and replaced it with the nucleus from an intestinal cell of a tadpole. Even though its genetic material came from a specialised intestinal cell, the altered frog's egg was still able to develop into all sorts of mature cells in an adult frog. Gurdon had thus demonstrated that all the information needed to regenerate all of the animal's cells is preserved during cell development. He had carried out the first cloning of a vertebrate.

These findings surprised the research community, and it took time before Gurdon's discovery became generally accepted. But his findings were confirmed, and most people have heard of Dolly, the world's first cloned mammal – a sheep that was produced according to the principle that Gurdon had used in his frog experiments.

More than 40 years after Gurdon's discovery, Shinya Yamanaka performed experiments that signified a new scientific breakthrough in the field. Gurdon had shown that the journey back to an immature state is possible. But could this journey take place in a mature cell, without the help of an egg cell? Was it instead possible to find genes that could start the return journey in a mature cell? Yamanaka selected genes that are important to immature so-called pluripotent stem cells and introduced them into mature skin cells. A combination of only four genes proved sufficient. These findings amazed the research world, since few could have imagined that such a simple recipe could return mature cells to the stem cell stage.

The publication of Yamanaka's findings in 2006 triggered amazingly rapid advances. Human skin cells can now be reprogrammed into stem cells, and in tissue cultures they can form nerve cells or heart muscle cells, for example. We now have access to entirely new tools for a better understanding of diseases and for the development of new diagnostics and therapies.

This year's Laureates have thus provided mature cells with a return ticket. They have thereby fundamentally changed our view of human development and cell specialisation.

Professor Gurdon and Professor Yamanaka,

Your groundbreaking research has demonstrated that it is possible to unlock the differentiated state and allow mature cells to return to an immature state from which all types of cells can be derived. Your discoveries have provided entirely new tools of immense value for the development of new diagnostics and therapies. On behalf of the Nobel Assembly at Karolinska Institutet, I wish to convey to you our warmest congratulations. May I now ask you to step forward to receive the Nobel Prize from the hands of His Majesty the King.

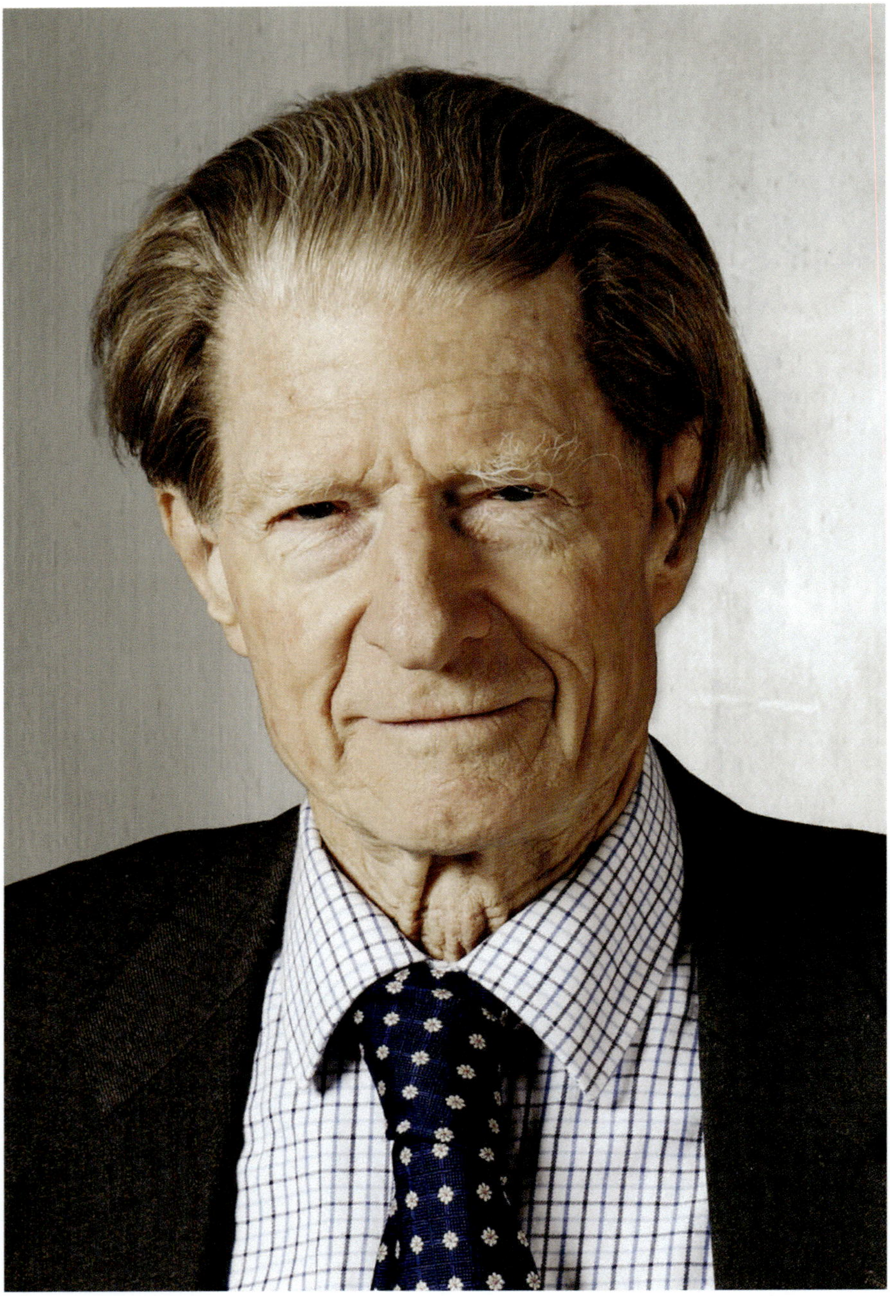

Sir John B. Gurdon. © The Nobel Foundation. Photo: U. Montan

Sir John B. Gurdon

FAMILY BACKGROUND

John Bertrand Gurdon (JBG), born 2 October 1933, was brought up in a comfortable home by his parents (fig. 1) on the Surrey/Hampshire border in a village, Frensham in South England, endowed with a large amount of National Trust heathland and ponds. His mother, Marjorie Byass, was from an East Yorkshire farming family. Brought up on a farm, and educated in that region, she became a physical training teacher working for some time in an American private school. When her son and daughter (Caroline, who trained as a nurse) had been raised, she gave much time to the regional administration of the "Women's Institute," a voluntary organisation for educating women.

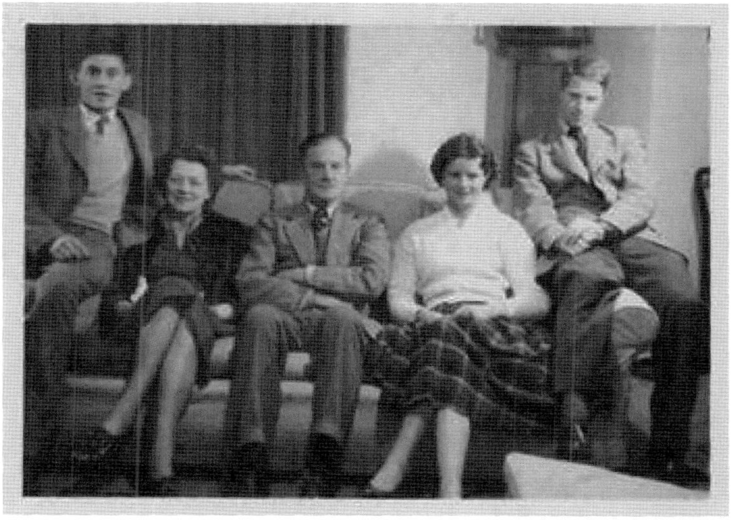

FIGURE 1. My cousin, Phil Gurdon; my mother, Elsie Marjorie Gurdon (nee Byass); my father, William Nathaniel Gurdon; my sister, Caroline Thompson (nee Gurdon); Myself, about 1960.

His father, William Gurdon, was from a longstanding Suffolk family whose ancestors go back to 1199 (fig. 2; Muskett, 1900; Cunnington, 2008); with the family motto "*virtus viget in arduis*" [virtue flourishes in adversity].

In The Roll of Battle Abbey, the earliest record of the principal families who came to England in 1066 with William The Conqueror, is the Norman adventurer Gurdon, the Seigneure of Gourdon near Cahors on the borders of Perigord.

His descendants are as follows;

Bertram de Gurdon: in 1199 shot King Richard the First (The Lion Heart) with an arrow from the walls of the Castle of Chalus in France, of which wound the King afterwards died, but he first forgave Bertram reflecting on his own avaricious undertaking.

Adam de Gurdon: d.1214, Kings Serjeant and mercenary for king John.

Sir Adam de Gurdon: d. 1231, Had land in Tystede.

Sir Adam de Gurdon: of Shropshire: d. 1310, Justice Itinerant. One of the most famous men of the Middle Ages, it has been said that the legend of Robin Hood has been based on part of de Gurdons life. He was Knighted on 28 May 1254 by king henry III. He was Baliff of Alton but was outlawed for treason and rebellion as one of the adherents of Simon Earl of Leicester. After the Battle of of Evesham he retired with his band of followers into the New Forest between Wilton and Fernham, from his base there no traveller was safe. In 1273 he was defeated in single combat by Prince Edward later King Edward I, in one of the most celebrated deeds of that age. Prince Edward who was pleased with de Gurdons bravery pardoned him. He was then appointed keeper of the Forest of Wolner and employed in high military commands. He resided at the Temple Selborne in Hampshire now occupied by the Earl of Selborne.

Robert Gurdon: d. 1345, Sheriff of London.

John Gurdon: d. 1385, Merchant in London.

Thomas Gurdon: d. 1436, of London and Kent, purchased Manor Clyne

John Gurdon of Kent: d. 1465

John Gurdon of Dedham: d. 1487

John Gurdon of Dedham: d. 1504

John Gurdon of Dedham: d. 1536, lord of Roushall near Clopton

Robert Gurdon of Waldingfield: d. 1578, High Sheriff of Suffolk, purchased Assington Hall and estate, one of the finest Elizabethan Houses in Suffolk. Destroyed by fire in 1957.

FIGURE 2. Paternal lineage of JBG.

John Gurdon of Assington: d. 1623, MP for Sudbury, High Sheriff of Suffolk.

Brampton Gurdon of Assington: d. 1647, High Sheriff of Suffolk. His wife Elizabeth descended from King Henry I.

John Gurdon of Assington: d. 1677, MP for Sudbury in the Long Parliament. His wife Anne descended from King Edward I. He was nominated to sit on Judgment of King Charles I, however he decided against signing the death warrant and this saved the Family on the Restoration of King Charles II. Oliver Cromwell was his guest at Assington during the siege of Colchester. His brother Colonel Brampton Gurdon led his Regiment of Suffolk Horse at the Battle of Naseby in the Civil War.

Rev. Nathaniel Gurdon DD: d. 1696

John Gurdon of Assington: d. 1758, MP for Sudbury.

John Gurdon of Assington: d. 1777

Rev. Philip Gurdon: d. 1817

John Gurdon of Assington: d.1863

John Gurdon of Assington: d.1869

Philip Gurdon of Assington and Tunbridge Wells, JP: d. 1942, Due to the repeal of the Corn laws he Sold Assington Hall and the estate to his cousin Sir William Gurdon KCMG.

William Gurdon DCM RE: d. 1977, late of Furnell House Frensham. His brother John won the Military cross in The Great War.

Professor Sir John Bertrand Gurdon FRS of Whittlesford.

FIGURE 2. (Cont.)

Many of them had distinguished careers in government and as regional administrators, including Sir Adam Gurdon [Muskett, 1900]. JBG's ancestors lived in a stately home, Assington Hall, in West Suffolk (fig. 3).

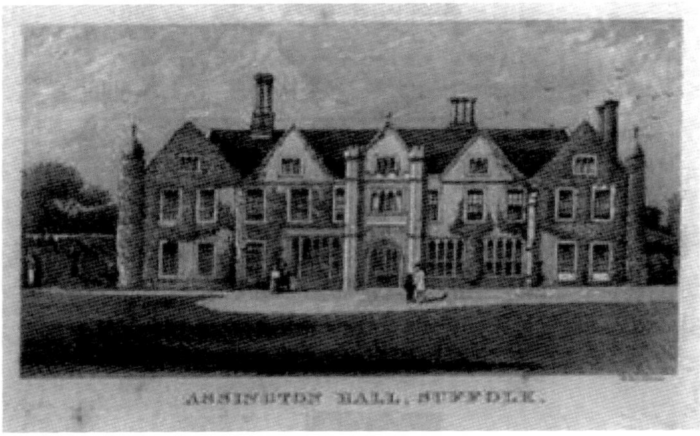

FIGURE 3. Assington Hall, Suffolk. Burnt down in 1957.

His grandfather had to leave the family home through lack of money to maintain it, due to repeal of the Corn Laws (1846) so that tenant farmers could no longer pay their rent, because of foreign imports. Assington Hall was requisitioned by the army during World War II, and was burnt down in a supposedly accidental fire in 1957. The remaining part of the house was partly restored and part of the original home, including its minarets, is still present in Assington. One of JBG's ancestors married again after his first wife died and the outcome of a second marriage yielded a distinguished lawyer who accepted the hereditary title of Baron Cranworth. JBG's father left school at the age of 16 and took a position in a rice broking firm in Burma. He was an early volunteer in the First World War and was decorated with the Distinguished Conduct Medal (DCM) before being commissioned to an officer rank. After that he led a career in banking in Assam and East India. He retired, in his forties, and in retirement, he gave much time to the transcribing of professional textbooks (especially legal) into Braille for the blind as voluntary work.

World War II started in 1939 when JBG was aged six. It was a time of austerity. Limited rations of food were managed by his mother, and the garden was used to raise chickens. He did not see luxuries like a banana or an orange until well after the end of the war. At the age of eight he was sent to a local private school, Frensham Heights. In an intelligence test at that age, he was asked to draw an orange. He started drawing the stalk by which the orange would hang from a tree, reasoning that an orange would not exist in space. The teacher tore up the piece of paper and reported to his parents that he was mentally subnormal and would need special teaching. The teacher meant to say, draw a circle. He was moved to another private school in the village, namely Edgeborough, where he thrived. At that age he had an intense interest in plants and insects. In most of his spare time he collected butterflies and moths and raised their caterpillars.

EDUCATION

At the age of 13, he started school at Eton as a boarder. He found life there intensely uncomfortable, because senior boys acted as despots, administering punishments for trivial misdemeanours. As a means of survival, he took up squash, and as a result of hard work rather than ability, he became eventually the school captain in this sport. While at school he continued his interest in Lepidoptera, raising large numbers of moths from their larval stage.

It was during his first term of being taught Science at the school, at the age of 15, that he received a totally damning report from the Biology master (fig. 4). This report resulted from JBG being placed in the bottom position of the lowest form in a group of 250 students of the same age. The report, sent to his house-master, resulted in him being taken off any further study of Science of any kind at the school. For the rest of his school days, for the next three years, he was given no Science teaching and was placed in a class which studied Ancient Greek, Latin and a modern language, a course intended for those judged to be unsuited for studying any subject in depth.

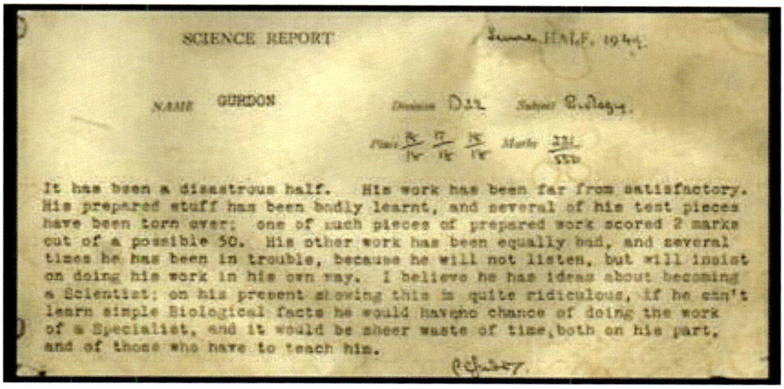

SCIENCE REPORT

NAME GURDON

It has been a disastrous half. His work has been far from satisfactory. His prepared stuff has been badly learnt, and several of his test pieces have been torn over; one of such pieces of prepared work scored 2 marks out of a possible 50. His other work has been equally bad, and several times he has been in trouble, because he will not listen, but will insist on doing his work in his own way. I believe he has ideas about becoming a Scientist; on his present showing this is quite ridiculous, if he can't learn simple Biological facts he would have no chance of doing the work of a Specialist, and it would be sheer waste of time, both on his part, and of those who have to teach him.

FIGURE 4. Eton school report for JBG from Biology master, 1949.

Entrance to University was a problem: having sat the Entrance examination in Latin and Greek, the Admissions tutor at Christ Church Oxford University told JBG that he would be accepted for Entrance on condition that he did not plan to study the subject in which he took the Entrance (Classics). Later the Admissions tutor admitted that he had under-filled the college and had his mind on other things; he was Hugh Trevor-Roper, later Lord Dacre, and author of *The Last Days of Hitler*. In due course it emerged that JBG's acceptance for Christ Church involved a complicated arrangement between JBG's uncle, at that time a Fellow of Christ Church, JBG's school housemaster and a friend of his uncle, Sir John Masterman, who was Master of Worcester College, Oxford and in charge of the wartime Enigma operation at Bletchley, agreeing to accept the housemaster's son. Such a manoeuvre, and admission to Oxford on those terms, could never happen now. At that time, 1952, it was not very easy to fill a college with paying students. Before entering University, JBG had to take a year off to learn elementary Biology with a private tutor, generously funded by his parents who had already paid several years of Eton fees. He was told that he could formally enter the Department of Zoology course at Oxford if he passed the elementary exams in Physics, Chemistry and Biology in a preliminary year. He survived this and started the course in Zoology at Oxford in 1953. The course was extremely oldfashioned, by today's standards. A major part of the teaching involved learning Palaeontology, and the names of skeletal parts of dinosaurs. JBG later became a personal friend of Sir Alister Hardy, the Head of that department, through his Oxford aunt (see later).

GRADUATE STUDENT WORK

As the Zoology course came to an end, JBG enquired about the possibility of doing a PhD in Entomology, in accord with his continuing interest in insects. While still a student, he had got permission to go to Oxford University's nature reserve, namely Wytham Woods, with his butterfly net. No butterflies were to be seen, but he caught the only moving thing, which was a kind of fly. He used the taxonomic reference works to try to identify this "fly." Having realised that the fly was a Hymenopteron, he was still unable to identify it. He therefore went to the Natural History Museum in London for help. They pronounced that it was in fact a species of sawfly new to Britain. This must have been intensely irritating to the Professor of Entomology, whose main research project was to identify animals and plants in Wytham Woods. JBG was later rejected for PhD work in Entomology. This was a great blessing because the work he would have done in Entomology was not well regarded and had very little, if any, analytical component to it. By his immense good fortune, he was invited to do a PhD with the Oxford University lecturer who taught Developmental Biology, Dr Michael Fischberg.

Fischberg was born in St Petersburg, Russia, in 1919. He was educated in Switzerland and was a PhD student of E. Hadorn. Hadorn in turn was a student of F. Baltzer, who was a student of H. Spemann, himself a student of T. Boveri. This German-Swiss lineage of eminent Developmental Biologists turns out to be the background of a great many of the successful Developmental Biologists of the mid-1950s. Most of those that did not have this background can trace their own training back to R. G. Harrison (1870–1959) of the USA, who pioneered cell culture. Having finished his PhD with Hadorn, Fischberg took a position in the Institute of Animal Genetics under Waddington in Edinburgh, from where he accepted his appointment in the Oxford Zoology department, headed by Professor Sir Alister Hardy, an eminent marine biologist [Royal Society memoirs].

Starting his PhD work in 1956, Fischberg suggested to JBG that he should try to carry out somatic cell nuclear transfer in *Xenopus*, a procedure for this having been recently published by Briggs and King (1952). The advisability and technical problems that arose at this point are described in the accompanying papers (Gurdon 2013 a,b). Once these technical obstacles had been overcome, largely as a result of good luck, JBG's work proceeded extraordinarily fast; strongly motivated by early success, he became an intensely hard worker. By the end of his PhD he had succeeded in obtaining normal development of intestinal epithelium cell nuclei transplanted to enucleated eggs of *Xenopus*. When these tadpoles had eventually reached sexual maturity, he was able to publish a paper entitled "Fertile intestine nuclei." This was the first decisive evidence that all cells of the body contain the same complete set of genes. This answered a long-standing and important question in the field of Developmental Biology. However it also showed very clearly, as was commented on in JBG's papers at the time, the remarkable ability of eggs to reprogram somatic cell nuclei back to an embryonic state. Eventually this phenomenon attracted increasingly large interest, and led to the idea of cell replacement using accessible adult cells, such as skin. A key future discovery was that of Martin Evans (Nobel Prize, 2006) that a permanently proliferating embryonic stem cell line could be established from mouse embryos. Under appropriate conditions these cells could be caused to differentiate into all different cell types. The combination of somatic cell nuclear transfer and the derivation of embryonic stem cells in mammals made it realistic to think of cell replacement for human diseases. A huge boost for this idea was later provided by Takahashi and Yamanaka (2006), with their discovery that the overexpression of certain transcription factors can also yield embryonic stem cells from adult somatic tissue. The accompanying Nobel lecture provides more detail of the later scientific part of JBG's career.

POST-DOCTORAL WORK

A visit by the Nobel Laureate George Beadle to the Fischberg Group in the Oxford Zoology department in 1960 led to an offer from the California Institute of Technology (CalTech) (previous chairman George Beadle) for JBG to do postdoctoral work there. Fischberg very wisely advised JBG to accept the CalTech offer of postdoctoral work rather than offers from other nuclear transplant labs. Stimulated by his mother's adventurous spirit, JBG decided to buy a secondhand Chevrolet in New York and drive across the USA to California, using the famous Route 66 (now replaced). He gave lectures as he travelled across the USA and stopped at laboratories of Briggs and King, Alexander Brink (paramutation) etc. He had hoped to become a post-doctoral student of R. Dulbecco at CalTech (Nobel Prize), but the chairman of that department advised against this because JBG had no training in virology. Therefore JBG did his postdoctoral work with Robert Edgar on Bacteriophage Genetics. JBG found he had no aptitude at all for Phage Genetics and decided to return to Britain after one year at CalTech. Nevertheless, that year at CalTech was extremely formative because it provided some acquaintance with Molecular Biology, which had so far entirely escaped his training. During that year he met Sturtevant, a student of Morgan, who pioneered the whole field of *Drosophila* Genetics. He also got to know Ed Lewis (future Nobel Laureate). Thanks to James Ebert (director of the Department of Embryology, Carnegie Institute of Washington, in Baltimore) JBG visited various labs in the USA at the end of his post-doctoral period and met Donald Brown in Baltimore on that visit. Meantime, the success of the nuclear transfer work in Oxford had led to Michael Fischberg being offered a head of department professorship in Geneva, Switzerland. JBG was offered the teaching position in Oxford vacated by M. Fischberg. JBG returned from California to England via Japan and many other countries over a two-month period. One month of that time he spent in Japan and met Tokindo Okada and made other friends in Japan, including M. Furusawa and subsequently Koichiro Shiokawa.

While doing graduate and postdoctoral work in Oxford, JBG made other contacts and friendships. His mother's sister lived in Oxford, and he spent much time at her house and visiting famous gardens, fostering a lifelong interest in plants. Through that connection he met Miriam Rothschild, and became a lifelong friend of hers (Van Emden and Gurdon, 2006). This friendship contained, through Miriam Rothschild's generosity, ski mountaineering holidays based in her house in Wengen. JBG had achieved the British ski club's Gold standard ski medal, again through relentless practice rather than any natural ability. Also, in accord with his interest in the open air and dogged determination, he became a reasonably accomplished ice figure skater.

ASSISTANT LECTURESHIP IN OXFORD, DEPARTMENT OF ZOOLOGY

On starting the job, JBG was immediately asked to do 24 lectures on Development. From then on his allocation of student lecturing duties went down progressively during his career until, in the end, he was only asked to do two such lectures per year. But the lectures seemed to go well because he attracted, almost immediately, some of the best students to do PhD work with him. Notable among these were C.F. Graham (later FRS) and R.A. Laskey (later FRS, Royal Medal and CBE). During his time in Oxford when he started his own research group, he was able to interact with many very senior scientists in other departments, notably R. R. Porter (Nobel), H. Harris and J. L. Gowans.

On return to Oxford, as an Assistant Lecturer in the Zoology department JBG was accorded a privileged position, at his Oxford College Christ Church, as a Research Fellow. He was given only minimal teaching duties, so that he could establish his own research group. At that time, he was fortunate to meet his future wife (fig. 5), Jean Elizabeth Margaret Curtis, eldest daughter of Mr H.J. Curtis who owned a successful business in Oxford in property and gravel. With his wife he had two children; his daughter Aurea has two of her own children His son, William, did not marry and has no issue.

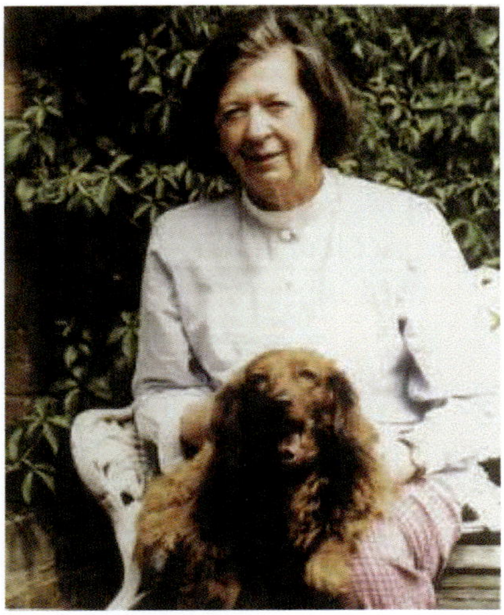

FIGURE 5. Jean Gurdon in the Master's Lodge, Magdalene College, Cambridge, 2000.

At fi he lived with his wife and children in a brew-house in Christ Church Oxford (fig. 6), then in a house they had built in his father-in-law's land.

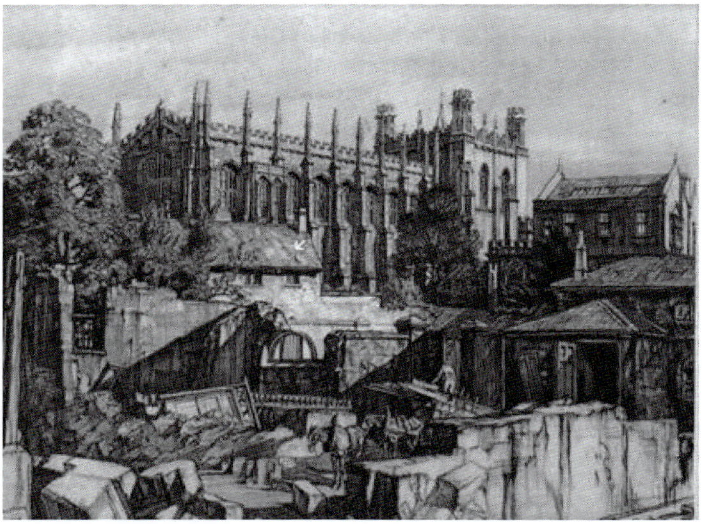

FIGURE 6. The Brew House in Christ Church, Oxford, 1970.

At this time he made, with his father-in-law, a crossing under the town of Oxford in a disused drain, the Trill Mill underground stream – now permanently closed (fig. 7).

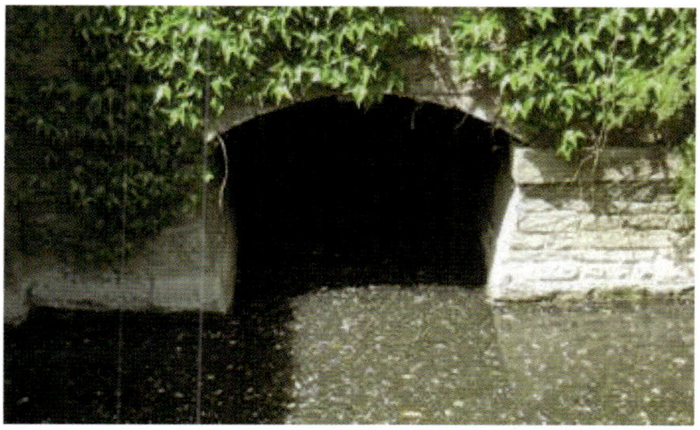

FIGURE 7. Trill Mill stream. Entry from Memorial Garden south of the College. Progresses under the town and emerges, after about two miles, in West Oxford.

On moving to Cambridge, he was able to acquire, largely through a successful property business of his wife, a large property with a 16th century house in the village of Whittlesford (fig. 8).

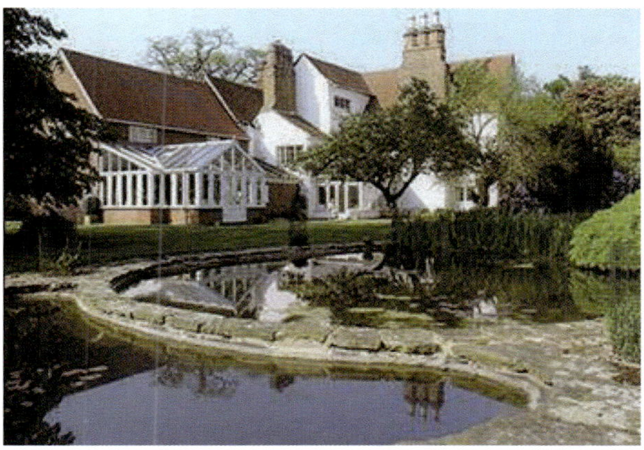

FIGURE 8. The Grove, Whittlesford, Cambridge.

CAREER MOVES

After nearly ten years (then 1972) as lecturer in the Zoology department, Oxford, JBG was given a very generous research grant by the MRC of four positions (3 Sci + 1 Tech). At the same time, Max Perutz of Cambridge MRC Molecular Biology lab offered him a position. Max Perutz had empty space that had (by MRC rules) to be filled externally. JBG accepted, and planned to move to Cambridge, very reluctantly by his wife because of our house and her family in Oxford). But senior professors in Oxford persuaded him to decline the offer, notably Rodney Porter (Biochemistry), James Gowan and H. Harris (Pathology). They tried hard to persuade his own (Zoology) Professor Pringle to give JBG the space needed for a now enlarging MRC "unit." But JBG said he could not manage with the very dispersed space offered. So JBG (eventually) accepted Max Perutz's offer, and moved to Cambridge LMB. After a few years, Rodney Porter (Biochemistry) offered JBG the Chair of Genetics in Oxford, a sub-department of Biochemistry, a position vacated by Professor Bodmer. By then JBG's wife and family were very settled in Cambridge and they decided not to move back to Oxford.

WELLCOME CRC INSTITUTE

After a further ten years (then 1982), Sir Gabriel Horn (Head of Zoology, Cambridge) offered JBG and Ronald Laskey professorships in his department. We both decided (RAL had by then also moved to LMB, Cambridge) to accept jobs in Zoology Cambridge, if they succeeded (as they did) in obtaining substantial support from the Cancer Research Campaign for a joint "unit" in Zoology, Cambridge. They were accommodated, very generously, by Professor Horn, in Zoology, Cambridge. At this time the Wellcome Trust had, thanks to Sir Roger Gibbs, become a major national funding agency. Ron Laskey and JBG were encouraged by the Wellcome Trust to bid for a small Institute to be built in Cambridge for their"unit" and to accommodate some other scientists. It was agreed that the Wellcome Trust and CRC would jointly fund an Institute costing £4M to include some two groups and four others for which we chose: Martin Evans, Janet and Chris Wyllie and Michael Akam. A new building was designed by Laskey and Akam, and they decided, generously, to have JBG as Chairman. We attempted to follow the administrative style of Max Perutz, whose LMB was widely regarded as the most successful research institute internationally. Our Institute thrived, and most particularly because Gabriel Horn, extremely generously, made our new Institute independent of his Zoology department. This arose, importantly by proposing that Group Leaders in our Institute should be affiliated with several different departments in Cambridge, and not all with Zoology. Their new appointments included Azim Surani, Daniel St Johnston, Steve Jackson and Tony Kouzarides (all later FRS). In the 1990s, the Institute had the chance to bid for a new building and more space. They were awarded a Wellcome Trust and CRUK building (£23M), located next to the new Biochemistry department in Cambridge (now 2000).

JBG was succeeded as Chairman by Jim Smith, and then, by Daniel St Johnston. By 2012 the Institute had 17 Group Leaders and had been joined by Anne McLaren. Its tally: one Dame, two Knights, two Nobels, four CBEs, eight FRS, importantly four home-grown.

CAMBRIDGE COLLEGE APPOINTMENTS

Soon after moving from Oxford to Cambridge in 1971 JBG was offered, on the recommendation of Professor Richard Keynes, a research fellowship at Churchill College. With no obligatory teaching duties, this was a very appealing college connection. Being a large college with over 100 fellows, this was a very welcome opportunity to meet a wide range of Cambridge academics. In 1985 JBG was offered by Lord Braybrooke, the College Visitor, the Mastership of Magdalene College. He accepted this position and this was a major blessing. Compared to two other colleges for which he had been unsuccessfully interviewed, Magdalene accepted that he would wish to keep his laboratory activities going while acting as Master of the College. He chose to decline the usual emolument of a Master so that it could be used to hire a professional fundraiser, thereby releasing JBG for his own laboratory work. The college required only minimal time and spared him much of the committee work normally expected. His wife took to the Master's wife job like a duck to water. She chose to entertain every undergraduate, every year, in the college to a sit-down Sunday lunch prepared and cooked by herself. She invited 20 students to lunch every Sunday in term. She got to know all the staff in the college and her complete involvement was enormously appreciated. With no internal frictions that he was aware of, the college seemed a happy place and a privileged existence for JBG and his family.

For other administrative jobs for which JBG had been proposed, fortunately he was not selected. In retrospect, any of these would have destroyed his remaining research career. He did however serve for 15 years as a Fellow (Governor) of Eton College where he met some outstanding individuals, including most notably Sir John Smith, the founder of the Landmark Trust, and also a benefactor to JBG's research. JBG also served for a long time on the Cancer Research Campaign (subsequently CRUK) research grant committee. Compared to many others this committee was very well run and promoted a very happy relationship among its members. This connection opened the door for eventual funding by the CRC/Wellcome Trust for a new Institute for him and his colleague Ron Laskey in Cambridge. JBG also served for a few years as a "Governor"(Board member) of the Wellcome Trust, under the chairmanship of Sir Roger Gibbs, who, as it later turned out, had in earlier years almost as undistinguished career as JBG at the same school.

OTHER ACTIVITIES

JBG sees himself as the ultimate non-intellectual. He prefers to do things himself rather than watch others. He never goes to the theatre or musical performances, and hates reading books. With the time thereby saved, he likes to take exercise, in earlier years through skiing and squash (later tennis). Throughout life he has travelled widely, with a special interest in going up mountains and seeing alpine plants. He has been to the top of many of the 14,000ers in Colorado, USA, the highest point in New Guinea, etc.

REFERENCES

Muskett, J.J. (1900), *Suffolk Manorial Families*, Wm Pollard & Co., Ltd, North Street, Exeter. Cunnington, B. (2008), *The Gurdon Family*, Cunnington, Bronwen. Beechwater, Australia, 3747.

Briggs, R. & King T.J. (1952), "Transplantation of living nuclei from blastula cells into enucleated frogs' eggs." *Proc. Nat. Acad. Sci.* **38**: 4 55–463.

Van Emden, H.F. & Gurdon J.B. (2006), "Dame Miriam Louisa Rothschild CBE 5 August 1908–20 January 2005." *Biogr. Mems Fell. R. Soc.* **52**: 315–330.

Gurdon, J.B. (2013a), "The egg and the nucleus: A battle for supremacy." *Development* **140**: 2449–2456.

Gurdon, J.B. (2013b) "The cloning of a frog." *Development* **140**: 2446–2448.

Takahashi, K. & Yamanaka S. (2006) "Induction of pluripotent stem cells from mouse embryonic and adult fibroblast cultures by defined factors." *Cell* **126**: 663–676.

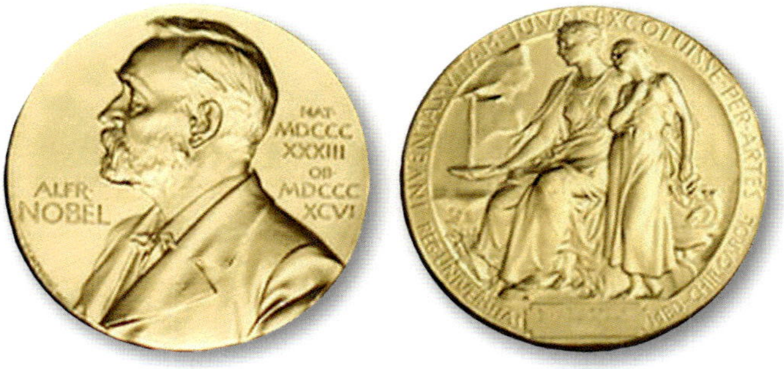

The Egg and the Nucleus: A Battle for Supremacy

Nobel Lecture, December 7, 2013

by Sir John B. Gurdon
Gurdon Institute, Cambridge, United Kingdom.

BACKGROUND

As a brand new graduate student starting in October 1956, my supervisor Michail Fischberg, a lecturer in the Department of Zoology at Oxford, suggested that I should try to make somatic cell nuclear transplantation work in the South African frog *Xenopus laevis*. There were good reasons for wanting to do this (see below). The very important question to be addressed at that time was whether all cell types in the body have the same set of genes. This question had been asked by embryologists since 1886 (Rauber 1886), and Spemann (1938) had demonstrated by an egg ligation experiment that the nuclei of an eight-cell frog embryo are developmentally totipotent. It was clear that a definitive experiment required the replacement of a zygote nucleus by a somatic cell nucleus, asking whether the somatic nucleus could functionally replace the zygote nucleus by eliciting normal development of the enucleated recipient egg (Fig. 1). Briggs and King (1952) had already succeeded in transplanting a blastula cell nucleus into an enucleated egg and obtaining normal tadpoles in the frog *Rana pipiens*. However, Briggs and King (1957) had also found that the nucleus of an endoderm cell from a neurula embryo could no longer support normal development (Fig. 2). They drew the reasonable conclusion that, as development proceeds from a blastula to a neurula stage (about 24 hours), some genes needed for normal development had either been lost or irreversibly repressed.

To this extent, the aim of my proposed PhD work had already been done and the answer to the primary question already obtained. Why then did it make

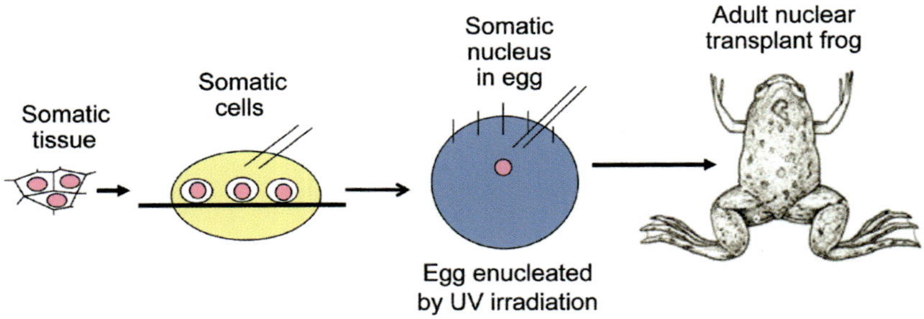

FIGURE 1. Design of a somatic cell nuclear transfer experiment using unfertilised eggs as first designed by Briggs and King (1952) for *Rana pipiens* and as used subsequently in *Xenopus*. In *Rana*, enucleation is by hand with a needle, and in *Xenopus* by ultraviolet light irradiation (Gurdon, 1960a).

sense for me to try to repeat this work on a related species? There appeared to be two possible outcomes. One was that I might obtain a different result from Briggs and King and so the primary question would be re-opened and subject to fruitful investigation. The other was that I might obtain the same result as Briggs and King and this would then open the important question of what the mechanism could be by which a somatic cell nucleus already committed to a specific (in this case endoderm) fate could not be reprogrammed by exposure to egg cytoplasm.

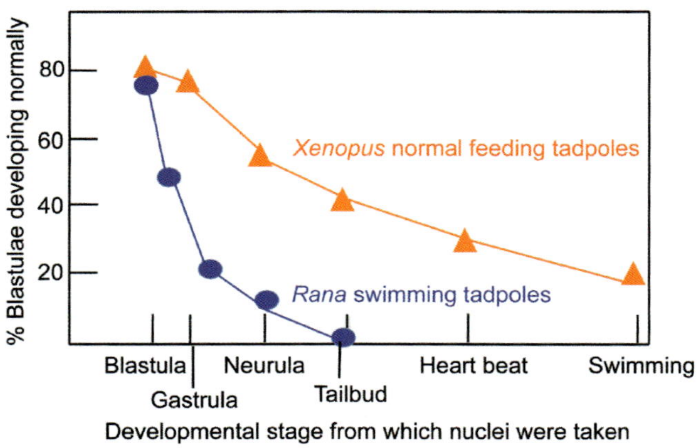

FIGURE 2. Survival of nuclear transplant embryos in *Rana pipiens* and *Xenopus laevis*. Even advanced donor cells from the endoderm have nuclei which can sometimes yield normal individuals after nuclear transfer (from Briggs and King 1957 [*Rana*] and Gurdon 1962 [*Xenopus*]).

Preliminary investigation showed that there would be substantial technical difficulties in achieving somatic cell nuclear transfer with *Xenopus*, in the way that Briggs and King succeeded for *Rana pipiens*. The first of these was that, unlike *Rana*, the *Xenopus* egg is covered with a dense and extremely elastic jelly, which is completely impenetrable by even the finest of micropipettes (Fig. 3). The second was that this jelly covering made it very hard, even if possible, to remove metaphase egg chromosomes by causing extrusion of them with a needle, the method used in *Rana pipiens*. There were, on the other hand, very good reasons to wish to make this technique succeed in *Xenopus*. How *Xenopus laevis*, a native of South Africa, came into use for Developmental Biology has an amusing and serendipitous history (Gurdon and Hopwood 2000). First, *Xenopus* would respond to the injection of commercially available mammalian hormone

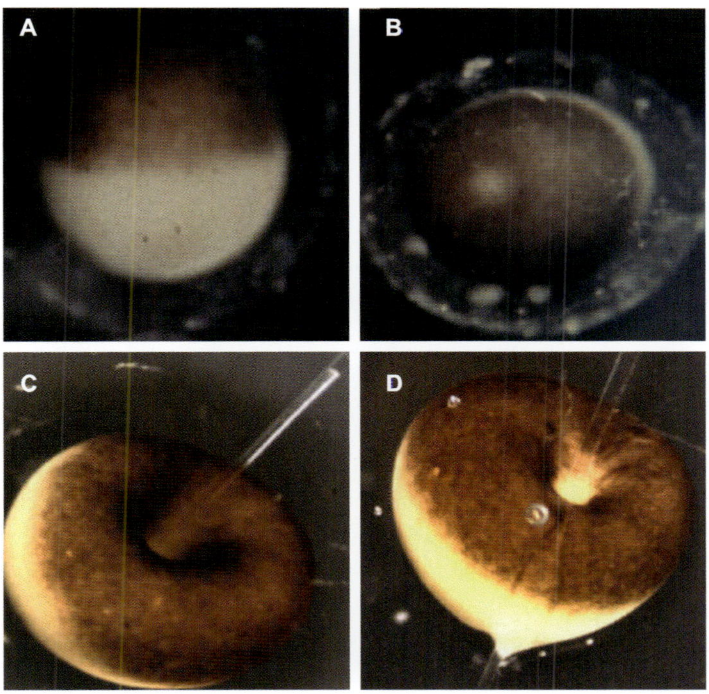

FIGURE 3. The Xenopus egg is surrounded by a dense elastic jelly so that it is not possible to penetrate into the egg cytoplasm with a micropipette, unless the jelly is removed or denatured by ultraviolet light.
(a) side view. (b) "animal" pole; the white area in the middle of the black area is where the egg chromosomes are located. (c) If the egg is not de-jellied, a micropipette depresses the jelly coat, eventually dragging the pipette, still surrounded by jelly, through the egg without entering the cytoplasm (d).

(Follicle Stimulating Hormone and Luteinizing Hormone) by laying eggs the next day and this procedure is effective throughout the year. In contrast, frogs of the European and North American *Rana* species will lay eggs only in the spring of each year unless they are injected with frog pituitary gland extract, and this requires about five pituitary glands from killed frogs to obtain one egg ovulation. In the past, European embryologists had the use of living frog eggs for only a month or two in the year and had to do other things, such as histology *etc*, for the rest of the year. *Xenopus*, in principle, permitted experiments on living embryos to be done throughout the year. Second, *Xenopus* is an aquatic frog and therefore easy to maintain in the laboratory in water tanks rather than having to clean a terrarium as was necessary with *Rana*. Furthermore, *Xenopus* species can be reared from the fertilised egg to sexual maturity in less than one year (compared to three to four years for *Rana*), thereby making it realistic to propagate genetic mutants and make use of them. A further advantage of *Xenopus laevis* is that this species lives in highly infected cattle sewage ponds and has built up an extraordinary resistance to infection and diseases. Michael Fischberg therefore concluded that it was sensible to have me try, at least for a while, to achieve successful somatic cell nuclear transfer in *Xenopus*.

The aim of this article is to recount the early history of nuclear transfer in *Xenopus* as a result of which the recent Nobel award was made (Jaenisch 2012). Further work in *Xenopus* that has led on from this up to the present time is covered only briefly, and has been reviewed elsewhere (Jullien *et al.* 2011; Pasque *et al.* 2011b).

THE TECHNIQUE OF NUCLEAR TRANSFER IN *XENOPUS*

There is no doubt that I was blessed with a considerable amount of luck. But the phrase that "luck favours the prepared mind" may well have been true. My supervisor had just acquired a microscope equipped with ultraviolet light illumination. There was reason to believe that ultraviolet light would destroy DNA in the egg chromosomes which, very fortunately, are located right on the surface of the animal pole of amphibian eggs. Aiming the ultraviolet light source onto the animal pole of unfertilised eggs was successful in destroying the egg chromosomes, as shown by fertilising such irradiated eggs with sperm and obtaining haploid embryos. If the egg chromosomes had not been located on the surface of a large amphibian egg, ultraviolet light (having very low penetration) would not have reached them (Gurdon 1960a). Perhaps even more fortunate was our finding that the particular ultraviolet lamp just bought for microscopy progressively denatured (dissolved) the elastic jelly around the egg. After ultraviolet

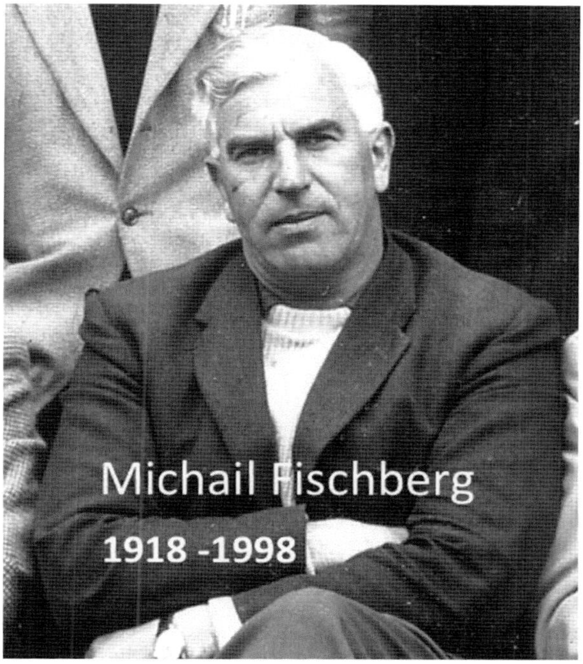

FIGURE 4. Michail Fishberg. Born in St Petersburg, educated in Switzerland and PhD under E. Hadorn. The education lineage traces back from Hadorn to Baltzer to Boveri. MF was my graduate supervisor in Oxford, England, from where he moved to Geneva.

light exposure, unfertilised eggs became easily penetrable by a micropipette, and this happened in a dose-dependent way, making it possible to enucleate the egg, leaving just enough jelly to help seal the penetration wound made by a micropipette. It was not known, at that time, that this egg jelly could be removed by an alkaline solution of cysteine hydrochloride, but good luck, or my supervisor's wisdom, or both, did not stop at this point. Crucial to the validity of these early experiments was proof that the egg chromosomes had in fact been destroyed and did not contribute to the development of the nuclear transplant embryos. Another PhD student of my supervisor, namely Sheila Smith, was studying the morphology of haploid development in *Xenopus*. She was advised to use a single nucleolus per nucleus as a measure of haploidy. She encountered an inexplicable result, namely that embryos carrying only one nucleolus per nucleus were diploid and developed entirely normally, whereas haploids (which have only one nucleolus per nucleus or chromosome set) always die as stunted early tadpoles. Most supervisors would have told the student to repeat the experiment the next week, starting with completely different material, to see if the result was reproducible. Michail Fischberg (Fig. 4), however, had the wisdom or intuition to tell the student to find out which frog had been used to give the eggs that yielded normal diploid one-nucleolated embryos. Amazingly, the student's result was reproducible. Michail Fischberg concluded that there must have been a mutation in one chromosome set so that it was unable to make a nucleolus (Elsdale *et al.* 1960). Later work showed that this strain of *Xenopus* had indeed lost all the ribosomal genes located in one nucleolus organizer and therefore that heterozygotes for this deletion would never carry more than one nucleolus per diploid chromosome set (Brown and Gurdon, 1964). This mutation gave us an extraordinarily valuable nuclear marker for nuclear transfer experiments (Fig. 5). Some years later, an albino strain of *Xenopus laevis* provided a more visually striking marker (Fig. 6).

Using the benefits of ultraviolet radiation, combined with a genetic marker, it was possible, rather rapidly, to show that somatic cell nuclear transfer in *Xenopus* worked well. Within one year of starting work, I had found that the nucleus of an endoderm cell from an advanced tadpole was able to yield some normal development up to the nuclear transplant tadpole stage. This was not in agreement with the results of Briggs and King (Fig. 2).

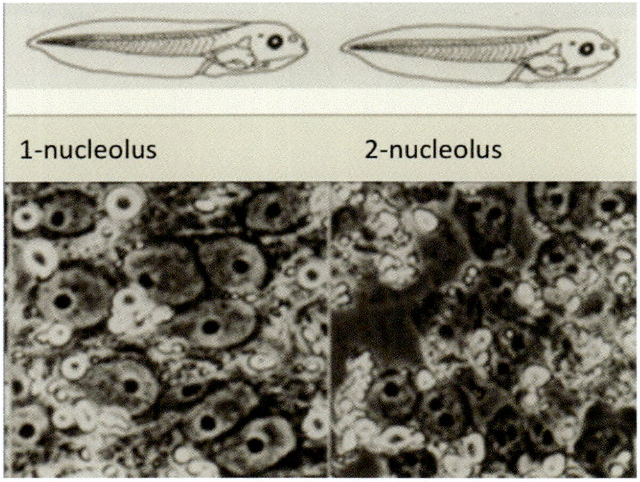

FIGURE 5. A nucleolar genetic marker for *Xenopus laevis* (Elsdale *et al.* 1960). Heterozygotes of the one-nucleolated strain have only one nucleolus per diploid nucleus (left), compared to the wild-type 2-nucleolated form most of whose nuclei have two nucleoli (right). The one-nucleolated strain has a deletion of ribosomal genes on one chromosome (Brown and Gurdon 1964).

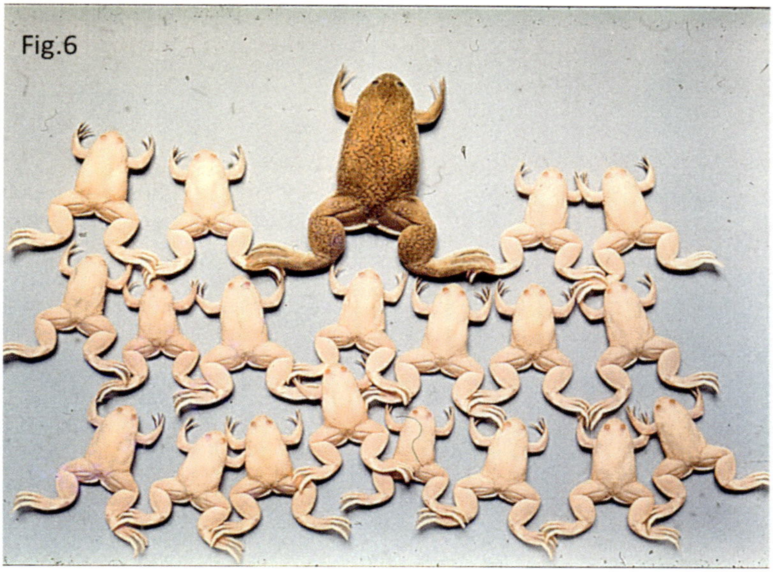

FIGURE 6. A clone of albino male frogs obtained by transplanting nuclei from cells of an albino embryo to enucleated eggs of the wild-type female shown. The albino frogs are genetically identical and will accept skin grafts from each other.

NORMAL DEVELOPMENT FROM THE NUCLEI OF DIFFERENTIATED INTESTINAL EPITHELIUM CELLS

Within another year, now 1958, I found that it was technically possible to transplant single nuclei from the intestinal epithelium of feeding tadpoles. I found it best to distort the donor cells to the least amount possible (Gurdon, 1960b), so that at least some of them had the nucleus in a ruptured cell wall, even though other such donor nuclei may have been transplanted in whole non-permeabilised cells, which however would not be able to respond to the egg cytoplasm or begin to cleave. It seemed important not to expose the nucleus of a ruptured cell to the simple saline medium used for nuclear transfer. It was later found that treating small donor cells with Streptolysin O was a great deal easier than cell rupture in a narrow pipette (Chan and Gurdon 1996).

The success of these intestinal epithelium nuclear transfers differed from one experiment to another. Moreover, some females supplying recipient eggs gave significantly better development than others. Egg quality was therefore a factor. Nevertheless, these results showed that starting with nuclei from differentiated intestinal epithelium cells, with a striated border, some of the nuclear transplant embryos developed entirely normally to the feeding tadpole stage and were progressing towards metamorphosis. Furthermore, these tadpoles carried only one nucleolus per nucleus with a diploid set of chromosomes. This showed that the transplanted nucleus that gave normal development did indeed derive from an intestinal epithelium cell. Although the percentage of intestinal epithelium cell nuclear transfers that yielded entirely normal feeding tadpoles was low (1.5%) (Gurdon 1962) many such individuals were obtained and they all carried the nuclear marker.

My supervisor and his assistant looked after my nuclear transplant tadpoles, which had by now metamorphosed into young frogs, during my absence for postdoctoral work in another field. On my return, these intestinal nuclear transplant tadpoles had become adult male and female frogs, and their fertility and ability to generate normal embryos was tested. This yielded, in 1966, our paper entitled, "Fertile" intestine nuclei (Gurdon and Uehlinger 1966). This therefore gave the opposite conclusion to that of the Briggs and King work with *Rana pipiens*. Of course, there was criticism that a graduate student, working almost alone, should not be able to repeat the results of well-established and highly-respected workers Briggs and King. The use of the one-nucleolated genetic marker was crucial in persuading scientists that this *Xenopus* work was valid. In the course of time, it became accepted in scientific circles that cells can undergo complete differentiation, to the point of making intestinal epithelium cells of a feeding tadpole, without any loss or stable inactivation, of genes needed for entirely unrelated cell lineages and indeed for every cell type.

After these early experiments, the main conclusion that, during the course of cell differentiation the genome is conserved and repressed quiescent genes can be reactivated, was confirmed. With various colleagues, and especially R. A. Laskey, we were able to obtain normal tadpoles from adult foot web skin and from a range of adult organs such as heart, lung, etc. from cells grown out in culture from these tissues (Laskey and Gurdon 1970). Although we were able to obtain normal sexually mature male and female adult animals from the intestinal epithelium cells of a feeding tadpole and we were able to obtain feeding tadpoles from the nuclei of adult cells, we never obtained a sexually mature adult animal starting from the nucleus of another adult cell. We think that the intensely rapid cell division and DNA replication enforced on an Amphibian transplanted nucleus by an activated egg has a high probability of introducing replication defects, as is seen in *Rana pipiens* (Di Berardino and King 1967) thereby greatly reducing the chance of obtaining entirely normal development from the nucleus of an adult cell.

EPIGENETIC MEMORY

In addition to the rapid DNA replication and cell division enforced on a transplanted somatic nucleus, there are other ways in which we may account for the progressively decreasing success rate of nuclear transfers from differentiating and differentiated cells. One of these is that there may be a memory of a pattern of gene expression characteristic of the differentiated state. One obvious possibility is that there could be a resistance to the reactivation of those genes which are needed for early development but which have become quiescent or repressed during cell differentiation. This possibility is discussed below under the heading of "Resistance."

Another interesting possibility is that there could be a memory of an active gene state. For example, those genes that are strongly expressed in specialised cells might fail to be switched off after nuclear transfer and might then interfere with new directions of lineage selection by nuclear transplant embryos. Methods that were not available when amphibian nuclear transfers were first carried out have now made it possible to test this idea. Nuclei were transplanted from muscle or other lineage-specific progenitor cells to make nuclear transplant embryos. Although many of the resulting nuclear transplant embryos developed abnormally, it was possible to collect enough material from partially cleaved embryos to carry out gene-specific transcript assays. The surprising result was obtained that a considerable memory of an active gene state persisted in these nuclear transplant embryos through many cell cycles of inactive transcription characteristic of early amphibian embryos. We found that the neurectoderm and endoderm lineages of nuclear transplant embryos derived from muscle progenitor nuclei often continued to express muscle genes to an excessive extent (Ng and Gurdon 2005). The memory was imperfect, in that about half of the nuclear transplant embryos from muscle progenitor cells showed an excessive, sometimes very large, overexpression of muscle genes in inappropriate tissues whereas the other half did not (Fig. 7). Genes characteristically expressed in a certain lineage became repressed for the early cleavage divisions of a nuclear transplant embryo but then became re-expressed throughout the embryo after the stage of transcriptional activation at the late blastula stage. This result was also found in other, non-muscle lineages (Ng and Gurdon, 2005). It was also found that this "memory" of an active gene state was associated with histone H3.3, an abundant protein in eggs and early embryos. The explanation offered for this phenomenon was that the very high level of histone normally present in oocytes and eggs (Cho and Wolffe 1994) enhances transcription of any gene

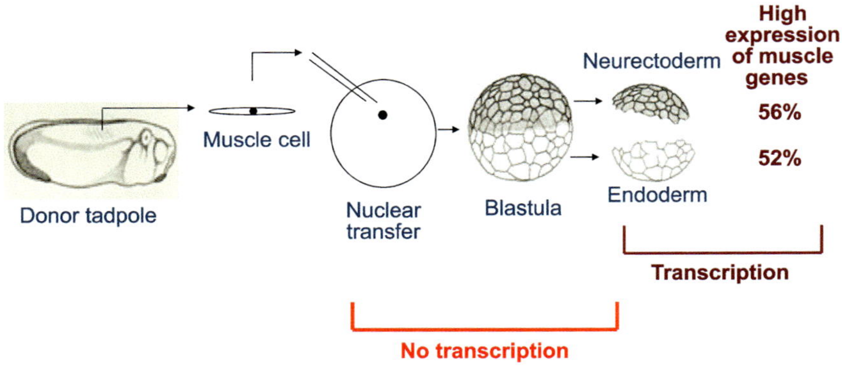

FIGURE 7. Epigenetic memory in nuclear transplant embryos. Nuclear transplant embryos derived from muscle nuclei were grown to the blastula stage, and then depleted of the mesoderm region (muscle lineage). The remaining regions (neurectoderm for nerve/skin cells and endoderm for intestine lineages) express the muscle gene marker MyoD to an excessive extent in about half of all such embryos (Ng and Gurdon 2008).

that is in an active state at the time of nuclear transplantation (Ng and Gurdon 2008). Histone H3.3 is known to be associated with active transcription. Memory of an active gene state was subsequently described in iPS experiments (Polo *et al.* 2010). The observation that about 50% of nuclear transplant embryos show this memory that is not seen in the other 50% exemplifies the concept (see later) that there is a conflict between components of an egg that are designed to restore gene expression to that characteristic of an egg and embryo and the resistance of the nucleus of determined or specialised cells to resist any change, thereby stabilising the pathway of differentiation on which an embryonic cell has set out.

NUCLEAR TRANSFER IN MAMMALS

For these early results in *Xenopus* to be reproduced in mammals took nearly 40 years (Campbell *et al.* 1996; Wilmut *et al.* 1997) in sheep. A very important feature of these first successful mammalian nuclear transfer in sheep was the use of unfertilised eggs, as was actually used in amphibia. Earlier work with mice (McGrath and Solter 1984) used fertilised eggs. Although fertilised eggs can be used (Egli *et al.* 2007), synchronisation between nucleus and egg is harder to achieve than with the use of unfertilised eggs. A very elegant and important experiment that confirmed the general principle that cell differentiation proceeds

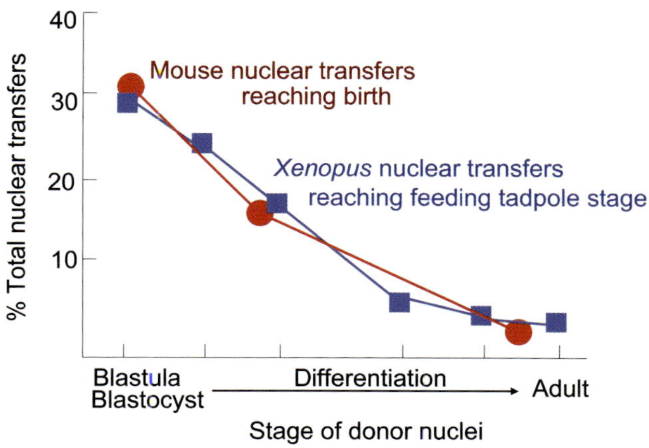

FIGURE 8. Survival of nuclear transplant embryos in *Xenopus* (Gurdon 1962) and the mouse (Wakayama *et al.* 1998).

with the retention of a complete set of genes was carried out using nuclei with a rearranged genome from mature mouse B or T donor cells (Hochedlinger and Jaenisch 2002). In the course of time, somatic cell nuclear transfer to eggs has been successful in the eggs of mice and other mammals (Wakayama *et al.* 1998). In each species there seem to be some technical requirements which have to be identified and overcome. In mammals, the early cell divisions after fertilisation are extremely slow compared to amphibians (20 hours from fertilisation to two-cell stage in the mouse). It is therefore unlikely that the chromosome damage seen in amphibian work (above) is important in mammals. Nevertheless the decreasing success rate of nuclear transplant embryo development is about the same in mice and frogs (Fig. 8). There must be other reasons for this resistance to reprogramming by eggs.

This brief history of successful somatic cell nuclear transplantation does not do justice to the many important contributions made after the early *Xenopus* work. For reviews of the early *Xenopus* work see Gurdon 1986. Subsequent reviews which also cover the early work have been published by McKinnell (1978), Di Berardino and Hoffner (1983) and Gurdon (2006).

MECHANISMS OF NUCLEAR REPROGRAMMING BY EGGS

The second question raised when embarking on a PhD thesis on nuclear transfer in *Xenopus* concerned mechanisms of reprogramming. There are two parts to this question. First, how does an egg reverse the differentiation state of a somatic nucleus to enable it to behave like a zygote nucleus when it leads to entirely normal development? The second question asks in what way do the nuclei of somatic cells become progressively resistant to the reprogramming conditions of an egg?

To approach these questions it was clearly necessary to focus on the transcription of individual kinds of genes. At that time, in the 1960s, genes had not been cloned and it was only possible to work with genes which were present in multiple copies per genome, such as 28S, 18S and 5S ribosomal genes. Working with ribosomal genes, transfer RNA genes, and the gross class of genes whose base composition resembled the average of the genome, it was shown that transplanted somatic nuclei in blastula and gastrula stages of nuclear transplant embryos had reverted to an embryonic pattern of transcription (Woodland and Gurdon 1969). However this did not lead to understanding the mechanism by which this rejuvenation took place. It took a few decades before single genes expressed in early *Xenopus* development had been cloned and the necessary probes and procedures developed by which the expression of these genes could be monitored in nuclear transplant embryos.

At this time it seemed useful to investigate the mechanisms that guide early embryo development when nuclear transplant embryos, especially from advanced donor stages, often develop very abnormally. I wondered whether the nuclear transfer techniques could be used to introduce purified macromolecules into an egg, and hence into embryonic cells. Thanks to my scientific friendship with Jean Brachet of Belgium, a major contributor to the field of Developmental Biology (Brachet 1957), I was able to acquire a small sample of purified globin mRNA from the laboratory of Dr Chantrenne. He was one of the first to purify any animal mRNA. Even a few micrograms of this was more precious than gold dust, and anything that came in contact with it had to be chromic acid cleaned for fear of RNAse. A highlight of my career at this time was the discovery that purified messenger RNA could be extremely efficiently translated into protein when injected directly into an egg or embryonic cell (Gurdon *et al.* 1971). Interestingly, this finding was completely unexpected because of the very high ribonuclease activity present in eggs. For this reason a grant application to permit such an experiment would not have succeeded. I was fortunate to have enough other funding to do this work without specific grant support. Amazingly it was possible to inject rabbit globin mRNA into the fertilised *Xenopus* egg, grow that egg to a tadpole stage and demonstrate that tissues such as muscle were still translating high levels of globin, wholly inappropriate to that cell type, without any interference in normal development (Woodland and Gurdon 1974). The injection of messenger RNA, and other macromolecules, into an egg has now become a very widely used procedure in developmental biology. I am still amazed at how well this works. We can now understand that the injection of an egg with a micropipette is sufficiently harmless that ribonuclease is not released from egg cytoplasm. It may be that the penetration of an egg with a micropipette is no more harmful than the penetration of an egg by sperm after fertilisation. mRNA injection led to the widespread use of mRNA injection for over- and under-expression experiments in developmental biology.

A key mechanism in early development is the concentration-dependent response of cells to signalling molecules, an area known as morphogen gradient interpretation. Even two-fold differences in ligand concentration are enough to make competent embryonic cells choose which cell type lineage to follow (Green and Smith 1990; Dyson and Gurdon 1998). We now know that small quantitative deficiencies in signalling can adversely affect nuclear transplant embryo development, as shown in cross species nuclear transplantation (Narbonne *et al.* 2011). Another particularly interesting aspect of concentration-dependent signalling is illustrated by the community effect (Gurdon 1988). Resulting from single cell transplantations, the concept developed by which a group of similar cells can contribute a high enough concentration of signal molecule to exceed a threshold never produced by a single cell. This community effect seems to contribute to the normal development of multicellular tissues in development. It later turned out that the principle behind the community effect had already been proposed, as "quorum sensing," to be involved in bacteria-dependent light emission in predatory fish and in other examples (Lamb 2012).

To progress with the analysis of reprogramming by egg cytoplasm, an obviously desirable route would be to achieve successful reprogramming of somatic nuclei by extracts of eggs; this could lead to the identification of such components by fractionation and selective depletion. Somatic nuclei transplanted to eggs are almost immediately induced to commence DNA replication (Graham *et al.* 1966). Extracts of eggs are remarkably successful in inducing DNA replication in isolated nuclei (Laskey *et al.* 1989; Mechali 2010) but such extracts are notoriously difficult to make in such a way that transcription proceeds meaningfully. This difficulty in making functional extracts of cells is in marked contrast to the long lasting success of injecting messenger RNA, genes, *etc.* into living cells. The injection of components into eggs and early embryo cells can be regarded as "living biochemical test tubes" (Gurdon 1974).

THE ANALYSIS OF NUCLEAR REPROGRAMMING BY OOCYTES

It was evident from the earliest amphibian nuclear transfer experiments that the replication of DNA and chromosomes in somatic nuclei transplanted to eggs is very often defective (Di Berardino and King 1967). Once penetrated and activated by sperm or an injection pipette, amphibian eggs immediately enter a phase of some ten or more rapid cell division cycles. It is very difficult for a somatic cell nucleus, which might normally divide once every two days, to switch immediately to a division cycle of 30 minutes. As a result, the DNA of transplanted nuclei or their daughters is often torn apart at cell division when incompletely replicated. This leads to major chromosome loss and other defects, especially when the nucleus of a slow-dividing somatic cell is transplanted. It was clear, at this point, that we had to find a way of analysing the reprogramming of somatic cell nuclei without the disadvantage and damaging effect of enforced rapid DNA replication and cell division. This led to the introduction of amphibian oocytes as somatic cell nuclear transfer recipients.

The amphibian oocyte is the growth phase of an early germ cell to a full-sized egg progenitor with lampbrush chromosomes over a period of several months (Callan 1982). These cells are in the prophase of first meiosis (Fig. 9).

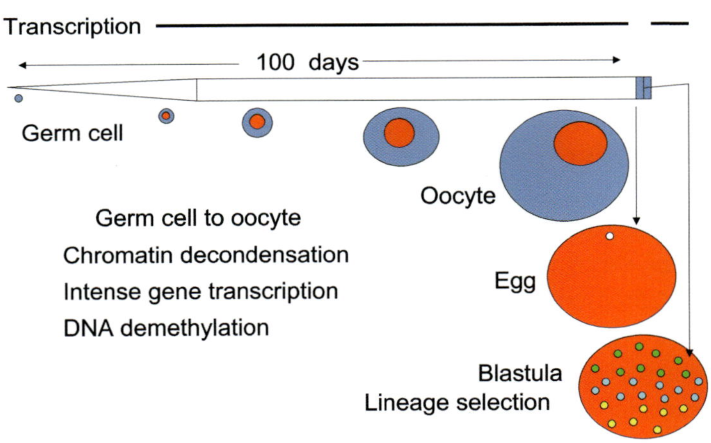

FIGURE 9. The *Xenopus* oocyte grows in the ovary from a germ cell over many months while it is in first meiotic prophase. When fully grown it can respond to hormones, such as progesterone, to complete first meiosis and arrest in second meiotic metaphase. Once fertilised, it progresses to the blastula stage in 8 hours and somatic lineages already start to appear.

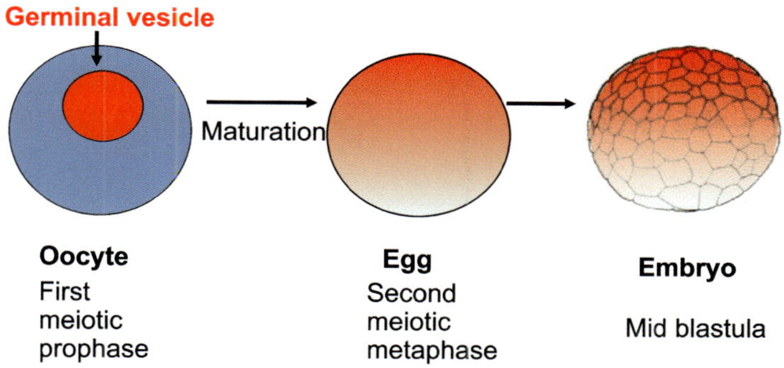

FIGURE 10. A *Xenopus* oocyte has a huge (420μ diameter) germinal vesicle, which includes its tetraploid chromosome set. After completion of meiosis, the germinal vesicle contents are distributed to the egg and subsequently to the embryo.

These full-sized egg progenitors are normally induced by hormone levels to complete first meiosis and progress to the metaphase of second meiosis, after which they can respond to fertilisation. While still in my PhD graduate work, I developed the use of *Xenopus* oocytes to analyse the origin of the DNA replication inducing capacity of eggs. Even sperm nuclei can be converted to lampbrush chromosomes after injection to oocytes (Gall and Murphy 1988). It became clear that somatic nuclei or even pure DNA would be efficiently and correctly transcribed when injected into the germinal vesicle (= nucleus) of an oocyte (Mertz and Gurdon 1977; Brown and Gurdon 1977). It is important to appreciate that the germinal vesicle of an amphibian oocyte contains an enormous reserve of developmentally essential components, which are distributed to the egg cytoplasm during completion of meiosis (Fig. 10). These reserves are necessary for normal embryonic development. Fortunately for developmental biologists, these components, specified by the intensely active lampbrush chromosomes, are accumulated in the specialised germinal vesicle where they represent a high concentration of components that later enter the egg cytoplasm. Since DNA replication and cell division do not take place in these growing oocytes, the oocyte germinal vesicle provides an accessible accumulation of transcriptionally-active components.

Somatic nuclei, chromatin, or DNA, of amphibian or mammalian origin, can, with practice, be injected into the invisible germinal vesicle of an intact oocyte (Halley-Stott 2010). Xenopus oocytes show selective transcription of somatic nuclei from unrelated species (De Robertis and Gurdon 1977). Transcription

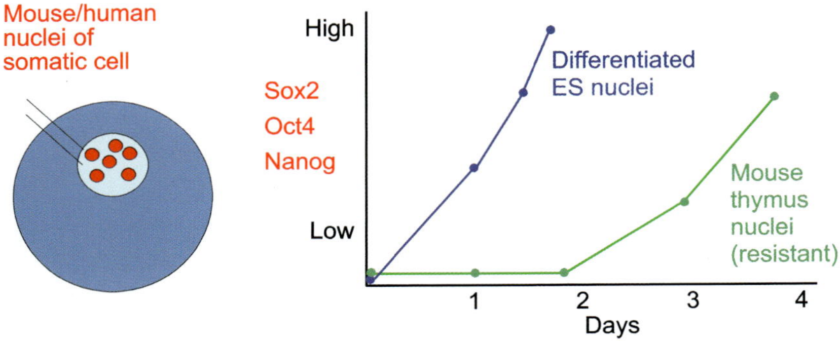

FIGURE 11. Somatic nuclei injected into the germinal vesicle of an oocyte transcribe genes that are quiescent in the donor cells but are rapidly transcriptionally activated. The most specialised donor nuclei (mouse thymus) showed temporal resistance to transcriptional activation.

of injected nuclei or genes takes place at a high rate, with as much as several hundred re-initiations of transcription on a gene per day. Two hundred to 300 somatic nuclei can be injected into one oocyte's germinal vesicle, so that one injected oocyte provides the same amount of nuclear material as 250 eggs injected with a single nucleus (Fig. 12). This makes it realistic to carry out on oocytes those molecular techniques that normally require large amounts of material. When injecting purified DNA, this becomes chromatinised (Wyllie *et al.* 1977). Oocytes continue to transcribe injected nuclei or chromatin for several days. It is possible to manually isolate the germinal vesicle from an oocyte, containing injected somatic nuclei, and to carry out antibody binding, FRAP assays etc. on individual transplanted nuclei. After injection into the germinal vesicle, somatic nuclei undergo a massive chromatin decondensation as does sperm in an egg. After transfer to oocytes, some genes are transcribed extensively, and continue to accumulate large numbers of transcripts. These activated genes include some of those that are active in embryos, including the well-known pluripotency genes, such as Oct4, Sox2, Nanog, etc. These characteristics make the injected first meiotic prophase oocyte of *Xenopus* very suitable for analysing both the activation of genes during reprogramming as well as the basis of resistance by the nuclei of differentiated somatic cells (Halley-Stott *et al.* 2010).

TRANSCRIPTIONAL ACTIVATION

Several necessary early steps have now been identified. The first of these is the movement of a special linker histone, known as B4 in amphibia or H1foo in mammals, into transplanted nuclei. This histone protein is very abundant in the germinal vesicle of amphibian oocytes and a large amount of it is incorporated into the chromatin of injected nuclei within 2–3 hours at 17°C. This step is necessary for subsequent transcriptional activation, as shown by the use of antibodies and overexpressed dominant negative forms of this histone which inhibit subsequent pluripotency gene activation (Jullien *et al.* 2010). When B4 histone invades transplanted nuclei, these nuclei lose the somatic form of linker histone. This substitution of linker histone in chromatin is likely to be an important part of the striking decondensation of chromosomes that takes place soon after nuclear injection. This early event is thought to give access of other oocyte components, including transcription factors, to injected chromatin. B4 histone is abundant in oocytes but is not present in normal development after the blastula stage (Smith *et al.* 1988). The next important events include the movement of another oocyte-specific histone, namely histone H3.3, into injected nuclei. Histone H3.3 is present in somatic cells but at a much higher concentration in oocytes, and is generally associated with active transcription. We have noted above that histone H3.3 may be causally associated with epigenetic memory in somatic nuclei transplanted to second metaphase eggs. If histone H3.3 has a general role of enhancing transcription, this would help to account both for epigenetic memory in nuclear transplant embryos as well as for the increasing level of transcription seen in somatic nuclei transplanted to oocytes (Gurdon 1986). A later event is the polymerisation of nuclear actin in oocytes and in nuclei transplanted to their germinal vesicles (Miyamoto *et al.* 2011). This seems to enhance the level of transcription of transplanted nuclei during the first two days. This sequence of events leads to a high level of transcriptional reprogramming, and takes place at a remarkably fast rate. Within two days, most of the somatic nuclei transplanted to oocytes have strongly activated transcription of the pluripotency gene Sox2; this happens at 17°C, the metabolic equivalent of 12 hours at 37°C.

Although the transcription of some genes, after nuclear transfer to oocytes, is enormously increased from a somatic level, up to 100 times for Sox2, the oocyte germinal vesicle does not cause a global transcriptional enhancement of all genes. RNA-Seq analysis shows that most genes in a mouse somatic cell are not changed in transcription, some remaining at a high level and others remaining at a repressed level. A minority of genes that were active in somatic cells become repressed after transfer to oocytes and a smaller fraction undergoes a great enhancement of transcription. Thus the reprogramming of somatic nuclei by the oocyte germinal vesicle is highly selective (Jullien *et al.* unpublished). Those genes that are transcriptionally activated include ones that are strongly

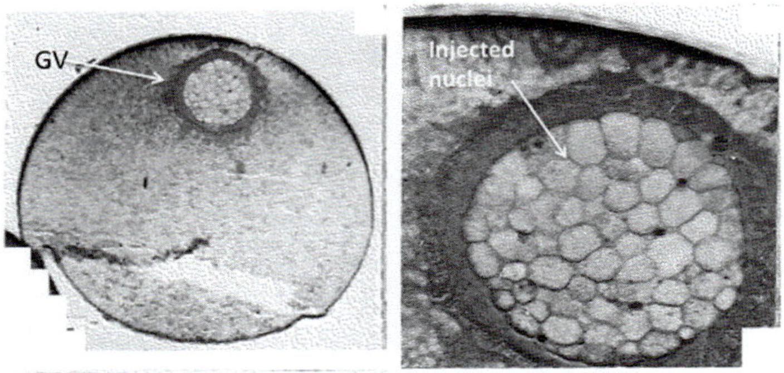

FIGURE 12. Multiple somatic nuclei can be injected into the germinal vesicle of an oocyte; whole oocyte (left) and germinal vesicle (right).

expressed and important in early mammalian development, including Sox2, Oct4, and Nanog. The germinal vesicle of an oocyte seems to be endowed with components that induce intense transcriptional activity, as seen in lampbrush chromosomes, for all genes that are accessible (Jullien *et al.* 2011). However some genes in somatic nuclei do not respond to the transcription-inducing conditions of the egg.

RESISTANCE TO REPROGRAMMING BY OOCYTES

To me, resistance to transcriptional activation is now the most interesting aspect of nuclear reprogramming. This increasing resistance associated with development seems to reflect the remarkable stability of cell differentiation (Fig 11). Hardly ever does a cell of one specialised type switch to another cell-type, or produce daughter cells that do so. Resistance to reprogramming is also evident in cell fusion experiments (Blau *et al.* 1983), and even more so in iPS work (Yamanaka 2012). The transplantation of mammalian somatic nuclei containing a repressed X chromosome has identified one kind of molecule responsible. Mouse embryo fibroblasts containing an inactive X chromosome are highly resistant to the transcription of these genes after nuclear transfer to oocytes. However, the nuclei of mouse embryo blastodisc cells that also contain an inactive X chromosome are strongly reactivated transcriptionally by oocytes. This difference between blastodisc and adult nuclei has turned out to be attributable to the chromosomal component macroH2A whose removal or inactivation in adult mouse embryonic fibroblast (MEF) nuclei results in transcription of pluripotency genes (Pasque *et al.* 2011a). At present, we envisage the female mammalian X inactivation process as a set of steps that progressively stabilise the inactive state. Thus, as development and cell differentiation proceed, successive levels of inactivation, involving histone modifications such as H3K27Me2/3 and macroH2A absorption into chromatin, and finally methylation of DNA, cause a gene to become stably repressed and highly resistant to reprogramming (Pasque *et al.* 2011b).

To analyse other ways in which genes become resistant to reprogramming, two experimental routes are likely to prove useful. One is to progressively remove components of isolated nuclei, and then test their transcription in injected oocytes until resistance is lost (Halley-Stott, unpublished). This procedure is proving successful in depleting nuclei of all RNA including non-coding RNA. Increasing concentrations of NaCl with Triton can progressively deplete isolated nuclei of chromosomal proteins. If resistance can be restored by adding back defined fractions of released proteins, this could lead to the identification of those chromosomal proteins that confer resistance on individual genes. Another potentially valuable experimental approach is to overexpress, by mRNA injection to oocytes, those enzymes that add or remove modifications to histones. It should then be possible to relate a particular histone or other chromosomal modification to the resistance of a gene to reprogramming by oocytes. By these methods, there is a prospect of understanding, in reasonable detail, the mechanisms of nuclear reprogramming and resistance in nuclei transplanted to amphibian oocytes.

OVERVIEW AND PROSPECTS

The process of nuclear reprogramming by eggs and oocytes can be seen as a conflict between the cytoplasm of an egg whose components are designed to promote rapid DNA replication and then transcription, and the components of differentiated cell nuclei whose function is to maintain a stable state. The cytoplasm of an egg is specially designed to activate the highly condensed and specialised nucleus of sperm, with 100% efficiency. Not surprisingly, the same components are effective at activating the nucleus of a somatic cell. The difference is that a somatic cell nucleus has become, during the process of cell differentiation, highly resistant to activation by egg cytoplasm in a way that is different from sperm nuclei. These nuclei of differentiated cells are provided with molecules that stabilise their differentiated state and resist reversal or rejuvenation. If differentiated cell nuclei could be too easily switched to an embryonic state, this could permit the reversal of differentiation and lead to cancer and other defects.

The experimental work described here has centred on the use of amphibian eggs and oocytes because of the abundance of material and ready availability offered by them, an advantage that was very clear to developmental biologists up to the 1950s. The general principles that have emerged from work on amphibia seem also to apply to mammals and other vertebrate species. A full understanding of nuclear reprogramming by amphibian eggs and oocytes may well facilitate nuclear reprogramming in mammals including humans, and hence contribute to the eventual therapeutic application of cell replacement.

REFERENCES

Blau, H.M., Chiu, C.P., Webster, C. (1983), "Cytoplasmic activation of human nuclear genes in stable heterokaryons," *Cell* 32:1171–1180.

Brachet, J. (1957), *Biochemical Cytology*. New York: Academic Press, 516pp.

Briggs, R. & King, T.J. (1952), "Transplantation of living nuclei from blastula cells into enucleated frogs' eggs," *Proc Natl Acad Sci USA*, 38:455–463.

Briggs, R. & King, T.J. (1957), "Changes in the nuclei of differentiating endoderm cells as revealed by nuclear transplantation," *J Morph*. 100:269–312.

Brown, D.D. and Gurdon, J.B. (1964), "Absence of ribosomal-RNA synthesis in the anucleolate mutant of *Xenopus laevis*," *Proc Natl Acad Sci USA*. 51:139–146.

Brown, D.D. and Gurdon, J.B. (1977), "High fidelity transcription of 5S DNA injected into *Xenopus* oocytes," *Proc Natl Acad Sci USA*. 74:2064–2068.

Callan, H.G. (1982), The Croonian Lecture, 1981, "Lampbrush chromosomes," *Proc R Soc London Ser. B* 214:417–418.

Campbell, K.H., McWhir, J., Ritchie, W.A., Wilmut, I. (1996), "Sheep cloned by nuclear transfer from a cultured cell line," *Nature* 380:64–66.

Chan, A.P. and Gurdon, J.B. (1996), "Nuclear transplantation from stably transfected cultured cells of *Xenopus*," *Int J Dev Biol*. 40:441–451.

Cho, H., Wolffe, A.P. (1994), "*Xenopus laevis* B4, an intron-containing oocyte-specific linker histone-encoding gene," *Gene* 143:233–238.

De Robertis, E.M. and Gurdon, J.B. (1977), "Gene activation in somatic nuclei after injection into amphibian oocytes," *Proc Natl Acad Sci USA* 74, 2470–2474.

Di Berardino, M.A., King, T.J. (1967), "Development and cellular differentiation of neural nuclear transplants of known karyotype," *Dev Biol*. 15:102–128.

DiBerardino, M.A., Hoffner, N.J. (1983), "Gene reactivation in erythrocytes: nuclear transplantation in oocyts and eggs of *Rana*," *Science* 219:862–864.

Dyson, S. and Gurdon, J.B. (1998), "The interpretation of position in a morphogen gradient as revealed by occupancy of activin receptors," *Cell* 93:557–568.

Egli, D., Rosains, J., Birkhoff, G., Eggan, K. (2007), "Developmental reprogramming after chromosome transfer into mitotic mouse zygotes," *Nature* 447:679–85.

Elsdale, T.R., Gurdon, J.B. and Fischberg, M. (1960), "A description of the technique for nuclear transplantation in *Xenopus laevis*," *J Embryol exp Morph.* 8:437–444.

Gall, J.G., Murphy, C. (1998), "Assembly of lampbrush chromosomes from sperm chromatin," *Mol Biol Cell.* 9:733–747.

Graham, C.F., Arms, K. and Gurdon, J.B. (1966), "The induction of DNA synthesis by frog egg cytoplasm," *Dev Biol.* 14:349–381.

Green, J. B., Smith. J.C. (1990), "Graded changes in dose of *Xenopus* activin A homologue elicit stepwise transactions in embryonic cell fate," *Nature* 374:391–394.

Gurdon, J.B. (1960a), "The effects of ultraviolet irradiation on uncleaved eggs of *Xenopus laevis*," *Quart J Micr Sci.* 101:299–312.

Gurdon, J.B. (1960b), "Factors responsible for the abnormal development of embryos obtained by nuclear transplantation in *Xenopus laevis*," *J Embryol exp Morph.* 8: 327–340.

Gurdon, J.B. (1962), "The developmental capacity of nuclei taken from intestinal epithelium cells of feeding tadpoles," *J Embryol exp Morph.* 10:622–640.

Gurdon, J.B. (1974), "Molecular biology in a living cell," *Nature* 248:772–776.

Gurdon, J.B. (1986), "Nuclear transplantation in eggs and oocytes," *J Cell Sci.* (Suppl.) 4, 287–318.

Gurdon, J.B. (1988), "A community effect in animal development," *Nature* 336:772–774.

Gurdon, J.B. (2006), "From nuclear transfer to nuclear reprogramming: the reversal of cell differentiation," *Ann Rev Cell Dev Biol.* 22:1–22.

Gurdon, J.B. and Hopwood, N. (2000), "The introduction of *Xenopus laevis* into developmental biology: Of empire, pregnancy testing and ribosomal genes," *Int J Dev Biol.* 44:43–50.

Gurdon, J.B. and Uehlinger, V. (1966), "'Fertile' intestine nuclei," *Nature* 210:1240–1241.

Gurdon, J.B., Lane, C.D., Woodland, H.R. and Marbaix, G. (1971), "The use of frog eggs and oocytes for the study of messenger RNA and its translation in living cells," *Nature* 233:177–182.

Halley-Stott, R.P., Pasque, V., Astrand, C., Miyamoto, K., Simeoni, I., Jullien, J. and Gurdon, J.B. (2010), "Mammalian Nuclear Transplantation to Germinal Vesicle stage *Xenopus* Oocytes—A method for Quantitative Transcriptional Reprogramming," *Methods* 51:56–65.

Hochedlinger, K. and Jaenisch, R. (2002), "Monoclonal mice generated by nuclear transfer from mature B and T donor cells," *Nature* 415:1035–1038.

Jaenisch, R. (2012), "Nuclear cloning and direct reprogramming: the long and the short path to Stockholm," *Cell Stem Cell*, 11:1–4.

Jullien, J., Astrand, C., Halley-Stott, R.P., Garrett, N. and Gurdon, J.B. (2010), "Characterization of somatic cell nuclear reprogramming by oocytes in which a linker histone is required for pluripotency gene reactivation," *Proc Natl Acad Sci USA.* 107:5483–5488.

Jullien, J., Halley-Stott, R.P., Miyamoto, K., Pasque, V. and Gurdon, J.B. (2011b), "Mechanisms of nuclear reprogramming by eggs and oocytes: a deterministic process?," *Nature Reviews Molecular & Cell Biology* 12:453–459.

Lamb, R.F. (2012), "Amino acid sensing mechanisms: an Achilles heel in cancer?," *FEBS J* 279:2624–31.

Laskey, R.A. and Gurdon, J.B. (1970), "Genetic content of adult somatic cells tested by nuclear transplantation from cultured cells," *Nature* 228:1332–1334.

Laskey, R.A., Fairman, M.P., Blow, J.J. (1989), "S phase of the cell cycle," *Science* 246:609–14.

McGrath, J., Solter, D. (1984), "Inability of mouse blastomere nuclei transferred to enucleated zygotes to support development *in vitro*," *Science* 226:1317–9.

McKinnell, R.G. (1978), *Cloning: nuclear transplantation in Amphibia*, University of Minnesota Press, Minneapolis, USA.

Mechali, M. (2010), "Eukaryotic DNA replication origins: many choices for appropriate answers," *Nat Rev Mol Cell Biol.* 11:728–38.

Mertz, J.E. and Gurdon, J.B. (1977), "Purified DNAs are transcribed after microinjection into *Xenopus* oocytes," *Proc Natl Acad Sci. USA* 74, 1502–1506.

Miyamoto, K., Pasque, V., Jullien, J. and Gurdon, J.B. (2011), "Nuclear actin polymerization is required for transcriptional reprogramming of Oct4 by oocytes," *Genes & Development* 25(9):946–958.

Narbonne, P., Simpson, D.E. and Gurdon, J.B. (2011), "Deficient induction response in a *Xenopus* nucleocytoplasmic hybrid," *PLoS Biology* 9(11):e1001197.

Ng, R.K. and Gurdon, J.B. (2005), "Epigenetic memory of active gene transcription is inherited through somatic cell nuclear transfer," *Proc Natl Acad Sci. USA*, 102:1957–1962.

Ng, R.K. and Gurdon, J.B. (2008), "Epigenetic memory of an active gene state depends on histone H3.3 incorporation into chromatin in the absence of transcription," *Nature Cell Biol.* 10(1):102–9.

Pasque, V., Gillich, A., Garrett, N. and Gurdon, J.B. (2011a), "Histone variant macroH2A confers resistance to nuclear reprogramming," *EMBO J.* 6;30(12):2373–87.

Pasque, V., Jullien, J., Miyamoto, K., Halley-Stott, R.P. and Gurdon, J.B. (2011b), "Epigenetic factors influencing resistance to nuclear reprogramming," *Trends in Genetics* 27(12):516–525.

Polo, J.M., Liu, S., Figueroa, M.E., Kulalert, W., Eminli, S. et al. (2010), "Cell-type of origin influences the molecular and functional properties of mouse induced pluripotent stem cells," *Nat Biotechnol.* 28(8):848–55.

Rauber, A. (1886), "Personaltheil und germinaltheil des individuum," *Zool. Anz.* 9, 166–171.

Smith, R.C., Dworkin-Rastl, E., Dworkin, M.B. (1988), "Expression of a histone H1-like protein is restricted to early *Xenopus* development," *Genes Dev.* 2:1284–1295.

Spemann, H. (1938), *Embryonic development and induction*, New Haven, Conn: Yale University Press.

Wakayama, T., Perry, A.C., Zuccotti, M., Johnson, K.R., Yamagimachi, R. (1998), "Full-term development of mice from enucleated oocytes injected with cumulus cell nuclei," *Nature* 394:369–74.

Wilmut, I., Schnieke, A.E., McWhir, J., Kind, A.J. and Campbell, K.H.S. (1997), "Viable offspring derived from fetal and adult mammalian cells," *Nature* 385:810–813.

Woodland, H.R. and Gurdon, J.B. (1969), "RNA synthesis in an amphibian nuclear-transplant hybrid," *Dev Biol.* 20:89–104.

Woodland, H.R., Gurdon, J.B. and Lingrel, J.B. (1974), "The translation of mammalian globin mRNA injected into fertilised eggs of *Xenopus laevis*. II. The distribution of globin synthesis in different tissues," *Dev Biol.* 39:134–140.

Wyllie, A.H., Gurdon, J.B. and Price, J. (1977), "Nuclear localization of an oocyte component required for the stability of injected DNA," *Nature* 268:150–152.

Yamanaka, S. (2012), "Induced pluripotent stem cells: past, present, and future," *Cell Stem Cell* 10:676–684.

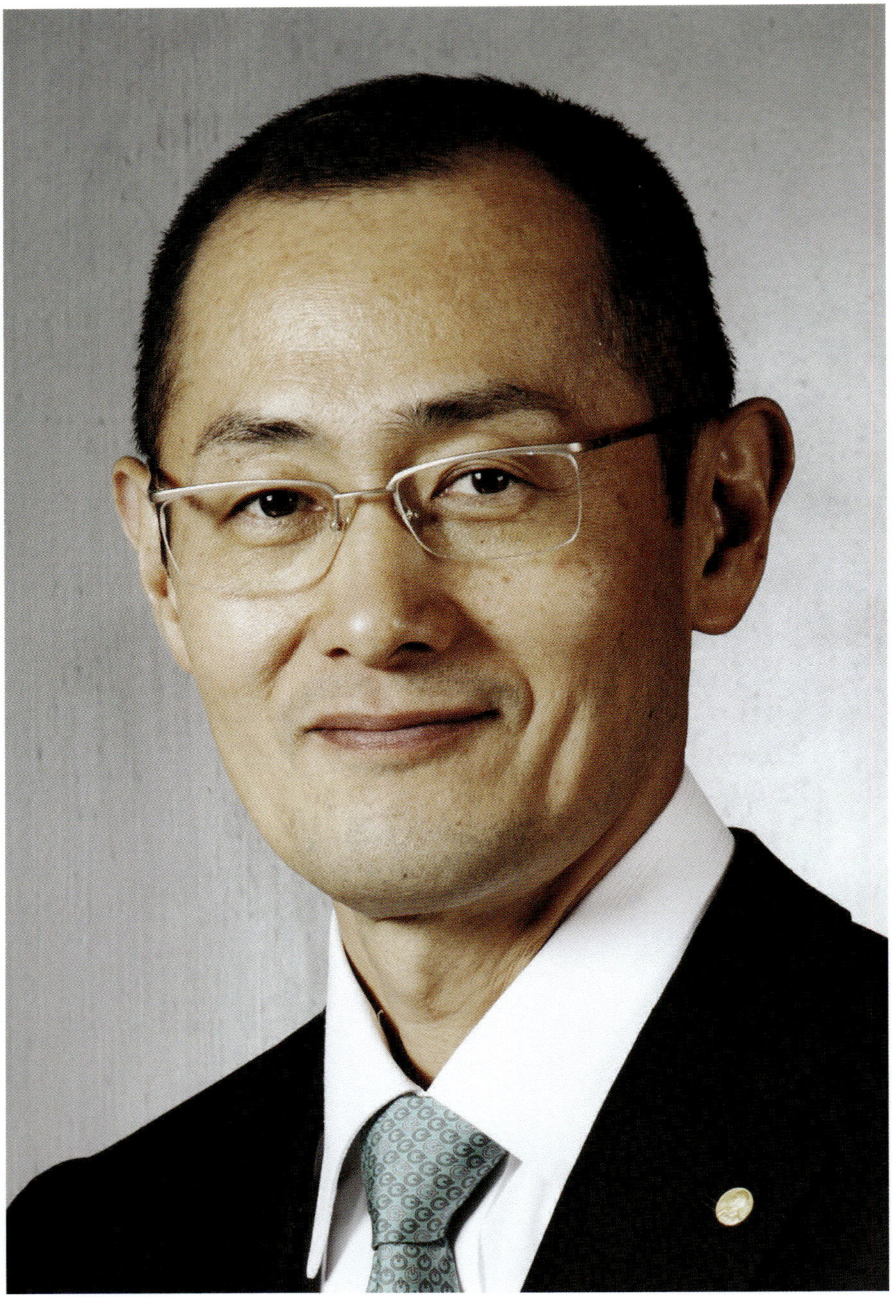

Shinya Yamanaka. © The Nobel Foundation. Photo: U. Montan

Shinya Yamanaka

I was born on September 4, 1962, in Osaka, Japan. My father, Shozaburo, ran a small factory in the city of Higashi-Osaka manufacturing components for sawing machines, which he took over in his early 20s after my grandfather passed away. Higashi-Osaka is well known for its cluster of highly skilled small and midsize manufacturers. Like other owners of small companies in the area, my father was an engineer who designed new products and made them by himself. My mother, Minako, helped him run the business, raising their two children, me and my older sister, Yumiko. Looking back on my childhood, I can see now that my father exerted a great influence on me. He did not force me to do or be anything, but, by showing diligence in his work, he taught me silently how meaningful it is to create something from the drawing board, and how interesting it is to seek for oneself a better way of achieving a goal.

SCHOOL DAYS

I remember that when I was a child, I found it very exciting to dismantle clocks and radios into small pieces and then try to assemble them again, though most of the time I ended up breaking them. Maybe I just copied what my father was doing. My childhood dream was to become an engineer like him. Science was one of my favorite classes at school. I liked reading a monthly scientific magazine for elementary school children. This magazine came with various kits for children to do experiments. I remember one time I was doing an experiment with an alcohol lamp that came with the magazine. It dropped onto a *kotatsu* heater table and the quilt over it caught fire. I was severely scolded by my mother.

I was educated at the Tennoji Junior High School/High School attached to Osaka Kyoiku University and received an excellent education, with many unique friends and teachers. Entering the junior high in 1975, I joined its judo team as my father recommended me. He thought I was too skinny and should become stronger. I devoted myself to judo and continued practicing it for several years until I quit it due to a serious injury in my second year at college. At the high school, there were some teachers who often told students that we should try to become a superman or superwoman, meaning that we should not only study hard but also try to experience many activities such as sports and activities in the student association. Inspired by them, I formed a folk song band with my classmates, called "Karesansui" ('Dry Garden Style'), and performed at the school's student festivals. I played the guitar and was a vocalist. I also committed to the school association as a vice president.

Throughout my school years, I was good at mathematics and physics. Thinking about my career, I considered studying basic sciences in college but decided to go to medical school, partly because my father used to advise me to become a physician instead of taking over his business. I don't know why that was his wish, but he may have thought that I was not cut out for business or may have wanted me to have a job more stable than running a small business that is easily affected by the economic climate. A book also pushed me to become a medical doctor. I was deeply inspired by Torao Tokuda, a physician who founded a hospital group in the 1970s that tried to revolutionize the Japanese medical care system. In 1981, I succeeded in my ambition of being accepted at Kobe University's School of Medicine. There again, I enjoyed playing judo and rugby, and suffered many broken bones while doing sports. In addition, I often suffered from severe pain in my legs due to over-training. These experiences made me interested in sports medicine and I decided to become an orthopedic surgeon.

RESIDENT AT A HOSPITAL

After receiving an M.D. from Kobe University in 1987, I served as a resident at the Osaka National Hospital for two years. During this period, two major events happened to me. I married Chika, whom I first met as a classmate at junior high school. She became a dermatologist and now runs a clinic in Osaka. The other unforgettable event was my father's death. He had long suffered from diabetes and also had hepatitis caused by a blood transfusion he had received a few years earlier to treat an injury. During his last two years, as a medical student and resident I gave him injections and administered intravenous drips, and he seemed happy to receive such treatments from his son.

Working at the hospital, I found that my surgical skills were not as good as I expected. One time it took me two hours to do a surgical operation which could have been completed in 30 minutes by other surgeons. My supervisors were very tough on new residents like me, and I lost confidence in my ability. In addition, treating many patients with intractable diseases and injuries such as rheumatoid arthritis and spinal cord injury, I realized that there were many diseases that even talented surgeons and physicians cannot cure. Even now, I recall clearly one female patient who had severe rheumatoid arthritis. There was a photograph of a cheerful woman on her bedside cabinet. I though it must be her sister or something. Learning that it was herself only a few years back, I was shocked that the patient looked totally different because of the disease. Painful and unforgettable bedside experiences finally drove me to switch my goal from becoming a surgeon who would help free patients from pain to becoming a basic scientist who would eradicate those intractable diseases by finding out their mechanisms and ultimately a way of curing them.

FROM SURGEON TO SCIENTIST

As the first step toward my new goal, I became a Ph.D. student in pharmacology at Osaka City University Graduate School of Medicine in 1989, working in Kenjiro Yamamoto's laboratory. During the next four years, I learned the essentials about how to design and conduct experiments and analyze data from my direct mentor, Katsuyuki Miura. The first instruction he gave me was to read as many papers as possible to help me think about a research theme. A few months later he assigned me to perform an experiment to study the role of a blood lipid named platelet-activating factor in lowering blood pressure in dogs.

Miura's hypothesis was that administering an inhibitor of another lipid, thromboxane A2, which is activated by platelet-activating factor, would prevent the blood pressure from going down. But my experiment showed a completely opposite result. I was so excited with the unexpected outcome that I became totally fascinated by basic science. Miura was also enthusiastic about the findings even though they were against his hypothesis. This study later became my Ph.D. dissertation, published in *Circulation Research* in 1993. There was an eye-opening moment when Miura told me that scientists have to compete with researchers around the world. When I was a resident, my rivals were other residents at the same hospital. As a scientist, I could win global recognition in a scientific field, albeit a small one, if my findings were published in high-profile journals. His words made me pay keen attention to research abroad.

POSTDOCTORAL FELLOW AT GLADSTONE

At the time, I was astonished by mouse transgenesis and gene targeting, which specifically induce or delete a single gene of interest, because no pharmacological agents could perform such miracles. After finishing my Ph.D. work in 1993, I applied for as many postdoctoral positions as I could in labs doing mouse molecular genetics because I wanted to obtain postdoctoral training and further skills including techniques to make knockout mice.However, it was very natural that a failed surgeon with little experience in molecular biology had a hard time finding a position. A turning point came when I got a fax from Thomas Innerarity at the Gladstone Institute of Cardiovascular Diseases in San Francisco. After a short telephone conversation, Tom was brave enough to give me a postdoctoral position in his lab! Working at Gladstone was one of the best decisions I ever made in my life. Gladstone provided an almost perfect environment for an ambitious new researcher like me thanks to its skillful technicians and the provocative discussions about science I had with enthusiastic colleagues.

When I joined Tom's lab, he had a hypothesis that forced expression in the liver of APOBEC1, the ApoB messenger RNA-editing enzyme, would lower plasma cholesterol levels and thus prevent atherosclerosis. To examine this hypothesis, I generated transgenic mice overexpressing Apobec1 in their livers. To our surprise, however, the transgenic mice developed liver tumors. We learned that Apobec1 is a potent protooncogene. Naturally, Tom was disappointed, but I became very interested in the molecular mechanisms of this totally unexpected result. Tom, despite the finding being against his hypothesis, encouraged me to continue studying the APOBEC1-mediated oncogenesis. Thanks to his support, I identified a novel target of Apobec1, Nat1, which was aberrantly edited in the transgenic mouse livers. I decided to generate Nat1-knockout mice to study the gene's function. Robert Farese at Gladstone and his research associate Heather Myers kindly taught me how to culture mouse embryonic stem (ES) cells and make chimeras.

Gladstone also provided me with the opportunity to acquire presentation skills and to learn a key idea for success as a scientist. One day, Robert Mahley, the then president of Gladstone, gathered about 20 postdocs and said that "VW" was a magic word to make us successful scientists. What he meant was that scientists need to have a clear vision and work hard toward it. I found myself not having a clear vision, although I was confident that I was one of the most hard-working postdocs at Gladstone at the time. I have since set my vision as being "to contribute to the development of new cures for patients through basic research." I still have the "VW" lesson in mind and often quote it to my students in my lab.

In 1996, my wife Chika and our two daughters, Mika and Miki, who were living in San Francisco with me, returned to Japan to enroll Mika in an elementary school in Osaka. About six months after they left, I went back to Japan as I missed them so much. Back in my home country, I eventually got an assistant professor position in the department of pharmacology at Osaka City University Medical School. Tom kindly let me continue the Nat1 work and shipped three chimeric mice I had made to Japan. The then chairman of the department, Hiroshi Iwao, was very supportive and allowed me to work on Nat1, which seemed to have little value in pharmacology. I found that Nat1 is required for early mouse development.

More importantly, I found that Nat1-null embryonic stem (ES) cells proliferate normally but cannot properly differentiate. These surprising findings changed the meaning of mouse ES cells for me from a research tool to a research subject. I became intrigued in how ES cells maintain their differentiation ability while rapidly proliferating.

POST AMERICA DEPRESSION

In Japan, however, I found myself suffering from Post America Depression or PAD. The environment for researchers in Japan was quite different in many ways from that in the U.S. At the medical school, very few scientists showed interest in the basic biology of mouse ES cells, and there was little thought-provoking discussion with my colleagues. Some of my colleagues advised me to work on something more related to medicine. Furthermore, I could not get enough funding and had to change the cages of the numerous mice by myself every week. What was worse, the Nat1 work was being rejected by many journals. I felt lonely and depressed, and I was about to give up my career as a scientist and return to the path of physician.

Fortunately, two events rescued me from PAD and from giving up on science. First, James Thomson of the University of Wisconsin-Madison and his colleagues announced that they had succeeded in generating human ES cells in 1998. His success taught me that ES cells have enormous potential in medicine and encouraged me to continue my research. Second, in December 1999, I got a new position as an associate professor with my own laboratory for the first time in my career at the Nara Institute of Science and Technology (NAIST) in

Nara Prefecture. This institute has brilliant investigators in basic and applied sciences, an excellent research environment and competent Ph.D. students. I was fortunate that several talented colleagues and students joined my laboratory.

RESEARCH AT NAIST

At NAIST, I was expected to establish a knockout mouse core facility. It was a difficult task, but thanks to an excellent technician, Tomoko Ichisaka, and to funding from NAIST, we were able to establish it within a few years. The first gene that we knocked out was Fbxo15, which we identified as a gene specifically expressed in mouse ES cells. One of my first Ph.D. students, Yoshimi Tokuzawa, with the help of Tomoko, successfully targeted the gene. However, we did not see any phenotypes in mice or ES cells lacking Fbxo15. We were disappointed, but this knockout mouse line turned out later to be useful in the generation of induced pluripotent stem cells or iPS cells.

As a principal investigator, I needed to set a long-term goal for my laboratory. Because of my interest in ES cells, because of the successful generation of human ES cells and because I had to use ES cells anyway in the knockout mouse core facility, I decided to list "ES cells" in the title of my lab website. At the time, most researchers focused on differentiating from ES cells into somatic cells. Human ES cells are associated with two major hurdles – ethical issues regarding the use of human embryos and immune rejection after they are transplanted into a human body. The use of human embryos has been an obstacle to the promotion of ES cell research in many countries, including the U.S. and Japan. To overcome these major hurdles, I decided nuclear reprogramming would be the goal of my lab. More precisely, I set my lab's goal as being to generate ES cell-like pluripotent cells from somatic cells, without using embryos.

Nuclear reprogramming was first proved by Sir John Gurdon in 1962, the year I was born. He reported the generation of new frogs by transferring tadpole intestine cell nuclei into enucleated eggs from the African clawed toad, *Xenopuslaevis*. Then, in 1997, Sir Ian Wilmut's team unveiled Dolly the sheep, the first cloned mammal created using a nuclear transfer method. These achievements showed that the genome DNA of mature cells theoretically have all the information needed to develop animals. A further advance came in a 2001 report by Takashi Tada of Kyoto University, who demonstrated that thymocytes acquire pluripotency upon electrofusion with mouse ES cells, which indicated that ES cells also contain factors that induce pluripotency in somatic cells.

However, I knew that making pluripotent cells from somatic cells would be extremely difficult, and when I started this project with my lab members at NAIST, I was not sure if the goal could be achieved in my lifetime.

My initial hypothesis was that factors that maintain the pluripotency of mouse ES cells might induce pluripotency in somatic cells. With the great help of the initial members of my lab – Tomoko, Yoshimi, and two other students, Kazutoshi Takahashi and Eiko Kaiho, and then Assistant Professor Kaoru Mitsui, my lab identified many factors that either are specifically expressed by or have important roles in mouse ES cells. Among them was the transcription factor Klf4, identified by Yoshimi. By 2004, with our own work and that of other groups, we had collected 24 initial candidate genes that might be able to induce pluripotency in somatic cells. We then needed a simple and sensitive assay system to evaluate these candidates, and the Fbxo15-knockout mice turned out to be such a system. Instead of simply deleting the gene, we knocked the neomycin resistant gene (neoR) into the Fbxo15 locus. Somatic cells derived from these mice do not express neoR and are sensitive to the antibiotic G418. Somatic cells that become ES cell–like pluripotent cells after transfection with some of our candidate genes should express neoR and become resistant to G418.

THE DISCOVERY OF IPS CELLS

In 2004, I moved to the Institute of Frontier Medical Sciences at Kyoto University as a professor. The major reason for the change was that I wanted to conduct experiments using human ES cells. NAIST did not have a medical school and a hospital attached, and therefore had no institutional review board to examine a study plan using human ES cells. At that time, Kyoto University was the only institute in Japan that had succeeded in culturing human ES cells. I came to Kyoto with the 24 candidate genes, the Fbxo15-neoR knock-in mice and many members of my lab, including Tomoko and Kazutoshi. I asked Kazutoshi to test the 24 candidates using the Fbxo15 knock-in mice. He was pleased to take over this very risky project and did a remarkable job. When Kazutoshi introduced each candidate into the Fbxo15-neoR reporter fibroblasts using retroviral vectors, no G418-resistant colonies emerged. However, when he introduced the mixture of all 24 genes via retroviral vectors, we observed several drug-resistant colonies in a Petri dish. These cells were similar to ES cells in morphology, proliferation and gene expression. When transplanted into nude mice, they formed teratomas containing a variety of tissues from all three germ layers, showing their pluripotency. Among the myriad combinations of the 24 factors, Kazutoshi found that four transcription factors – Oct3/4, Sox2, Klf4 and c-Myc – are essential.

In 2005, we succeeded in generating ES-like cells with the four factors, and I named the resulting cells "induced pluripotent stem cells or iPS cells." I was anxious about whether they were really the pluripotent cells that we were looking for because the method used to generate the iPS cells was much simpler than I had expected. In addition, after hearing about a big scandal involving a Korean researcher who falsely reported the successful generation of human ES cells by cloning at around that time, I thought we should repeat our experiments to make sure of the result so that no researcher could cast doubt on our findings. In 2006, we published a paper in *Cell* on the successful generation of mouse iPS cells using the four factors. Some researchers seemed surprised at the finding that only four genes are needed to reprogram somatic cells into the embryonic state. But in the following months, a few labs at MIT and Harvard demonstrated that they had been able to produce mouse iPS cells using our protocol, and an increasing number of researchers have since started working on the new technology.

Right after we generated mouse iPS cells, my team began to work on reprogramming human somatic cells. In November 2007, we reported the generation of human iPS cells from human fibroblasts by introducing the same quartet of genes via viral vectors. On the same day, Thomson's lab announced in *Science* that they had also succeeded in making human iPS cells using a different set of four factors – Nanog, Lin28, Oct3/4 and Sox2. I remember that I worked day and night to publish our paper as quickly as possible after I heard a rumor in the summer that a U.S. group had submitted an article on the successful generation of human iPS cells. My lab members continued to improve the induction and selection methods. Keisuke Okita, with the help of Tomoko, succeeded in making iPS cells that are competent for production of adult chimeras and germline transmission. Masato Nakagawa and Michiyo Koyanagi then showed that iPS cells can be generated without c-Myc, an oncogene. Takashi Aoi showed that iPS cells can be generated not only from fibroblasts but also from adult mouse hepatocytes and gastric epithelial cells.

With the ability to differentiate into virtually all types of cell and to grow robustly like ES cells, iPS cells have enormous potential for pharmaceutical and clinical applications. Patient-specific iPS cells can be used to produce disease model cells in which the pathological process can be studied. Thousands of chemicals and natural products can be tested on such cells, some of which we hope will become new effective medicines for intractable diseases.

CENTER FOR IPS CELL RESEARCH AND APPLICATION

The Ministry of Education, Sports, Science and Technology of Japan has since supported iPS cell research in cooperation with other government agencies by providing sufficient funding. Encouraged by this support, in January 2008, about two months after we reported the generation of the human iPS cells, Kyoto University founded the Center for iPS Cell Research and Applications (CiRA), the world's first organization solely focusing on iPS cell technology, under the auspices of the Institute for Integrated Cell-Material Sciences (iCeMS). I was appointed as the Director of CiRA. I had given up my career as a physician, but I had found a powerful tool that could help develop new cures for disease. This center is designed not only to progress with basic research to improve fundamental iPS cell technology but also to use the technology in clinical applications. In April 2010, CiRA became independent of iCeMS as a full-fledged institute in a newly opened research building. At the inauguration ceremony for the new CiRA research building, I publicly pledged to achieve four goals over the first ten years:

CiRA's Goals for the First 10 Years

1. Establish basic iPS cell technology and secure intellectual property.
2. Create an iPS cell stock for clinical use in regenerative medicine.
3. Conduct preclinical and clinical studies on such diseases as Parkinson's disease, diabetes and blood diseases.
4. Contribute to the development of therapeutic drugs using patient-derived iPS cells.

Since the discovery of human iPS cells, I have seen iPS cell technology advancing at an amazing speed. Owing to its simple and reproducible method, numerous laboratories inside and outside Japan are now working on iPS cell research, and protocols have been developed for direct reprogramming, whereby somatic cells are directly converted into mature cells of a different type. My lab developed a method to generate safer iPS cells without integrating viral vectors into the cell genome, which was one of the major safety concerns. Now CiRA is promoting the iPS cell stock project, in which we make clinical-grade iPS cell lines from blood cells donated by healthy HLA-homozygous individuals. The iPS cell lines will be distributed to other institutes so that they can differentiate them into various types of cell for use in transplantation therapy. Scientists at CiRA have succeeded in recapitulating a number of abnormalities in the cells of patients with such diseases as amyotrophic lateral sclerosis (ALS) and chronic infantile neurologic cutaneous and articular (CINCA) syndrome, which I hope will contribute to development of new therapeutic drugs. I have a small laboratory at Gladstone since I was offered a senior investigator position in 2007 and the lab members are also working hard. Working for Gladstone is a great pleasure for me as it means I can make some contribution to the institute where I received excellent training as a young scientist.

Running CiRA with some 250 staff, I have come to spend less time discussing their data with my colleagues and students, and have been absorbed by my duties as the "chief executive officer" of CiRA, including devising strategies to advance both basic and applied research and to obtain sufficient funding. Anxious about the lack of financial resources for the future to allow us to continue hiring research support staffers, I even ran the full Kyoto Marathon in 2012 to raise online donations from the public. It was hard but helped us raise more than 10 million yen. Now I hope that receiving the Nobel Prize in Physiology or Medicine will consolidate long-term support from the government and the general public for iPS cell research nationwide.

THANK YOU FOR YOUR SUPPORT!

Looking back at my life, I have been very fortunate that I have encountered many talented students and colleagues who have supported and encouraged me on many occasions, including my lab members in the past and the present. In addition to my direct mentors, I also owe much not only to the great scientists who made breakthrough discoveries in biology but also to countless predecessors who have contributed to the development of nuclear reprogramming and stem cell biology. I am deeply thankful to my wife and our two daughters, who have supported my hectic life as a scientist for years. Finally I am grateful to my parents. I was glad that my mother was able to take part in the award ceremony of the 2012 Nobel Prize in Stockholm. My father wanted me to become a physician who helps a lot of patients. Although I gave up my career as a surgeon, I still hope to help people suffering from serious diseases and injuries. With iPS cell technology I will continue to work hard together with my colleagues to achieve this goal as quickly as possible.

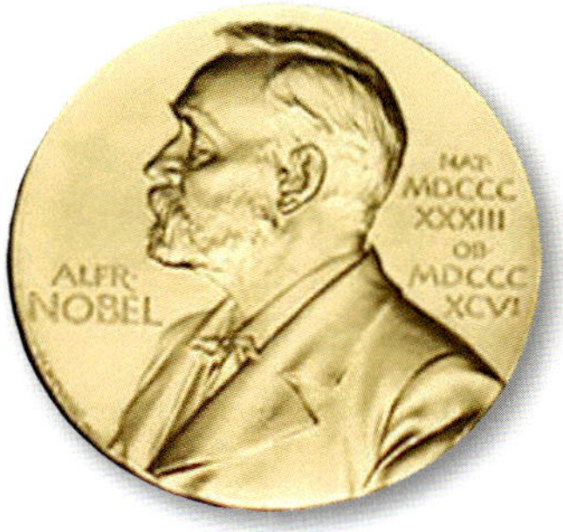

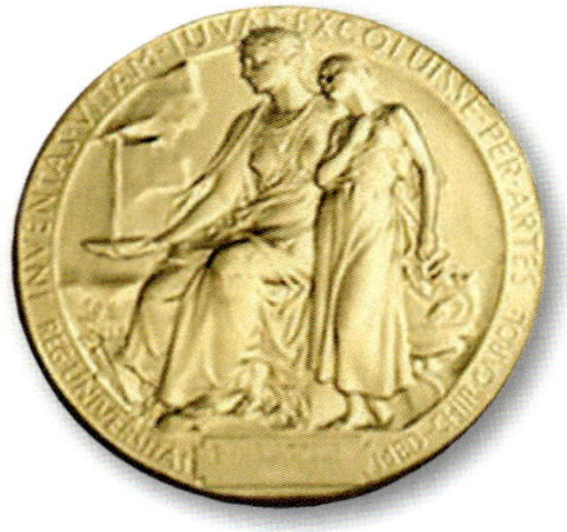

The Winding Road to Pluripotency

Nobel Lecture, December 7, 2012

by Shinya Yamanaka
Center for iPS Cell Research and Application (CiRA), Kyoto University, Kyoto 606-8507, Japan.
Gladstone Institute of Cardiovascular Disease, San Francisco, CA 94158, USA.

INTRODUCTION

John Gurdon received recognition for his landmark achievement in 1962, which provided the first experimental evidence of reprogramming by the transplantation of amphibian somatic cell nuclei into enucleated oocytes [1]. This breakthrough in technology introduced a new paradigm; that each nucleus of a differentiated cell retains a complete set of blueprints for the whole body, while oocytes possess a certain potential for reprogramming.

Inspired by this paradigm shift and subsequent research achievements, we identified four transcription factors that could induce pluripotency in somatic cells by their forced expression and successfully consolidated effective reprogramming methods in mouse cells in 2006 [2] and in human cells in 2007 [3]. The established reprogrammed cells were named "induced pluripotent stem (iPS) cells." I would like to provide an overview focusing on the experimental background of the generation of iPS cells, and the future perspectives regarding iPS cell research, which has been developing rapidly.

MY EARLY DAYS AS A SCIENTIST

I graduated from Kobe University School of Medicine, Japan, and obtained my medical license in 1987. I decided to become an orthopedic surgeon and started my training as a resident in Osaka, Japan. During my school days, I had practiced

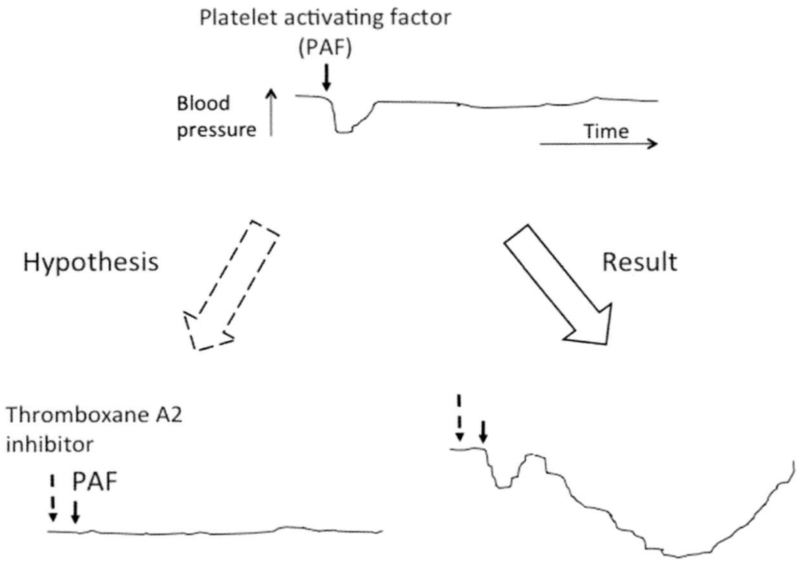

FIGURE 1. My first experiment as a graduate student. Intravenous injection of a vasoactive molecule platelet activating factor (PAF) caused a transient decrease in blood pressure in dogs (upper panel). We hypothesized that this hypotension would be blocked by pretreatment with a thromboxane A2 inhibitor (lower left panel). Unexpectedly, we observed a profound hypotension (lower right panel).

judo and played rugby, and injured myself many times, including more than 10 fractures throughout my body. It was thus natural for me to have become interested in orthopedic surgery. I especially wanted to treat patients suffering from sport injuries and overtraining.

In 1989, however, my life took a new turn from clinical medicine in orthopedic surgery to basic science research for two reasons. First, I found that I was not a very talented surgeon. Second, I saw many patients suffering from intractable diseases and injuries, which even highly talented surgeons and physicians were not able to cure. For example, I had encountered patients suffering from spinal cord injuries, amyotrophic lateral sclerosis and osteosarcomas. Furthermore, I lost my father due to liver cirrhosis during my residency. Basic medical research is the only way to find cures for these patients. For these reasons, I decided to go back to school. I became a Ph.D. student at Osaka City University Medical School in April of 1989.

Among the many departments at the school, I applied to the Department of Pharmacology, directed by Dr. Kenjiro Yamamoto. At the interview, I was not able to answer many questions about pharmacology, because I had not studied pharmacology well enough when I was a medical student. Instead, I tried to convince the interviewer, Dr. Fumihiko Ikemoto, that I really wanted to do basic medical research, despite my lack of knowledge. I am so grateful that Dr. Ike-moto accepted me into the department. Dr. Ikemoto repeatedly told me that we should not perform research that simply reproduced somebody else's re-sults. Rather, we should do something unique and new. During my training as a scientist, I was very fortunate to have two types of teachers: namely, great men-tors and unexpected results from my experiments.

My direct mentor at the graduate school was Dr. Katsuyuki Miura. In my first few months as a Ph.D. student, Dr. Miura told me to read as many manuscripts as possible and propose new projects. I felt like I was given a blank canvas and told that I could draw whatever I wanted. This mentorship was very different from what I had experienced during my residency. At the hospital, I'd had little freedom, and had to follow instructions from senior physicians and textbooks. I thought "wow, I like this system!" Another thing that Dr. Miura often told me was that we were competing worldwide. Whatever project you chose, you will compete with other scientists throughout the world, mostly in the U.S. or Europe, on the same or similar projects. This was again very different from my experience at the hospital, where I was competing only with other residents at the same hospital. The idea of "worldwide" competition had never entered my mind when I was working at the hospital. For all of these reasons, I found that basic research was a more suitable career, based on my interests and temperament.

In the summer of 1989, I was still struggling to find my project. Dr. Miura proposed a simpler project to begin my research studies. He suggested that I examine the role of a vasoactive molecule, platelet activating factor (PAF), in dogs to study the regulation of blood pressure (Fig. 1). Because it was known that the intravenous injection of PAF into dogs caused a transient decrease in blood pressure (transient hypotension), Dr. Miura hypothesized that this decrease in blood pressure would be mediated by another vasoactive molecule, thromboxane A2. If that hypothesis was correct, then pretreatment with a thromboxane A2 inhibitor should block the PAF-induced transient decrease in blood pressure. My first experiment, where I treated dogs with an inhibitor of thromboxane A2, was performed based on his hypothesis, and I had expected no decrease in the blood pressure in the pretreated dogs. It should have been a simple experiment suitable for a beginner. However, the result was totally unexpected. In the beginning, the thromboxane A2 inhibitor did not seem to be effective, with subsequent PAF treatment inducing the normal transient decrease in the blood pressure. Surprisingly, however, a few minutes after the treatment, a profound and prolonged decrease in blood pressure was observed, which we had never observed following treatment with PAF alone (Fig. 1). I got so excited! I ran into Dr. Miura's office to report this result excitedly. Although the result did not support his hypothesis, Dr. Miura responded with excitement, too, and encouraged me to explore the finding further. I spent another two years uncovering the mechanism responsible for this unexpected result [4, 5]. I was extremely lucky to obtain this kind of unexpected result in my very first experiment as a graduate student.

The fact that I got very excited with the result clearly told me that I had found the correct career. During my thesis work, however, I was often frustrated by my scientific approach, which relied on pharmacological tools, such as inhibitors and agonists. No drug can be 100% specific or effective, so there are always non-specific activities or incomplete blockade of the targets. In contrast, I was fascinated by the emerging gene engineering technologies being demonstrated in mice, especially the knockout mouse technology, by which any gene of interest could be deleted with 100% specificity and efficacy. There were a few groups in Japan who brought the technology from the U.S. or Europe to their pharmacological studies. This technology seemed like a miracle to me. I really wanted to utilize the knockout mouse technology in my own research. Therefore, in order to learn about the genetic engineering of mice, I decided to become a postdoctoral fellow in the U.S., where the technology was being widely used in many laboratories. I check advertisements in journals such as *Nature*, *Science* and *Cell*, and applied to as many laboratories as possible. The very first person who replied to my application was Dr. Thomas (Tom) Innerarity at the Gladstone Institute of Cardiovascular Disease, San Francisco (Fig. 2). After a short interview by telephone, Tom offered me a position. In April 1993, I crossed the Pacific Ocean with my wife and two little daughters.

In Tom's laboratory, I started working on the mechanisms underlying the gene expression of Apo B (Apolipoprotein B), which is a constituent of LDL (low-density lipoprotein) and thought to be important in cholesterol regulation. In particular, we focused on an mRNA editing factor, APOBEC1 (Apo B mRNA editing catalytic subunit 1) to analyze its gene function. Our original objective was to explore the possibility of using gene therapy for familial hypercholesterolemia to prevent atherosclerosis. Tom hypothesized that the overexpression of APOBEC1 in the liver would lower the plasma cholesterol levels, and he planned to examine this possibility using transgenic mice that overexpressed APOBEC1 in a liver-specific manner. I worked very hard and was able to quickly generate transgenic mouse lines. However, we observed totally unexpected results. We found that there was abdominal expansion of transgenic mice as if they

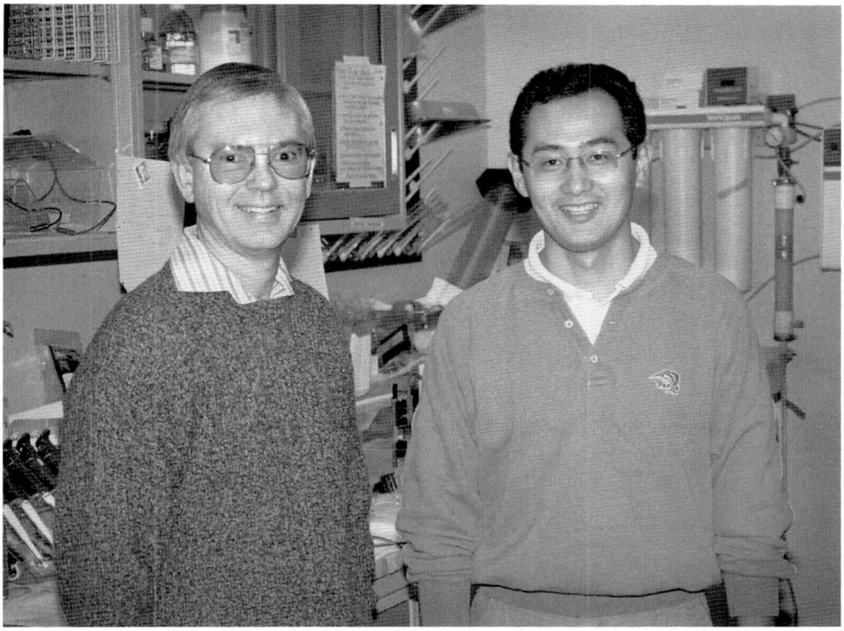

FIGURE 2. Days at the Gladstone Institute as a Postdoctoral Fellow. A picture taken with Dr. Thomas Innerarity in his laboratory (1995, Gladstone Institutes).

were pregnant, regardless of whether they were male or female. An exceptionally high incidence of liver tumor in these mice was confirmed by autopsy (Fig. 3) [6]. It turned out that APOBEC1 is a very potent oncogene. Therefore, we can never use this gene for gene therapy. Again, I got very excited about this unexpected result, although it indicated that APOBEC1 could not be used to prevent atherosclerosis, thereby effectively halting my previous line of research. Although it contradicted his hypothesis, Dr. Innerarity kept supporting me while I decided to work on liver cancer, showing a similar excitement as Dr. Miura did in response to the unexpected results. He encouraged me to keep working on APOBEC1 to elucidate the mechanism by which it led to cancer formation. I became the only person who worked on liver cancer at the Gladstone Institute of Cardiovascular Diseases.

I met another person who ended up being very important in my life at Gladstone. It was the then president of the institute, Dr. Robert Mahley. He once told us (postdoctoral fellows) about how to become successful in science. He said the secret was "VW." He had and still has a Volkswagen car, but in this case, VW did not mean Volkswagen. Instead, he meant vision and hard work. Dr. Mahley

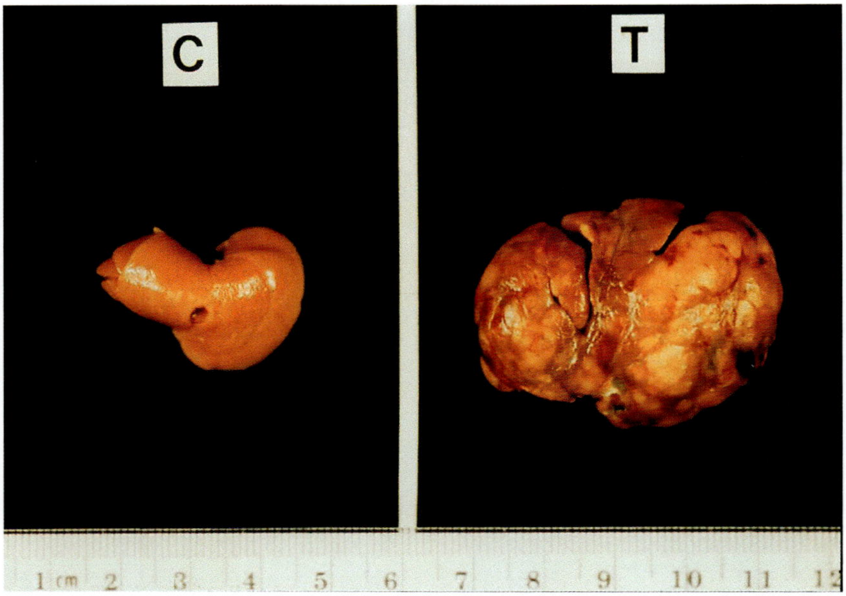

FIGURE 3. Hepatocellular Carcinoma in APOBEC-1 transgenic mouse. Livers from non-transgenic control mouse (left) and transgenic mouse (right). [6] (© 1995, the National Academy of Sciences)

told us to have a clear vision and then work hard toward that goal. I was working very hard day and night. However, I realized I did not have a clear vision. Why am I doing many of my experiments? Why did I quit working at hospitals to become a postdoctoral fellow in the U.S.? I then realized that my vision or motivation for doing science was to contribute to patient health and longevity. Of course, we cannot immediately help any patients by doing experiments in laboratories. However, basic medical research has the potential to help thousands of patients suffering from intractable diseases and injuries.

As noted above, I very was fortunate to have two types of great teachers in my early days as a scientist. First, my mentors, including Dr. Miura, Dr. Innerarity and Dr. Mahley, encouraged me to continue my projects despite the fact that the results contradicted their hypotheses. They served as models of good mentors for me to follow. The other great teacher was nature itself, which gave me totally unexpected results that led me to completely new research themes. Without these two types of great "teachers," I could have never initiated my research that led to the generation of iPS cells.

THE RESEARCH THAT LED TO THE PRODUCTION OF IPS CELLS

What brought me to cell reprogramming biology was another set of totally unexpected experimental results and an encounter with ES (embryonic stem) cells through my research experience, along with related scientific streams. While trying to elucidate the molecular mechanisms underlying the carcinogenesis induced by APOBEC1, I discovered an interesting molecule that was a novel target of APOBEC1. I named this molecule NAT1 (Novel APOBEC1 Target #1) [7]. We found that the overexpression of APOBEC1 resulted in aberrant editing at numerous sites of the NAT1 mRNA, including those that generated premature termination codons. Consequently, the NAT1 protein levels were markedly reduced. I also found that the NAT1 protein was similar to eukaryotic translation initiation factor (eIF) 4G and likely functioned as a translational regulator. Based on these observations, I hypothesized that NAT1 could function as a tumor suppressor gene. In order to examine this hypothesis, I decided to generate NAT1 knockout mice. At that time, I had learned the skills necessary for generating knockout mice, including the preparation of targeting vectors and cultivation of mouse ES cells from Dr. Robert Farese Jr., a friend of mine who established the ES cell and knockout core laboratory at Gladstone. This was how I first encountered ES cells.

Again I worked very hard. Three years had passed since I joined Gladstone, and my wife had to go back to Japan because we decided to send our elder daughter to an elementary school there. After my family left San Francisco, I worked even harder. I really wanted to find out the function of NAT1, the gene I had identified myself. Without my family at home, I did not have anything else to do. I literally worked day and night. I generated a targeting vector quickly and was able to obtain targeted ES cell clones. I asked the knockout core laboratory to inject the targeted ES cells into mouse blastocysts to generate chimeric mice. I was happy about the scientific progress I was making.

At the same time, however, I felt lonelier and lonelier without my family. The only way to live with my family was to go back to Japan. However, I was unable to find a good position in Japan. Fortunately, I obtained a fellowship from the Japanese Government and decided to go back to Japan for a second postdoctoral fellowship. Owing to the invaluable help and generosity of Dr. Innerarity, I was able to continue the research on NAT1 after I returned to Japan at Osaka City University Medical School. The following year, I became an assistant professor and continued working on NAT1.

The generation of the NAT1 knockout mice went smoothly. We obtained good chimeric mice, and subsequently, F1 heterozygous mutant mice. Tom sent those F1 mice to me. However, I could not obtain homozygous mutant mice from intercrossing the heterozygous mutants, thus suggesting that NAT1 was indispensable for mouse development. I then struggled with the analyses of mutant embryos, since neither I nor anyone around me had ever worked on mouse embryogenesis. I learned how to dissect embryos by reading textbooks. With great encouragement from my colleagues, including Dr. Katsuyuki Miura, I finally showed that NAT1 mutant embryos died around the time of implantation.

In order to further characterize the functions of NAT1, I generated homozygous deletion mutant ES cells. In found that NAT1-null ES cells proliferated normally when they were maintained on undifferentiated feeder cells. However, when they were cultured without feeder cells or leukemia inhibitory factor, I observed marked differences. Under these conditions, the wild-type ES cells rapidly differentiated in terms of their morphology and gene expression. In contrast, mutant ES cells showed resistance to differentiation. This meant that NAT1 is essential for maintaining the pluripotency of ES cells [8]. This was the pivotal moment when ES cells became my main research subject. My future career developed from merely a research tool (knockout mouse construction), thanks to the unexpected results of the NAT1 functional analysis. This unexpected result changed my project again—from cancer to ES cells.

Mammalian ES cells were first derived from mouse embryos in 1981 by Dr. Martin Evans, and also by Dr. Gail R. Martin. ES cells have two important properties [9, 10]. The first is their rapid proliferation, which can be considered to provide them with immortality. The other important property is pluripotency, the ability to differentiate into virtually all types of somatic and germ cells that exist in the body. NAT1 is essential for pluripotency, but not for the rapid proliferation of mouse ES cells. Because of the important role of NAT1, I became very interested in the biology of ES cells.

Although I was obtaining important results about the molecular functions of NAT1, I started to become frustrated and wondered whether my basic research could eventually contribute to clinical medicine, which was my true goal. I was working at the medical school, where most of my colleagues participated in medical research projects, such as drug development or understanding the pathophysiology of diseases. My vision was (and still is) to contribute to the lives of patients through basic research, but I was not sure whether working on NAT1 and mouse ES cells could realize my vision. At that time, my colleagues often told me that, "Shinya, those mouse cells may be interesting, but you should do something more closely related to human disease and human medicine." Very luckily, however, two events happened in the late 90s, which encouraged me to continue working on ES cells.

The first event was the generation of human ES cells by Dr. James Thomson at the University of Wisconsin in 1998 [11]. Immediately after this paper was published, the ES cell research field began to draw public attention because of its potential value in regenerative medicine. Human ES cells have the two same properties as mouse ES cells, rapid proliferation and pluripotency. Human ES cells can be expanded indefinitely, and they can be used to generate various types of human somatic cells, such as dopaminergic neurons, neural stem cells, cardiac cells, and so on. These human cells should then be able to be used to treat patients suffering from various diseases and injuries, such as Parkinson's disease, spinal cord injuries, etc. So again, it turned out that ES cells themselves could help patients, not mouse patients, but human patients. When I first read the landmark paper by Dr. Thomson, I got very excited—I still remember that moment. However, the generation and use of human ES cells is associated with an ethical obstacle regarding the use of human embryos. In Japan, we were not allowed to use human ES cells. Thus, human ES cell research was a distant and forbidden world to me then.

The other event that encouraged me was my promotion. I had a chance to organize my own laboratory. In 1999, I moved to the Nara Institute of Science and Technology (NAIST) as an associate professor. In 1998, I found an advertisement for that position in a Japanese scientific magazine. It said that the institute was seeking a scientist at the associate professor level who would run his or her own laboratory while organizing a core facility for mouse genetic engineering for the institute. It seemed a perfect position for me, and I decided to apply for the position. I did not expect to be chosen, since I had only published a few papers using the technology. Surprisingly, however, I was provided an opportunity to give a job seminar at the institute, and more surprisingly, I got the position!

In December of that year, I entered through the main gate of the NAIST with excitement and nervousness. The NAIST is one of only a few national universities that only have graduate schools in Japan (most also have medical and dental schools). It has a beautiful campus, good equipment, talented faculty members, and, most importantly, highly motivated and brilliant graduate students. My frustration disappeared unconsciously. Because of these two events, the generation of human ES cells and my promotion to associate professor at the NAIST, I was able to continue my research on ES cells.

Then the word "VW" came to my mind again. Now that I was starting my own laboratory, I decided that I needed to have a clear vision or long term goal that I was going to share with future lab members. Many laboratories working on ES cells, including those famous in the field, were working on *in vitro* directed differentiation of cells into various lineages, such as cardiac myocytes and neuronal cells. I did not think it would be wise to compete with these laboratories, since my lab was very small and new. I decided to do the opposite. I decided that the goal of my laboratory would be to establish ES cell-like pluripotent stem cells that were not derived from embryos, but from differentiated somatic cells. By achieving this goal, we would be able to overcome the obstacles facing the development of medicine using human ES cells, namely, the use of human embryos and immune rejection after transplantation. I thus started trying to reprogram somatic cells back into the embryonic state.

I knew reprogramming was possible, at least in theory. Somatic cell reprogramming techniques had been developed by several groups. For example, Dr. Ian Wilmut succeeded in generating a first cloned mammal, "Dolly" the sheep, by transplanting the nucleus of a fully developed cell into an enucleated egg [12]. However, the efficiency of the method was extremely low. In addition, it had been pointed out that this system was technically quite difficult to apply to primates, including humans. Another example was the cell fusion technique between ES cells and somatic cells to attain pluripotency [13]. However, the resultant fused cells did not seem to be suitable for application in a clinical setting due to the generation of tetraploid cells. However, the fact that somatic cells were able to attain pluripotency following nuclear transplantation or fusion with ES cells provided a lot of scientific encouragement, because it led us to hypothesize that oocytes or ES cells contain intrinsic factors that can reprogram somatic cells into a pluripotent state.

In addition to this background, there were also other discoveries of master transcription factors involved in vertebrate development, such as Antennapedia in the fly [14] or MyoD in the mouse [15]. From these findings, it was a simple logical step to deduce that a combination of factors should be able to induce pluripotency in somatic cells. I just did not know which or how many factors were required. When we first started our research, it could have been one, several, one hundred or even more, and we thought at that time that the project would take 10, 20, 30 years or even longer to complete.

I hypothesized that many of the reprograming factors are expressed predominantly in eggs and ES cells. In order to search for factors that are specifically expressed in ES cells, we planned to utilize an EST (expressed sequence tag) database, which is a kind of catalog of genes that are expressed in each tissue or organ, obtained by random sequencing of cDNA libraries made from tissues or organs in various species. In a timely fashion, large quantities of mouse EST data were disclosed by RIKEN [16]. Furthermore, a program that analyzed EST databases to predict the expression pattern of each gene became available from the National Center for Biotechnology Information (NCBI) [17]. I utilized this program, designated an *in silico* differential display, to compare EST libraries from mouse ES cells and those from various somatic tissues. I was immediately able to identify multiple genes that were highly and specifically expressed in undifferentiated mouse ES cells and early embryos. Among them, we particularly focused on the genes with the highest enrichment. These included well-known genes, such as Oct3/4 [18, 19], Utf1 [20] and Rex1 [21], which had been experimentally identified as ES cell-specific markers. This confirmed the usefulness of this approach. We designated other ES cell-enriched genes "ES cell-associated transcripts" (ECATs). We confirmed the ES cell-specific expression of ECATs by performing northern blot analyses [22–24].

I characterized the functions of ECATs in ES cells and mice with the new members who had joined my lab, including three graduate students, Eiko Kaiho, Yoshimi Tokuzawa and Kazutoshi Takahashi. I was lucky to have these talented and hard-working students with me from the beginning. Furthermore, I was very fortunate to have Tomoko Ichisaka in my lab, as a technical staff member of the core facility for mouse molecular engineering. I believe that Tomoko is one of the best technicians in terms of the manipulation of mouse embryos in Japan, and maybe in the world. Thanks to Tomoko and the core facility, we were able to generate knockout mice to examine many ECATs.

The first gene we knocked out in mice at the NAIST was ECAT3, also known as Fbox15. These mice were part of Yoshimi Tokuzawa's project. Yoshimi, Tomoko and I were very happy when we obtained the first targeted ES line, the first chimeric mice and then germ-line transmission. However, when we generated homozygous mutant mice lacking the functional ECAT3 gene, we did not observe any obvious phenotypes [22]. Because of its specific expression in mouse ES cells and embryos, we expected that its disruption would result in early lethality during embryogenesis. Furthermore, we showed that Fbox15 is a direct target of Oct3/4 and Sox2, another transcription factor essential for the maintenance of pluripotency [25]. On the contrary, we obtained homozygous mutant mice in accordance with the Mendelian law from heterozygous intercrosses. Yoshimi then generated homozygous mutant ES cell lines, hoping that she would observe drastic phenotypes. However, again, we did not see any significant changes. ECAT3-null ES cells proliferated normally and showed normal differentiation potentials. Thus, both the ECAT3 knockout mice and ES cells were apparently normal. This often happened with other ECATs. These experiences reminded us that science is often tough.

An exception was ECAT4, a transcription factor that was later re-named Nanog. We and others found that Nanog played important roles in the maintenance of pluripotency in mouse ES cell [24, 26]. Nanog was also essential for mouse embryonic development before implantation. In addition to Nanog, Yoshimi Tokuzawa identified another transcription factor, Klf4 that played important roles in mouse ES cells. Another group reported the important role of the well-known oncogene, c-Myc, in pluripotency. By 2004, we had identified a total of 24 factors, including Oct3/4, Sox2, c-Myc, Nanog, other ECATs and Klf4, as candidate reprogramming factors.

What we then needed was a sensitive and rapid assay system to screen these candidate factors. It turned out that the Fbox15-null knockout mice provided such an assay system. When we made knockout mice of Fbox-15 and other ECATs, we utilized a gene trap strategy, in which we knocked the neomycin resistance gene into the gene of interest. Thus, in ECAT3 knockout cells, the neomycin resistance gene is expressed from the enhancer and promoter of ECAT3, which was active only in ES cells and early embryos, but not in somatic cells. Somatic cells, such as mouse embryonic fibroblasts (MEFs) derived from the ECAT3 knockout mice are sensitive to G418, whereas ECAT3 knockout ES cells were resistant to high concentrations of G418. Based on these results, we expected that if any of the 24 candidates could actually induce pluripotency in ECAT3 knockout MEFs, the reprogrammed cells would become resistant to G418. We confirmed this strategy by using a fusion reprogramming system. The ECAT3 knockout mice that showed few phenotypes and thus disappointed Yoshimi and me turned out to provide a very useful assay system to evaluate candidate reprogramming factors.

My lab moved to Kyoto University in 2005, with the 24 gene candidates, the ECAT3-based assay system and Tomoko Ichisaka and Kazutoshi Takahashi. In Kyoto, I asked Kazutoshi Takahashi to examine the 24 factors by using the assay system [2]. To tell the truth, we did not expect that we had the answer among these 24 factors. We thought we had to screen many more factors, and had already started to prepare cDNA libraries from mouse ES cells and testes. Nevertheless, Kazutoshi introduced each of the 24 candidate genes, one by one, into ECAT3 knockout MEFs by retroviral transduction. As, in a sense, expected, we did not obtain any drug-resistant colonies using any single factor, thus indicating that no single candidate gene was sufficient to elicit reprograming and induce pluripotency. In addition to the single factor transduction, Kazutoshi proposed to transduce all 24 factors together into ECAT3 knockout MEFs as a practice for performing a cDNA library screening. It was like a mini-library consisting of 24 cDNAs. To our surprise, four weeks after transduction, we obtained several G418-resistant colonies. I thought this might be some kind of mistake, such as contamination with ES cells. I asked Kazuthoshi to repeat the experiment again and again. It always worked. Kazutoshi picked up the G418-resistant colonies for expansion. We found that these cells were expandable and showed a morphology similar to that of mouse ES cells. A reverse transcription PCR (RT-PCR) analysis revealed that the iPS-MEF24 clones expressed ES cell markers, including Oct3/4, Nanog, E-Ras, Cripto, Dax1, Zfp296 [24] and Fgf4 [27].

Next, to determine which of the 24 candidates were critical, Kazutoshi examined the effects of withdrawal of individual factors from the pool of transduced candidate genes. ES cell-like colonies did not form when either Oct3/4 or Klf4 was removed. The removal of Sox2 resulted in only a few ES-like colonies. When he removed c-Myc, the ES cell-like colonies did emerge, but these had a flatter, non-ES-cell-like morphology. Removal of the remaining factors did not significantly affect the colony numbers or characteristics. We finally showed that a combination of four genes, Oct3/4, Klf4, Sox2 and c-Myc was sufficient to produce ES cell-like colonies. These data demonstrated that pluripotency could be induced from MEF culture by the introduction of four transcription factors; Oct3/4, Sox2, c-Myc and Klf4. I designated the new pluripotent stem cells "iPS cells," short for induced pluripotent stem cells.

We examined the pluripotency of iPS cells by the teratoma formation assay in animals. We obtained tumors from iPS cells after subcutaneous injection into nude mice. A histological examination revealed that the iPS cells differentiated into all three germ layers, including neural tissues, cartilage and columnar epithelium. We also examined the ability of iPS cells to produce adult chimeras. We injected iPS cells into mouse-derived blastocysts, which we then transplanted into the uteri of pseudo-pregnant mice. We obtained adult chimeras from those injected iPS cells as determined by the coat color of the resulting pups. From these chimeras, we were able to obtain F1 mice through germline transmission. Based on these results, we concluded that iPS cells are comparable to ES cells in terms of their pluripotency [28].

The following year, we reported the generation of iPS cells from human fibroblasts using the same factors [3]. In the case of ES cells, it took 17 years to move from the mouse to human cells. This was in part because, although mouse ES cells and human ES cells share many similar features, they are very different in many aspects, including the culture conditions and morphology. In the case of iPS cells, it took much less time. This was because we already knew both how to culture human pluripotent stem cells and what they should look like. In other words, we could have never generated human iPS cells without the previous reports on human ES cells.

The generation of iPS cells was an exceptional experience in my scientific career, in that everything went smoothly. In all other cases, my career has been full of failures. This luck resulting from the dedicated work of young researchers, especially three people, Kazutoshi Takahashi, Yoshimi Tokuzawa and Tomoko Ichisaka. It was these three who generated the iPS cells. Without these three young lab members, we could have never generated the iPS cells in my laboratory. Therefore, I am extremely grateful to these three and the other members of my lab for their tireless efforts.

When I initiated my basic research 25 years ago, I did not imagine at all that I was going to work on stem cells in the future. It was the unexpected results from PAF, APOBEC1 transgenic mice and the NAT1 knockout mice that brought me to the new field. The encouragement from my mentors, including Drs. Yamamoto, Miura, Innerarity and Mahley was essential for me to continue my work as a scientist. I am grateful to my two types of teachers, these mentors and nature itself.

THE POTENTIAL APPLICATIONS OF IPS CELLS

One of the advantages of the iPS cell technology is its simplicity and reproducibility. We can now generate human iPS cells not only from skin fibroblasts, but also from other somatic cells, including peripheral blood cells. Hundreds of laboratories all over the world are now working on iPS cells, trying to apply the technology in medicine and in the pharmaceutical industry (Fig. 4). Without the iPS cell technology, it would be difficult to obtain sufficient numbers of somatic cells, such as heart cells or brain cells, from patients suffering from diseases affecting the heart or brain. With the iPS cell technology, all that is needed is a tiny

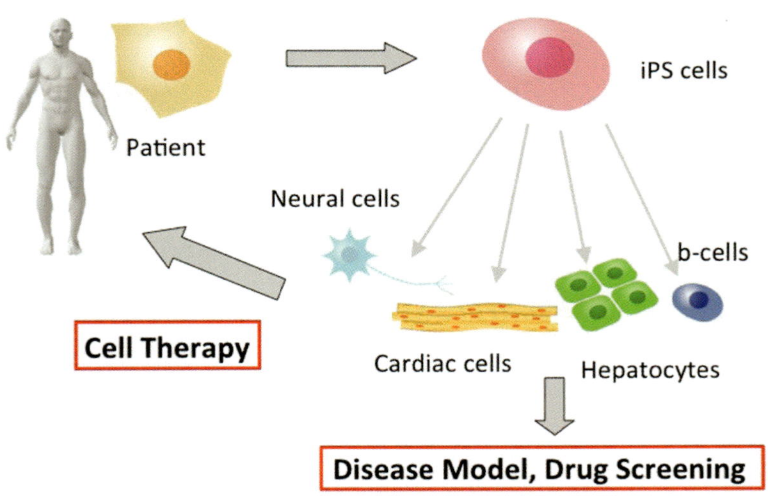

FIGURE 4. Potential Applications of iPS Cells.

amount of blood cells from the patients. We can then generate iPS cells, expand the cells as much as we want, and then make heart cells or brain cells to specifically study the affected tissues. These cells have the same genetic information as the patients and will provide unprecedented opportunities for predicting the toxicity of drugs, making disease models in petri dishes, performing drug screening and for cell transplantation therapies.

Many effective drugs have been withdrawn from the market because of side effects such as cardiac arrhythmia and liver toxicity. The best known cardiac toxicity is long QT syndrome, as characterized with prolonged intervals between the Q and T waves in electrocardiograms, which often cause lethal arrhythmia. Since human heart cells are hard to obtain, pharmaceutical companies have been using non-cardiac cancer cell lines, into which only one cardiac gene has been transfected, to predict the development of long QT syndrome and other types of cardiac toxicity of their drug candidates. However, this artificial system suffers from both false positive and false negative results. Now, human cardiac myocytes derived from iPS cells are commercially available from multiple companies. Pharmaceutical companies are now beginning to use these cells to predict cardiac toxicity. Similar approaches can be taken to predict the side effects in the liver and brain. These new types of medical application of the iPS cell technology are considered to be just around the corner.

I believe that the biggest potential of this technology resides in disease modeling and drug screening. Hundreds of diseases can be studied this way. Progress has been made in modeling intractable diseases while searching for new drugs with patient-derived iPS cells by many groups all over the world. To my surprise, it has been shown that iPS cells can be used to recapitulate the phenotypes of not only monogenic diseases, but also some late-onset polygenic diseases, such as ALS (amyotrophic lateral sclerosis, widely known in the U.S. as Lou Gehrig's disease) and Alzheimer's disease [29, 30].

ALS is a late-onset motor neuron disease. Most cases of ALS are sporadic, and are not caused by a mutation in a single gene. It has been more than 100 years since this disease was first recognized. However, there is still no effective treatment, despite numerous scientific efforts. In many diseases, animal models have been useful to understand the mechanisms and identify effective drugs. In the case of ALS, animal models do exist and many drugs have been developed that are effective on those animal models. However, the same drugs are not effective in human ALS patients. Therefore, drug screening for ALS needs to be conducted with human cells, but it has been difficult to obtain sufficient numbers of motor neurons and other affected cells from patients.

Now that iPS cells can be utilized to produce the cells of interest, many scientists have been generating iPS cells from ALS patients and producing large numbers of motor neurons having the same genetic information as the patients. Among them is Dr. Haruhisa Inoue at our institute (CiRA, the Center for iPS Cell Research and Application) [29]. Dr. Inoue demonstrated that motor neurons from patients had significantly shorter projections, which are necessary for signal transduction from the brain to muscles, than did those from healthy control individuals (Fig. 5). He also found that a histone acetyltransferase inhibitor, called anacardic acid, reverted the abnormal ALS motor neuron phenotype. In addition to ALS, scientists at the CiRA have been working on other intractable diseases, such as FOP (fibrodysplasia ossificans progressiva) and CINCA (chronic infantile neurological cutaneous and articular) syndrome [31]. The findings of their studies have shown that patient–derived iPS cells can provide a useful tool for elucidating the disease pathogenesis and for screening drug candidates.

Stem cell therapy is another promising medical application of iPS cells. In Japan and other countries, researchers are conducting pre-clinical studies to prove the efficacy and safety of iPS cells for treating various diseases and injuries, such as Parkinson's disease, macular degeneration, cardiac failure, spinal cord injury and platelet deficiency [32]. The iPS cell technology has progressed rapidly in the last five years. We and others have reported an integration-free method that can be used to generate human iPS cells using episomal vectors [33]. We also have shown that p53 shRNA[34], L-Myc [35] and Glis1 [36], when strongly expressed, can replace the oncogene c-Myc, and efficiently generate human iPS cells. We have also developed systems to evaluate iPS cells. We believe that the technology is getting closer to clinical trials. Dr. Masayo Takahashi at the Riken Center for Developmental Biology (CDB) has already applied for permission to conduct an iPS cell-based clinical trial for macular degeneration from the Japanese Ministry of Health and Labor.

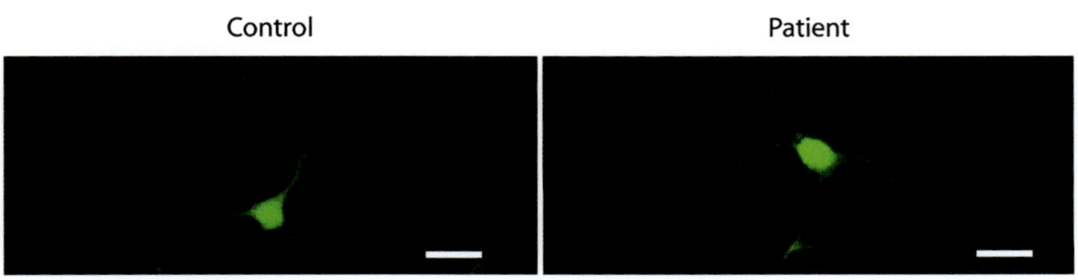

FIGURE 5. Disease Modeling of Motor Neuron from ALS Patient-Derived iPS Cells. Microscopic images of motor neurons that were differentiated from iPS cells derived from a control donor (left) and an ALS patient (right). [29] (© 2012, American Association for the Advancement of Science).

Some of these clinical trials will initially begin with autologous iPS cells derived from the patients' own somatic cells. However, for larger scale trials and more standard therapies, preparing autologous iPS cells from each patient may not be practical, since it will be time-, labor- and cost-intensive. Generating, expanding and differentiating iPS cells under a good manufacturing protocol are expensive. In addition, these processes take several months. In the case of spinal cord injuries, it has been shown that the best result can be expected when cells are transplanted within a month after the onset of injury. Therefore, if the generation, expansion and differentiation of iPS cells is started after a patient is injured, the cells will never be ready in time. To overcome these practical problems, we are now trying to establish iPS cell stocks for regenerative medicine purposes. To minimize immune-mediated rejection, our plan is to generate iPS cells from donors with HLA homozygous alleles. In Japan, we estimate that iPS cell lines from 140 HLA homozygotes will cover up to 90% of the Japanese population.

SCIENTIFIC STREAMS TOWARD THE FUTURE

I receive this prize on behalf of numerous researchers and scientists who have contributed to the generation and rapid progress of the iPS cell technology. As I described, iPS cells were established on the basis of three preexisting scientific streams (Fig. 6).

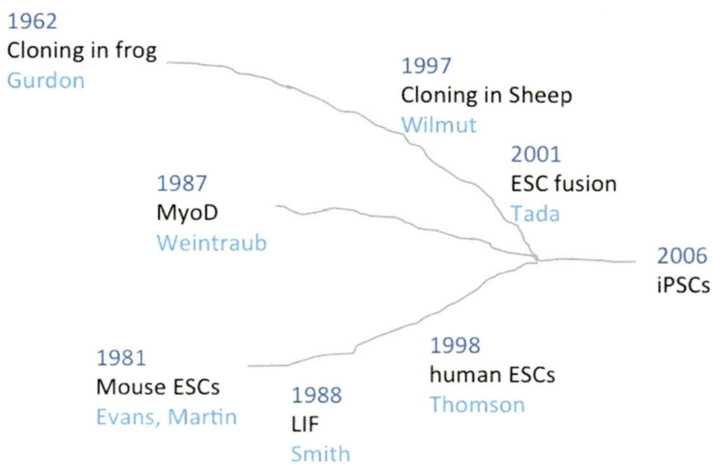

FIGURE 6. Three Scientific Streams That Led to the Development of iPS Cells. Shown are landmark events with the name of senior authors and publication years.

The first stream was nuclear reprogramming, initiated by Dr. John Gurdon more than 50 years ago. A nucleus from a fully differentiated intestinal cell of a tadpole was transplanted into an unfertilized egg in which the nucleus had been destroyed by ultraviolet light. The egg with the transplanted nucleus developed into an adult frog, thus achieving cloning [1]. A few decades later, Dr. Ian Wilmut succeeded in the somatic cloning of a mammal, a sheep, for the first time in 1997 [12]. Although nuclear transfer in mammals is more technically demanding due to the smaller cell size and physiological adjustment of the egg's cell cycle, his team demonstrated the birth of a lamb by nuclear transfer from an adult mammary gland or differentiated fetal cells into an enucleated sheep egg. Their successes in somatic cloning demonstrated that even differentiated cells contain all of the genetic information required for the development of entire organisms, and that oocytes contain factors that can reprogram somatic cell nuclei. In 2001, Dr. Takashi Tada demonstrated that mouse ES cells also contain reprogramming factors by showing that the fusion of somatic cells and ES cells can induce reprogramming in somatic nuclei [13]. This scientific stream was essential for me to initiate our project that led to the development of iPS cells.

The second important stream was factor-mediated cell fate conversion, first demonstrated by Dr. Weintraub [15]. His team converted mouse fibroblasts into myoblasts by forced expression of one of the myoblast-specific transcription factors, "MyoD." These results led to the concept of a "master" transcription factor that determines the fate of the cell lineage.

The third essential stream was ES cell research, which was initiated by Dr. Martin Evans and Dr. Gail Martin in 1981 [9, 10]. Until then, pluripotent cell lines had been obtained only from teratocarcinoma cells. They established pluripotent cell lines with a normal karyotype, which had been isolated directly from mouse early embryos *in vitro*. Dr. Austin Smith and others identified (and are still identifying) many factors which are essential for pluripotency, including Oct3/4 and Sox2 [19, 37, 38]. In 1998, Dr. James Thomson succeeded in generating human ES cells with optimal culture conditions, which are very different from those for mouse ES cells [11]. All of these findings were indispensable for providing ideas about the existence of reprogramming factors, the factor combinations and culture conditions for pluripotent cells, eventually leading to the generation of iPS cells.

New scientific streams have already emerged from the iPS cell studies (Fig. 7). In 2007, Dr. Rudolf Jaenisch provided the first proof of concept of iPS cell-based cell therapy in mouse models [39]. They demonstrated that mouse models of sickle cell anemia can be treated by transplantation with hematopoietic progenitors, which were obtained *in vitro* from gene-corrected autologous iPS cells.

In 2008, Dr. George Daley [40] and Dr. Kevin Eggan [41] first generated iPS cells from patients. Dr. Daley established iPS cells from patients with a variety of intractable diseases, such as adenosine deaminase deficiency-related severe combined immunodeficiency (ADA-SCID), Shwachman-Bodian-Diamond syndrome (SBDS), Gaucher disease type III, Duchenne (DMD) and Becker muscular dystrophy (BMD), Parkinson's disease, Huntington's disease, juvenile-onset type 1 diabetes mellitus, Down syndrome, Lesch-Nyhan syndrome, X-linked adrenoleukodystrophy, dyskeratosis congenita, Hurler syndrome, fragile X syndrome and NEMO deficiency [40, 42–45]. Dr. Eggan produced patient-specific iPS cells directly from an elderly (82-year-old) familial ALS patient, and successfully differentiated the iPS cells into motor neurons [41].

Another important scientific stream that emerged from the iPS cell technology is "direct reprogramming", which was first shown by Dr. Douglas Melton's group in 2008 [46]. They reported that the cell fate can be directly transdifferentiated *in vivo*, in living mice, by introducing just a small number of transcription factors. They identified a combination of transcription factors which converted differentiated pancreatic exocrine cells into endocrine cells that secreted insulin.

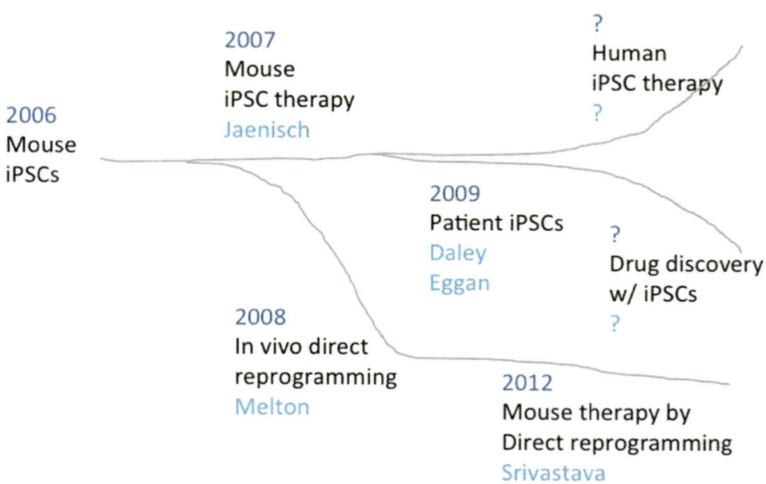

FIGURE 7. New Scientific Streams Derived from iPS Cells.

Many studies have followed, and in 2012, Dr. Deepak Srivastava provided the first proof of concept of therapies based on direct reprogramming in mice [47]. They succeeded in directly converting cardiac fibroblasts into cardiac myocytes *in situ* after coronary ligation. Their results showed decreased infarct size and recovery of some cardiac functions.

The history of iPS cell research has only just begun, and this technology has a remarkable potential for use in cell therapy, drug screening and personalized medicine. Unexpected results have opened up an entirely new research field. I hope that iPS cells will be utilized by many scientists in multiple research areas related to medicine or biology, and that some of those researchers will also receive a Nobel Prize for their excellent work in the near future.

ACKNOWLEDGEMENT

I would like to express my sincere gratitude to all of the members of the Center for iPS Cell Research and Application at Kyoto University, and the Gladstone Institutes in San Francisco for their continuous support of my scientific research and life. I wish to thank all of the previous and current colleagues in my laboratory for their dedicated and tireless efforts.

My deepest gratitude goes to my family for their unflagging support throughout my life. I could not be here today without them. Although my father, who talked me into pursuing a career in medicine, and my father-in-law, who showed me how to be a good doctor, are no longer with us, I believe they all share our happiness and joy in heaven. I sincerely wish to help make this iPS cell technology a clinical reality before I meet both of my fathers again in the future.

REFERENCES

1. Gurdon, J.B., "The developmental capacity of nuclei taken from intestinal epithelium cells of feeding tadpoles," *J Embryol Exp Morphol*, 1962. **10**: p. 622–40.
2. Takahashi, K. and S. Yamanaka, "Induction of pluripotent stem cells from mouse embryonic and adult fibroblast cultures by defined factors," *Cell*, 2006. **126**(4): p. 663–676.
3. Takahashi, K., et al., "Induction of pluripotent stem cells from adult human fibroblasts by defined factors," *Cell*, 2007. **131**(5): p. 861–72.
4. Yamanaka, S., et al., "Putative mechanism of hypotensive action of platelet-activating factor in dogs," *Circ Res*, 1992. **70**(5): p. 893–901.
5. Yamanaka, S., et al., "Effect of the platelet-activating factor antagonist, TCV-309, and the cyclo-oxygenase inhibitor, ibuprofen, on the haemodynamic changes in canine experimental endotoxic shock," *Br J Pharmacol*, 1993. **110**(4): p. 1501–7.

6. Yamanaka, S., et al., "Apolipoprotein B mRNA-editing protein induces hepatocellular carcinoma and dysplasia in transgenic animals," *Proc Natl Acad Sci U S A*, 1995. **92**(18): p. 8483–7.
7. Yamanaka, S., et al., "A novel translational repressor mRNA is edited extensively in livers containing tumors caused by the transgene expression of the apoB mRNA-editing enzyme," *Genes Dev*, 1997. **11**(3): p. 321–33.
8. Yamanaka, S., et al., "Essential role of NAT1/p97/DAP5 in embryonic differentiation and the retinoic acid pathway," *Embo J*, 2000. **19**(20): p. 5533–41.
9. Evans, M.J. and M.H. Kaufman, "Establishment in culture of pluripotential cells from mouse embryos," *Nature*, 1981. **292**(5819): p. 154–6.
10. Martin, G.R., "Isolation of a pluripotent cell line from early mouse embryos cultured in medium conditioned by teratocarcinoma stem cells," *Proc Natl Acad Sci U S A*, 1981. **78**(12): p. 7634–8.
11. Thomson, J.A., et al., "Embryonic stem cell lines derived from human blastocysts," *Science*, 1998. **282**(5391): p. 1145–7.
12. Wilmut, I., et al., "Viable offspring derived from fetal and adult mammalian cells," *Nature*, 1997. **385**(6619): p. 810–3.
13. Tada, M., et al., "Nuclear reprogramming of somatic cells by in vitro hybridization with ES cells," *Curr Biol*, 2001. **11**(19): p. 1553–8.
14. Schneuwly, S., R. Klemenz, and W.J. Gehring, "Redesigning the body plan of Drosophila by ectopic expression of the homoeotic gene Antennapedia," *Nature*, 1987. **325**(6107): p. 816–8.
15. Davis, R.L., H. Weintraub, and A.B. Lassar, "Expression of a single transfected cDNA converts fibroblasts to myoblasts," *Cell*, 1987. **51**(6): p. 987–1000.
16. Kawai, J., et al., "Functional annotation of a full-length mouse cDNA collection," *Nature*, 2001. **409**(6821): p. 685–90.
17. "Digital Differential Display," http://www.ncbi.nlm.nih.gov/UniGene/ddd.cgi
18. Nichols, J., et al., "Formation of pluripotent stem cells in the mammalian embryo depends on the POU transcription factor Oct4," *Cell*, 1998. **95**(3): p. 379–91.
19. Niwa, H., J. Miyazaki, and A.G. Smith, "Quantitative expression of Oct-3/4 defines differentiation, dedifferentiation or self-renewal of ES cells" *Nat Genet*, 2000. **24**(4): p. 372–6.
20. Okuda, A., et al., "UTF1, a novel transcriptional coactivator expressed in pluripotent embryonic stem cells and extra-embryonic cells," *Embo J*, 1998. **17**(7): p. 2019–32.
21. Rogers, M.B., B.A. Hosler, and L.J. Gudas, "Specific expression of a retinoic acid-regulated, zinc-finger gene, Rex-1, in preimplantation embryos, trophoblast and spermatocytes," *Development*, 1991. **113**(3): p. 815–24.
22. Tokuzawa, Y., et al., "Fbx15 is a novel target of Oct3/4 but is dispensable for embryonic stem cell self-renewal and mouse development," *Mol Cell Biol*, 2003. **23**(8): p. 2699–708.
23. Takahashi, K., K. Mitsui, and S. Yamanaka, "Role of ERas in promoting tumour-like properties in mouse embryonic stem cells," *Nature*, 2003. **423**(6939): p. 541–5.
24. Mitsui, K., et al., "The Homeoprotein Nanog Is Required for Maintenance of Pluripotency in Mouse Epiblast and ES Cells," *Cell*, 2003. **113**(5): p. 631–42.

25. Masui, S., et al., "Pluripotency governed by Sox2 via regulation of Oct3/4 expression in mouse embryonic stem cells," *Nat Cell Biol*, 2007. **9**(6): p. 625–635.
26. Chambers, I., et al., "Functional expression cloning of nanog, a pluripotency sustaining factor in embryonic stem cells," *Cell*, 2003. **113**(5): p. 643–55.
27. Yuan, H., et al., "Developmental-specific activity of the FGF-4 enhancer requires the synergistic action of Sox2 and Oct-3," *Genes Dev*, 1995. **9**(21): p. 2635–45.
28. Okita, K., T. Ichisaka, and S. Yamanaka, "Generation of germ-line competent induced pluripotent stem cells," *Nature*, 2007. **448**: p. 313–7.
29. Egawa, N., et al., "Drug screening for ALS using patient-specific induced pluripotent stem cells," *Sci Transl Med*, 2012. **4**(145): p. 145ra104.
30. Yahata, N., et al., "Anti-Abeta Drug Screening Platform Using Human iPS Cell-Derived Neurons for the Treatment of Alzheimer's Disease," *PLoS One*, 2011. **6**(9): p. e25788.
31. Tanaka, T., et al., "Induced pluripotent stem cells from CINCA syndrome patients as a model for dissecting somatic mosaicism and drug discovery," *Blood*, 2012. **120**(6): p. 1299–308.
32. Takayama, N., et al., "Transient activation of c-MYC expression is critical for efficient platelet generation from human induced pluripotent stem cells," *J Exp Med*, 2010.
33. Okita, K., et al., "A more efficient method to generate integration-free human iPS cells," *Nat Methods*, 2011. **8**(5): p. 409–12.
34. Hong, H., et al., "Suppression of induced pluripotent stem cell generation by the p53-p21 pathway," *Nature*, 2009. **460**(7259): p. 1132–5.
35. Nakagawa, M., et al., "Promotion of direct reprogramming by transformation-deficient Myc," *Proc Natl Acad Sci U S A*, 2010. **107**(32): p. 14152–7.
36. Maekawa, M., et al., "Direct reprogramming of somatic cells is promoted by maternal transcription factor Glis1," *Nature*, 2011. **474**(7350): p. 225–9.
37. Smith, A.G., et al., "Inhibition of pluripotential embryonic stem cell differentiation by purified polypeptides," *Nature*, 1988. **336**(6200): p. 688–90.
38. Avilion, A.A., et al., "Multipotent cell lineages in early mouse development depend on SOX2 function," *Genes Dev*, 2003. **17**(1): p. 126–40.
39. Hanna, J., et al., "Treatment of Sickle Cell Anemia Mouse Model with iPS Cells Generated from Autologous Skin," *Science*, 2007. **318**(5858): p. 1920–3.
40. Park, I.H., et al., "Disease-Specific Induced Pluripotent Stem Cells," *Cell*, 2008. **134**(5): p. 877–886.
41. Dimos, J.T., et al., "Induced Pluripotent Stem Cells Generated from Patients with ALS Can Be Differentiated into Motor Neurons," *Science*, 2008. **321**: p. 1218–1221.
42. Jang, J., et al., "Induced pluripotent stem cell models from X-linked adrenoleukodystrophy patients," *Ann Neurol*, 2011. **70**(3): p. 402–9.
43. Agarwal, S. and G.Q. Daley, "Telomere dynamics in dyskeratosis congenita: the long and the short of iPS," *Cell Res*, 2011. **21**(8): p. 1157–60.
44. Urbach, A., et al., "Differential modeling of fragile X syndrome by human embryonic stem cells and induced pluripotent stem cells," *Cell Stem Cell*, 2010. **6**(5): p. 407–11.
45. Guan, X., et al., "Derivation of human embryonic stem cells with NEMO deficiency," *Stem Cell Res*, 2012.

46. Zhou, Q., et al., "In vivo reprogramming of adult pancreatic exocrine cells to beta-cells," *Nature*, 2008. **455**(7213): p. 627–632.
47. Qian, L., et al., "In vivo reprogramming of murine cardiac fibroblasts into induced cardiomyocytes," *Nature*, 2012. **485**(7400): p. 593–8.

Physiology or Medicine 2013

James E. Rothman, Randy W. Schekman and Thomas C. Südhof

"for their discoveries of machinery regulating vesicle traffic, a major transport system in our cells"

The Nobel Prize in Physiology or Medicine

Speech by Professor Juleen Zierath of the Nobel Assembly at Karolinska Institutet.

Your Majesties, Your Royal Highnesses, Esteemed Laureates, Ladies and Gentlemen,

Imagine this Nobel Prize Award Ceremony without any of the beautiful flowers that you can see here around me. These flowers are transported to Stockholm each year from Sanremo in Italy. But imagine if they were missorted and ended up in Copenhagen. Without a functioning transport system, this could easily be a reality. To avoid chaos, we are totally dependent on fine-tuned transport systems, where cargo is loaded into the right vehicle and transported to the right destination at the right time.

The cell, with its different compartments, faces a similar transport challenge. Each cell in the body functions like a factory, producing molecules, which are delivered to specific locations at exactly the right moment. Bubble-like vesicles carry the molecules between different compartments in the cell. One of the great mysteries of cell physiology was how these vesicles could be delivered to the right destination at the right time. And how was this process controlled with temporal precision?

In the 1970s, Randy W. Schekman was fascinated by these questions. He studied vesicle transport using yeast as a model. He identified yeast cells with defective transport machinery. These cells showed a resemblance to a poorly planned public transport system: similar to a situation in a bustling city, when trains cannot depart from the station due to rail defects. Consequently some passengers pile up at the station and others get routed to new destinations. In Schekman's experiments, vesicles piled up in certain parts of the cell. He found that the cause of this congestion was genetic and went on to identify the mutated genes. By these groundbreaking experiments, Schekman provided new insight into the tightly regulated machinery that mediates vesicle transport in the cell.

James Rothman was also intrigued by the nature of the cell's transport system. While studying vesicle transport in the 1980s and 1990s, he discovered a protein complex that enables vesicles to dock and fuse with target membranes. In this fusion process, proteins on both the vesicle and the target membrane bind to each other like two sides of a zipper. The fact that there are many such proteins and that they bind only in specific combinations guarantees that cargo is delivered to the right destination. In these elegant experiments, Rothman revealed how vesicles, using this zipper-like function, are able to locate the correct docking site in the cell. Cargo, like these flowers around me, could be delivered to the right location!

But questions still lingered. How are molecules released from vesicles in such a precise manner? Thomas Südhof was interested in how nerve cells communicate with one another in the brain. The signalling molecules, neurotransmitters, are released from vesicles using the machinery discovered by Rothman and Schekman. In the 1990s, Südhof searched for calcium sensitive proteins that control this process. He identified molecules that sense calcium ions and trigger vesicle fusion. This allows the zipper to open so that cargo can be released. Südhof's electrifying discovery explained how vesicles can rapidly release their cargo on command. Neurotransmitters are delivered with temporal precision from nerve cells, just like these flowers could be delivered to this Nobel Ceremony on the right day.

The 2013 Nobel Laureates have discovered a truly fundamental process in cell physiology. Their discoveries have had a major impact to advance our understanding of how molecules are correctly routed to appropriate destinations in the cell with timing and precision. Without this wonderfully precise mechanism, we would not survive. This process is required for sending neurotransmitter substances from one nerve cell to another, as well as for the release of hormones, such as insulin, to control blood sugar after a meal.

Professors Rothman, Schekman and Südhof,

With brilliant experiments, you have solved one of the great mysteries of cell physiology. Your discoveries represent a paradigm shift in our understanding of how the cell organises the routing of molecules packaged in vesicles to various cellular destinations. Specificity and timing in the delivery of molecular cargo are essential for our survival.

On behalf of the Nobel Assembly at Karolinska Institutet, I wish to convey to you our warmest congratulations. May I now ask you to step forward to receive the Nobel Prize from the hands of His Majesty the King.

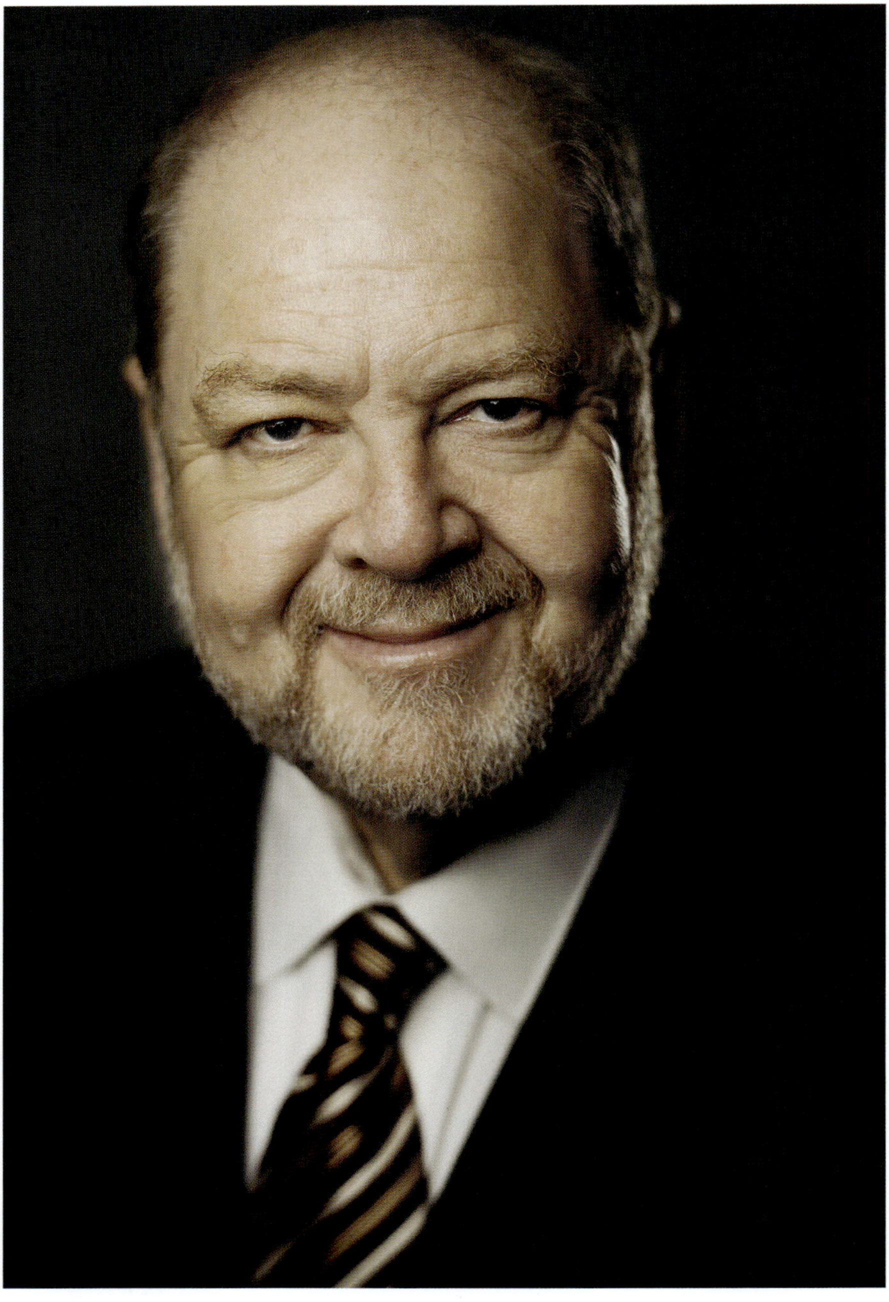

James E. Rothman. © Nobel Media AB. Photo: A. Mahmoud

James E. Rothman

This autobiographical sketch of a life in science mainly focuses on a question I am now often asked—when and how did you know you wanted to be a scientist, and how did you become one? I am also asked by young scientists for advice I could impart from my own experiences and observations. With this in mind, this essay essentially provides bookends of my life until now, and I hope it may be of interest less from the particulars and more from generalizations that may emerge in the eyes of a reader, especially a young scientist. My Nobel lecture complements this essay, focusing mainly on what happened in between the bookends.

CHILDHOOD

From the earliest time I can remember I wanted to be a scientist, especially a physicist. I am not entirely sure where this came from, but at least in part it must have come from my parents (Fig. 1) who deeply valued education, especially in science and medicine. I was really fortunate and owe my parents a lot—they made me feel that I could do anything, and they provided the resources to enable me a privileged education unencumbered by financial needs.

My mother Gloria, with her enormous focus and drive, would in today's world have been a high-powered executive. But she grew up in an earlier era where women had far fewer options. She ran the home and my Dad's pediatric practice and taught me how to organize and manage. My father Martin was an intellectually oriented small-town physician who had wanted to do medical research as a young man, but had graduated in the Great Depression and then been caught up in World War II. He was always keen to involve me in the things he did. At perhaps the age of eight (Figure 2, left), I remember accompanying him on nocturnal house calls, at other times to the hospital; assisting him at

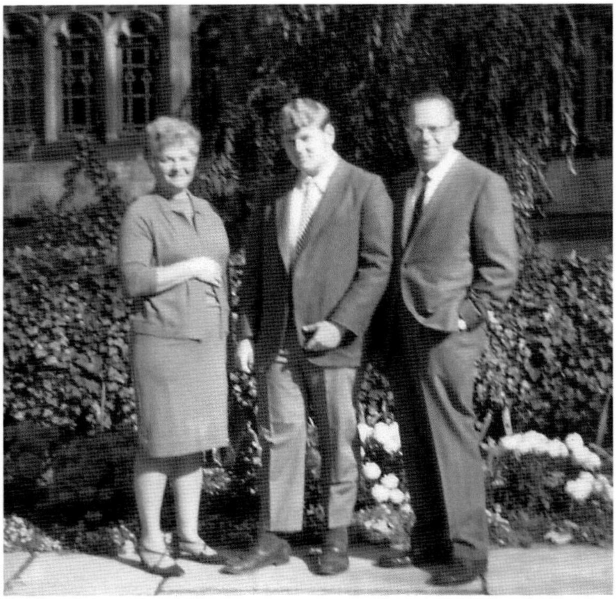

FIGURE 1. My parents Gloria and Martin Rothman bringing me to Yale as a freshman (1967). Photograph taken in front of Branford College, where I lived as an upper classman, and where my wife Joy Hirsch and I now live as Resident Fellows. Our children Matthew and Lisa both lived in Branford College, graduating from Yale in 2000 and 2004, respectively.

home by measuring the intervals in his patients' electrocardiograms; and helping him perform blood analyses in the small lab behind his office.

But I believe that my focus on science came at least as much from the times during which I grew up, and the values that I and other Americans internalized from the society around us. In the 1950s and 1960s science and technology were viscerally understood and applauded by most Americans as mainstays of economic and political power following the victories of World War II. This era began with the polio vaccine eradicating a dread disease and with atomic energy (for better and for worse). It ended with the transistor, the digital computer, and the first men on the Moon.

In such an environment, and with my supportive family, and with an abundance of curiosity and a natural talent for mathematics, it is not surprising that I was designing and building electronics and launching rockets while still in elementary school. Rockets were a big thing for me as a boy (Figure 3). I taught myself basic trigonometry in 7th grade so I could triangulate the height of the rockets, and then calculus two years later so I could better understand the physics involved. As I began to study more advanced physics and mathematics

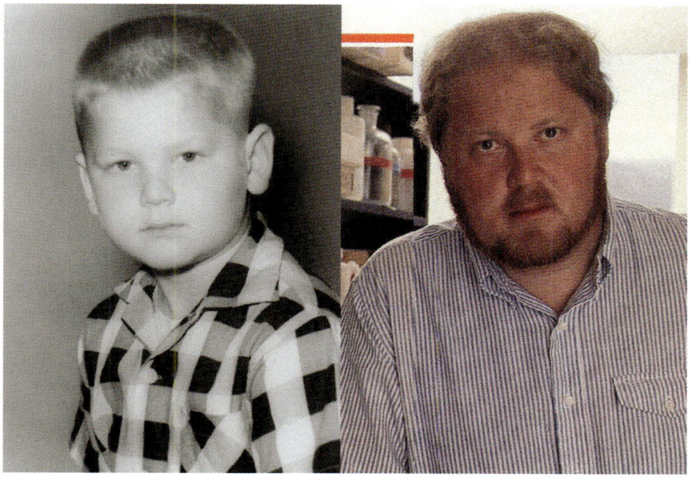

FIGURE 2. Photographs of the author in 1958 (age 8) and much later in 1984 in my laboratory at Stanford University, the same month that our three pivotal papers appeared in *Cell* describing cell-free transport between Golgi stacks.

formally in high school, I devoured the subject and challenged myself far outside the excellent curriculum at my secondary school (Pomfret School), so much so that I was graduated after my junior year. Entering Yale College in 1967, I was absolutely committed to theoretical physics.

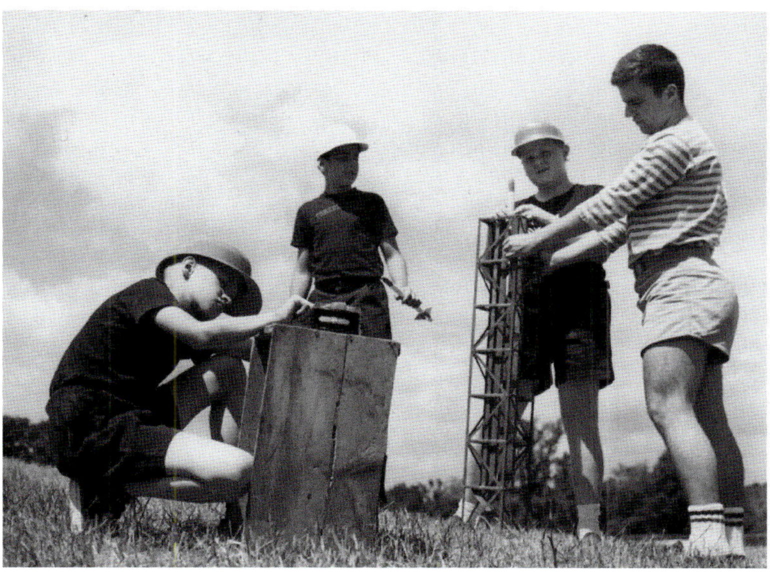

FIGURE 3. The author, second from the right, preparing to launch a model rocket, age 12. I was entranced by mathematics, physics, and technology.

YALE

Yale provided the perfect environment in which a committed young scientist could develop while also immersed in the broader culture. Yale was big enough to provide every opportunity, yet organized into relatively intimate units (Colleges) small enough to foster the individual. The students had all varieties of interests, and my friends were drawn largely from outside the sciences, providing breadth to complement my personal scientific focus (these friendships continue today with annual summer reunions of the "812 Club," named after a room in Branford College). I also studied and especially internalized from my friends a great deal about art, philosophy, and history.

As an entering freshman, I was accepted into an "Early Concentration" program which rapidly enabled me to focus deeply on mathematics and physics at an advanced level. Physics taught me how to rigorously analyze the components of a problem by first imagining the form a solution would take. This can be a useful approach when engulfed in the fog that envelopes the uncharted waters of biology.

As I began my junior year, perhaps with fatherly concerns about the poor employment prospects for physicists at that time, my Dad strongly encouraged me to at least give biology a try. I was not especially open-minded, as there was a well-understood intellectual pecking order that every budding physicist was soon informed of. Theoretical physicists were the brightest. Experimental physicists were failed theoreticians, but nonetheless useful for confirming theories. Chemists were not so bright, but still socially acceptable. Biologists were said to be even less bright, and generally not worth mentioning. But, even at the very first lecture in the general biology course, I was amazed that (in contrast to the highly structured field of physics) the research frontier in molecular biology seemed instantly accessible, and yet could be equally rigorous and structure-based.

Thus began a multi-year process in which I gradually learned to think like a biologist, while still retaining the orthogonal way of thinking like a physicist. I believe this mindset was critical not only in my choice of the problem whose solution was recognized by this Nobel Prize, but also in providing me the means to solve it (as elaborated in my Nobel lecture). Therefore, I will devote some detail here to this process of transition from physics towards biology.

The transition came in stages, initially via self-taught physical chemistry (though I never formally studied this subject or many others—in fact, I have completed only one term of college chemistry and biology and most of what I have learned in science and medicine has been self-directed). In physics, I had gravitated to statistical mechanics, probably because unlike quantum mechanics you can visualize it in simple terms. Statistical mechanics served as my intellectual bridge to biology. For example, consider that the three dimensional conformations of polymers (a classic problem in statistical physics and thermodynamics) such as polypeptides are a fundamental determinant of their biochemical mechanisms. A term of research (junior year) with the theoretical chemist Marshall Fixman on the statistical mechanics of polymers equipped me with a fluid way of visualizing individual versus ensemble behavior of molecules that to this day guides my thinking in biochemistry and cell biology.

The next stage in my transition (also junior year) came via Harold Morowitz, introduced by Fixman, a theoretical biophysicist with equal interest in science as in philosophy. Harold was a broad intellectual who has had many interests, but just then he was especially interested in the hotly debated question of the basic structure of biological membranes. His laboratory had just done some influential experiments demonstrating thermal phase transitions in the membrane of microorganisms mimicking the behavior of isolated lipid bilayers. In retrospect, I was attracted by a combination of the familiar (thermal physics and conformational changes of a polymer [fatty acid chain] in the phase transition) and Harold's personal warmth and charm. Soon I was working in his lab with a postdoctoral fellow, designing and building an instrument to measure the phase transitions, and was deeply engaged.

Harold had a way of collecting interesting people around him, including his former PhD student Donald Engelman. Harold advised me to go to the research seminar that Engelman was to give during an upcoming visit to Yale. This was the first seminar I had ever attended, and as it turned out it was a "job seminar" resulting in Don joining the faculty of Molecular Biophysics and Biochemistry soon thereafter. He spoke about his now classic experiments with Maurice Wilkins (Nobel Prize, 1962) demonstrating the lipid bilayer in biological membranes using an elegant combination of microbiology and X-ray diffraction. I think Harold asked Don to take me under his wing, where in a sense I have been ever since (Don remains one of my closest friends and happily we are both now at Yale). We took on the problem of how cholesterol buffers the fluidity of the lipid bilayer, extinguishing the thermal phase transitions, and my earliest publications came from this. Don taught me by his example how to dissect each morsel of data to get the most from it.

In doing this, I learned another important lesson—the central importance of numbers. My students sometimes seem surprised that there are a lot of numbers that I have at my disposal whenever I may need them; this is true, and it is no accident. From Yale onwards, I have always made a point of remembering key numbers, and I have learned to do this automatically every time I hear a new one. For example, π and e in mathematics; Boltzmann's constant in physics; absolute zero temperature, the diameter of a hydrogen atom, and the density of various materials in chemistry; the size of proteins and their secondary structure motifs, and the sizes of viruses, organelles and so on in biology; and the rates of fundamental processes (for example, diffusion in water, lipid bilayers; the rate of cell locomotion and so on). Ready knowledge of scale and rates allows one to quickly see if a hypothesis or a result or an experimental design is reasonable.

At that time Yale had an unusual program for a dozen or so seniors called Scholar of the House (sadly this wonderful program has been discontinued). This program allowed me to spend senior year fully in research (with Harold and Don) with no formal course work, and to graduate solely on the strength of a thesis, if it was accepted (if it was not I would need to repeat senior year conventionally). The thesis was evaluated by a committee of Yale's most eminent scholars drawn mainly from the humanities. With so much riding on this, I was mortified when Harold playfully showed me the evaluation of my work he had written fully in limericks—I was sure I was doomed; but apparently it was just right for the humanists, and I was graduated (with the award for the best thesis).

During that last year at Yale I became a scientist.

HARVARD

My father had convinced me that I should go to a medical school rather than directly to a PhD program. At that point my knowledge of biology was as narrow as my knowledge of physics was deep, and it would have been impossible to make an informed choice of which discipline in biology to focus on. Therefore, I entered Harvard Medical School (in 1971) with the idea of learning biology and then doing research, rather than ever practicing. I succeeded in the former, ultimately leaving the MD program more or less after the basic sciences (but with enough clinical exposure to gain a lifetime of respect for clinical medicine).

The first year at Harvard Medical School easily proved to be the greatest didactic experience of my life because HMS offered an unencumbered platform for self-directed learning with wonderful access to first-class research professors built on a broad and well-organized curriculum. I still rely on the many things I learned in that first year or so.

In particular, it was as a first year medical student in histology that I first learned about the secretory pathway, at a time when the discoveries of George Palade (Nobel Prize, 1974) were still fresh and remarkable. What an astonishing process—how could cells make vesicles from membranes? How could each vesicle know where to go? How could it fuse? It was particularly amazing because at the time it was not even possible to begin to imagine the form a molecular solution might take. This captured my imagination, but not enough was known to productively take up the problem then. But it would ultimately become a lifelong focus when I started my own laboratory at Stanford in 1978.

My PhD thesis (initially as part of Harvard's MD-PhD program) was with Eugene Kennedy, a master of membrane biochemistry. Kennedy, who was a brilliant intellectual and an original thinker, taught me how to formulate a complex problem in biochemical terms. Some of this work was in collaboration with John Lenard, whom I will soon mention. We established how lipid bilayers in cell membranes are formed by asymmetric biosynthesis, following on the PhD thesis work of Roger Kornberg (Nobel Prize, 2006), which had at that time just established the basics of the physical dynamics of lipids in membranes.

Harvard, therefore, is where I became an experimentalist and in particular a professional biochemist. Everything that happened afterwards followed from that.

Deep and enduring scientific friendships

A life in research provides many opportunities to meet remarkable people as a student and afterwards around the world. It is hard to over-emphasize the importance of several formative, warm and enduring friendships for my development and success as a scientist. Some evolved from what we would today call mentoring relationships, initially with somewhat older (but still young) scientists who were nonetheless more established than me. This group included (in the order of our first acquaintance) Donald Engelman, John Lenard, Qais Al-Awqati, Roger Kornberg and Per Peterson. I first met each of these extraordinary individuals essentially as teachers. I have already mentioned Engelman.

John Lenard was a young full professor at Rutgers when we met in 1974. He took me into his lab (and his home) while I was still a graduate student so we could understand the topology of lipids in viral envelopes. We worked day and night together and we soon bonded personally. Though we never collaborated experimentally again, many ideas and personal decisions have been subject to John's wise counsel. We wrote several review articles together over the decades, and in each case he taught me how to improve the framing of ideas and my writing style. Happily, we see each other regularly for dinners, museums, and theatre in Manhattan.

Qais Al-Awqati was my teacher in renal physiology when I was a second year medical student (1972) and he was junior faculty at Mass General. We met again much later (1986) when coincidently we both were at Cold Spring Harbor Laboratory summer lab courses, and we had many lovely evening walks together discussing books and occasionally science. We have been close ever since. Qais is not only one of the world's best physicians and cell biologists, but without doubt one of the most intelligent and cultured people I have ever met. What a privilege it is to continue to learn from and enjoy him, whether we talk about science or he guides me through the Metropolitan (be it the art museum or the opera).

Roger was an assistant professor in the department of Biological Chemistry at Harvard Medical School and I met him as a PhD student. We had a common interest in membranes, but soon we were discussing ever-widening scientific terrain because of his deep and penetrating mind. He broadened and sharpened my perspective on biochemistry, first as a student and then soon as faculty colleague at Stanford. At Stanford we met many times a week, and I turned to him for criticism and inspiration. After I left Stanford (1988) this of course diminished in frequency, but never in intensity. I also suspect that Roger's endorsement after "road-testing" me at Harvard somehow figured importantly in the job offer from his father Arthur Kornberg (Nobel Prize, 1959) and the other faculty to join their Biochemistry department, which came while I was still in the MD-PhD program in 1976.

Per Peterson, as he puts it, "discovered me" at a membrane meeting in Heidelberg (1980). Per is a cellular immunologist, and was at that time the director of the Wallenberg Laboratory in Uppsala (Sweden). As he told me, my findings were good raw material, but needed polishing. Of course, he was correct. He has been trying, with occasional modest success, to improve me ever since. Per has a rare combination of great analytical power with a genuinely sympathetic understanding of human nature. This has enabled him both to contribute centrally to science, and to build and run large and successful organizations, most recently as the Chairman of Research and Development at Johnson & Johnson. During his evolution Per has kept me at his side, and taught me a tremendous amount about the dynamics of industry and approaches to management that have proven very useful to me. He continues to inspire me and help me focus on what really matters.

Other important friendships started on more personal terms but soon evolved into long-term informal intellectual or actual collaborations where new ideas could be debated with absolute intellectual honesty in friendly ways and often in nice settings as well. I met Graham Warren (Figure 4, top) in 1976 when

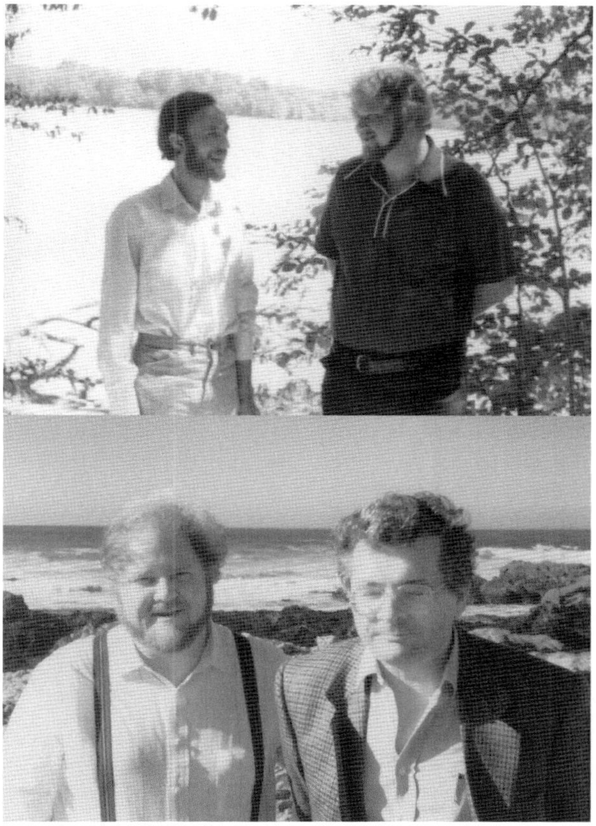

FIGURE 4. Top: the author with Graham Warren in 1976, photographed in Haverhill, Massachusetts, my home town shortly after we first met when he was visiting Harvard and I was still a PhD student there. Many of my formative ideas took shape in discussions with Graham, and later ones as well. Bottom: with Felix Wieland in 1987, photographed in Half Moon Bay, California, taken during the period of his pivotal sabbatical in my Stanford laboratory. Felix is a consummate enzymologist and taught me much.

he was a postdoctoral fellow at Cambridge (UK) on an extended visit to Harvard, and we immediately hit it off, his reserve a complement to my exuberance, Graham harboring a well-known (merciless) intellectual rigor salved by his gracious humor. Graham and his family spent a summer at Stanford in 1978, so we could work together (actually starting my lab jointly) on what turned out to be a bold but ultimately ill-conceived hypothesis that we had convinced ourselves was the key to the sorting problem. Although in the past few years, with his responsibilities directing the Max Perutz Institute in Vienna, and mine at Yale, our contact has been less, we have seen each other numerous times every year and many of my best ideas have often drawn on our discussions.

I met Felix Wieland (Figure 4, bottom) in 1985 at Regensburg (Germany) where he was then an assistant professor. He came up to me after my lecture on cell-free reconstitution with the idea of spending two years at Stanford trying to figure out how membrane fusion worked. As with Graham, we also immediately hit it off, though in Felix's case it was his contagious Bavarian exuberance and humor synergizing with mine. Soon, he was in Palo Alto. Wieland was a real enzymologist who taught me (and the rest of my lab) how the business is really done, having himself learned at the hands of a master (his uncle) Fyodor Lynen (Nobel Prize, 1964). Without Felix, I doubt there would have been NSF, SNAP,

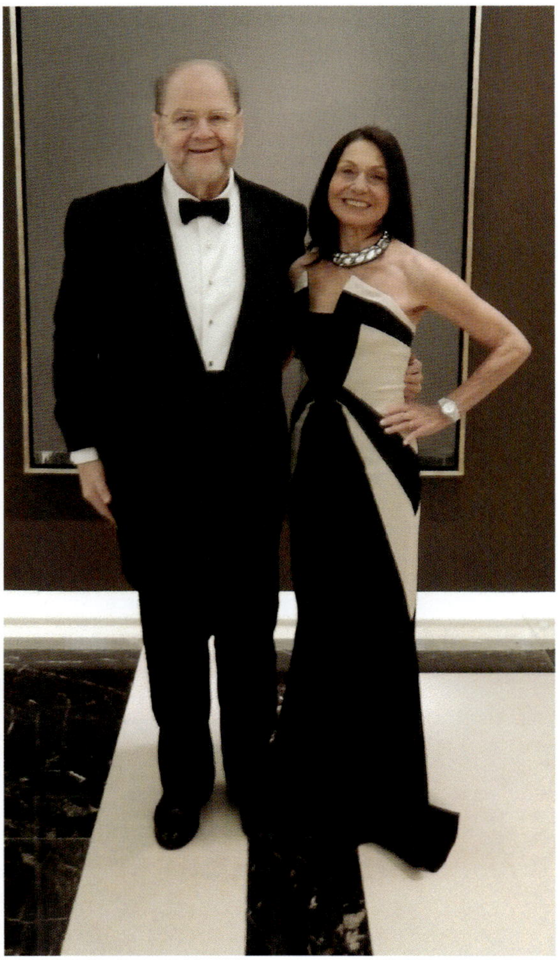

FIGURE 5. With my wife, Joy Hirsch, in the lobby of the Four Seasons Hotel in Washington D.C. on November 19, 2013, just after the meeting of the American Nobel laureates and spouses with President Obama, en route to the dinner at the Swedish Embassy.

SNAREs or coatomer, and even if there were they would not have been as much fun. By 1987 Felix moved back to Germany (at Heidelberg) but we still see each other frequently. I look forward to our annual escapes with our wives to Bad Drei Kirchen (Bolzano), and the Rothman and Wieland children continue their childhood friendships to this day.

Without a doubt the most important, deepest, and most vital relationship is of course with my wife, Joy Hirsch (Figure 5). In addition to the personal side, Joy is also my scientific partner. She is my sounding board on every subject, and has been my critic and supporter through the many early years when my work was not accepted as it is now. Joy comes from a successful farming family in Salem, Oregon and from this very American background is imbued with the Yankee attitude that every problem can be solved if you think about it enough and try hard enough. Joy also lives by this belief in her research. She is also a Professor at Yale, and is gifted scientist who is renowned for her fundamental studies of human cognitive processes and related diseases.

Observations on style from a life in science

As a closing bookend, I will offer some observations that may be of interest to others, especially younger scientists. This is not necessarily to impart specific advice, which would be disingenuous as I rarely followed the advice I was given as a young man; it is more to offer the use of some of my personal experiences as a springboard for generalizations that may apply to the reader. Some of these thoughts will be familiar to several generations of my students, who may recall having heard one or another as a frequently trodden-out aphorism. Some are from my own teachers.

Science and art. Science at the edge is an art form as much as a strictly logical development of ideas. The rare artists and the rare scientists capable of performing at the edge have a lot in common. They both have an intuitive vision carrying strong emotional content. Neither is easily discouraged from their work, even with strong obstacles in their path. These are essential traits.

Choosing a problem. As a new junior faculty member at Stanford, I asked Arthur Kornberg why he chose to understand DNA synthesis in the early 1950s. He said that the problem was of the greatest importance; that everyone else assumed it could not be done; but that he thought it could be. I listened very carefully when he said this.

The importance of a clear hypothesis. I often tell people in my lab "if you want to hit a home run, you have to be in the ball park. If you are outside the ball park you can swing all day but you will never hit a home run." This idea comes from physics where computationally complex problems are approached by making simplifying "ball park" assumptions so that the main variables can be identified. To do this in biology, you imagine you are designing the system and therefore how you would design it for the required function. This provides a model—a hypothesis—of the form that a likely solution will take. You are now in the ball park, because you can now design specific tests of the model. Your exact model is almost certain to be wrong in detail (evolution rarely works by Cartesian rules) but is likely to be correct in spirit, and this will allow you to get to the truth faster. This process is very basic to my approach to science, as I described in my Nobel lecture (Figure 9 in the published lecture).

Troubles Are Good For You (TAGFY). The "TAGFY Philosophy" was first enunciated by the master enzymologist Ephraim Racker, and I pass it on. TAGFY has proven true for me over and over again. For example, after Erik Fries and I first published cell-free transport, we had great difficulty repeating our exact results, and it would have been easy to be discouraged. But TAGFY meant that we were really about to discover something basic that we had no idea about. Indeed, in resolving the "trouble" we found that we had reconstituted intra-Golgi vesicular transport, a process not previously known to exist (as documented in the Nobel lecture). TAGFY can give you strength in hard times.

If you are hitting your head against a brick wall, find a new wall. It is so human to try that experiment one more time hoping for a better result. It almost never pays. Try a new approach. Remarkably, most people don't.

It is much harder to stop a project than to start one. To do so takes real intellectual honesty and a complete disregard of ego. Worse, stopping involves a huge sunk cost of time and emotion, but if you don't, then the next phase (which may hold success) will be only further away.

Don't be afraid to be "stupid." If you don't understand it, it is probably unclear. If you don't know how to do something, ask. It is far better than losing days in the lab because you didn't. It is amazing how many people don't ask. I always did and it made a difference.

Smart is good; lucky is better. Eugene Kennedy always said this, and he was right. In other words, in spite of any and all, don't over-think and be open to chance.

Additional personal history

In addition to me (1950) my parents Gloria Rothman (née Hartnick, born 1923) and Martin Rothman (1915–2005) had two children, Richard (1953) and John (1955). My brother Richard is an MD-PhD who recently retired from the NIH after many years as a leading researcher in neuropharmacology, and is now in practice in Psychiatry. John is a successful attorney specializing in mediation. I am married to Joy Hirsch (Figure 5) who is an eminent professor at Yale in Neurobiology and Psychiatry. She is a graduate of the University of Oregon (BS) and Columbia (PhD). We reside in New York and New Haven. I am always dazzled by her beauty and elegance but equally by her brilliance and compassion. Joy is the glue that holds together our wide circle of personal and scientific friends, and our extended family. She has also been an exceptional stepmother to our children, and we are very proud of their accomplishments. Matthew (1977;

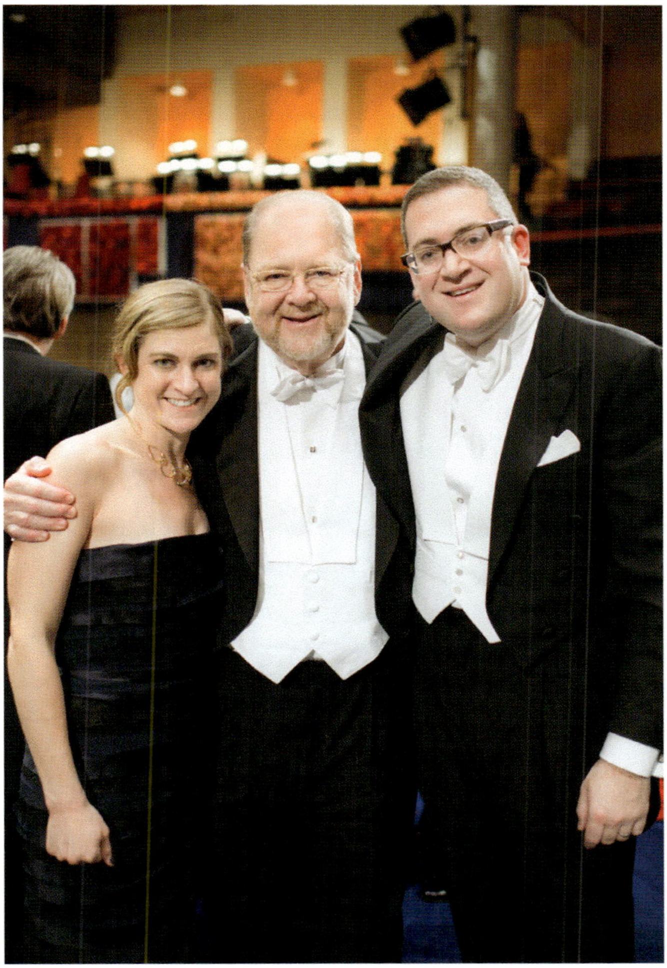

FIGURE 6. With my children, Lisa and Matthew on the stage in the Concert Hall in Stockholm, immediately after the conclusion of the Nobel Prize Ceremony, December 10, 2013. (Courtesy of the Alexander Mahmoud and the Nobel Foundation).

Figure 6) graduated from Yale (BA) and Columbia (MBA) and is a senior executive in a major investment firm. He is married to the former Sarah Levinson, a senior executive in a national public relations firm. Sarah and Matthew are superb parents to our two delightful grandchildren, Alexandra (2010) and George (2012). Lisa (1982; Figure 6) graduated from Yale (BA) and Columbia (MD) and soon will start her residency in Dermatology at NYU. She is married to the former Jeannie Chung, an attorney in a major Manhattan law firm.

Curriculum vitae

James Edward Rothman was born on November 3, 1950 in Haverhill, Massachusetts (U.S.A.). He went to public schools in Haverhill, Massachusetts for elementary school through 8th grade, and then to Pomfret School (Pomfret, Connecticut) in 1964, from which he graduated in 1967. He then matriculated at Yale College, graduating *summa cum laude* in 1971 with a B.A. in Physics, having been Scholar of the House. Rothman then matriculated at the Harvard Medical School as an MD student, then joined the MD.-PhD program there. Ultimately, he graduated with a PhD in Biological Chemistry (thesis advisor, Eugene P. Kennedy) in 1976. He then joined the laboratory of Harvey F. Lodish in the Department of Biology at M.I.T. as a Damon Runyan postdoctoral fellow (1976–1978). In 1978 he joined the Department of Biochemistry at Stanford University as an assistant professor, and was promoted to associate professor with tenure (1981) and then full professor (1984). Rothman moved in 1988 to Princeton University in the Department of Molecular Biology where he held the E. R. Squib Chair of Molecular Biology. In 1991 he moved to the Memorial Sloan-Kettering Cancer Center where he founded and chaired the Cellular Biophysics and Biochemistry department, served as a Vice-Chairman of the Sloan-Kettering Institute for Cancer Research, and held the Paul Marks Chair. In 2004, Rothman joined the Columbia University College of Physicians and Surgeons as a professor in the Department of Physiology and Cellular Biophysics, where he also directed the Columbia Genome Center and held the Clyde and Helen Wu Chair of Chemical Biology. Then, in 2008 he returned to Yale and at the time of this writing is the Wallace Professor of Biomedical Sciences and Chair of the Department of Cell Biology and a Professor of Chemistry.

Prior to the Nobel Prize, Rothman's contributions to cell biology, biochemistry, and neuroscience were recognized by numerous prizes and honors. These include: the Eli Lilly Award for Fundamental Research in Biological Chemistry, U.S.A. (1986); the Passano Young Scientist Award, U.S.A. (1986); the Alexander Von Humboldt Award, Germany (1989); the Heinrich Wieland Prize,

Germany (1990); election as Member, U.S. National Academy of Sciences (1993); the Rosenstiel Award in Biomedical Sciences, U.S.A. (1994); election as Fellow, American Academy of Arts and Sciences (1994); the Fritz Lipmann Award, U.S.A. (1995); elected as Member, Institute of Medicine, National Academy of Sciences, U.S.A. (1995); Honorary Degree, University of Regensburg, Germany (1995); elected as Foreign Associate, European Molecular Biology Organization (1995); the Gairdner Foundation International Award, Canada (1996); the King Faisal International Prize in Science, Saudi Arabia (1996); the Harden Medal of the British Biochemical Society, U.K. (1997); the Lounsbery Award, National Academy of Sciences, U.S.A. (1997); the Feodor Lynen Award, U.S.A. (1997); honorary MD and PhD degrees, University of Geneva (1997); the Jacobæus Prize, Denmark (1999); the Heineken Prize for Biochemistry, The Netherlands (2000); the Otto-Warburg Medal, German Biochemical Society, Germany (2001); the Louisa Gross Horwitz Prize, U.S.A. (2002); the Lasker Basic Research Award, U.S.A. (2002); elected as Honorary Member, Japanese Biochemical Society (2005); the Beering Award U.S.A. (2005); elected as Fellow, American Association for the Advancement of Science (2007); the E.B. Wilson Medal, American Society for Cell Biology (2010); the Kavli Prize in Neuroscience, Norway (2010); and the Massry Prize. U.S.A.

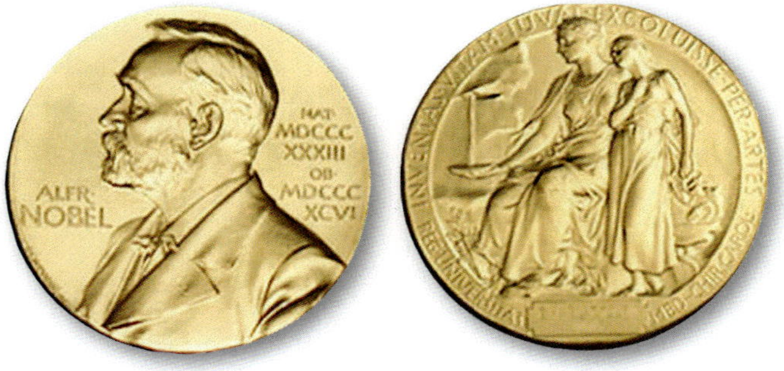

The Principle of Membrane Fusion in the Cell

Nobel Lecture, 7 December 2013

by James Edward Rothman
Yale University, New Haven, CT, USA.

By 1970 the already-classic work of George Palade (Nobel Prize, 1974; Figure 1) had made it evident that secreted proteins are carried from the endoplasmic reticulum (ER) to the cell surface in specialized containers, or transport vesicles, that bud from one membrane and fuse with the next, transiting the Golgi stack *en route* (Figure 2). We now know that such intracellular protein transport is a universal process in all eukaryotes. Many kinds of vesicles traverse the cell, laden with many kinds of cargo for delivery. The result is a choreographed program of secretory, biosynthetic and endocytic protein traffic that serves the cell's internal physiologic needs, propagates its internal organization and allows it to communicate with the outside world and to receive nutrients and signals from it.

All vesicle transfer processes can be thought of as having two basic steps: budding (when the vesicle pinches off from a 'donor' membrane) and fusion (when the membrane of the vesicle merges with the 'acceptor' membrane of the intended target). The membrane fusion process has special importance for both intracellular and extracellular physiology (Figure 3). Fusion of vesicles within the cell must be done with exquisite specificity to prevent one organelle from taking on another's functional properties. Fusion with the cell surface (plasma) membrane (exocytosis) results in the release of the vesicle's contents, almost

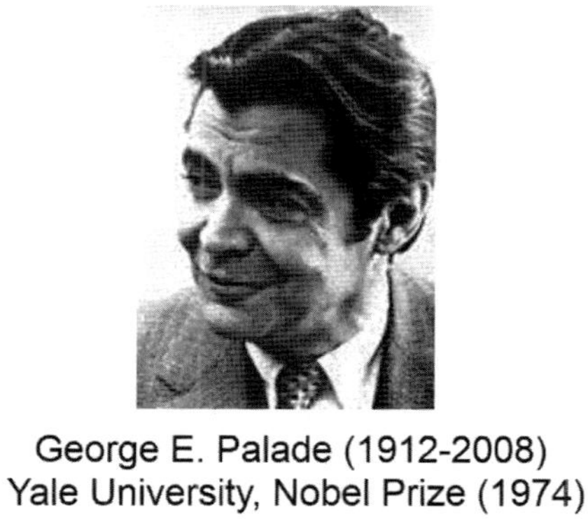

FIGURE 1. The generally-agreed founder of modern cell biology, George E. Palade. He was a recipient of the 1974 Nobel Prize in Physiology or Medicine, when he was at Yale University, where he founded what is now the Department of Cell Biology, which I chaired when I received the Nobel Prize.

always consisting of highly active substances, and therefore must be exquisitely regulated. Exocytosis is used by almost every cell and tissue in the body. The dizzying array of signaling molecules secreted by exocytosis affords a veritable tour of physiology and, frequently, related diseases: neurotransmitters and their ion channel receptors, endocrine hormones like insulin, transporters for

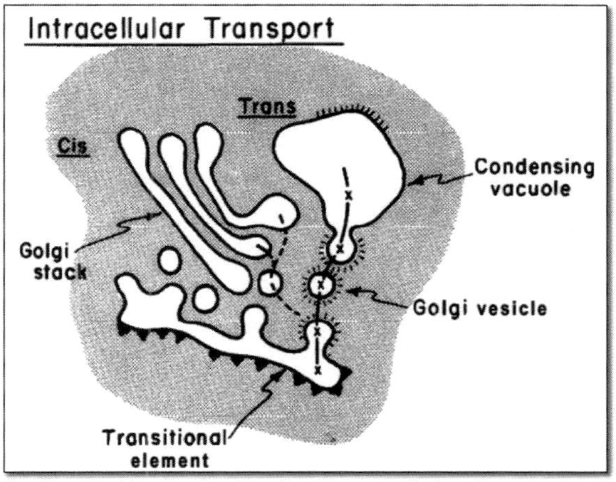

FIGURE 2. The concept of intracellular transport as laid out by Palade in his Nobel Lecture (1974). Fundamental unanswered questions included how the proposed transport vesicles form and how they can fuse specifically with their target membranes to deliver the right cargo to the right place at the right time. This figure is reproduced from the published lecture (Palade, 1975).

glucose and other nutrients, systemic mediators such as histamine and adrenaline, growth factors, and many others.

SETTING THE STAGE

From the earliest time I can remember I wanted to become a scientist, especially a physicist. I am not sure where this came from. Certainly in part from a family that deeply valued education, and especially science and medicine. My mother Gloria, with her enormous focus and drive, would in today's world have been a high-powered executive. She ran the home and my Dad's pediatric practice and

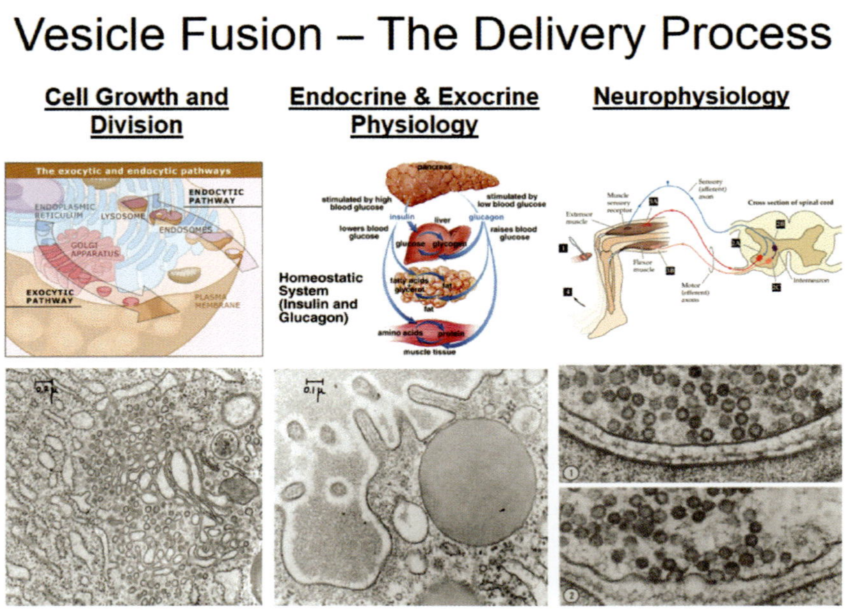

FIGURE 3. Membrane fusion is the fundamental process that allows specific cargo delivery, Fusion of vesicles carrying diverse cargo underlies a great variety of fundamental processes in cell and organismal physiology, ranging from the distribution of specific sets of proteins to designated compartments in the cytoplasm including signaling receptors at the plasma membrane (cell growth and division; top left panel), secretion of hormones and other signaling molecules (endocrine and exocrine physiology; top middle panel), and synaptic transmission (top right panel), a special case of inter-cellular communication. Electron micrographs (bottom panels) illustrate (left to right) the transport vesicles linking the ER to the Golgi in the early secretory pathway (exocrine pancreatic acinar cell), larger secretory storage vesicles containing insulin before and after fusion (endocrine pancreatic beta cell), and synaptic vesicles (containing neurotransmitters) before (above) and (below) after release is triggered by change in the membrane potential (neuromuscular junction).

by example taught me how to organize and manage. My father Martin was an intellectually oriented small-town doctor who had wanted to do medical research as a young man, but had graduated in the Great Depression then been caught up in events of World War II. He was always keen to involve me in the things he did. At perhaps the age of ten, I remember accompanying him on nocturnal house calls, sometimes to the hospital; assisting him in measuring QT intervals in his patients' electrocardiograms; and helping him perform blood analyses in the lab behind his office.

But I believe that my focus on science came at least as much from the ecosystem I grew up in. In the 1950s and 1960s science and technology were viscerally understood by Americans to be mainstays of economic and political power following the victory of World War II. This era began with the polio vaccine eradicating a dread disease and with atomic energy (for better and for worse). It ended with the transistor, the computer, and the first men on the Moon. The best-known of the scientists and practitioners were public heroes: Salk, Einstein, Oppenheimer, and the first astronauts (Figure 4).

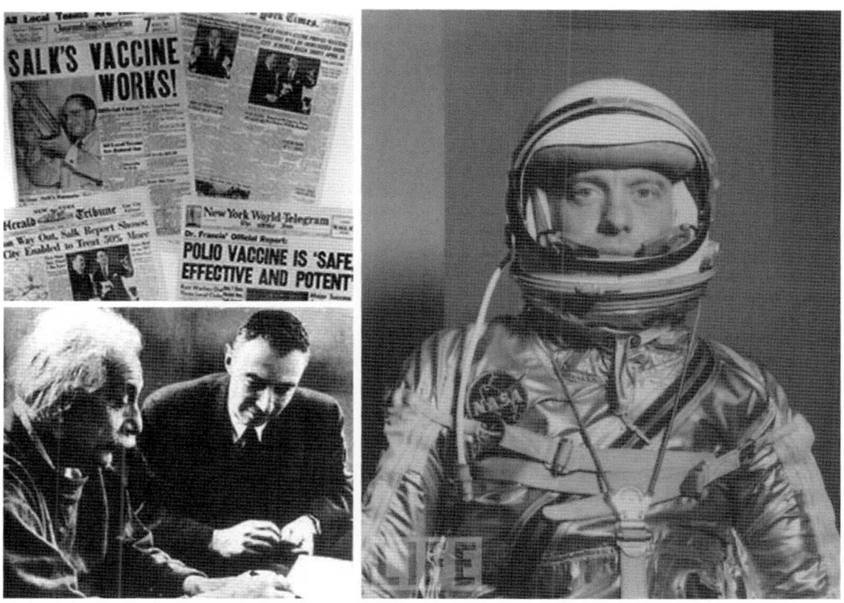
SALK'S VACCINE WORKS!
New York World-Telegram
POLIO VACCINE IS 'SAFE EFFECTIVE AND POTENT'

FIGURE 4. The period 1950–1965, when I grew up, was in many respects the height of the era of physics. The era of biology had already begun but was not fully underway. Top left, Jonas Salk succeeded in producing the first widely available vaccine to prevent polio. Bottom left, the physicists Albert Einstein and J. Robert Oppenheimer at the dawn of nuclear energy. Right, the Mercury astronaut Alan Shepard preparing for launch.

In such an ecosystem, and with my supportive family, and with an early talent for mathematics, is it surprising that I was building electronics and launching rockets while still in elementary school (Figure 5)? Rockets were a big thing for me. I taught myself basic trigonometry in 7th grade so I could triangulate the height of the rockets, and then calculus a bit later so I could better understand the physics involved. As I studied physics and mathematics formally in high school and beyond, I devoured the subject and read far outside the curriculum at my secondary school (Pomfret School), so much so that I was graduated after my junior year. Entering Yale College in 1967, I was absolutely committed to theoretical physics.

While that isn't how it ended up, physics taught me how to rigorously analyze the components of a problem by first imagining the form a solution would take. This can be a useful approach when engulfed in the fog that envelopes the uncharted waters of biology. A last minute and nearly instantaneous conversion to biology (following my father's suggestion/insistence that I try some biology instead of all physics) occurred during my junior year at Yale. Even at the very first lecture in the general biology course (by the charismatic and brilliant biophysicist Frederic Richards), I was amazed that—in contrast to the highly structured field of physics—the research frontier in molecular biology seemed instantly accessible, and yet could be equally rigorous and structure-based.

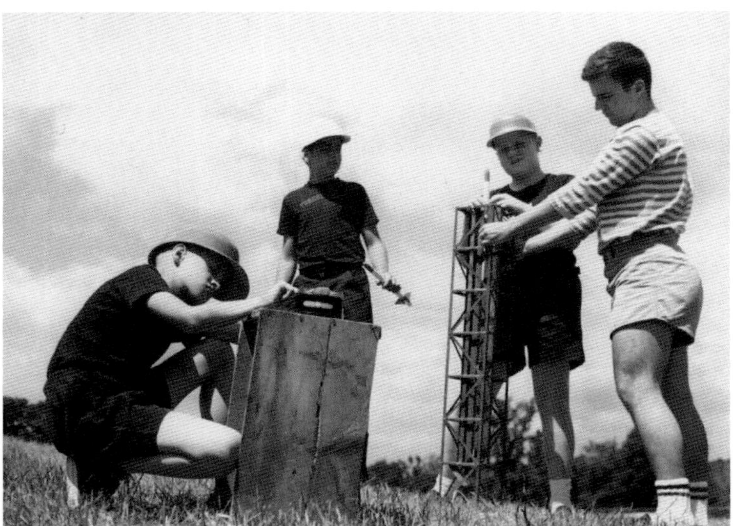

FIGURE 5. The author, second from the right, preparing to launch a model rocket, age 12. I was entranced by mathematics, physics, and technology.

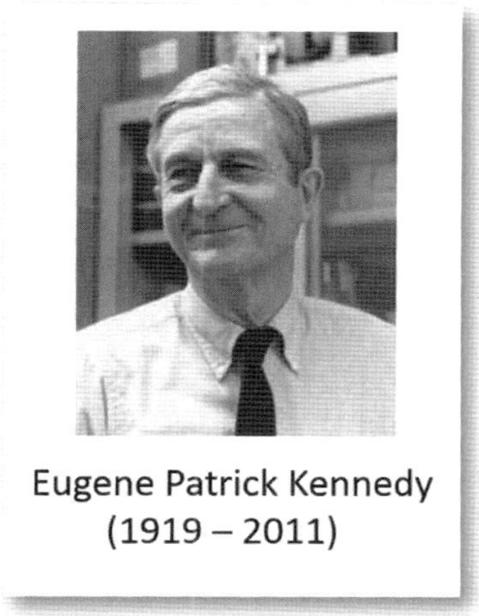

FIGURE 6. My PhD thesis adviser, Gene Kennedy, a master of membrane biochemistry.

A series of events then led me to Donald Engelman, then a new assistant professor of biophysics at Yale, and so my imprinting in experimental science was in the biophysics of membranes. Yale allowed me to drop all formal course work (and yet still graduate; they do not permit that anymore . . .) to pursue full-time research, for which I will always be grateful. That year, I learned from Engelman how to dissect each morsel of data to get the most from it, and I became a scientist. Next, I entered Harvard Medical School (in 1971) with the idea of learning biology broadly (rather than practicing). I succeeded in the former, leaving the MD program more or less after the basic sciences (but with enough clinical exposure to gain a lifetime of respect for clinical medicine).

It was as a first year medical student in histology that I first learned about the secretory pathway, at a time when George Palade's discoveries were still fresh and remarkable. What an astonishing process—how could cells make vesicles from membranes? How could each vesicle know where to go? How could it fuse? It was particularly amazing because at the time it was not even possible to begin to imagine the form a molecular solution might take. This captured my imagination, but not enough was known to productively take up the problem then.

My PhD thesis (as part of Harvard's MD-PhD program) with Eugene Kennedy (Figure 6) at Harvard Medical School, a master of membrane biochemistry, established how the lipid bilayer is formed by asymmetric biosynthesis. Kennedy, a brilliant intellectual and an original thinker, taught me how to formulate a complex problem in biochemical terms.

THE KEY ELEMENTS FOR A BREAKTHROUGH

Looking back, it is easy to see that many elements combined in fortunate ways to enable me to make the discoveries recognized by the Nobel Prize. I took up the sorting problem in the late 1970s with a broad background outside the field that proved helpful in itself and that left me sufficiently naive to be uninhibited. Other key factors included the training and perspective I was equipped with as a young scientist (outlined already); a working environment in a department that encouraged risk-taking; stable federal research funding over a decade that enabled innovation; an astute choice of problem (at the right time, still difficult but not impossible and yet impactful); a unique and productive way of approaching the problem (in my case through the simplifying mind-set of physical chemistry, as I will describe); the right (brilliant) students at the right times; and of course hard work and persistence to develop a method that works in the wake of many painful failures.

First, an ideal working environment: I was very fortunate to receive an offer to join the biochemistry department at Stanford while still a medical student, an opportunity I could not pass up because it provided the rare chance to start my own research in the remarkable environment created by Arthur Kornberg, one of the great biochemists of the 20th century (Figure 7). Happily Stanford was prepared to wait a year or so for me to do a postdoctoral fellowship, so I left Harvard Medical School (with a PhD) in 1976 for MIT and Harvey Lodish, with Stanford much in mind. Lodish taught me how to work with complex cell-free

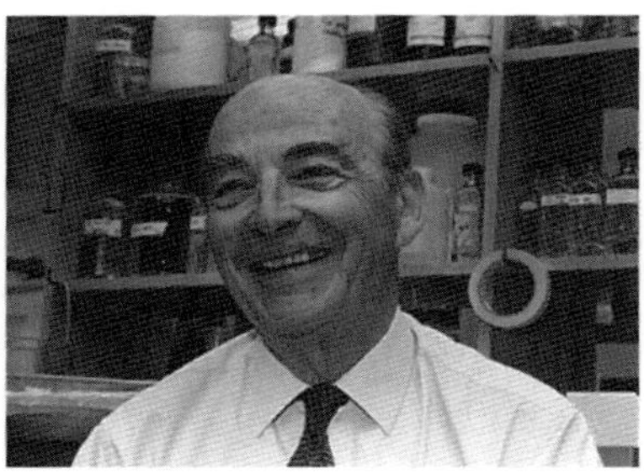

Arthur Kornberg (1918- 2007)
Stanford University, Nobel Prize (1959)

FIGURE 7. Arthur Kornberg, a master of enzymology, founded the Department of Biochemistry at Stanford University and was still its *de facto* leader when I joined as an assistant professor in 1978. In the next door laboratory, he taught me by example how a great scientist equipped with Buchner's world view attacks a complex biological process.

systems (translocation across membranes coupled to protein synthesis) and (frankly) how a large laboratory can be run boldly and energetically.

With the move to Stanford in the summer of 1978 a new era of my development as a scientist began. From Kornberg I learned two critical things at a critical time: how to formulate the strategy for a successful biochemical dissection of a complex system; and a deep faith that no matter how complex the problem, biochemistry would (eventually) succeed and would indeed provide the only sure route to the underlying molecular mechanisms. Kornberg's preaching on this subject was convincing because it stood on very solid ground. After all, cell-free reconstitution had been the central experimental approach of all biochemistry since its founding with the discovery of alcoholic fermentation in yeast extracts by Eduard Buchner (Nobel Prize, 1907) at the end of the nineteenth century, who founded what became modern biochemistry (Figure 8). And by the late 1970s, the core principles of ATP synthesis, DNA replication, RNA transcription, protein synthesis and even the genetic code were all relatively fresh 'trophies' of the reconstitution approach, which effectively strips away the subtleties of physiologic regulation to show the robust core machinery beneath.

The choice of the right problem at the right time: focusing deeply on the central rather than a peripheral aspect of a problem that is impactful and ripe for the right approach. As noted above, I was smitten by the "sorting problem" (as it was then called—how newly made proteins were distributed from ribosomes to their specific destinations in the cell) even as a medical student in the early

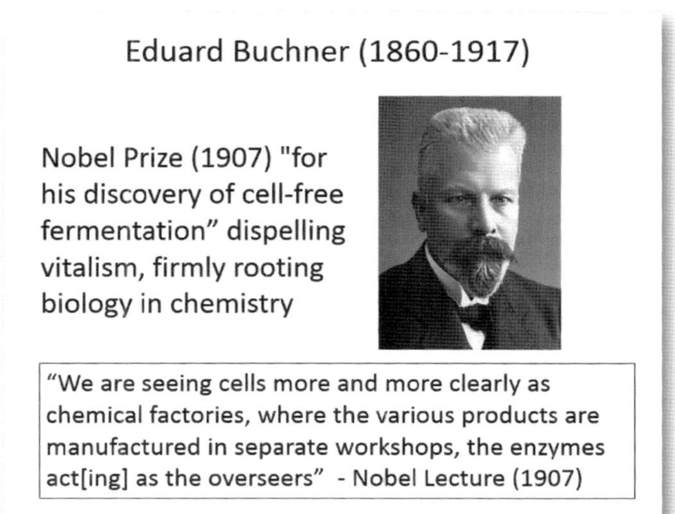

FIGURE 8. Eduard Buchner can be regarded as the founder of modern biochemistry.

1970s, but it was not ripe for attack until the late 1970s. The situation changed dramatically because of several key findings that together allowed the sorting problem to be posed in much more precise terms. Günter Blobel (Nobel Prize, 1999) had by then discovered that these proteins carry built-in signals that direct them into the ER and by implication that proteins quite generally have signal sequences that specify their location in the cell, now a basic principle. Michael Brown and Joseph Goldstein (Nobel Prize, 1985), in the course of elucidating basic mechanisms of cholesterol homeostasis, had just provided the first clear demonstration that selective transport between compartments is mediated by vesicles involving receptors specific for these signals in the transported cargo (particles of low density lipoprotein, LDL). They found that "coated vesicles" (first discovered by the great morphologist Keith Porter in 1964 (Roth and Porter, 1964), and first purified by Barbara Pearse in 1976 (Pearse, 1976) thus discovering the first protein (clathrin) coating vesicles budding from the plasma membrane. Clathrin-coated vesicles carry out the endocytosis of plasma lipoproteins, allowing their cholesterol to be released in lysosomes for re-use by cells. These vesicles garner lipoproteins from the medium by means of a receptor (LDL receptor) localized to the coated regions of membrane involved in budding. As a result of all of this, it became evident that solving the sorting problem essentially required understanding how each type of vesicle targets to and fuses with the correct target membrane in the cell.

A unique way of approaching the problem: Applying the mindset of a physicist to the complexities and mysteries of cell biology afforded me such a perspective and the approach to productively tackle the problem. Physicists seek universal laws to explain all related processes on a common basis, and achieve this by formulating the simplest hypothesis to explain the facts. The prevailing opinion among cell biologists was without doubt that the anatomical arrangement of the endomembrane systems in the cell—for example the fact that the transitional ER (from which vesicles bud to carry secretory products to the Golgi) is placed near the Golgi—is vital to ensure the delivery of cargo. As seen in Figure 9 (left side) in a classic micrograph from Palade, the ER seems almost to "force-feed" vesicles to the entry (cis side) of the Golgi stack, consistent with the idea that anatomy dictates specificity. But the simplest idea is rather the opposite—that intrinsic chemical specificity enables specific cargo delivery, and that the observed anatomy arises as the consequence of chemical specificity in operation. (Figure 9, right side).

The more common and more complex idea, that anatomy dictates specificity would mean that accurate vesicle traffic could never take place in the absence of pre-existing cellular organization. This strong prejudice—deeply rooted in

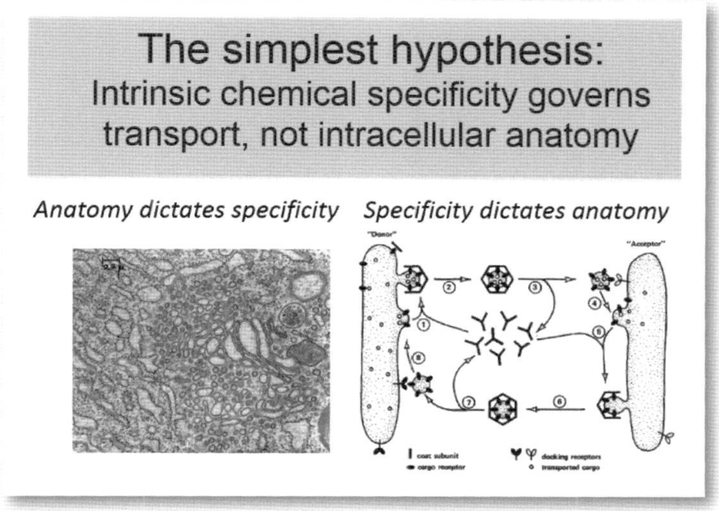

FIGURE 9. My thinking in 1978 on which the cell-free reconstitution approach was attempted. The model at bottom left (published in the 1982 Cold Spring Harbor Symposia on Quantitative Biology, Volume XLVI) was drawn long before any of the protein machinery was known. The logical organization of the pathway was correct, even though the responsible (then hypothetical) proteins were not yet identified.

cell biology from its origin as a branch of microscopic anatomy—no doubt accounted for much of the skepticism with which our reconstitution experiment was to be received for many years.

On the other hand, the great virtue of the simpler idea is the remarkable prediction it makes: that accurate vesicle traffic can in principle take place accurately in cell-free extracts, which would open the door to Kornberg-style enzymology. Once reconstituted, cell-free transport could be used as an assay to permit the underlying enzyme proteins to be discovered and purified according to their functional requirements.

Finally, the right partner to attack the problem, who was my first postdoctoral fellow, Erik Fries (Figure 10, right). Erik, a young Swedish scientist who had just arrived at Stanford from the new European Molecular Biology Lab in Heidelberg, Germany. Erik had worked with Ari Helenius and Kai Simons, providing key insights that led to their uncovering the mechanism of viral entry into cells. As a result, Erik brought with him a deep understanding of both cell biology and of physical biochemistry, and his own rigorous and quantitative style. He also had a rare combination of being adventurous and at the same time persistent, which enabled him to sign on to what most everyone thought would be a hopeless effort.

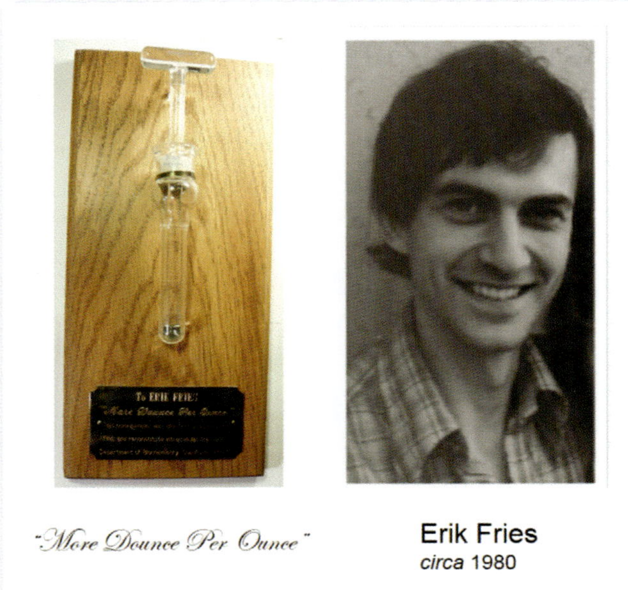

FIGURE 10. At left, the Dounce homogenizer used by my first post-doctoral fellow Erik Fries and me in 1979 to successfully reconstitute "intracellular" transport in a cell-free extract, now in the Nobel Museum. Initially it was mounted as a going-away gift to Erik (pictured at right during this era). Erik is now a professor at Uppsala University, and it was my pleasure to introduce him at my Nobel Lecture.

CELL-FREE RECONSTITUTION OF VESICLE TRANSPORT

Our goal was therefore to detect transport of a protein between membrane-bound compartments in a cell-free extract. As it was not yet possible to express cloned genes in animal cells, we studied the transport of a membrane glycoprotein (G protein) that is copiously expressed during infection by vesicular stomatitis virus (VSV), then a very popular system that I had learned in Harvey Lodish's laboratory. The processing of G protein's oligosaccharide chains during passage through the Golgi also provided a necessary biochemical handle to follow potential transport in homogenates. The detailed pathway by which Asn-linked oligosaccharide chains are matured by processing had then only recently been uncovered by Stuart Kornfeld and others.

As shown in Figure 11, oligosaccharide processing entails the initial addition of a precursor oligosaccharide to the protein in the ER, followed by the sequential removal of certain glucose and mannose residues, and then the addition of the "terminal" sugars *N*-acetyl-glucosamine (GlcNAc), galactose, and

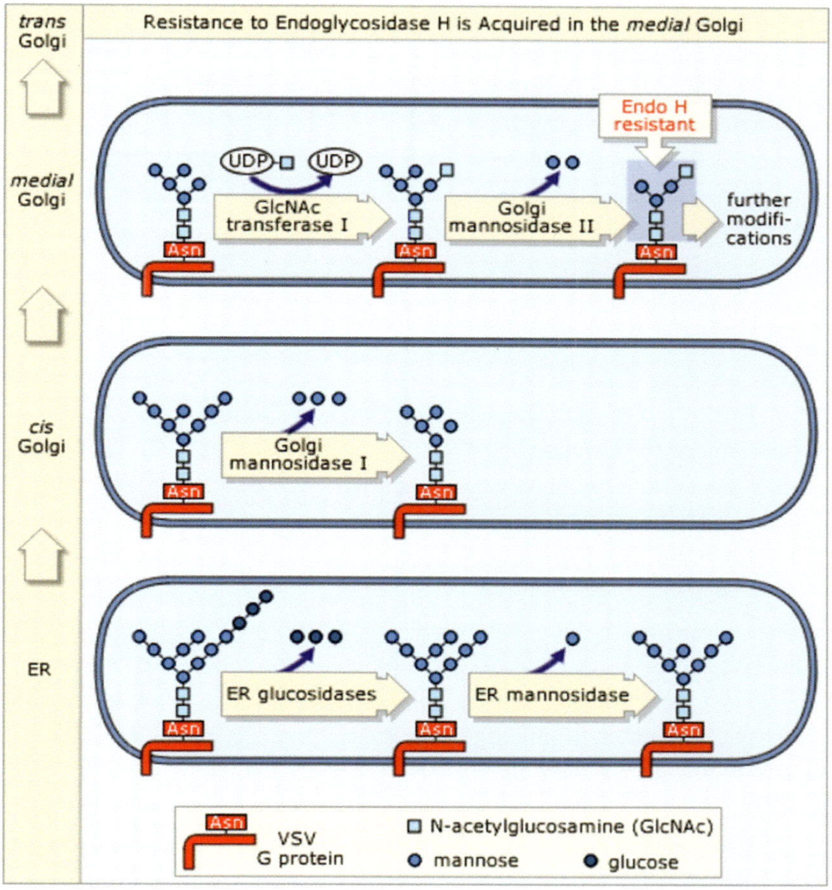

FIGURE 11. The pathway of processing in the Golgi of the Asn-linked oligosaccharide chains of ER-derived glycoprotein, elucidated in 1976–1978 most notably by Stuart Kornfeld. Figure 1. Processing of N-linked oligosaccharides in the secretory pathway. N-linked complexes become resistant to cleavage by Endoglycosidase H following addition of N-acetylglucosamine by GlcNAc transferase I and subsequent release of mannose residues by Golgi mannosidase II in the medial Golgi.

sialic acid at successive locations within the Golgi stack. Phillips Robbins had just worked out a neat shortcut for following saccharide processing using SDS protein gels that exploits an unusual microbial endoglycosidase (Endo H) that cleaves the precursor and immature saccharide chains characteristic of the ER and early Golgi, but which cannot cleave processed chains containing GlcNAc or other terminal sugars added later in the Golgi. Since the saccharide chain (except for the single inner GlcNAc that is directly linked to Asn) is removed, the overall molecular weight of the glycoprotein is noticeably reduced and its band shifts on an SDS gel (to the G_S position). When only part of the population of G protein has entered and been processed in the Golgi, two bands are observed: the parent band (G_R, resistant to Endo H) and the shifted band (G_S, sensitive to EndoH). Earlier methods for analysis of saccharide chains, which involved multiple steps of fragmentation and chromatography that required days, were prohibitive for the routine enzyme assay we imagined that reconstitution of transport might become.

Erik began by radiolabeling VSV-infected hamster cells in tissue culture with ^{35}S-methionine for what we knew would be enough time (about 5 minutes) to allow newly synthesized G protein to enter the ER while hardly entering the Golgi. Then, we disrupted the cells (with the very Dounce homogenizer pictured in Figure 10, left), incubated the homogenate with ATP, and determined whether any of the Endo H-sensitive G protein present at the outset of the cell-free incubation in the ER had become Endo H-resistant (which would indicate transport from the ER to the Golgi).

Little, if any, G_R was produced. When we extended the labeling time, a small signal (G_R produced in the homogenate) did appear but it was quickly dwarfed by the ever-increasing amount of G_R present in the homogenate at the outset of cell-free incubation due to increasing amounts of G protein entering the Golgi in the cell. No amount of tinkering with the cell-free conditions improved this picture. Worse yet, we could not even be sure that our small signal represented transport taking place in the homogenate. The extra G_R produced *in vitro* could merely have resulted from completion of processing on G protein that had already reached the Golgi before cell disruption.

Facing this quandary led to the breakthrough. I realized that a mutant hamster cell line (clone 15B) defective in a specific glycosylation step in the Golgi could be harnessed in a variation of the above experiment, both to eliminate the background of Endo H-resistant G protein at the outset of the incubation and to ensure that any glycosylation during the incubation could only result from transport. That mutant, clone 15B, had been isolated by Stuart Kornfeld on the basis of its resistance to an ordinarily toxic plant lectin. It lacks the enzyme *N*-Acetyl-Glucosamine Transferase I (NAGT-I; also known as GlcNAc transferase), normally found in the central cisternae of the Golgi stack (Figure 11). As a result of their enzyme deficiency, 15B cells cannot process G protein to Endo H-resistance although they transport the partially processed G protein normally to the cell surface. G protein therefore remains Endo H-sensitive in the ER, Golgi, and in the plasma membrane of 15B cells. So, when homogenates of ^{35}S-methionine-labeled, VSV-infected 15B cells are incubated, the G protein in their membranes will always remain Endo H-sensitive, even if it were to undergo further transport.

The critical variation (Figure 12) was simply to incubate two homogenates together—one (the "donor") produced from *VSV-infected* 15B mutant cells, and the other (the "acceptor") produced from *uninfected* wild-type cells. Now it is possible for Endo H-sensitive G protein (originating in donor 15B membranes) to be processed by NAGT-I (present in acceptor wild-type cell membranes) and thereby be made Endo H-resistant. For example, if vesicles carrying the G_S protein were to bud off from donor ER membranes and fuse with the Golgi membranes from the acceptor homogenate, then the transported G_S would be converted to G_R. A *bona fide* signal in this revised cell-free reaction explicitly requires that proximity relationships in the cell are not essential for transport, since transport would take place between organelles derived from separate cells. So any signal would suggest that inherent chemical specificity is the key to sorting, not intracellular anatomy.

With this new "complementation assay" design, we could indeed find *in vivo* labeling conditions that allowed cell-free processing at about the same rate and with about the same efficiency as transport in the cell (Figure 13b). As in the cell, cell-free "transport-coupled glycosylation" is ATP-dependent and occurs between closed membrane-bound compartments, the latter shown by the resistance of the lumenally-oriented spike portion of G protein to external proteolytic attack (Fries and Rothman, 1980). The first successful *in vivo* labeling

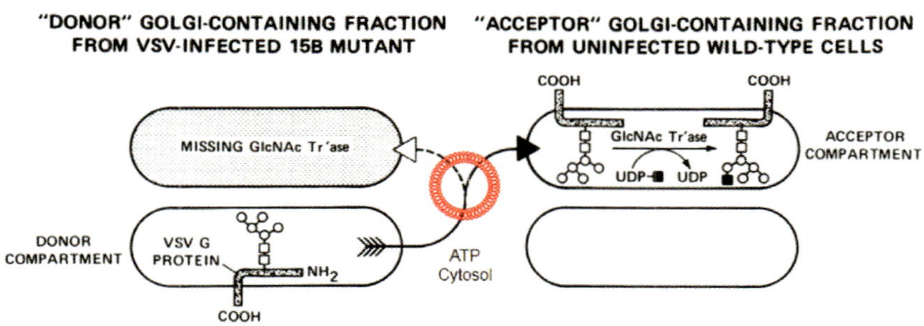

FIGURE 12. The "complementation" method that finally gave successful results. Assay for transport of VSV G protein to the medial Golgi. 15B cells lack GlcNAc transferase I; thus, proteins in these cells never acquire Endo-H resistance, although they are transported through the secretory pathway. To assay for transport, the Golgi-containing fraction from (radiolabeled) VSV-infected 15B cells is incubated with the Golgi-containing fraction from uninfected wild-type cells (plus ATP and cytosol). Acquisition of Endo-H resistance by G protein is a measure of the extent of its transfer from donor compartments to the medial Golgi. The red-walled circle between the two Golgi stacks indicates that transport vesicle that we inferred to bud and fuse in order to account for our results.

(a)

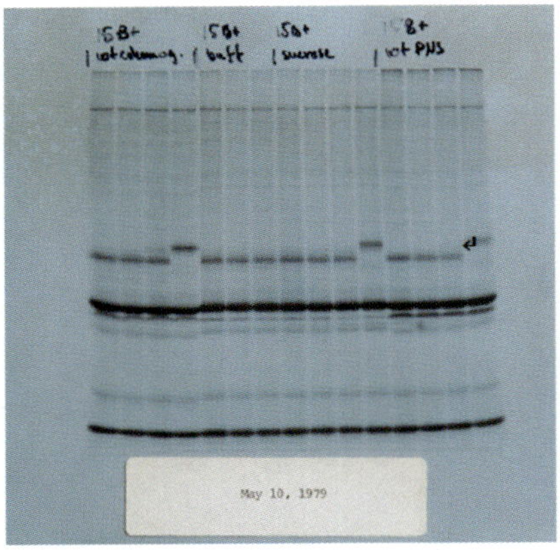

(b)

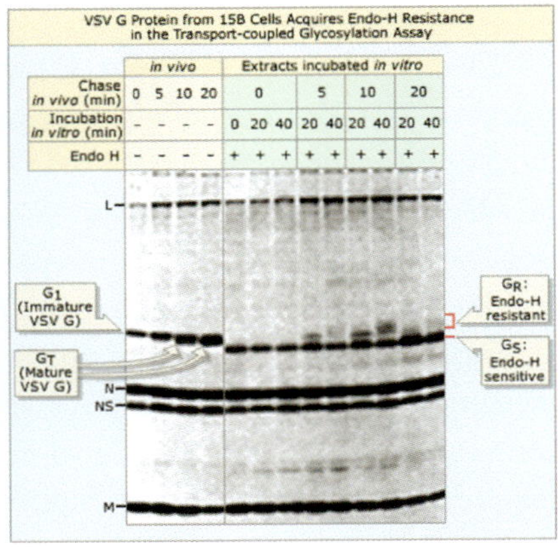

FIGURE 13 A). The first successful reconstitution of cell free transport. From Erik Fries' laboratory notebook of May 20, 1979. The faint band above the main VSV G band in the second lane from the far right (arrow) is due to maturation of the G protein (derived from donor membranes) in the acceptor Golgi compartment. b) Further optimization of incubation conditions improved the yield of the significant Endo H-resistant band for the published work. Figure 4. Left panel: VSV-infected 15B cells were pulse-labeled with ^{35}S-methionine for 5 minutes, then incubated in medium with unlabeled methionine for 0, 5, 10 or 20 minutes, and homogenized. Extracts were applied directly to the gel. Note that in 15B cells the mature G protein has a slightly lower apparent molecular weight than the immature G protein. L, N, NS and M are non-secreted VSV proteins. Right panel: VSV-infected 15B cells were pulse-labeled, and the radioactivity was chased as indicated for the samples in the left panel. Cells were homogenized, and the Golgi-containing fraction was incubated with the Golgi-containing fraction from uninfected, unlabeled wild-type cells for 0, 20 or 40 minutes, then treated with Endo-H. Note that by 5 minutes chase in vivo and 20 minutes incubation in vitro, Endo-H resistant G protein is detected. Adapted from Fries and Rothman (1981).

conditions involved a short "pulse"-label with ^{35}S-methionine followed by a 20-minute period of "chase" with unlabeled methionine in the presence of a proton ionophore "uncoupler" that stops transport by inhibiting ATP synthesis in mitochondria (Figure 13a). That ATP (or other NTP) is required for transport had been found in 1968 by James Jamieson and George Palade, who used a similar protocol to block exit from the ER at its "transitional elements," specialized regions where vesicles appear to bud off from the Golgi. With this background, the simplest working hypothesis was that we had reconstituted transport from transitional elements of the ER (from 15B cells) to the Golgi (from wild-type cells). However, we also recognized that the identity of the donor compartment was not firmly established as the ER and could be a later compartment (Fries and Rothman, 1980).

Indeed, the latter proved to be the case. We subsequently found (Fries and Rothman, 1981) that transport could be reconstituted without ATP depletion simply by extending the *in vivo* chase period by enough time (5–10 minutes) to allow the ^{35}S-labeled G protein to reach the 15B cell Golgi before homogenization. This implied that the donor is the Golgi—not the ER or its transitional elements. Since the acceptor is also a Golgi membrane, it followed that transport between two Golgi stacks, one from the 15B cells and the other from the wild-type cells, had been reconstituted.

This was very surprising because it was then textbook knowledge that the Golgi cisternae flow across the stack from its "immature" or "forming" (now termed "cis") face to its "mature" (now termed "trans") face. This view had been based on anatomical observations rather than functional evidence. (Now, more than three decades later, it is increasingly clear that transport across the Golgi stack in animals indeed mainly the result of vesicle transport, though some still adhere to cisternal flow models). The straightforward interpretation of our data was that transfer between Golgi compartments can be mediated by vesicles, and that we had reconstituted this process. Unfortunately, this put us in the unenviable position of having reconstituted a process not then known to exist, a dual burden that slowed acceptance of the significance of these results for many years until we (Wilson et al., 1989) ultimately found that one of Randy Schekman's yeast secretion genes (Novick et al., 1980) was the protein required for vesicle fusion in cell-free extracts, NSF.

We did, however, have some powerful criteria to suggest that specific membrane fusion was important for the assay signal. As seen in Figure 13b, Endo H-resistance was observed in samples that had been labeled with a 5-minute pulse followed by a 5-minute chase *in vivo* before homogenization and incubation with acceptor membranes. At this time point, much of the labeled VSV G is known to be present in the Golgi. However, no Endo H resistant G protein is produced *in vitro* when cells were disrupted right after the 5-minute pulse (no chase); at this time point, the labeled VSV G is still in the ER. And importantly, with longer times of chase, as G protein is progressively depleted from the donor Golgi as it transfers to the plasma membrane before cell disruption, and cell-free transport is correspondingly attenuated. Re-examination of our first experiments confirmed that even though energy production was poisoned, this did not occur instantly, and transport had continued during the several minutes required for the cell to use all of its existing ATP. This period was ample to permit much of the G protein to enter the Golgi, thereby reconciling the two experiments. (It now turns out that transport requires only about 10 mM ATP whereas cells normally maintain ATP in the low millimolar range, so transport can continue until the cell has used up most of its ATP.)

The strong dependence of the efficiency of cell-free transport on the presence of VSV G protein in Golgi vs. other cellular membranes convinced us that this was a *bona fide* reconstitution, and not the result of non-specific membrane fusion. More detailed analysis (Balch et al., 1984a; Balch, Glick, and Rothman, 1984b; Braell et al., 1984) soon confirmed this interpretation and provided key improvements. Adding UDP-[^{3}H]GlcNAc (the donor of GlcNAc for glycosylation by NAGT-I) marks each transported G protein with a fixed quantity of radioactivity as it arrives in the acceptor Golgi. Transport is then simply measured by the amount of [^{3}H]-G protein produced. This improvement, made together with then-postdoctoral fellow William Balch (Balch et al., 1984a), massively improved the signal-to-background and the dynamic range of the assay, and made

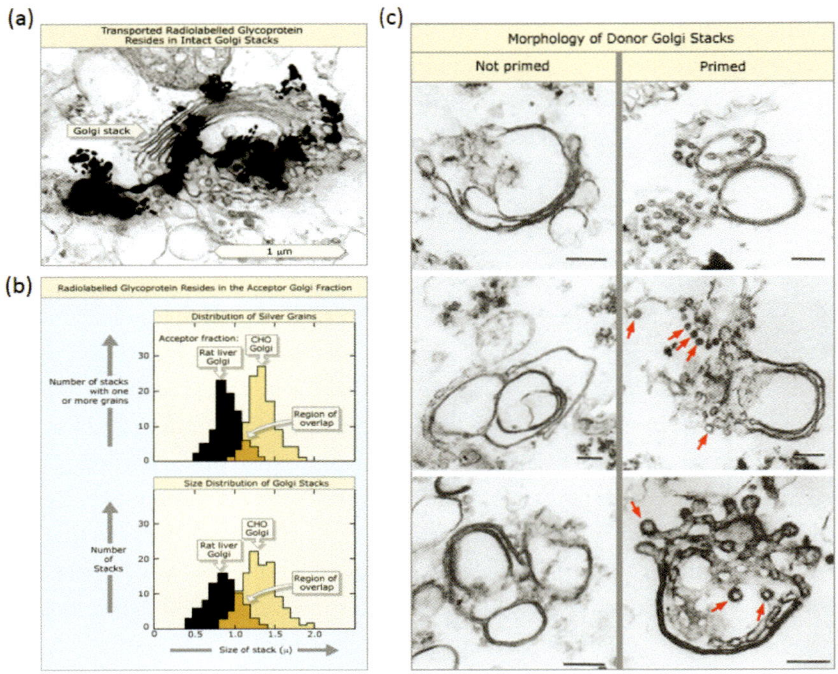

FIGURE 14. (a) Electron microscope autoradiograph showing that protein containing ^{3}H-GlcNAc is associated with Golgi stacks. The Golgi-containing fraction from VSV-infected 15B cells was incubated with the Golgi-containing fraction from wild-type cells that had taken up UDP-^{3}H-GlcNAc, and the mixture prepared for electron microscope autoradiography. Adapted from Braell et al. (1984).

it possible to accurately measure initial rates. This, in turn, made the assay a practical springboard for enzymology to guide the purification and discovery of required components.

With ^3H to indicate the transported G protein, we could now use autoradiography of electron microscope sections to localize the acceptor site where the labeled protein resides (Figure 14a). This analysis, performed by postdoctoral fellow William Braell (Braell et al., 1984), confirmed that the glycosylated G protein resides in morphologically-intact Golgi stacks derived from the acceptor homogenate. Thus, the donor- and acceptor-derived Golgi stacks remain as two distinct and unaltered populations, and the processed G protein resides exclusively in the acceptor-derived Golgi population (Figure 14b, forcefully implying that G protein is transferred between them by vesicles. We then discovered by electron microscopy that 70–90 nm-diameter vesicles containing G protein form at the donor Golgi stacks (Figure 14c) (Balch, Glick, and Rothman, 1984b). Later work, with Lelio Orci of the University of Geneva, directly demonstrated that these vesicles (now termed COPI-coated vesicles) contain VSV G protein and are captured by the acceptor stacks and thereby equilibrate between the two populations (Orci et al., 1989).

THE BASIC PRINCIPLE OF VESICLE BUDDING

Having reconstituted for the first time the process of vesicle budding, we could now apply the methods of enzymology to identify the responsible proteins and learn their mechanism of action. This in turn required the ability to visualize budding intermediates to enable the site of action of responsible proteins to be established.

By good fortune, having just read our three back-to-back papers in *Cell* (December, 1984) describing biochemical intermediates and the first images of vesicles formed in cell-free extracts, the great electron microscopist Lelio Orci (Figure 15) reached out to me in a phone call over the Christmas holidays. Thus began what turned out to be a long-term and exceptionally productive collaboration which made it possible to use electron microscope immunocytochemistry to more precisely delineate the nature and composition of the intermediates in transport. Soon, together with a graduate student, Benjamin Glick, we confirmed that the budding transport vesicles contained VSV G protein in their membranes and found that they had a coat on their cytoplasmic surface distinct from the then-known clathrin coat (Orci et al., 1986).

The essential step in establishing the budding mechanism stemmed from my finding (during a brief sabbatical in William Balch's lab, then at Yale) that

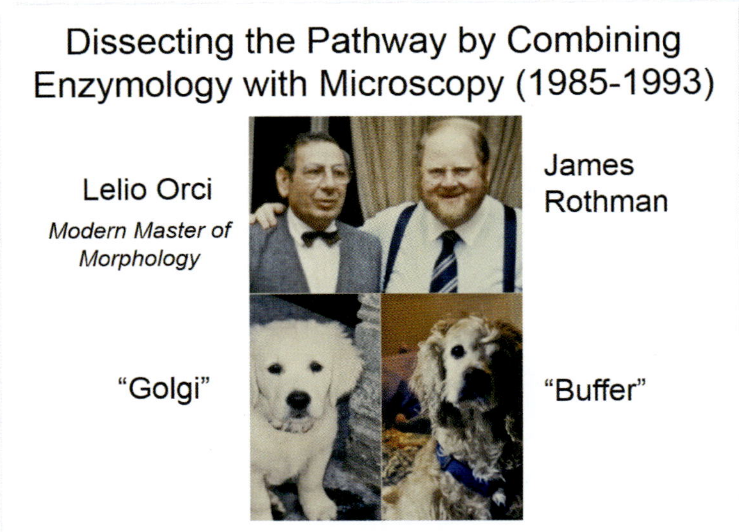

FIGURE 15. My long-term collaborator and friend Lelio Orci, the modern master of morphology. Together, between 1985 and 1993 we combined morphology and enzymology using the cell-free system to dissect a cycle of vesicle transport and in the process discovered COPI-coated vesicles and the GTPase switch mechanism that governs transport vesicle budding and uncoating for fusion. Below us our our treasured dogs whimsically named in the midst of this period to connote the interface between biochemistry (our dog "Buffer") and morphology (his dog "Golgi").

transport was inhibited by a non-hydrolyzable analog of GTP, GTPγS (Figure 16). Lelio and I and a postdoctoral fellow, Paul Melancon, then found (Melancon et al., 1987) that GTPγS blocks uncoating, so that the 'COP-coated' transport vesicles (as we termed them, now re-named COPI to later make way for Randy Schekman's COPII vesicles (Barlowe et al., 1994)) massively accumulate, which enabled their purification (Figure 17) by Vivek Malhotra and Tito Serafini (Malhotra et al., 1989). From the isolated vesicles came two central findings: the seven subunit 'coatomer' (Waters et al., 1991) that assembles to constitute the coat; and the discovery that the GTPase ADP Ribosylation Factor (ARF) is present along with coatomer in stoichiometric amounts, explaining the previously mysterious effect of GTPγS. The latter observation also pointed the way to the basic principle underlying the budding mechanism (Serafini et al, 1991; Tanigawa et al., 1993; Ostermann et al., 1993): GTP-bound ARF recruits the coatomer to the Golgi (triggering coat assembly and vesicle budding), and releases it back to the cytosol after it hydrolyzes the GTP (uncoating).

Incubation	$[^3H]$ GlcNAc Incorporated into VSV-G Protein	
Complete	3500 cpm	
- ATP	50	
- Cytosol	75	
- Golgi membranes	95	
+ GTPγS (10 μM)	420	Transport Vesicles Accumulate
NEM-membranes	225	

FIGURE 16. The requirements for cell-free transport of VSV G protein between Golgi stacks, using the simplified assay developed with Bill Balch (Balch et al., 1984). In later work, with Lelio Orci, we found two specific inhibitors of transport (GTPγS and NEM) which accumulate transport vesicle intermediates at distinct stages of maturation.

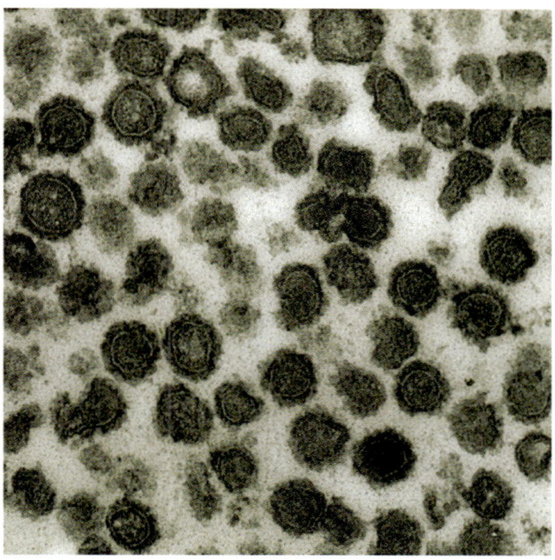

FIGURE 17. Inhibition of transport by GTPγS accumulates intermediate ~ 70 nm diameter transport vesicles encased in a protein coat (originally termed COP-coated vesicles and now termed COPI) containing the cargo VSV G protein. A pure fraction of COPI-coated vesicles produced in cell-free incubations of Golgi membranes (Malhotra et al, 1989) made possible by the blockage of uncoating by non-hydrolyzable analogues of GTP. This key development allowed the discovery of the coat protein subunits (coatomer) and the role of the GTPase switch of ARF protein in triggering sequential assembly and disassembly of the coat (Figure 18).

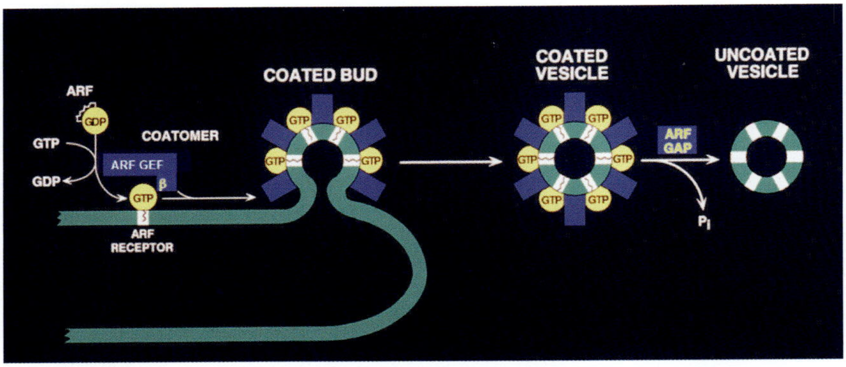

FIGURE 18. The GTP-switch mechanism for sequential budding and uncoating of transport vesicles for membrane fusion. Rothman, Orci and co-workers 1991–1993. See text for details.

By 1993, the validity of this simple and intuitive mechanism was confirmed using pure proteins (Orci et al., 1993). ARF is charged with GTP at the Golgi surface, 'switching on' budding by recruiting coatomer from the cytosol. Coatomer, now locally concentrated and oriented on the membrane surface, self-assembles by polymerization into the coat, including ARF [GTP]. The growing coat acts as a mechanical device to sculpt the applied membrane into the shape of a vesicle whose size is determined by the inner diameter of the coat. The coat now forms an exoskeleton that must be shed to enable the enclosed vesicle to fuse, which occurs when ARF hydrolyzes GTP (Figure 18).

The same principle extends to clathrin-coated vesicles (Stamnes et al., 1993) and to COPII-coated vesicles budding from ER, as found by Orci and Schekman (Barlowe et al., 1994) The particular ARF GTPase family member used and the species of coatomer varies, allowing diversity in physiologic regulation (by GTP exchange/hydrolysis) and in cargo selection (by binding subunits of the coat). But in all cases cycles of GTP binding and subsequent hydrolysis promote unidirectional (vectorial) cycles of vesicle budding and uncoating for membrane fusion.

THE CYTOSOLIC PROTEINS ENERGIZING MEMBRANE FUSION

The identification of the first proteins needed for membrane fusion also stemmed directly from the cell-free reconstitution of protein transport. This part of the story begins in 1987 with the finding by my graduate student Benjamin Glick

(Glick et al., 1987) that cell-free transport is blocked (Figure 16) by low concentrations of the sulfhydryl alkylating reagent N-ethylmaleimide (NEM). Felix Wieland (then on a sabbatical from Regensburg) and a postdoctoral fellow, Mark Block, then purified the N-ethylmaleimide-sensitive factor (NSF) from cytosol of CHO cells based on its ability to restore transport following NEM inactivation (Block et al., 1988). Electron microscopy and other tests revealed that NSF is required for fusion since vesicles accumulate after NEM inhibition (Figure 19; Malhotra et al., 1988). We soon appreciated that NSF is an ATPase and that NSF and ATP hydrolysis are required for vesicle fusion at many compartments in the cell, and that it is extremely well conserved in evolution. As noted above, our identification of NSF as the animal equivalent of Schekman's Sec18 yeast gene was pivotal because it cemented the physiologic relevance of the mechanistic results from the cell-free system and foreshadowed the universality of the fusion mechanism (Wilson et al., 1989).

Because NSF is a soluble cytoplasmic protein, it must bind to membranes to function in the fusion process. How this happens was clarified with the identification of *S*oluble *NSF* *A*ttachment *P*rotein (SNAP) which was purified according to its ability to bind NSF to Golgi membranes (as diagrammed in Figure 20) by my graduate student Douglas Clary (Clary et al., 1990).

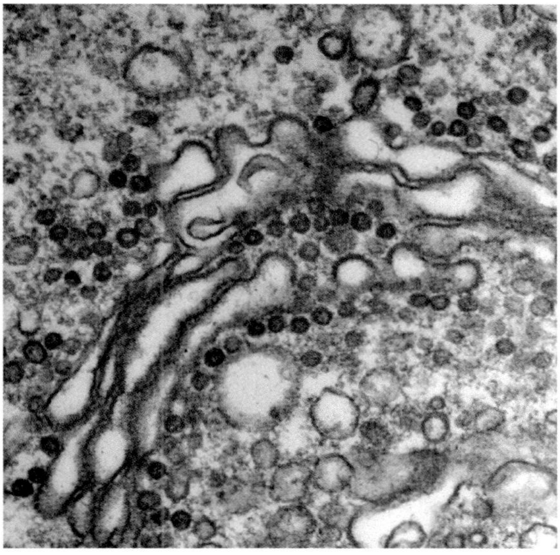

FIGURE 19. NEM inhibition accumulates ~ 70 nm diameter uncoated vesicles containing VSV G protein that fail to fuse. From Malhotra et al. (1988).

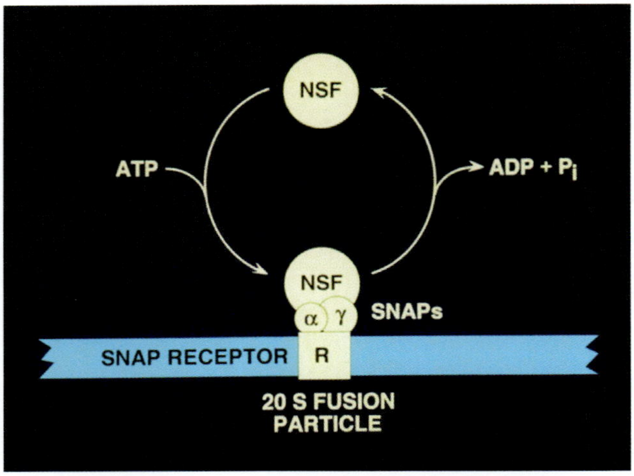

FIGURE 20. Cycle of 20S particle assembly and disassembly. NSF, SNAPs and SNAREs form hetero-oligomeric complexes, then termed 20S particles. ATP hydrolysis by NSF dissociates the 20S particles, regenerating the individual components for another round of membrane fusion.

THE DISCOVERY OF THE SNARE COMPLEX

How, then, does SNAP—which is also a cytosolic protein—bind to membranes? SNAP binds to one or more saturable, high affinity "*SNA*P *RE*ceptors" ("which we termed SNAREs") on Golgi membranes before binding to the ATP-bound form of NSF. This complex of NSF, SNAP and SNAREs sediments as a 20S particle after extraction from membranes with mild detergents. When NSF hydrolyzes the ATP, it releases itself from the complex (Wilson et al., 1992).

It seemed likely that SNAREs would be directly inserted into membranes because the SNAP receptors retain their ability to bind SNAP, even after extraction of membranes with strong alkali, a harsh treatment that removes all but integral membrane proteins (Weidman et al., 1989). That put purification of this membrane protein(s) at the very top of our agenda because of the expectation that lipid bilayer fusion would require membrane-anchored proteins. The SNARE proteins thus became the prime candidates for the fusion proteins.

At this critical juncture in 1991, I was joined by Thomas Söllner, (Figure 21, right), a gifted scientist who had just arrived in New York City at Sloan-Kettering, where I had just then moved to found the Cellular Biochemistry and Biophysics Department. Thomas had just completed foundational work identifying

Purification of SNAP Receptor (SNARE) Proteins

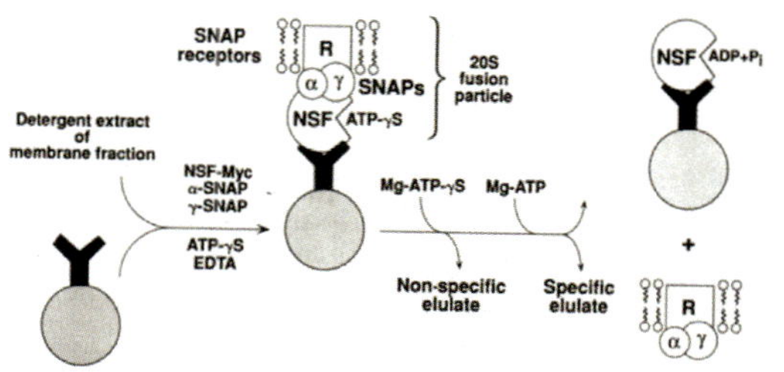

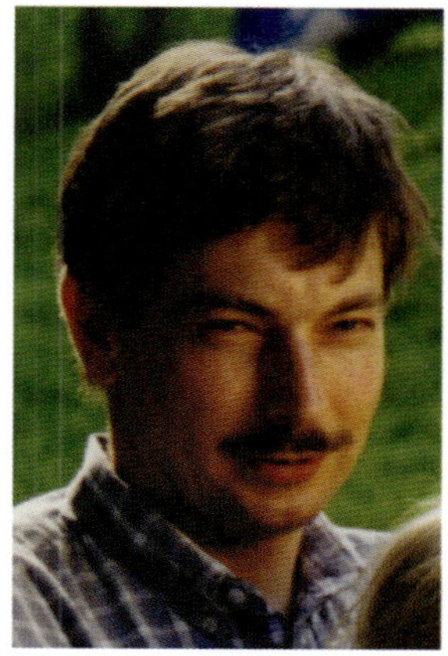

Söllner *et al.* Nature,1993

Thomas Söllner
circa 1993

FIGURE 21. Purification of SNARE proteins. At left, recombinant SNAP, and epitope-tagged NSF were assembled into 20S particles together with SNAREs derived from detergent-solubilized membrane fractions in the presence of the non-hydrolizable ATP analogue, ATPγS. The 20S particles were then immobilized on beads via an antibody directed to the epitope-tagged NSF, washed in the presence of MgATPγS ("non-specific eluate") and then disassembled in the presence of MgATP, releasing SNAPs and SNAREs ("specific eluate"). NSF remains bound via the antibody to the beads. At right, Thomas H. Söllner (circa 1993), who joined me at Sloan-Kettering and with whom I discovered the SNARE complex and enjoyed a productive collaboration in the ensuing decade that established the SNARE hypothesis for specific membrane fusion. Thomas is now a professor of Biochemistry at the University of Heidelberg. It was my pleasure that he could join the Nobel lecture, and that I could introduce him on that occasion.

key proteins in the mitochondrial outer membrane needed for protein import, learning biochemistry as a PhD student with Walter Neupert in Munich. This was another very fortunate event, and the beginning of a very productive collaboration that was to last a decade during which we would suggest and then test the tenets of the SNARE Hypothesis.

The meaning of the seemingly futile cycle (Figure 20) of membrane binding and ATPase-driven release of NSF was unclear at the time Söllner joined the Rothman lab. Then, we had imagined that energy from hydrolysis of ATP somehow activated the membrane-anchored SNAREs to power fusion. However, the existence of the binding-release cycle had a huge impact on our strategy for identifying the SNAREs. The assembly and disassembly of 20S particles, involving binding and release of NSF from SNAP, respectively, could be exploited as sequential affinity purification steps to isolate SNAREs (Figure 21, left). Previous experiments had shown that standard chromatographic methods and a single affinity step were inadequate for isolating SNAREs; the 20S ATPase cycle would add a second level of biological specificity.

SNARE (i.e. SNAP-binding) activity could be found in crude membrane fractions from homogenates of various cell lines and animal tissues, in addition to the purified Golgi membranes in which it was originally detected. It turned out that brain homogenates have the highest specific SNARE activity of the tissues that were tested, and large quantities of SNAREs could be easily obtained. These are, of course, the classic criteria for choosing a source for protein purification, but in our case the choice of brain would soon prove to have been most fortunate for unexpected reasons. Grey matter was homogenized, the total membrane fraction was isolated by centrifugation, and then a "soluble" protein extract was prepared by treating the membrane pellet with a detergent. This detergent extract contained SNARE activity as well as the bulk of integral membrane proteins now "solubilized"; i.e., distributed among micelles of the detergent.

The assembly arm of the NSF cycle was then utilized on a preparative scale as the first of two biologically specific steps, depicted in Figure 20. The idea was that SNAREs would be sequestered from the bulk of membrane protein by incorporation into 20S complexes formed with exogenously added, purified recombinant (bacterially-expressed) NSF and SNAP proteins. This incubation would be done in the presence of ATPγS (a non-hydrolyzable analogue of ATP) and in the absence of free magnesium ion (Mg^{++} is required for hydrolysis of ATP by NSF) to promote 20S particle assembly. The recombinant NSF was expressed with a short peptide epitope from myc to allow the 20S particles to be isolated with a monoclonal antibody (immobilized on beads) directed against this myc tag.

The second biologically-specific step recapitulated the disassembly of 20S particles. As depicted in Figure 21 (left), SNAREs would be released when the beads are incubated with magnesium ion and ATP to allow NSF to hydrolyze ATP. Recombinant myc-tagged NSF would remain bound to the beads by the antibody, but the recombinant SNAP proteins would be released along with the SNAP binding proteins from the brain membranes.

Because vesicle fusion occurs at many membrane compartments, we had suspected that cells would have a large family of SNARE proteins, related in sequence and differing in location. We were therefore surprised when the SNAREs

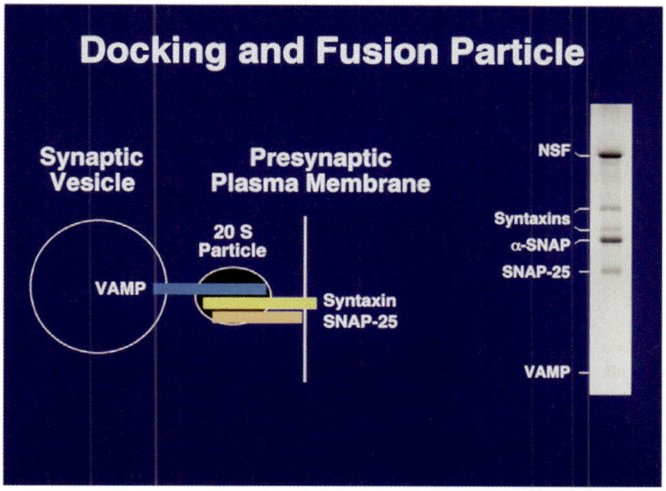

Söllner et al. Nature,1993

FIGURE 22. The SNARE complex, known at the time of its discovery as the docking and fusion particle. At right, the specific MgATP-eluate was analyzed by polyacrylamide gel electrophoresis. Proteins were revealed by staining with Coomassie blue and then identified by amino acid sequencing and mass spectroscopy. The bands at the top of the gel were also observed in the nonspecific eluate. At left, our interpretation on which a complex of the SNARE proteins links the synaptic vesicle to the plasma membrane to firmly dock the vesicle and initiate fusion.

derived from whole brain yielded a remarkably simple protein pattern (shown in Figure 22, right) consisting of only four proteins, each present in the specific (MgATP) eluate and absent from the non-specific (MgATPγS) eluate (Söllner et al., 1993a).

The identity and purity of these membrane proteins was established by micro-sequencing and by mass spectroscopy of peptides derived from the very small amount of material we had isolated, made possible by the expert protein chemistry of Paul Tempst at Sloan-Kettering. Amazingly enough, all four SNAREs turned out to be proteins found in synapses (Figure 22, right). Although they had all previously been cloned and sequenced, their function was still unknown. Two are isoforms of syntaxin, a plasma membrane protein independently identified by Richard Scheller (Bennett et al., 1992) and Kimio Akagawa (Inoue et al. 1992). The third SNARE protein is SNAP-25, short for synaptosome-associated protein of 25 kDa, cloned by Michael Wilson (Oyler et al., 1989). SNAP-25 mainly resides in the plasma membrane and was originally identified because of its abundance in synapses. Its connection to syntaxin and to membrane fusion was a surprise, as was the coincidental relationship of its acronym to that of the soluble NSF attachment protein, SNAP.

VAMP/Synaptobrevin-2 was the last SNARE protein to emerge. It had been cloned independently by Pietro DeCamilli and Reinhard Jahn, and by Scheller (Baumert et al., 1989; Elferink et al., 1989). In contrast to SNAP-25 and syntaxin, VAMP resides mainly in synaptic vesicles.

The discovery of VAMP in the complex was the lynchpin observation because it immediately suggested how the complex of SNARE proteins (perhaps with NSF and SNAP) could be important for membrane fusions. Since VAMP protrudes from the vesicle membrane into the cytosol, and syntaxin and SNAP-25 likewise protrude from the plasma membrane, a complex involving all three integral membrane proteins could bring the vesicle to the plasma membrane, placing their lipid bilayers within molecular contact range (Figure 22, left).

THE SNARE HYPOTHESIS AND THE BASIC PRINCIPLE OF MEMBRANE FUSION

Instead of limiting ourselves to the special point-of-view of synaptic vesicle exocytosis we chose to interpret the SNARE complex more speculatively from a very broad perspective (Söllner et al., 1993a).

First principles require that vesicles and targets somehow be marked to indicate which vesicles will fuse where. This, in turn, indicates that vesicle and target markers must be matched pairwise. We suggested that the simplest mechanism for matching is self-assembly, in which only matching pairs of "cognate" vesicle ('v') and target ('t') markers bind each other between membranes, thereby forming a 'v-t' complex prerequisite for membrane fusion.

Based on our cognate vesicle and target marker concept, we proposed the "*SNARE hypothesis*" in which the SNAREs are the vesicle and target markers, which we termed v–SNAREs and t-SNAREs (Figure 23). VAMP is the v-SNARE of the synaptic vesicle; syntaxin and SNAP-25 are the subunits of the cognate t-SNARE in the plasma membrane. The SNARE hypothesis provides the framework to generalize our results. We suggested that each type of vesicle in the cell would have its own characteristic v-SNARE, a homologue of VAMP, and that each target membrane in the cell would be marked by a characteristic t-SNARE, having subunits homologous to syntaxin and SNAP-25. In addition, we suggested that "In the simplest view, that is, if there were no other source of specificity, only when complementary v-SNARE and t-SNARE pairs engage would a productive fusion event be initiated" (Söllner et al., 1993a).

Consistent with our simple model, VAMP and syntaxin are membrane-anchored proteins with cytoplasmic domains, and SNAP-25 is anchored to the cytoplasmic side of the plasma membrane via covalently-attached fatty acids. Close to equimolar amounts of VAMP, syntaxin (its two isoforms considered together) and SNAP-25 were recovered in the isolated complexes. Furthermore,

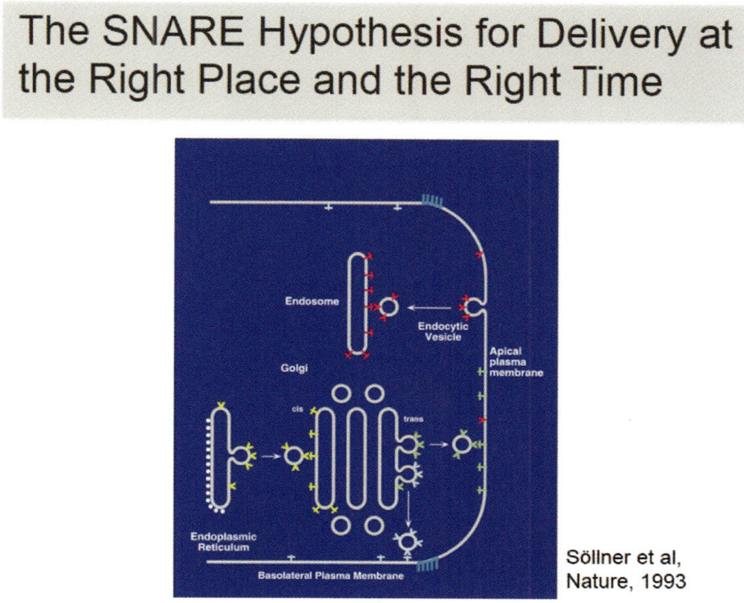

FIGURE 23. The SNARE Hypothesis as initially proposed, explained in the text.

the SNARE proteins were isolated because they bind to and form a 20S particle with NSF and SNAPs, which are known to function in fusion, implying that SNAREs also function in fusion. The SNARE complex progressed from first discovery to final publication in a dizzying sweep lasting only 5 weeks.

At the time of this experiment, membrane fusion seemed complex and confusing because a conceptual framework with which to organize the continuously increasing list of genes and sequences was lacking. A great many genes and proteins of yeast and animal cells, including neurons, were implicated as being somehow involved in the overall process of vesicle transport or fusion or its regulation. It was readily appreciated that many of these genes and proteins belong to evolutionarily-conserved families affecting different transport steps (reviewed by Bennett and Scheller, 1993). A dozen or more proteins were known to reside in the synaptic vesicle alone. But it was guess work as to which proteins could catalyze fusion or provide for its specificity, as distinct from affecting fusion indirectly at the level of cellular regulation, and many proteins had been considered to be candidates for fusion, including at one time or another synaptophysin, synaptoporin and SV2. Interestingly, although VAMP and syntaxin were seen to be important players, they were not highlighted in this context and not suggested to form a complex, and SNAP-25 was not connected to exocytosis.

The primary impact of our paper stemmed from its combination of an unexpected discovery—the SNARE complex—and a broad and clearly-stated concept—the SNARE hypothesis—deduced from it. Its impact was amplified because the discovery of the SNARE complex firmly linked three fields (cell biology (vesicle transport), physiology (endocrine and exocrine secretion), and neurobiology (synaptic transmission)), three disciplines (cell-free biochemistry, yeast genetics, and electrophysiology), and many favorite cells and organisms. As a result our paper changed the focus of cell biology, away from differences in physiology and regulation and on to core machinery and universal mechanisms.

In follow-up work we found that NSF and SNAP function to disrupt the SNARE complex using energy derived by ATP hydrolysis (Söllner et al, 1993b), and it was later shown by William Wickner that SNAP and NSF are not directly involved in bilayer fusion (Mayer et al., 1996). This focused attention on the simplest remaining possibility, that the SNARE complex is all that is needed to mediate fusion. However, NSF and SNAP play a critical role in sustaining ongoing fusion. They separate v-SNAREs from t-SNAREs after fusion (i.e., when they reside in the *same* bilayer), but not during fusion (i.e., when they are paired *between* bilayers) (Weber et al., 2000). This allows NSF and SNAP to recycle SNARE complexes after fusion while sparing fusion in progress.

The SNARE complex is extraordinarily stable, resisting heat denaturation up to 90°C (Hayashi et al., 1994). The rod-like structure of the SNARE complex, with its membrane anchors at one end, implies that it could bring two membranes into close contact and it was suggested that the binding energy from SNARE assembly could drive bilayer fusion (Hanson et al., 1997).

A direct test of the possibility that the SNARE complex is the active principle of fusion could only come from assessing this function in the absence of all other proteins. Reconstituting recombinant exocytic/neuronal SNAREs into liposomes established that the pairing of cognate SNARES between lipid bilayers indeed results in spontaneous membrane fusion (Weber et al., 1998) (Figure 24). Thus, when complementary v-SNARE and t-SNARE pairs engage, a productive fusion event is not only initiated—as we had first imagined—but it is also completed.

The ability to observe fusion by isolated SNAREs opened the door to a very direct test of the central tenet of the SNARE hypothesis, that specificity for membrane fusion is encoded in the physical chemistry of the isolated SNARE proteins (McNew et al., 2000; Parlati et al., 2000; Fukuda et al., 2000; Paumet et. al, 2001; Parlati et al., 2002). A total of 275 combinations of the potential v-SNAREs and t-SNAREs encoded in the genome of yeast, representing ER,

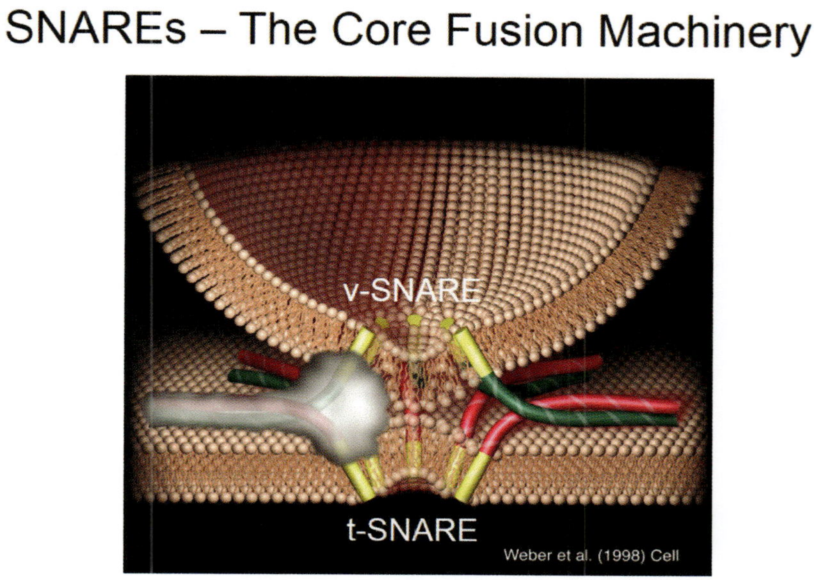

FIGURE 24. v-SNAREs (in green) on a vesicle bind to their cognate t-SNAREs (in red) on the target membrane, forming specific SNAREpins that then fuse the two membranes. For simplicity, the t-SNARE is shown as a single elongated rod, although it is now known to contribute three alpha helices to a four-helix v-t-SNARE bundle. Other proteins regulate the assembly and disassembly of SNAREpins and thus control membrane fusion.

Golgi, plasma membrane, endosomes, and vacuoles (lysosomes), have been tested for fusion. Of these, only 9 combinations (~3%) are fusogenic and all but one (~0.4%) correspond to known transport pathways (Figure 25). Virtually without exception, fusion only takes place with the rare combinations of v- and t-SNAREs that are drawn from compartments connected by vesicle shuttles in the living cell. Put differently, a physical chemist armed only with the DNA sequence of yeast and the SNARE hypothesis could test isolated SNAREs to read out the fusion potential and transport pathways allowed in the cell with at least 99.6% accuracy.

THE MECHANISM OF LIPID BILAYER FUSION BY SNAREPINS

The physical chemical mechanism of fusion was strongly suggested by the X-ray crystal structure of the SNARE complex elucidated by Axel Brunger and Reinhard Jahn later that year (Sutton et al, 1998). It revealed a bundle of four parallel alpha helices that forms a pin-like arrangement forcing the two bilayers together as the SNARE complex "zippers up" to result in fusion (Figure 26). We termed these "SNAREpins." Very recently, in collaboration with Yale colleague

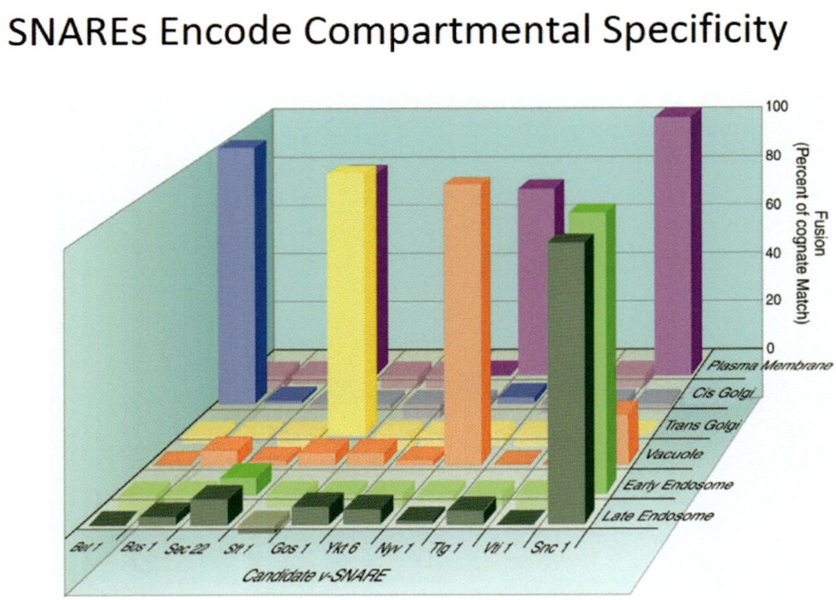

FIGURE 25. Proof that SNAREs encode compartmental specificity was obtained from a large scale experiment (200–2002) in which the complement of SNAREs encoded in the yeast genome was tested for its fusion potential in many combinations in reconstituted lipid vesicles. See text for details.

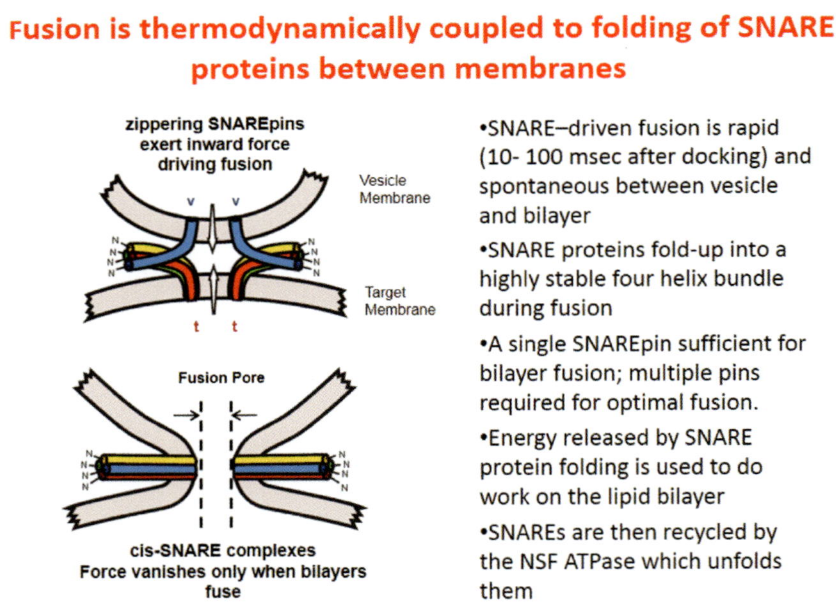

FIGURE 26. Summary of current knowledge of the fusion mechanism. Adapted from Südhof and Rothman (2009).

Yongli Zhang, we have directly measured the force that fuses the bilayers in single molecule experiments (Figure 27) in which a SNARE complex is literally pulled apart and the allowed to zipper back up again—the power stroke of fusion—which it does in two discrete steps (Gao et al., 2012).

The half-zippered intermediate provides a natural pause point that can be stabilized by binding to other proteins to permit regulation of membrane fusion after vesicle docking. An important example is provided by the protein complexin (McMahon et al., 1995), discovered by Thomas Südhof, along with the calcium ion sensor synaptotagmin (Geppert et al., 1994)) to be a key regulator of neurotransmitter release in synaptic transmission. In a recent collaboration with Yale colleague Karin Reinisch (Kümmel et al., 2011), we found that complexin stabilizes exactly this half-zippered state (Figure 28), explaining how synaptic vesicles can be ready to release neurotransitters much in < 1 msec, much faster than the time (50–100 msec) required for the overall process of fusion by isolated SNAREs after initial docking by the SNAREpin (Karatekin et al., 2010).

With my current laboratory colleagues in the Department of Cell Biology at Yale (Figure 29) I am primarily hoping to better understand how SNARE proteins are regulated in exocytosis and the still debated details of the dynamics of protein sorting in the Golgi stack.

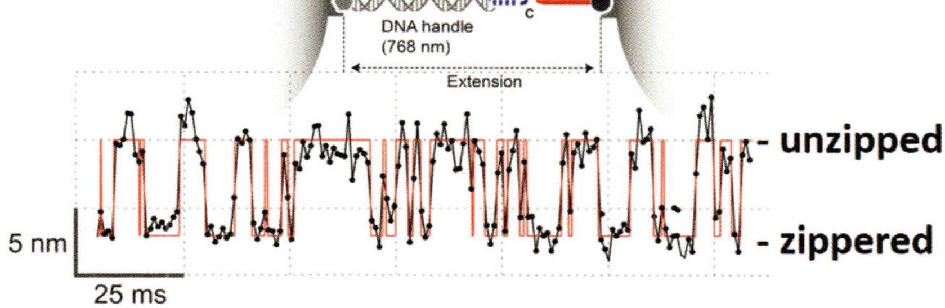

FIGURE 27. The modular structure of the SNARE complex. When pulled apart with optical tweezers, the C-terminal (membrane-proximal) half of the four helix bundle (CTD) unzips and re-zips in an all-or-none fashion, demonstrating a half-zippered intermediate in SNARE-dependent fusion. From Gao et al (2012).

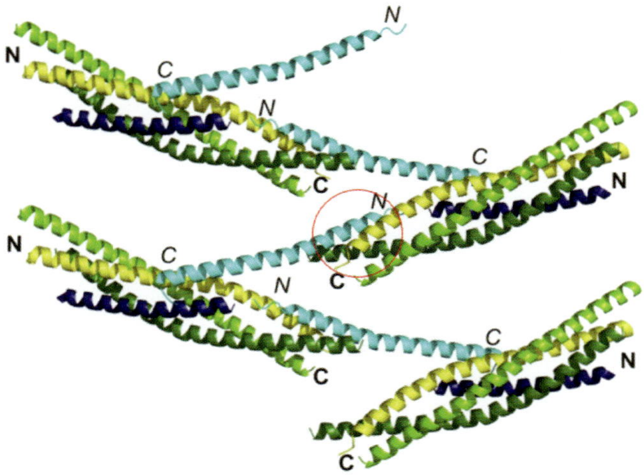

FIGURE 28. Complexin (helices in magenta) trans-clamps half-zippered SNAREpins to synchronize neurotransmitter release to enable rapid synaptic transmission. The accessory helix of complexin reaches across from one SNAREpin to insert into the membrane-proximal portion of another (red circle). Here the accessory helix binds to the t-SNARE (green and yellow helices) in the same place where the v-SNARE (blue) would otherwise bind to complete membrane fusion. Thus, complexin stabilizes the otherwise transient half-zippered intermediate seen with the optical tweezers (Figure 27). From Kümmel et al. (2011).

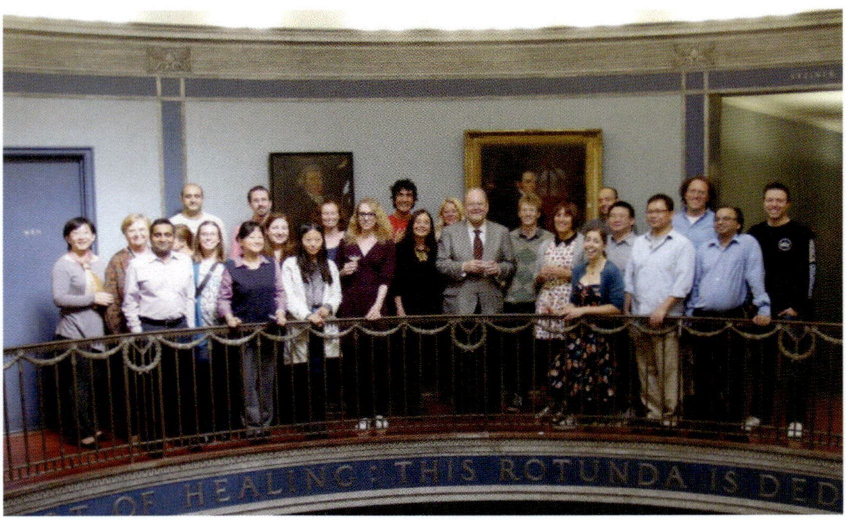

FIGURE 29. My laboratory and I assembled under the rotunda above the Yale Medical School Historical Library on the morning of the announcement of the Nobel Prize. My wife Professor Joy Hirsch is on my right.

FINAL THOUGHTS

How membranes flow in the cell was a fundamental problem in biology that seemed unapproachable three decades ago. Yet, today we have an understanding of the main features of this vital process at the physical chemical level. This is simply testimony to the power of the reductionist method of science, espoused so insightfully and so early by Eduard Buchner at the very dawn of modern biochemistry more than a century ago (Figure 8).

In writing this lecture, which affords a rare opportunity to look back over decades at one's own contributions, increasingly I see how my work prospered because of the scientific culture (or ecosystem). As Sir Hans Krebs (Nobel Prize, 1953) wrote, "scientists are not so much born as made by those who teach them" (Krebs, 1967). In this excellent article Krebs explains his origins as a scientist in terms of a lineage of great organic chemists and biochemists, each of whom successively trained the next, spanning nearly a century, a chain that is to this very day unbroken, going back to the dye chemist von Baeyer, virtually all Nobel laureates (Figure 30). There are many similar lineages in other fields such as genetics, physiology, microbiology and investigative medicine. Such extraordinary ecosystems have a major temporal component that makes them hard to establish, and correspondingly valuable to the rare societies that possess them,

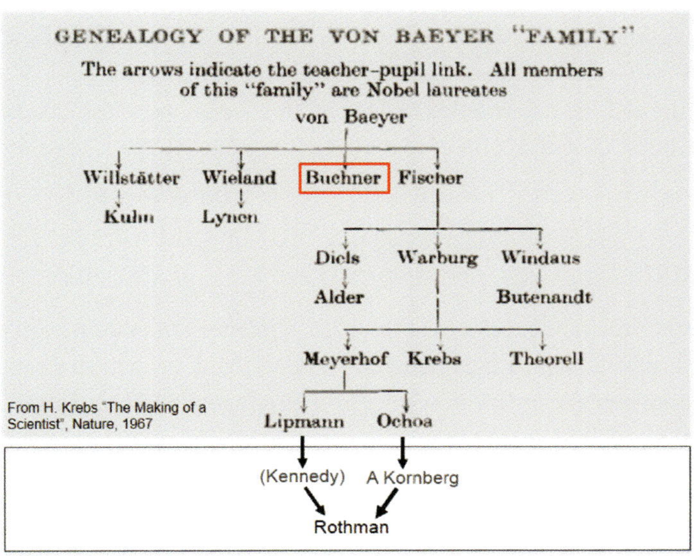

FIGURE 30. A century-long scientific ecosystem—from dye chemistry to enzymology to modern cell biology. The shaded portion is reproduced from H. Krebs "The Making of a Scientist" Nature (1967).

> "We must never let ourselves fall into thinking *"ignorabimus"* ("We shall never know"), but must have every confidence that the day will dawn when even those processes of life which are still a puzzle today will cease to be inaccessible to us natural scientists." - E. Buchner

from the Nobel Lecture December 11, 1907

FIGURE 31. Buchner's early faith in reductionism proved to be well-founded, and his words still ring true today.

not only for the knowledge and technologies they generate but also for the economic benefits they provide. Scientific ecosystems can only thrive in societies that sustain science over the very long term.

I am deeply humbled by the insights and accomplishments of these predecessors. As Buchner enunciated in his time (Figure 31), we share the deep conviction, now evidenced by the results of more than a century of discoveries, that there is no process in biology that, at its very core, is not physical-chemical in nature. As the direct consequence, we can expect that, in due course, all of life—even human thought and emotion—will be understood as emergent from physics and we will understand ourselves in health and in disease as complex, organically composed self-determining machines. This is a perspective that may frighten some, but it should not because it offers our species the best hope for the long term.

ACKNOWLEDGMENTS

Though it is often frustrating, Science at the edge combines fun and discovery equally (whimsically illustrated in Figure 32). I wish to thank my personal ecosystem for helping to make my life in science both productive and fun. This includes an enormous debt of gratitude to the many students and postdoctoral fellows who have contributed to this body of work over more than three decades, most of whom have not been specifically mentioned. It also includes the great exemplars and teachers I have apprenticed with as noted in the text; the wonderful environments in which I have been privileged to work, most especially in the earlier years at Stanford and at Sloan-Kettering under Paul Marks' leadership; many close long-term personal and scientific friends who have enriched my life

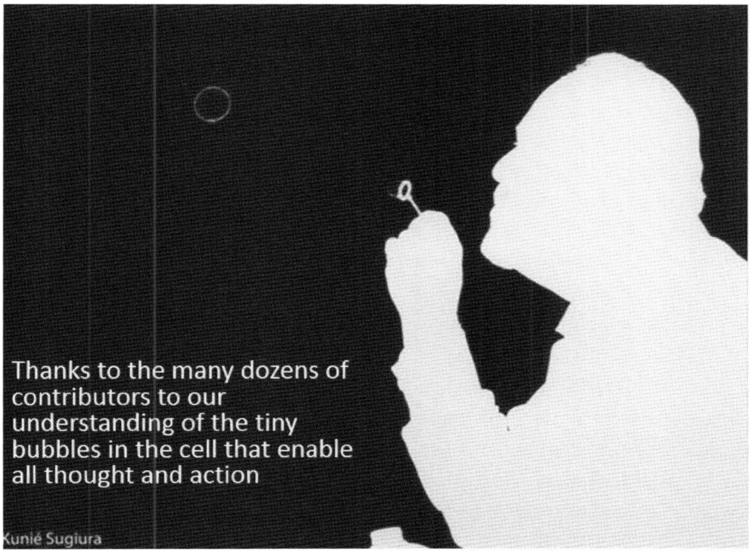

FIGURE 32. Bubbles symbolize vesicles in the cell but also the fun and freedom of good science. So, when I was asked about ten years ago by the Japanese photographer Sugiura to pose for one of her unique photograms while doing something to illustrate my scientific work, I chose to blow bubbles.

and my work; and most especially my wife, soul-mate and intellectual partner, Joy Hirsch; and my children, Lisa and Matthew.

In preparing the written form of this Nobel Lecture I have drawn liberally on my own language previously published in connection with earlier awards, notably the Lasker Award and the Kavli Prize, and also from two publications in the Great Experiments series, a web-based publication from 2001 that is unfortunately no longer available. Finally, a special mention to Willa Bellamy who for 22 years at three academic institutions was my executive assistant, retiring this year.

REFERENCES

Balch, W., Dunphy, W., Braell, W.and Rothman, J. (1984a). "Reconstitution of the transport of protein between successive compartments of the Golgi measured by the coupled incorporation of N-acetylglucosamine." *Cell* **39**, 405–16.

Balch, W., Glick, B. and Rothman, J. (1984b). "Sequential intermediates in the pathway of intercompartmental transport in a cell-free system." *Cell* **39**, 525–36.

Barlowe C., Orci L., Yeung T., Hosobuchi M., Hamamoto S., Salama N., Rexach M., Ravazzola M., Amherdt M., and Schekman R. (1994). "COPII: a membrane coat formed by Sec proteins that drive vesicle budding from the endoplasmic reticulum." *Cell* **77**, 895–907.

Baumert, M., Maycox, P. R., Navone, F., De Camilli, P., and Jahn, R. (1989). "Synaptobrevin: an integral membrane protein of 18,000 daltons present in small synaptic vesicles of rat brain." *EMBO J.* **8**, 379–84.

Bennett, M., and Scheller, R. (1993). "The molecular machinery for secretion is conserved from yeast to neurons." *Proc. Natl. Acad. Sci. U.S.A.* **90**, 2559–63.

Bennett, M., Calakos, N., and Scheller, R. (1992). "Syntaxin: a synaptic protein implicated in docking of synaptic vesicles at presynaptic active zones." *Science* **257**, 255–9.

Block, M., Glick, B., Wilcox, C., Wieland, F. and Rothman, J. (1988). "Purification of an N-ethylmaleimide-sensitive protein catalyzing vesicular transport." *Proc. Natl. Acad. Sci. U.S.A.* **85**, 7852–56.

Braell, W., Balch, W., Dobbertin, D., and Rothman, J. (1984). "The glycoprotein that is transported between successive compartments of the Golgi in a cell-free system resides in stacks of cisternae." *Cell* **39**, 511–24.

Clary, D., Griff, I. and Rothman, J. (1990). "SNAPs, a family of NSF attachment proteins involved in intracellular membrane fusion in animals and yeast." *Cell* **61**, 709–21.

Elferink, L., Trimble, W., and Scheller, R. (1989). "Two vesicle-associated membrane protein genes are differentially expressed in the rat central nervous system." *J. Biol. Chem.* **264**, 11061–4.

Fries, E. and Rothman, J. (1980). "Transport of vesicular stomatitis virus glycoprotein in a cell-free extract." *Proc. Natl. Acad. Sci. U.S.A.* **77**, 3870–74.

Fries, E. and Rothman, J. (1981). "Transient activity of Golgi-like membranes as donors of vesicular stomatitis viral glycoprotein *in vitro*." *J. Cell Biol.* **90**, 697–704.

Fukuda, R., McNew, J., Weber, T., Parlati, F., Engel, T., Nickel, W., Rothman, J., and Söllner, T. (2000). "Functional architecture of an intracellular membrane t-SNARE." *Nature* **407**, 198–202.

Geppert, M., Goda, Y., Hammer, R., Li, C., Rosahl, T., Stevens, C., and Südhof, T. (1994). "Synaptotagmin I: a major Ca2+ sensor for transmitter release at a central synapse." *Cell* **79**, 717–27.

Glick, B. and Rothman, J. (1987). "A possible role for acyl–coenzyme A in intracellular protein transport." *Nature* **326**, 309–12.

Gao, Y., Zorman, S., Gundersen, G., Xi, Z., Ma, L., Sirinakis, G., Rothman, J. and Zhang, Y. (2012). "Single Reconstituted Neuronal SNARE Complexes Zipper in Three Distinct Stages." *Science* **337**,1340–43.

Hanson, P., Roth, R., Morisaki, H., Jahn, R., and Heuser, J. (1997). "Structure and conformational changes in NSF and its membrane receptor complexes visualized by quick-freeze/deep-etch electron microscopy." *Cell* **90**, 523–35.

Hayashi, T., McMahon, H., Yamasaki, S., Binz, T., Hata, Y., Südhof, T. C., and Niemann, H. (1994). "Synaptic vesicle membrane fusion complex: action of clostridial neurotoxins on assembly." *EMBO J.* **13**, 5051–61.

Inoue A., Obata K., Akagawa K. (1992). "Cloning and sequence analysis of cDNA for a neuronal cell membrane antigen, HPC-1." *J. Biol Chem.* **267**, 10613–9.

Karatekin, E., Di Giovanni, J., Iborra, C., Coleman, J., O'Shaughnessy, B., Seagar, M., and Rothman, J. (2010). "A fast, single-vesicle fusion assay mimics physiological SNARE requirements." *Proc. Natl. Acad. Sci. U.S.A.* **107**, 3517–21.

Krebs, H. (1967). "The Making of a Scientist." *Nature* **215**, 1441–45.

Kümmel, D., Krishnakumar, S., Radoff, D., Li, F., Giraudo, C., Pincet, F., Rothman, J., and Reinisch, K. (2011). "Complexin Cross-links prefusion SNAREs into a Zig-Zag Array." *Nat. Struct. Mol. Biol.* **18**, 927–33.

Malhotra, V., Serafini, T., Orci, L., Shepherd, J., and Rothman, J. (1989). "Purification of a novel class of coated vesicles mediating biosynthetic protein transport through the Golgi stack." *Cell* **58**, 329–36.

Malhotra, V., Orci, L., Glick, B., Block, M. & Rothman, J. (1988). "Role of an N-ethylmaleimide-sensitive transport component in promoting fusion of transport vesicles with cisternae of the Golgi stack." *Cell* **54**, 221–27.

Mayer, A., Wickner, W., and Haas, A. (1996). "Sec18p (NSF)-driven release of Sec17p (alpha-SNAP) can precede docking and fusion of yeast vacuoles." *Cell* **85**, 83–94.

McMahon H., Missler, M., Li, C., Südhof, T. (1995). "Complexins: cytosolic proteins that regulate SNAP receptor function." *Cell* **83**, 111–9.

McNew, J., Parlati, F., Fukuda, R., Johnston, R., Paz, K., Paumet, F., Söllner T., and Rothman, J. (2000). "Compartmental specificity of cellular membrane fusion encoded in SNARE proteins." *Nature* **407**, 153–59.

Melançon, P., Glick, B., Malhotra, V., Weidman, P., Serafini, T., Gleason, M., Orci, L., and Rothman, J. (1987). "Involvement of GTP-binding "G" proteins in transport through the Golgi stack." *Cell* **51**, 1053–62.

Novick, P., Field, C., and Schekman, R. (1980), "The identification of 23 complementation groups required for post-translocational events in the yeast secretory pathway." *Cell* **21**, 205–15.

Orci, L., Glick, B. and Rothman, J. (1986). "A new type of coated vesicular carrier that appears not to contain clathrin: Its possible role in protein transport within the Golgi stack." *Cell* **46**, 171–84.

Orci, L., Malhotra, V., Amherdt, M., Serafini, T., and Rothman, J. (1989). "Dissection of a single round of vesicular transport: Sequential intermediates for intercisternal movement in the Golgi stack." *Cell* **56**, 357–68.

Orci, L., Palmer, D., Amherdt, M., and Rothman J. (1993). "Coated vesicle assembly in the Golgi requires only coatomer and ARF proteins from the cytosol." *Nature* **364**, 732–34.

Ostermann, J., Orci, L., Tani, K., Amherdt, M., Ravazzola, M., Elazar, Z., and Rothman, J. (1993). "Stepwise assembly of functionally active transport vesicles." *Cell* **75**, 1015–25.

Oyler, G., Higgins, G., Hart, R., Battenberg, E., Billingsley, M., Bloom, F., and Wilson, M. (1989). "The identification of a novel synaptosomal-associated protein, SNAP-25, differentially expressed by neuronal subpopulations." *J. Cell Biol.* **109**, 3039–52.

Palade, G. (1975). "Intracellular aspects of the process of protein synthesis." *Science* **189**, 347–58.

Parlati, F., McNew, J., Fukuda, R., Miller, R., Söllner, T., and Rothman, J. (2000). "Topological restriction of SNARE-dependent membrane fusion." *Nature* **407**, 194–8.

Parlati, F., Varlamov, O., Paz, K., McNew, J., Hurtado, D., Söllner, T., and Rothman, J. (2002). "Distinct SNARE complexes mediating membrane fusion in Golgi transport based on combinatorial specificity." *Proc. Natl. Acad. Sci. U.S.A.* **99**, 54424–29.

Paumet, F., Brügger, B., Parlati, F., McNew, J., Söllner, T., and Rothman, J. (2001). "A t-SNARE of the endocytic pathway must be activated for fusion." *J. Cell Biol.* **155**, 961–68.

Pearse, B. (1976). "Clathrin: A unique protein associated with intracellular transfer of membrane by coated vesicles." *Proc. Nat. Acad. Sci. U.S.A.* **73**, 1255–59.

Roth, T. and Porter, K. (1964). "Yolk protein uptake in the oocyte of the mosquito." *Aedes Aegypti* L., *J. Cell Biol.* **20**, 313–32.

Serafini, T., Orci, L., Amherdt, M., Brunner, M., Kahn, R., and Rothman, J. (1991). "ADP-ribosylation factor is a subunit of the coat of Golgi-derived COP-coated vesicles: A novel role for a GTP-binding protein." *Cell* **67**, 239–53.

Söllner T., Whiteheart, S.W., Brunner, M., Erdjument-Bromage, H., Geromanos, S., Tempst, P., and Rothman, J. (1993a). "SNAP receptors implicated in vesicle targeting, and fusion." *Nature* **362**, 318–24.

Söllner, T., Bennett, M., Whiteheart, S., Scheller, R., and Rothman, J. (1993b). "A protein assembly-disassembly pathway in vitro that may correspond to sequential steps of synaptic vesicle docking, activation, and fusion." *Cell* **75**, 409–18.

Stamnes, M. and Rothman, J. (1993). "The binding of AP-1 clathrin adaptor particles to Golgi membranes requires ADP-ribosylation factor, a small GTP-binding protein." *Cell* **73**, 999–1005.

Sutton, R., Fasshauer, D., Jahn, R. and Brunger, A. (1998). "Crystal structure of a SNARE complex involved in synaptic exocytosis at 2.4 Å resolution." *Nature* **395**, 347–53.

Südhof, T. and Rothman, J. (2009). "Membrane Fusion: Grappling with SNARE and SM Proteins." *Science* **323**, 474–77.

Tanigawa, G., Orci, L., Amherdt, M., Ravazzola, M., Helms, J., and Rothman, J. (1993). "Hydrolysis of bound GTP by ARF protein triggers uncoating of Golgi-derived COP-coated vesicles." *J. Cell Biol.* **123**, 1365–71.

Waters, M., Serafini, T., and Rothman, J. (1991). "'Coatomer': A cytosolic protein complex containing subunits of non-clathrin-coated Golgi transport vesicles." *Nature* **349**, 248–51.

Weber, T., Parlati, F., McNew, J., Johnston, R., Westermann, B., Söllner, T., and Rothman, J. (2000). "SNAREpins are functionally resistant to disruption by NSF and alphaSNAP." *J. Cell Biol.* **149**, 1063–72.

Weber, T., Zemelman, B., McNew, J., Westermann, B., Gmachl, M., Parlati, F., Söllner T., and Rothman, J. (1998). "SNAREpins: Minimal machinery for membrane fusion." *Cell* **92**, 759–772.

Weidman, P., Melancon, P., Block, M., and Rothman, J. (1989). "Binding of an N-ethylmaleimide-sensitive fusion protein to Golgi membranes requires both a soluble protein(s) and an integral membrane receptor." *J. Cell Biol.* **108**, 1589–96.

Wilson, D. W., Whiteheart, S. W., Wiedmann, M., Brunner, M., and Rothman, J. (1992). "A multisubunit particle implicated in membrane fusion." *J Cell. Biol.* **117**, 531–8.

Wilson, D., Wilcox, C., Flynn, G., Chen, E., Kuang, W., Henzel, W., Block, M. R., Ullrich, A., and Rothman, J. (1989). "A fusion protein required for vesicle-mediated transport in both mammalian cells and yeast." *Nature* **339**, 355–9.

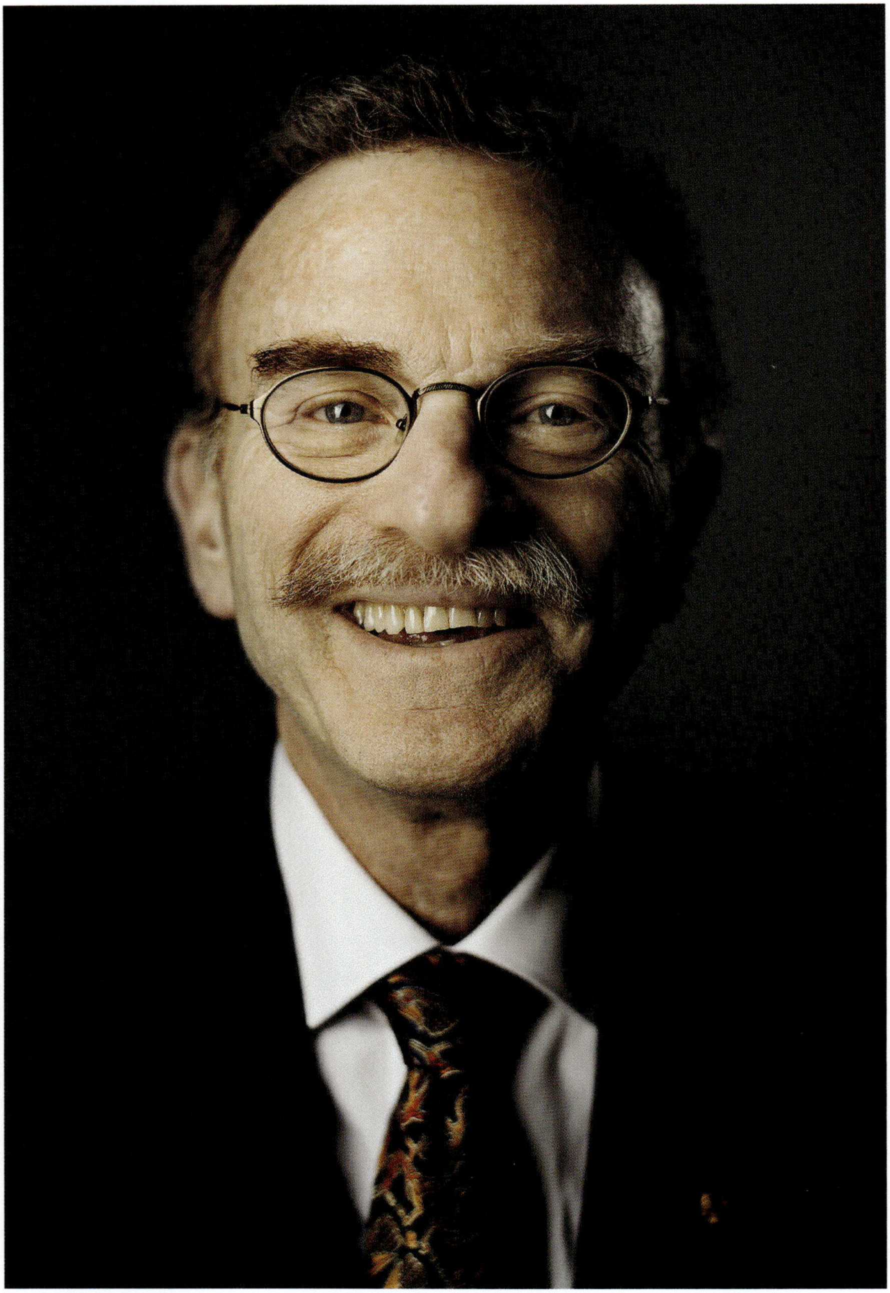

Randy W. Schekman. © Nobel Media AB. Photo: A. Mahmoud

Randy W. Scheckman

ANCESTORS

The Russian Revolution and the growing influence of the Soviet empire stimulated a migration of Jews to America and Israel. My father's father, Norman, followed his brother Nathan to Massachusetts where he enlisted in the British foreign brigade to fight in Palestine. He returned to the US and settled in Minnesota, along with a growing Jewish community in the Twin Cities. He met and married my grandmother, Rose, after whom I was given the name Randy, or Ruvain in Hebrew. My grandparents raised their children, my aunt Helen, my father Alfred, born in 1927, and my uncle Arthur in St. Paul. My grandfather had several careers; one I recall hearing about was as a traveling salesman selling clothing to farmers in the agricultural areas around the Twin Cities. My grandmother Rose died tragically of a stroke just as my father met and dated Esther Bader, a young high school student living on the north side of Minneapolis, then an enclave for Jewish immigrants from Eastern Europe. They married in 1947 at the tender ages of 20 for my father and just 18 for my mother.

My mother's parents, Raymond and Ida, grew up in a village in Bessarabia, which at the time was part of Romania, but which is now Moldova. My grandfather became a tailor, my mental image of which will always be fixed by the character Motel from "Fiddler on the Roof." He was drafted onto the Romanian Army as a tailor and then by some stroke of good fortune won a lottery to immigrate with my grandmother to the US in 1927. Most of the members of their families were slaughtered in the Nazi takeover of Eastern Europe in the early years of WWII, but some managed to escape to Israel where a branch of our family lives today. My grandparents landed in Providence, Rhode Island and found their way to New York City. My grandmother was uncomfortable in a big city, so they sought out an adopted member of my grandmother's family who had previously migrated to Minneapolis, where they ultimately settled and had two daughters, my aunt Mary and then one year later in 1929, my mother

Esther. The family struggled to get by in the Depression, made worse by the illness of my grandmother who contracted tuberculosis and was taken to a sanitarium for a couple of years, during which time my mother and her sister were sheltered in an orphanage so that my grandfather could work as a tailor to cover the family expenses. Many decades later, years after my mother died, I learned from Rodney Rothstein, a fellow yeast geneticist, that his mother had befriended my mother and aunt during their years in the orphanage. I had the surreal experience of meeting Mrs. Rothstein at a special occasion where Rodney was honored and she recounted her memories, some 70 years later, of my mother during that tim2e4i1n the early 1930s. I will never forget embracing Mrs. Rothstein as a living memory of the mother I so cherished.

EARLY YEARS IN MINNESOTA

My parents took an apartment in St. Paul and I was born a year later in 1948. We then moved to another small apartment on the north side of Minneapolis, probably so that my mother could be closer to her parents. My sister Wendy was born in 1950 and my earliest memories are of the two of us as infants in cribs in that small apartment. My sister and I occupied the one small bedroom and my parents slept in the living room, which doubled as the dining room. My aunt Mary married Marshall Kopman, and for two years they lived together in the second bedroom of my grandparent's home, probably no more than a mile away from our family apartment.

My oldest cousin Michael was born around that time and I am told – but do not recall – that I walked by myself to my grandparent's home to see him, much to the horror of my parents. In the first years of my life, it was clear that I was shorter than my peers so my mother, who was quite combative as a child, decided that I needed to learn self-protection. She claimed, but again I do not recall, that she tried to teach me to hold up my fists in a threatening gesture, but it may have backfired when I resorted to the use of the top of a garbage can when I fought with a local child.

We remained in that apartment for several years. My father then designed and had built a small three-bedroom home of less than 1000 sq. ft. a couple of miles away, but still in the north side area just a block away from a home my uncle Marshall had built for his family. During the six years we lived on Upton Avenue, the Schekman family grew with two more boys, my brothers Murry and Cary, and the Kopman family grew with two girls, Jodi and Robin. We were a close knit family with daily activities revolving around playtime with my cousins and friends from the neighborhood, school at the Jewish community center and John Hay Elementary School, and afternoon Hebrew lessons at a religious school just down the block from my grandparents. The regular highlights were Friday evening Sabbath dinners at my grandparents' home, holidays at the synagogue, a conservative congregation that my grandparents joined. My fondest memories are of drives to the countryside for an ice cream cone, occasional sleep overs on the porch at my grandparent's home, but most of all, our annual trips to a cottage on a lake in Northern Minnesota, where my grandfather would take us fishing in a boat in pursuit of sunfish, walleye, crappie and the special treat of early morning trolling for northern pike. We lived and associated exclusively with other Jewish families and I was unaware of anti-Semitism until one day on my way to the Jewish Community Center, an older kid slugged me in the stomach when he learned where I was headed.

I have fewer memories of my father's family. We would occasionally see his father and new wife, Evelyn, a dear woman who was sweet to the children and whom I grew to love in later years on a high school trip to Florida where she and my grandfather moved for retirement, and then later, after my grandfather died, on a visit to her sisters and their families in the New York area. My father's younger brother Arthur lived with us briefly in the Upton Avenue house. We had more social occasions with Arthur and my aunt Carol and their children, Scott, Ronnie and Lorrie when they moved to Southern California in the 1960s. My father's sister Helen moved to Columbus, Georgia and raised a family of five boys, whom I am sorry to say we almost never met for family events, other than one trip with my wife and son and my parents to a meeting in Atlanta in 1987.

I have only vague memories of any particular academic interest during those years in Minnesota. My father was a mechanical engineer working at General Mills. He was drafted after the war, but never left the country after boot camp and had attended the University of Minnesota on the GI bill. My mother worked part time in a department store during and after high school, but did not attend college. It was clear that the family valued learning and college for all the children was always an expectation, but any particular professional goals beyond college never entered my mind. I remember a casual interest in astronomy and I still have some electron microscope (EM) pictures of bacterial viruses that my father took which were used in particle size calibration at work. My casual reading was almost always of boy's adventure stories. I briefly belonged to a troop of cub scouts, but that sort of regimented activity had little appeal. Correspondingly, my most unpleasant memory of that time was of a military outfit that my parents bought for one of my birthdays.

WESTWARD TO CALIFORNIA

In 1959, my father answered an ad for an engineering position in Southern California. On returning home from Los Angeles he announced that we would move at the end of the year to the great frontier of the Golden State. Neither of my parents had known anything other than Minnesota and yet my father somehow knew his future lay in the burgeoning computer industry of Southern California. My mother was traumatized by the move. She was emotionally dependent on her parents and could not bear the thought of such a geographic separation. For years after the move, she was inconsolable – when visits to Minnesota and/or of her parents to us in Southern California came to an end.

For me however, the move was a great adventure. We packed up the car and drove off in the deep cold of December 1959, traveling through snow flurries in the Midwest over the 2,000 miles to Los Angeles. The weather delayed our excursion and when we finally arrived on December 31, the reservation my father had made at a motel was cancelled and we had to scrounge for a single unheated room where the children bundled into one bed for warmth on New Year's Eve. Still, Southern California was a dream with the network television studios just down the block from the motel we occupied for several weeks before moving to a rental home in Pacoima. I still recall with awe my first glimpse of the vast Pacific Ocean and the maze of freeways, not yet impassable with the choked traffic of today.

In 1960, my father purchased a new tract home in Rossmoor, then a new development in western Orange County, just adjacent to Long Beach. I had the privilege of my own bedroom where I hung out for long hours listening to the daily radio broadcasts of the LA Dodgers and their famous – and still active – announcer Vin Scully. My hero, indeed the hero of the entire Jewish community, was Sandy Koufax, the greatest pitcher of his generation. Those great World Series championships, especially the shutout of the Yankees in the 1963 World Series, are cherished memories that an impressionable child can never forget. On the other hand, although I have now lived in the San Francisco Bay Area for most of my life, I can never forgive the Giants and their infamous pitcher Juan Marichal who took a bat to the head of the Dodger's great catcher Johnny Rosboro during a tense moment in a game at Chavez Ravine in 1965. I was a baseball nut but not at all athletic. My one year in little league ended ignominiously with a strike out on a bad pitch that I never should have swung at.

My father expected his children to be industrious and to work for extra money. I baby sat for the children of my parents' friends, mowed lawns and held a paper route delivering news for the now defunct Los Angeles Examiner. My memories of school are not particularly strong. I remember the expectation of academic performance instilled by my parents, but until around 7th grade, I recall no particular interests or ability at the end of elementary and beginning of junior high school. That began to change when I received a toy microscope and collected a jar of pond scum from a local creek. I recall with amazement the rich microbial life seen in a drop of that pond scum, even just from squinting into the plastic lens of that toy.

THE MICROBIAL WORLD

In the spring of 7th grade, I attended the school science fair and was captivated by the dozens of projects that the older students had assembled. The vivid memory of that simple event resonated somehow in a way that nothing else in my experience in school ever had. Here were simple but clearly individual efforts on display for recognition by fellow students, teachers and parents. In retrospect, this may have been the single event in my youth that fixed my path in science. In the following year, I spent countless hours looking into or projecting an image onto a sintered glass screen of paramecia and rotifers gliding or crawling across my field of view.

I built a science project display based on my simple observations for my first entry in 8th grade, and although I recall no particular recognition for that work, I was nonetheless hooked, and the annual science fair became my one abiding academic passion through junior and high school. Another revealing moment came that year when I recounted my excitement about these protozoa in a family conversation at the dinner table. My father, perhaps recalling his own experience with EM images of bacterial viruses, was dubious that anything of value could be seen in my toy microscope. At that point, I resolved to save and buy a student professional microscope using the money from my odd jobs.

Time went on, but I never seemed to reach my goal of $100 because my mother would borrow the money for family expenses. One Saturday I became so upset that after mowing a neighbor's lawn, I bicycled to the police station and announced to the desk officer that I wanted to run away from home because my mother took my money and I couldn't use it to buy a microscope. My father was called in and words were exchanged behind a closed door, the net effect of which was that we purchased my microscope at a pawnshop in Long Beach that afternoon! That microscope became my treasured possession for the rest of my years at school, but it was inevitably put aside as I went ahead to college and graduate school. Fortunately, my parents saved it and sent it up to my current home in the San Francisco Bay Area, where it languished in the dust for decades until the call from Stockholm at which point I realized it might be more interesting to visitors at the Nobel Museum. My old microscope is now on display, together with the tale of how it was acquired in a fit of childhood pique.

In 9th grade, a friend of my parents who worked in a hospital lab in Long Beach took an interest in my budding passion for microbes. She provided me with simple training in the classification of bacteria and valuable assistance in acquiring simple ingredients I would need to grow bacteria at home. I assembled a homemade incubator whose temperature was controlled by a light bulb hooked to a rheostat. I purchased simple supplies of glass petri plates, flasks and agar. Through my friend at the hospital, I was given units of spent human blood, which proved to be a rich source of nutrients for the growth of bacteria that were the subjects of my science fair projects over the next several years. I used my mother's pressure cooker to sterilize and melt the agar and stored the spent human blood and my fresh medium in her refrigerator. In truth I didn't really know what I was doing most of the time, but it certainly stimulated my reading of as many books on the microbial world as I could lay my hands on.

Just before I entered high school, my future biology teacher, Jack Hoskins, introduced himself as I stood in front of my project at the county science fair. Jack became my mentor during the next three years, and though his knowledge of experimental science was limited, he became a valuable source of encouragement outside of my family, who had much less knowledge of or interest in science. Indeed, we remained in contact through all the years since then – through to the morning of the Nobel Prize announcement when he sent a congratulatory message, expressing delight that he had lived to see this day. Back in high school, the peak of my effort was a fifth place prize in the senior life science division at the California State Science Fair, and an on-TV interview by Vin Scully, whose velvet voice of the LA Dodgers had entertained me for so many years.

As I dreamed of my future in college, I read such books as The Microbial World by Adelberg, Doudoroff and Stanier, and Bacterial Viruses by Gunther Stent. Indeed, as I explored the annual catalogue of courses at UC Berkeley I recognized the authors of these books as faculty members and wondered what opportunities I might have to learn directly from such individuals. The cost of college was foremost in the mind of my mother who thought it would be good enough if I lived at home and attended the local State College in Long Beach. However, I was certain that I wanted the more vigorous experience and peer group of a selective University, so I compromised on distance and applied to just one school, UCLA. In truth, UCLA also appealed because of the great basketball teams coached by John Wooden who had just recruited the best high school player of all time, Lew Alcindor (now Kareem Abdul Jabbar).

STIRRINGS OF THE LIFE OF A SCHOLAR

In the fall of 1966, I drove my motorcycle the 30 miles to UCLA where I took up residence in the student co-op dormitory along with my high school buddy Peter Wissner. The timing was perfect because just one week earlier my mother had given birth to my youngest brother, Tracey, and as hectic as college was, it would have been even more disruptive with a new baby back home. I threw myself into my studies and spent every waking hour in class or in study in a library. My courses were generally wonderful, particularly freshman chemistry then taught by a brilliant lecturer, Kenneth Trueblood, who received a standing ovation at the end of the term. I did well enough in that course to be admitted to an honors section for the third term, a course taught by Willard Libby, a Nobel Laureate who had won the prize for C14-radiodating of ancient materials.

The students in this class were clearly a cut above the others in my courses, and as a result I enjoyed my first taste of serious scholarship. Although it was inspiring to be taught by such a renowned chemist, Libby was not the effective lecturer we had experienced in Trueblood. But what made this class special was that each student was assigned to work in a Chemistry Department lab for the term. By chance, I was assigned to the lab of a new assistant professor, Michael Konrad, who had worked as a graduate student with Stent at Berkeley. Konrad assigned me to read a new book just off the press, entitled The Molecular Biology of the Gene, by James Watson. The book was a revelation to me and I read its paragraphs and chapters as though they came from a new bible of life. My project in the Konrad lab was simple enough: I hydrolyzed a sample of DNA and determined the base composition by chromatographic separation and UV absorption.

Although I had started UCLA with an aspiration to attend medical school and become a pathologist, the experience of my first year changed my outlook completely. I was disappointed that most of my pre-medical classmates were more interested in getting high marks than in the science itself. In contrast, the one term experience in Konrad's lab combined with Watson's book convinced me that my future lay in experimental science, preferably as an academic in a research university. The summer after my first year in college I worked with my father at his computer data firm. He had hoped to enthuse me about writing computer code, but I found it boring and my mind turned to how to pursue a basic molecular biology research project when I returned to UCLA for my second year. I cooked up an idea to look at the effect of a mild organic solvent, DMSO, on the uptake of viral DNA by bacterial protoplasts. After a couple of disappointing approaches to various faculty members, I found another new assistant professor, Dan Ray, of the then Zoology Department who was willing to gamble on me.

A PATH TO DISCOVERY OF MOLECULAR MECHANISMS

Dan had trained with Phil Hanawalt at Stanford studying bacterial DNA repair and then with Peter Hofschneider in Munich studying the replication of a small circular chromosome of the phage M13. I puttered around for a term trying to learn how to perform the experiments necessary to test M13 phage DNA uptake into E. coli protoplasts. Dan took me under his wing and gradually turned me to the interests he had in the mechanism of replication of the duplex form of M13 in cells infected with the phage. I was captivated by the idea that an experimentalist could use physical techniques such as velocity and density gradient separation of chromosomes extracted from infected cells to test models of chromosome strand inheritance during replication. Dan offered me a summer job and then generously listed me as a co-author on two papers he had prepared for publication.

Not many UCLA undergraduates worked in a research lab during that time, but I was happy to work alone well into the evening. Although my coursework was also going well, I increasingly began to feel that I was perhaps misplaced at UCLA, and that I might benefit by transfer to a school such as the University of Chicago that had a reputation for serious scholarship at the undergraduate level. James Watson himself had been an undergraduate at Chicago. Indeed, in the fall of 1967 I read Watson's The Double Helix, which as much as his textbook had steeled my determination to live the life of a scholar in pursuit of a basic understanding of life. But as a simpler and much less expensive alternative, I learned of the University of California education abroad program and I applied and was accepted for a year at the University of Edinburgh.

I was excited to travel to Britain – I had never been out of the US – and in anticipation I asked a professor who taught a graduate course in genetics whom I might approach on the faculty in Edinburgh. I learned that the prominent bacterial geneticist William Hayes, had just started a new Medical Research Council unit in this research topic. I wrote to Hayes and he welcomed me to join the new unit, though he mistakenly believed that I would spend the year as a sabbatical visitor. I arrived to find that I had been listed on the opening program as a visiting faculty member from UCLA and was assigned my own laboratory space. They quickly realized their error but graciously provided me an opportunity to learn bacterial genetics from a Lecturer, John Scaife. I managed also to continue my studies on M13 phage and took the biochemistry course in the medical school in downtown Edinburgh. The year provided a wonderful opportunity to travel on the continent during the term breaks. However, I was ill prepared for the British style of examination that consisted of one comprehensive exam followed by an interview with the Biochemistry faculty. I survived by the skin of my teeth, but was appropriately upbraided by the faculty who relished the opportunity to take an arrogant Yank down several notches in my exit interview.

The most enduring influence of my year in Edinburgh was my acquaintance with Leonard ("Len") Kelly, a graduate student in the lab next door in the Molecular Biology Department. Len shared correspondence with his brother Regis ("Reg") who was then a postdoctoral fellow in the laboratory of Arthur Kornberg, whom I knew to be the leading DNA enzymologist of this era. Reg had discovered that the DNA polymerase was capable of removing thymine dimers from UV-irradiated DNA in a repair-like replication reaction. The work was elegant and precise in a way that I had not experienced; I resolved to learn biochemistry from a master such as Kornberg. In the months before I left Edinburgh to return to the US, I considered summer opportunities in the US prior to my senior year at UCLA. One possibility was the Undergraduate Research Program at Cold Spring Harbor (CSH). I would have relished the total immersion of that program, and the timing could not have been better with the discovery of the E coli DNA polymerase mutant by John Cairns who was then the director of the CSH lab. However, the summer stipend they offered was just enough to live on and I had to save money to pay for my remaining year of college. Instead, I took a summer position with David Denhardt in the Biological Laboratories at Harvard. The ferment of the Bio labs was intense with the Walter Gilbert and James Watson labs just down the hall. But the bickering and contentiousness of the atmosphere left me with a bad feeling about what it would be like to do PhD work in such a hypercompetitive environment. Nonetheless, I had a wonderful time in Denhardt's lab and learned much to affirm my resolve to pursue a more biochemical approach to the study of DNA replication in graduate school. I left having done enough work to publish a first author paper in the Journal of Molecular Biology the following year.

PERSONAL GROWTH, LOSS AND CHALLENGES IN COLLEGE AND GRADUATE SCHOOL

My last year at UCLA brought emotional highs and lows. On the upside, I had the opportunity to meet Arthur Kornberg and to discuss my interest in the biochemistry of DNA replication and then in the spring of the next year, I was admitted to Kornberg's department at Stanford for graduate school. But before that, just as I returned home from my summer at Harvard, I was greeted by my mother at the Los Angeles airport with the news that my sister Wendy had been diagnosed with acute leukemia and was given just months to live. Wendy's rapid decline and our family's anguish at her loss left a scar that is never far removed from my thoughts, even 45 years after her death. My mother was tortured by the loss of her one daughter and never fully recovered from the emotional blow.

Perhaps in reaction to this trauma in my life, I threw myself into the work back in Dan Ray's lab at UCLA and didn't bother with many of the lectures in classes that I had to complete in order to graduate. As a result, my grades declined and I was placed on academic probation for the second of the three terms of the year. Indeed, I failed German twice and left UCLA without actually having graduated. The registrar at Stanford took a dim view of this gap in my record and it was not until a sympathetic Dean back at UCLA waived that requirement – thus allowing me to graduate – that I was able to look ahead to my graduate career.

My personal life at Stanford was also a mix of highs and lows. Although I was thrilled to be in such an exciting environment, my immaturity led to personal isolation. Most of my fellow PhD students came from elite private universities and I felt insecure as one of the few students from a public university. Kornberg once asked me why I hadn't enrolled in a "better" school, to which I responded that it was the best my family could afford. But looking back at what I was able to accomplish then, and now after nearly 40 years at UC Berkeley, I can state with confidence that I had the best preparation and that our great public institutions, the University of California in particular, offer educational and real life experiences that are second to none.

After a period of personal decompression (I was placed in small lab room by myself as penance for my obnoxious behavior), I slowly developed great friendships that have lasted a lifetime. Costa Georgopoulis, a postdoctoral fellow in Dale Kaiser's lab, took pity on me and invited me to join a group for a camping trip in a nearby state park.Costa deflated my ego by calling me a turkey, a term of endearment that seemed to fit and which stuck for some years. But my greatest friendship came when Bill Wickner joined the Kornberg lab in 1971. Although we were in a somewhat competitive situation in the first months of his time at Stanford, I will never forget the favor he did me when, after I made an aggressive remark, he lifted me from the floor by the front of my shirt and told me to settle down!

But Bill did more than that for me. After a few more months of intense and close cooperation, he could see that my personal life was going nowhere so he and his wife Hali conspired to find a suitable mate for me. After one failed effort at matchmaking, Bill had a call from a former girlfriend, Nancy Walls, whom he had dated in Boston. Nancy had completed her training as a nurse at Massachusetts General Hospital and decided to make a clean break to the West Coast. Feeling lonely herself, she called Bill at Stanford but learned that he had in the meantime married Hali, but he had a lab partner who needed distraction. I still remember our first date at a Greek restaurant in San Francisco and our first kiss goodnight. Nancy and I grew close quickly as these things happen when you are young. We moved into a small duplex home in Palo Alto and Nancy took a job as a nurse at Stanford Hospital. We would meet for a goodnight kiss while she was on a night shift and I worked into the wee hours of the morning in the lab. Nancy and I married in a '70s style outdoor wedding in Huddart Park in Woodside, near the Stanford campus. Our years at Stanford were fulfilling in every way. I grew emotionally secure in a loving relationship and even with the intense and sometime acrimonious battles I had with Kornberg, I left graduate school equipped with the intellectual and technical skills that made my subsequent career possible.

Nancy took classes at a local community college with the goal of obtaining a BA in nursing. As we considered our next move for my postdoctoral training, she felt we should remain in California where her course credits would be recognized by a state school. I arranged a postdoctoral position with SJ Singer at UC San Diego and we moved south for what would be a short two-year stay in San Diego. In spite of the issue of course credit, Nancy enrolled at private school, the University of San Diego, and completed the requirements for her BA degree. She worked as an intensive and coronary care nurse, but we both missed Northern California, so when the opportunity came for a position at Berkeley, we moved back north and have remained ever since.

FAMILY LIFE AND CAREER AT BERKELEY

We settled into a family life in El Cerrito, a bedroom community just north of Berkeley. Nancy took a job at Alta Bates Hospital in Berkeley and we saved as much as possible to afford a home which we purchased in 1977 – and where have lived to this day. Our son Joel was born at Alta Bates in March of 1978, and our daughter Lauren was born in Basel, Switzerland in November 1982, during a sabbatical year in Basel that Bill Wickner, I and our wives had arranged for the year after I was granted tenure at Berkeley. Both of our children inherited a talent and taste for classical music from Nancy, who had played the saxophone in school and her mother Beatrice, who played the violin, so it seemed natural to expose the children to piano and other forms of musical training. The years of our family life sped by, enriched by the music of our talented children who filled our home with beautiful sound. Joel took up the clarinet and never let go. His passion grew into a career as a classical musician, currently in the Grand Rapids, MI Symphony Orchestra.

Lauren sang in youth choirs that traveled the world, but she found more of a calling in economics, management and the business world, though she remains active in a semi-professional choir where she lives in Portland, Oregon.

Nancy worked full-time and then part-time when the children were young, and she may have remained active in nursing, but life intervened and at the relatively young age of 48, she was diagnosed with Parkinson's Disease (PD). In her case, the disease progressed quite slowly and was effectively controlled by medication, but inexorably the physical symptoms worsened. In 2009, she had neurosurgery to implant electrodes in a treatment called Deep Brain Stimulation. This procedure worked remarkably well, and together with medications, her physical symptoms are unusually mild for someone now 18 years post-diagnosis. Unfortunately, this awful disease comes with other disabilities and in her case, dementia set in, which has slowly but inexorably sapped her memory and independence. Two years ago, her dementia was diagnosed as an atypical form of PD called Diffuse Lewy Body Disease for which no effective treatment exists. Life continues and we remain devoted to each other after nearly 42 years of marriage, but I fear for the future as her condition worsens year by year.

My parents rejoiced in the birth of my children, their first grandchildren, and our occasions together were filled with pride in the musical accomplishments of Joel and Lauren. As my career flourished, my parents tagged along to every special event and award ceremony and they fully expected to include a trip to Stockholm at the end of the rainbow. But in 1996, my mother was diagnosed with an inoperable brain tumor, which took her life two years later at the age of 69.

This loss struck my father even more deeply than the loss of his daughter/my sister. However, with time he recovered and with the help of a support group he met a wonderful woman, Sandy, who had lost her husband to heart disease. They were married within two years and continue to live happily together in a new home in Southern California.

Sandy and my Dad were the first people I called on that fateful early Monday morning of October 7, 2013. Among the many thrills of our memorable trip to Stockholm, I will never forget having my father rise to receive my appreciation in front of the thousand people who attended my Nobel Lecture. He never faltered in his certainty that I would someday receive that recognition. In honor of my sister and mother, I donated my Nobel Prize funds to create an endowed chair, the Esther and Wendy Schekman Chair in basic cancer research at UC Berkeley.

AN APPRECIATION

In my Nobel essay, I described in detail the contributions of my students and postdoctoral fellows that led to our dissection of the secretory pathway in yeast and the many molecular insights that developed from our discovery of the SEC genes and their protein products.

I had the good fortune to attract some of the finest young scholars from around the world to join in that effort. But I owe at least as much to the many colleagues at Berkeley who taught me how to be a constructive citizen of science. Among them, I wish to offer a special tribute to Dan Koshland, Howard Schachman, Bruce and Giovanna Ames, Bob Tjian, Jeremy Thorner and Mike Botchan. They offered counsel and friendship that has enriched my life as a scholar and teacher.

During that nearly 40-year adventure, I observed a sea change in the attitudes and acceptance of women as scholars in the academic community. Gone are the days when women were relegated to "adjunct" status in couples seeking academic appointments. Instead, I found women who joined our department and my laboratory who had the highest standards and drive for achievement.

Several who stand out in my experience are Susan Ferro-Novick, who was and continues to be as ambitious as they come, Linda Hicke, whose experiment I detailed in my Nobel Lecture as one of the most memorable in my experience at Berkeley, Nina Salama, who completed the detection and purification of the

COPII proteins, Sabeeha Merchant, who came for a brief sabbatical and has remained a best friend and confidant ever since, and Liz Miller, who solved the mystery of cargo selection by the COPII coat. Science will never be the same now that women have taken a proper role in creative scholarship.

It is hard to believe that nearly 40 years has elapsed since that first day when I walked into the Biochemistry building to begin my career at Berkeley. The memories of all those years could fill a book, but I must bring this biography to a close with an appreciation of all that my family, friends, students and colleagues have done to make this a "Wonderful Life", as the director Frank Capra so movingly captured in the movie of that title. I am not a religious person but I feel that I have been blessed with opportunities and people who have enriched my life immeasurably. This essay is dedicated to those who have passed on and to the love of those who now sustain me.

Genes and Proteins that Control the Secretory Pathway

Nobel Lecture, 7 December 2013

by Randy Schekman

Department of Molecular and Cell Biology, Howard Hughes Medical Institute, University of California, Berkeley, USA.

INTRODUCTION

George Palade shared the 1974 Nobel Prize with Albert Claude and Christian de Duve for their pioneering work in the characterization of organelles interrelated by the process of secretion in mammalian cells and tissues. These three scholars established the modern field of cell biology and the tools of cell fractionation and thin section transmission electron microscopy. It was Palade's genius in particular that revealed the organization of the secretory pathway. He discovered the ribosome and showed that it was poised on the surface of the endoplasmic reticulum (ER) where it engaged in the vectorial translocation of newly synthesized secretory polypeptides (1). And in a most elegant and technically challenging investigation, his group employed radioactive amino acids in a pulse-chase regimen to show by autoradiograpic exposure of thin sections on a photographic emulsion that secretory proteins progress in sequence from the ER through the Golgi apparatus into secretory granules, which then discharge their cargo by membrane fusion at the cell surface (1). He documented the role of vesicles as carriers of cargo between compartments and he formulated the hypothesis that membranes template their own production rather than form by a process of de novo biogenesis (1).

As a university student I was ignorant of the important developments in cell biology; however, I learned of Palade's work during my first year of graduate school in the Stanford biochemistry department. Palade was a close friend of my graduate advisor Arthur Kornberg, who won the Nobel Prize in 1959 for his discovery of DNA polymerase, the first enzyme found to take its instructions from a DNA template (2). At first glance Kornberg and Palade had little in common. Palade was a classical anatomist and physiologist who used the electron microscope as his primary tool of analysis. Kornberg was a classical biochemist who cared deeply about the chemistry of life, which he probed exclusively through the study of pure enzymes. However, in the late 1960s as the study of DNA synthesis began to focus on the possible role of a membrane surface in organizing the segregation of replicating chromosomes, Kornberg took a keen interest in membrane biochemistry and in 1969, the year before I started graduate school, Kornberg traveled to several laboratories of membrane biologists including Palade's, who was then at The Rockefeller University. On return to Stanford, Kornberg turned his attention to membrane enzymes in the hope that a membrane surface may provide a crucial link to the problem of DNA replication. Just then, in the summer of 1969, the field of DNA replication was shaken with the discovery by John Cairns, then Director of the Cold Spring Harbor laboratory, that Kornberg's DNA polymerase was not required for chromosome replication. I visited Cold Spring Harbor that summer and was swept up in the excitement of the Cairns isolation of an *E. coli pol1* mutant, lacking polymerase activity, but which grew normally and yet was sensitive to UV irradiation, a clear sign that the classic polymerase could not be the enzyme responsible for replication but instead played a role in DNA repair (3).

THE POWER OF GENETICS AND BIOCHEMISTRY COMBINED

Kornberg was a dominant figure with a powerful personality and intellect. His focus on enzyme chemistry shaped a generation of students of DNA enzymology, including several former postdoctoral fellows and associates who joined him to form the core of what was to become the preeminent biochemistry department in the country at Stanford Medical School, where he moved from Washington University, St. Louis in 1959, the year in which he was awarded his Nobel Prize. With the pure DNA polymerase, Kornberg proved that it took its instructions from a template strand and copied DNA in an antiparallel direction, as predicted from the Watson-Crick model of the DNA duplex (4). The most persuasive evidence that it could be the replication enzyme came in1967 with the demonstration that polymerase alone copied the circular single stand template of the bacteriophage φX174 to make a complementary strand, which then also served as a template to make infectious viral strand DNA (5, 6). Thus the enzyme could faithfully take instructions from a template of around 5500 nucleotides and form, essentially error-free, a complement to reproduce the viral infectious cycle in a living cell.

However, several features of the polymerase left some investigators skeptical that it was the authentic replication enzyme. DNA chain elongation by the polymerase was quite slow in comparison to the progression of a chromosome replication fork. The enzyme had properties that suggested an ability to repair DNA damage, for example in the excision of thymine dimers on DNA isolated from cells exposed to UV light (7). Another puzzling feature was the requirement for a complementary oligonucleotide that forms a short duplex, which serves to launch the polymerase from a 3'OH provided by the primer (5). Nonetheless, an enzyme much like the *E. coli* polymerase is encoded by the T4 bacteriophage and in that case phage mutations in the polymerase gene show that it is clearly required for viral chromosome replication (8).

Quite independently, bacterial geneticists found genes essential for chromosome replication by the isolation and characterization of temperature sensitive (*ts*) mutations that arrest DNA synthesis in cells warmed at 42 C (9, 10). Cells carrying the *dna* mutations can grow at 30 C but cease growing at 42 C. The "*dna*" genes thus represented candidates for the authentic replication machinery quite distinct from the *pol1* gene identified as non-essential in the Cairns mutant. A grand union of the genetics and biochemistry first developed through a twist of fate with the discovery by Tom Kornberg, Arthur's middle son, then a graduate student in the laboratory of Malcolm Gefter at Columbia University, of another replication activity detected in lysates of the Cairns mutant (11). Gefter and Kornberg went on to discover that the authentic polymerase is encoded by the *dnaE* gene, one of the approximately half-dozen genes then known to be required for chromosome replication (12).

In 1970 I joined Arthur's lab powerfully influenced by the two strands of investigation, enzymology as practiced by the Kornberg school, and molecular biology and genetics, as best described in James Watson's textbook *Molecular Biology of the Gene* (13). I had read and reveled in the details in the first edition of this book when I was a freshman at UCLA, and although I was drawn to the Kornberg approach for graduate training, I was mindful that genetics and cellular physiology must inform the biochemistry.

A stunning precedent for the value of a combined genetic and biochemical approach came from the pioneering work of Robert Edgar, a bacterial geneticist who dissected the process of T4 phage assembly with the isolation of mutations in the genes that encode subunits of the phage coat (14), and William Wood, a new faculty colleague of Edgar's at Cal Tech. Wood had trained with Paul Berg, a former post-doctoral fellow of Kornberg's and then a colleague in the new Biochemistry Department at Stanford. At Cal Tech in the fall of 1965, Wood and Edgar joined forces to perform one of the classic experiments in molecular biology. Edgar had found that some of the viral coat mutants accumulated incomplete viral heads and tails within infected cells. Edgar used the standard cis-trans genetic complementation test, first developed by Seymour Benzer for the characterization of phage rII genes (15), to characterize the genes involved in T4 phage morphogenesis. Wood imagined that biochemical complementation might be achieved by mixing extracts of different phage assembly mutant-infected cells. Indeed, starting with separate extracts that had essentially no detectable infectious virions as assayed by the phage plaque test, Edgar and Wood found that mixing lysates of genetically complementing mutants (i.e. biochemical complementation) produced a thousand-fold increase in infectious particles (16). The team went on to identify functional assembly intermediates and to map the pathway of virus assembly. Clearly, this approach had the potential to dissect complex pathways and to reveal molecular details that might not otherwise be elucidated by a strictly genetic or biochemical analysis.

In 1971, Doug Brutlag, a talented graduate student in Arthur's lab, discovered that the conversion of the M13 phage single stand circle to the double strand replicative form was blocked in infected cells by an inhibitor of the transcription enzyme RNA polymerase, this in spite of the fact that no viral or host gene expression is required at the first stage of chromosome replication. Brutlag and Kornberg suggested that RNA polymerase might provide the missing primer to initiate the growth of a DNA chain (17). Brutlag then established a replication reaction in a concentrated lysate of uninfected *E. coli* cells and found that this faithfully reproduced the requirement for RNA polymerase in the conversion of M13 single strand template to the duplex replicative form (18). A similar concentrated extract of *E. coli* had been developed in the laboratory of Friedrich Bonhoeffer in Tübingen Germany, and found by one of Bonhoeffer's postdoctoral fellows, Baldomero Olivera, to be capable of replicating φX174 single strand circular template (20). Both concentrated lysates contained membranes and cytosolic proteins and it seemed possible that the reaction would require a membrane contribution. However, at the same time, Bruce Alberts, then at Princeton University, found that soluble cytosolic lysates of T4 phage infected cells replicated T4 DNA and applying the logic of Wood and Edgar, Jack Barry and Alberts showed biochemical complementation of soluble protein fractions obtained from different T4 replication mutant cells (21). At Stanford, a new postdoctoral fellow in the Kornberg group, William (Bill) Wickner, found that the lysate capable of replicating M13 DNA could be centrifuged to produce a soluble fraction with no loss of replication activity (18). All interest in membranes and DNA replication seemed to evaporate with that result.

I joined the effort initiated by Brutlag and Kornberg, first on the replication of M13 DNA and then using the cell-free reaction Doug Brutlag had developed, I found that φX174 double strand formation was insensitive to the drug that blocks the standard RNA polymerase, suggesting perhaps an alternative RNA polymerase for primer synthesis (18, 19). David Denhardt at Harvard University, with whom I had worked for a summer, had reported that φX174 double strand formation was dependent on the *E. coli dnaB* gene; thus it seemed possible that the cell-free reaction might provide a functional assay for the purification of the dnaB protein and for the remaining dna proteins. Indeed, it did, and this reaction permitted the detection and fractionation of the full set of *E. coli* chromosome replication proteins (22). One of the Dna proteins, DnaG, was found to catalyze a novel RNA synthesis reaction that provides the primer for φX174 as well as for *E. coli* chromosome fork replication. Going forward I was confident that the combined genetic and biochemical approach could prove crucial in the elucidation of other complex cellular processes.

The cell division cycle represented one such complex pathway that was just beginning to be probed by molecular genetic approaches. I was particularly taken by the efforts of Leland Hartwell who had exploited the classical genetic tools available for baker's yeast, *Saccharomyces cerevisiae*, to probe the essential series of events that lead to yeast cell division. The key was a set of genes, identified by the isolation of *ts* lethal mutations that focused attention on crucial control elements in the progression of the cell cycle (23). Subsequent molecular genetic discoveries by Paul Nurse, Tim Hunt and others illuminated the molecular basis of cell cycle control. Here again, the molecular insights that started with a classical genetic approach proved crucial to the discovery of a protein kinase that controls the decision to initiate the cell division cycle and then acts repeatedly in transitions throughout the division cycle. A billion years of evolution conserved a similar pathway in mammals. From this it seemed most likely that studies on yeast could pave the way for a mechanistic understanding of many, if not all, other essential eukaryotic intracellular processes.

INVESTIGATING BIOLOGICAL MEMBRANES AS A MACROMOLECULAR ASSEMBLY

Although the replication reactions he investigated were not directly connected to membranes, Kornberg remained interested in the problem of how to purify membrane enzymes and thus he was eager to welcome an experienced membrane enzymologist, Bill Wickner, who joined the lab as a postdoctoral fellow in 1971. Bill had trained as a medical student with Eugene Kennedy at Harvard Medical School where he lost interest in clinical medicine but gained an abiding passion for biological membranes. He and I shared endless hours in conversation about our work but importantly, I learned a great deal from him about what was or was not known about how membranes are put together. In this context, I read the work of Palade and his associates David Sabatini and Phillip Siekevitz who were then exploring the mechanism of vectorial membrane translocation of secretory proteins as they are made on ribosomes associated with the ER (24,25). The Stanford biochemistry department was a focal point for visits by all the leading figures in modern biology. I met Hartwell and two other memorable men who represented different approaches to the study of membrane function: Efraim Racker who shared Arthur's passion for enzymes in his dissection of the mechanism of mitochondrial oxidative phosphorylation and Daniel Koshland, who had exploited a genetic approach pioneered by Julius Adler to probe the mechanism of bacterial chemotaxis, a process intimately linked to the detection of chemical gradients at the bacterial cell surface.

As I considered my future research career directions, I was motivated by a desire to break away from the field of DNA replication but to appropriate the tools and logic that had propelled the Kornberg group to a successful resolution and reconstitution of the enzymes of the replication process. As I concluded graduate work in 1974, the beginnings of a revolution in genetic engineering and recombinant DNA were just emerging, largely from the work of Stanford biochemists Dale Kaiser and Paul Berg, Stanford microbiologist Stanley Cohen and the UCSF biochemist Herbert Boyer. The tools of molecular cloning were in prospect, thus it was appealing to consider how they may be applied to uncover essential genes in any number of cellular processes.

And yet I was uncomfortable with the frenzy of activity that focused on all things DNA. I did not enjoy the pressure of competing with other laboratories doing the same experiments. I nervously unwrapped each new issue of the Proceedings of the National Academy of Sciences (PNAS) to see if our competitors had beaten us to key discoveries. Basking in the glow of Kornberg's influence had its advantages, but in facing my own independent career I resolved to strike off in a new direction where I might have the chance to establish my own identity and not be dependent on or overshadowed by Kornberg's reputation.

In making a choice for future research, I was impressed with the work of S. Jonathan Singer at UC San Diego, particularly with his greatly influential paper on the Fluid Mosaic Model of Membrane Structure (26). Here was a grand synthesis that provided a conceptual framework to think about how a membrane might be constructed. Singer's lab had assembled tools to explore the topology of membrane proteins using electron microscopy. His associate Kiyoteru Tokuyasu had developed an impressive cryoelectron microscopic approach to the detection of antigens on membranes (27). They had demonstrated that glycans on glycoproteins and glycolipids are asymmetrically displayed on the extracellular surface of red cells and on the luminal surface of the ER membrane, thus fulfilling the prediction that transbilayer movement of hydrophilic proteins and glycans was thermodynamically unlikely, but at the same time explaining how the asymmetry of the plasma membrane may be achieved at the outset of the secretory pathway (28). Singer enjoyed the warm support of my mentors at Stanford so I set off with my bride Nancy, whom I had met through my friendship with Bill Wickner, to join Singer's lab as a postdoctoral fellow in the fall of 1974.

Singer was so different from Kornberg that I experienced a bit of culture shock while trying to identify a research project of mutual interest. Although he made his career as a physical chemist, he had evolved into a cell biologist focusing on questions of cellular organization. I was keen to use the reconstitution approach of Kornberg to probe some aspect of membrane assembly or endocytosis but Singer pressed me to pursue a morphological study using electron microscopy. Of course it was important to learn a new discipline as well as a different approach so I took up a project to investigate the unusual behavior of neonatal human erythrocytes, which unlike mature red cells are able to internalize antibody or lectin molecules clustered on the cell surface (29). I found the work frustrating, and in spite of Tokuyasu's patience, my technical skills in thin section electron microscopy left much to be desired. It took two years to obtain one precious Rh control sample of newborn cord blood. The prospect of a satisfying molecular understanding of this process seemed remote and my dependence on cord blood from the local labor and delivery ward slowed progress to a snail's pace. I was spoiled by my previous experience with microorganisms and the slow and cumbersome approaches then available for work with human samples or even with cultured mammalian cells simply could not compare. So I had time to read and think, which was perhaps the greatest benefit of my postdoctoral years.

Shortly after I started in Singer's lab, the annual meeting of the American Society for Cell Biology (ASCB) convened in San Diego. At the time the ASCB was a small and quite personal organization, much more of a cottage industry than was the larger and more influential American Society for Biological

Chemistry (ASBC), subsequently renamed the ASBMB. Palade had just returned from Stockholm to deliver a special lecture to an adoring crowd who rose to a standing ovation at the end of his presentation. Although I knew then, and learned even more so later, how brilliant and broad Palade was in his scholarship, I came away from the meeting feeling that cell biology had yet to enter the molecular world of biochemical mechanism. Here was an enormously complex pathway of membrane transformation in the secretory pathway and yet not a single protein had been ascribed a specific role in this essential process.

The first crucial breakthrough that delivered Palade's pathway into the molecular era came with the report in 1975 by the Palade protégé Günter Blobel, of a cell-free system that reproduced the initiation and translocation of a secretory precursor protein into the interior of isolated ER membranes. Two papers in the Journal of Cell Biology by Blobel and Dobberstein paved the way to a mechanistic understanding of the link between protein synthesis and the vectorial discharge of secretory proteins through what must surely be a hydrophilic channel protein in the ER (30, 31). Although earlier work by Sabatini and Palade had demonstrated the completion of the translocation event *in vitro* using rough microsomes isolated from pancreatic tissue, Blobel's breakthrough allowed the entire process to be replicated with the discovery of an essential role for the N-terminal signal peptide in guiding the nascent chain to a special site on the ER membrane. The signal hypothesis and the beautiful work that followed garnered a Nobel Prize for Blobel in1999.

Singer was quite excited by the Blobel discovery because it supported his view that the establishment of protein asymmetry in the membrane must depend on a special channel in the ER that would convey hydrophilic protein sequences through the hydrophobic bilayer. And yet, Singer remained skeptical that a biochemical reconstitution approach would yield an essential understanding of the process. But to me, this was precisely the way forward, though my own efforts in that direction would await an opportunity to take the initiative.

Increasingly, I believed a unique opportunity lay in the evaluation of plasma membrane assembly in *S. cerevisiae* and my reading of the literature focused on what was known before 1975, which outside of the work of Gottfried Schatz and Walter Neupert on mitochondrial biogenesis was essentially nil. I read about the organization of the yeastcell surface, particularly at the nascent division site, which had an intriguing intermediate filament ring abutting the cytoplasmic surface of the bud neck membrane and a unique deposition of chitin in a ring embedded within the cell wall polysaccharide (32, 33). Vesicles implicated in secretion were seen by thin section electron microscopy to localize to the cytoplasm of an early cell bud and then to appear near the cytokinesis furrow later in the cell cycle (Fig. 1) (34, 35). It seemed reasonable to suppose that these vesicles were responsible for secretion and localized plasma membrane assembly. These ideas excited me a great deal more than the tedious work I was doing on human neonatal erythrocytes.

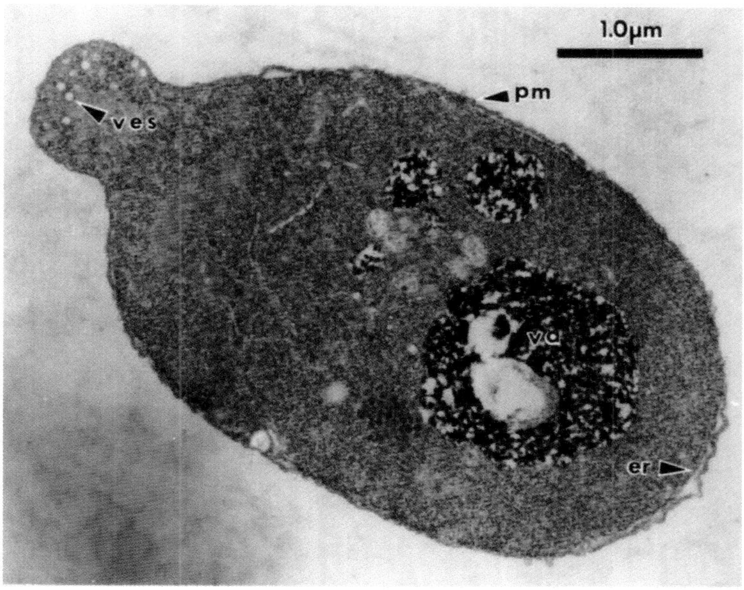

FIGURE 1. Thin section of wild-type yeast cell showing endoplasmic reticulum (er), vacuole (va) and secretory vesicles (ves).

FREE SPEECH AND FREE INQUIRY AT UC BERKELEY

Just as I left Stanford on my way to San Diego, I became aware of an Assistant Professor opening in the Biochemistry Department at University of California, Berkeley. Although I had no postdoctoral training, I decided to apply for this position just in case the Berkeley faculty would see my graduate record as an indication of my interests and abilities. Fortunately for me, the first person to whom they offered the job, turned it down, and in a call I will never forget, Michael Chamberlin, a Paul Berg-trained Stanford Biochemistry graduate and then Chair of the Berkeley search committee, conveyed the good news that I had the job. I was so excited that I foolishly accepted over the phone with no further negotiation! And so within the first few months of my postdoctoral training, I had the luxury of planning my future career without the responsibilities of the job.

The Berkeley Biochemistry Department was a perfect place for my interests. Daniel Koshland served as Chair and the faculty included a distinguished group of classical biochemists such as Esmond Snell, Jesse Rabinowitz, Clinton Ballou, Jack Kirsch and Howard Schachman, as well as a group with broader interests in genetics and molecular biology such as Allan Wilson, Stuart Linn, Ed Penhoet, Chamberlin, and Bruce and Giovanna Ames. Jeremy Thorner, a close friend from my Stanford years, had taken up a study of yeast pheromone biology as a beginning faculty member in the bacteriology and immunology department at Berkeley. Ballou was an expert in carbohydrate chemistry with a particular interest in the yeast cell wall. Koshland, whom I had met at Stanford, and Ames were most appealing because they blended genetics and biochemistry in a way that I found compatible with my temperament. I believed that my future colleagues would allow me the freedom to explore a new direction quite different from my graduate or postdoctoral work.

In the remaining time of my postdoctoral work, I completed a project and published a paper but all my thoughts were directed to my future at Berkeley. Of course, I had no experience with yeast and knew essentially no genetics so I planned to spend three weeks at the yeast genetics course offered at Cold Spring Harbor and taught by Fred Sherman and Gerald Fink. Sherman and Fink were master geneticists and were able to draw on all the major figures in the yeast community who dropped by to teach and remain for a day or two. It was a thrill to meet Lee Hartwell and to share my thoughts about how yeast cells may grow by vesicle traffic. On the other hand, like with thin section electron microscopy, my skills in yeast tetrad dissection were inadequate. I believe I held the record for fewest tetrads dissected until several years later when James Rothman took the course.

HOW TO STUDY SECRETION IN YEAST

As the time approached for the move to Berkeley, I worked feverishly to craft an NIH grant proposal that included a range of ideas on how to study secretion and membrane growth in yeast. Published evidence suggested that secretion was localized to the bud portion of the dividing cell but there were no tools available to study the localization of a newly synthesized plasma membrane protein. My ideas were fanciful but in the cold light of day, the NIH reviewing panel found my experience inadequate (I had no preliminary data) and my ideas unproven. The rejection was crushing and my colleagues must have wondered if their gamble on me was about to crash. Adding insult to injury, I was denied a Basil O'Connor starter grant from the March of Dimes where the interviewer found me intelligent but regretted that I had not proposed to work on cell division in Lesch Nyhan syndrome! Fortunately, the NSF, and friendly reviews from Lee Hartwell and Susan Henry, a young yeast geneticist who studied phospholipid regulation, rescued me with a grant in the princely amount of $35,000 for two years. With this and a small internal University grant, a modest effort took shape.

What to do first? In the fall of 1976, two graduate students joined my lab: Janet Scott and Chris Greer. Janet had transferred from another lab so she had to find something that would work quickly. I felt that in order to study the yeast plasma membrane it would be necessary to have a clean way to remove the cell wall avoiding the use of crude snail gut enzymes, Glusulase, that were used to convert cells to spheroplasts. Another lytic enzyme secreted by a soil bacterium, *Oerskovia xanthineolytica*, seemed a good source to begin a purification effort. Janet perfected the conditions of induction and purification of an enzyme we called lyticase (36). Subsequently the bacterial gene was cloned and lyticase is still used as a recombinant enzyme for experiments that require undamaged membranes. Chris also wanted to pursue a biochemical project, so I set him off on an effort to purify yeast actin, which at the time seemed a logical choice for a protein that may be involved in vesicle traffic. Chris completed the project but it was not until years later that Peter Novick, then a postdoctoral fellow in David Botstein's lab, showed that an actin *ts* mutation delayed and mislocalized secretion at a restrictive growth temperature (37).

With a small lab, a little money and time free from other responsibilities, I started a couple of my own projects to look at the localization of secretion with a focus on chitin, a polysaccharide in the division septum, and invertase an enzyme secreted into the cell wall. My first undergraduate research student, Vicki Brawley (now Chandler), helped me to study an unexpected surge in chitin synthesis that accompanied the arrest of the yeast cell division cycle in response to the mating pheromone α-factor. That work resulted in my first independent publication, a PNAS paper that was critically edited and communicated by my colleague Clint Ballou (38). The notion of localized deposition and activation of the plasma membrane enzyme chitin synthase seemed tractable but the subject excited little interest outside of a small and contentious community of yeast investigators. Fortunately, a breakthrough in the study of invertase secretion reinforced in my mind the importance of investigating a topic of general interest.

Within a few months, Peter Novick joined the group for his thesis work. Peter was quiet, focused and technically superior. His background was impressive, having trained as an undergraduate at MIT and during summers as a research student in the lab of Arthur Karlin at Columbia University where Peter's father was a Professor of Physics. Peter focused his studies on invertase, an enzyme that hydrolyzes sucrose to glucose and fructose and which yeast cells use to mobilize hexose for uptake by active transport at the cell surface. Invertase synthesis is repressed in cells growing on a medium containing high (2%) glucose and is derepressed when cells are shifted to low glucose (0.1%). Peter found that secretion of invertase is rapid: The pool of intracellular intermediates in the secretion of invertase is depleted within five minutes after the addition of cycloheximide to block new protein synthesis. He then looked at chemical agents that were reported to block secretion in animal cells to see if they could be used in yeast. My first thought was to find a way to block the fusion of secretory vesicles at the cell surface to see if both secretion and plasma membrane growth were arrested. Those experiments failed and we were faced with a question of how to find secretion mutants.

During that first year, I followed up on an intriguing observation made by Susan Henry, then at Albert Einstein Medical School, who showed that starvation of a yeast inositol auxotroph led to cell death and a rapid arrest in cell growth. She demonstrated that starved cells increase in buoyant density, suggesting an imbalance in macromolecule biosynthesis and net cell surface growth (39). I tested the possibility that inositol may be required for secretion and cell surface growth by assaying invertase activity in intact cells, a measure of enzyme in the cell wall (yeast cells are impermeable to and can not transport sucrose), and in detergent lysed spheroplasts from which the cell wall material had been removed, a measure of intracellular intermediates in secretion. Another dead end; I found that inositol starvation did not block secretion.

SECRETION MUTANTS

During my postdoctoral years, I kept a box of cards with ideas about what to pursue in my lab at Berkeley. One of many ideas was a search for secretion mutants. In retrospect, we could have initiated that search right away, but I was not a geneticist and just did not think that way. And when Novick's work inevitably turned to that approach, we assumed that a block to secretion would be lethal and that one would require a selection procedure to find what might be a rare *ts* lethal mutation. But what advantage could a dying secretion defective cell have over a viable one? One thought was to select against cells that could take up a toxic substance through a newly synthesized cell surface permease, one whose export would be blocked in a secretion mutant such that the mutant cell would survive exposure to the toxin. We settled on the yeast sulfate permease, which fails to discriminate sulfate and chromate. Under the right conditions, chromate kills cells that express the sulfate permease. Indeed in a screen of mutants that survived exposure to chromate at 37C, a standard non-permissive temperature for yeast, Peter found a *ts* lethal mutation that also blocks invertase secretion. However, on reconstructing the conditions of the selection, he found that this mutant died at 37C even more rapidly than the wild type strain in the presence or absence of chromate. So this was no selection at all! From this we concluded that the mutations may not be so rare after all and that a Hartwell style search among a set of random *ts* lethal mutations might turn up more secretion specific lesions.

The mutant, *sec1*, that came from the aborted attempt at a selection, turned out to conform to all the predictions we had made. At a permissive temperature, 24C, mutant cells behaved like wild type cells in growth and rapid secretion of invertase and another conveniently assayed secreted enzyme, acid phosphatase. The induction and appearance of sulfate permease was also normal. However, on shift to 37C, *sec1* mutant cells arrested secretion of invertase and acid phosphatase (Fig. 2), which accumulated to a high level within dying cells, and the sulfate permease failed to appear in intact cells. These blocks were reversible and on return to 25C, the accumulated invertase and acid phosphatase were secreted even in the absence of new protein synthesis. Thus, we concluded that the mutant Sec1 protein must be thermally, but reversibly, unstable.

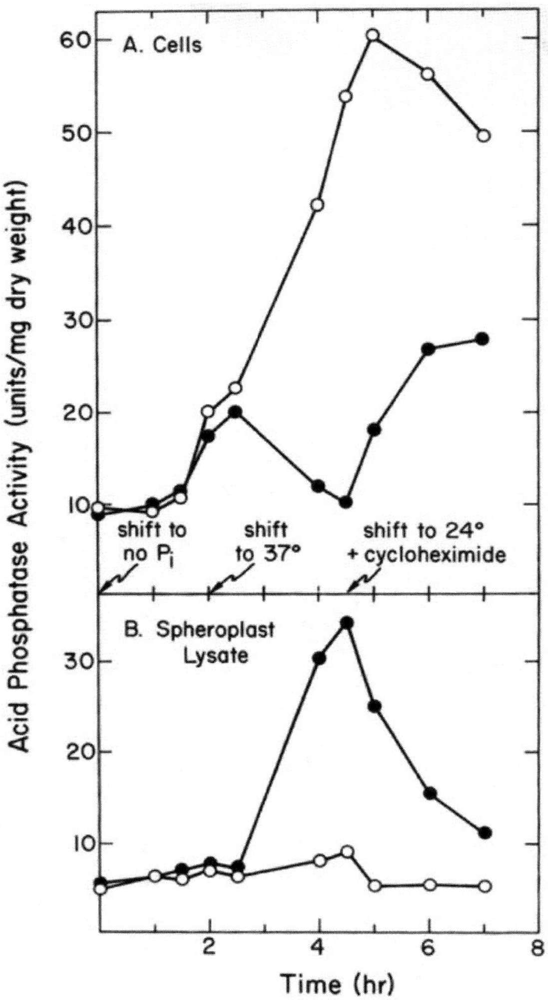

FIGURE 2. Secretion and accumulation of acid phosphatase in wild-type cells (open circles) and sec1 (closed circles) mutant cells (A) and spheroplasts (B). Reproduced from reference #40.

In May of 1978, George Palade visited Berkeley for two lectures in a series sponsored by the pharmaceutical company Smith, Kline and French. This was the first opportunity I had had to meet Palade personally and it was a thrill to be able to share with him what we were doing to study secretion in yeast. He was not aware that yeast cells secrete glycoproteins. The graduate students hosted Palade for dinner and in the course of the conversation, Peter Novick spoke of his new results on the *sec1* mutant. Palade encouraged Peter to examine the mutant by thin section microscopy. Shortly thereafter, Peter called my office from the EM lab in the basement of the Biochemistry building, urging that I come inspect the images of *sec1* mutant cells. The picture was stunning; cells chock full of vesicles filling the entire cytoplasmic compartment (Fig. 3). An enzyme-specific cytochemical stain for acid phosphatase showed all the vesicles carried this enzyme and likely other proteins secreted by yeast cells. Mutant cells grown at 24C behaved just like wild type cells did, with a small cluster of vesicles in the bud portion of the cell. Short of the moments I witnessed the birth of my children, nothing in my life compares to the excitement of that image in the EM room in the summer of 1978.

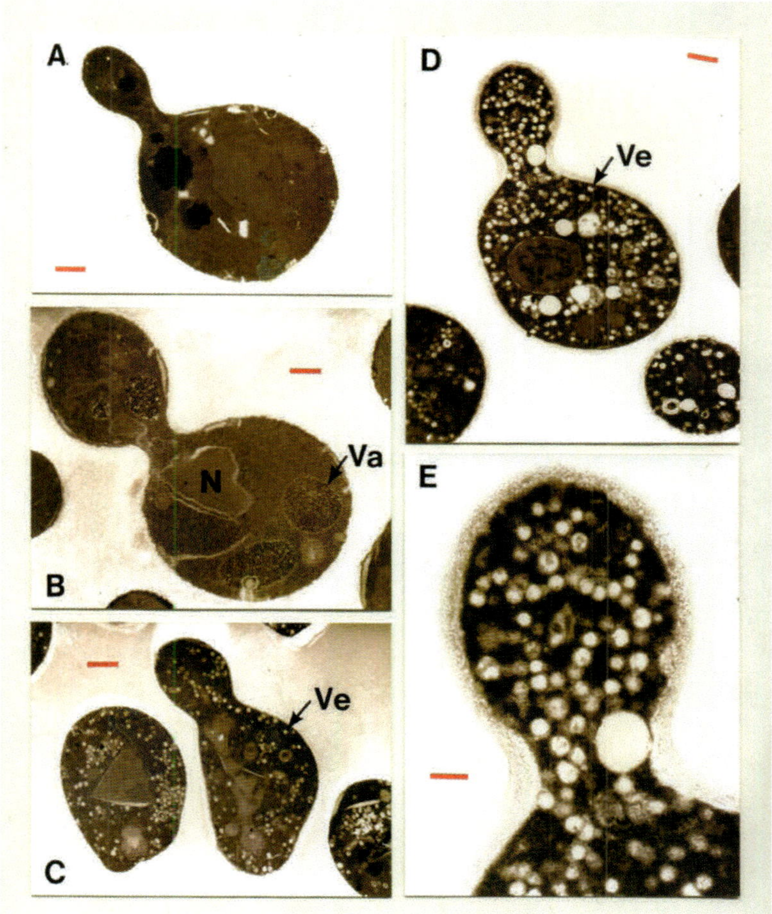

FIGURE 3. Wild-type (A) and sec 1 mutant cells at 24C (B) or 37C after 1h (C) or 3h (D, E). Reproduced from reference #40.

Peter and I assembled a paper for publication in the PNAS, which was communicated by Dan Koshland (40), and we continued a quest for more mutants of this sort because surely with a procedure that was unfavorable for the selection of *sec1*, many more genes might be found with no selection whatsoever. Peter collected 100 random *ts* mutant colonies by a standard mutagenesis protocol and found one more mutant, *sec2*, which phenotypically resembled *sec1* in accumulating a uniform population of vesicles. Thus at least two proteins were implicated in some step in the delivery of vesicles to a target membrane, possibly the plasma membrane. But surely there must be more such genes and the prospect of generating thousands of *ts* colonies in a time before the robotic approaches we now enjoy, was a bit daunting.

For the next of what would be a brilliant string of observations, Peter noticed that *sec1* mutant cells fail to enlarge, fail to divide and become phase refractile during an hour or more of incubation at 37C. This contrasts with the behavior of Hartwell's cell cycle *ts* mutants that arrest with a unique cell morphology characteristic of the cell cycle stage that is blocked, but that continue to enlarge into misshapen structures. Peter reasoned that secretion defective cells may continue to produce macromolecules but by failing to enlarge their buoyant density may increase, just as I had expected of the inositol auxotroph of Susan Henry. Peter then performed a beautiful experiment to test his theory. Mutant cells were constructed with a constitutively expressed form of acid phosphatase and an aliquot was incubated at 37C. A corresponding wild type cell sample with a normally repressed phosphatase gene was mixed in a ratio of 100:1 with the mutant cells and the mixed cells were centrifuged on a self-forming gradient of Ludox, a colloidal silica suspension that was then marketed as a commercial floor polish. Susan Henry had exploited the same preparation of Ludox to separate inositol-starved and normal cells. Fractions of the gradient plated on rich medium formed colonies that were then stained with a phosphatase-specific histochemical reagent to reveal the distribution of phosphatase-constitutive and -repressed colonies. The result was an absolute separation of *sec1* mutant cells at the bottom of the gradient and wild type cells at the top (Fig. 4). This density gradient then provided the opportunity Peter needed to enrich and screen many more *ts* colonies for additional *sec* mutants.

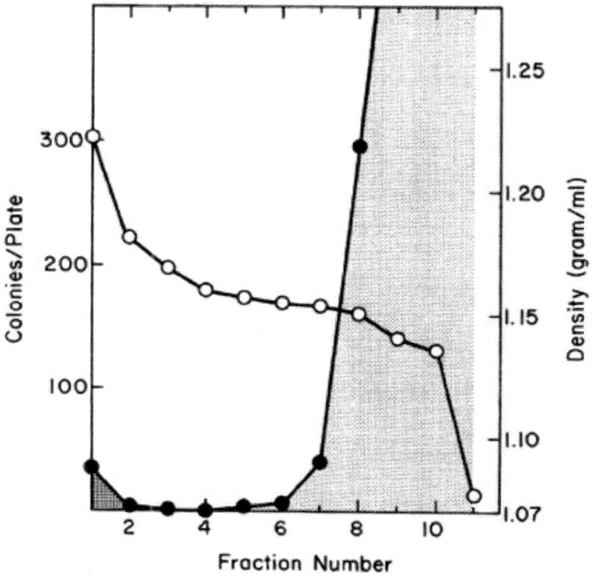

FIGURE 4. Ludox gradient of wild-type (light stipples) and sec1 mutant cells (heavy stipples) separated from bottom (high density) to top (low density) of centrifuge tube. Reproduced from ref. #41.

Over the next 18 months, Peter with Charles Field, a technician who was an expert in yeast genetics, repeated the mutagenesis on a large scale with different mutagens and assembled a large collection of density enriched *ts* colonies, 220 of which proved to be defective in secretion. Genetic complementation tests uncovered 23 genes among these mutants and the distribution of alleles suggested yet more genes were likely to be discovered. Electron microscopic inspection revealed three different phenotypic categories of organelle disruption: Mutations in 10 genes, like *sec1* and *2*, accumulated secretory vesicles, mutations in another 9 genes caused accumulation and distortion of the ER membrane, and another two caused a toroid-shaped organelle, which Novick called the "Berkeley body", to proliferate. One concern we had was that the *sec* mutations might not represent components of the secretory machinery, but merely defective biosynthetic cargo proteins that interfere with secretion. However, the simple complementation tests used to establish the genes showed all the alleles to be genetically recessive, and thus unlikely to represent dominant inhibitors of the process. Novick and Field completed a morphological and physiological characterization of selected alleles of each of the 23 genes, and we put together a comprehensive paper for the relatively new journal, Cell, which through the force of the personality of the Editor, Benjamin Lewin, was changing the way life science research was evaluated and promoted (41).

In the following year, Novick and Susan Ferro, who later became Susan Ferro-Novick (the first of many marriages within my laboratory), teamed up to apply a classic genetic epistasis test to establish the order in which the *SEC* genes exert their function. In the course of this work Peter found that one of the mutants *sec7* that accumulates the odd "Berkeley bodies" appeared to define a stage equivalent to that of the Golgi apparatus in mammalian cells. Quite by chance he found that this structure irreversibly blocked secretion unless cells were incubated in medium containing low glucose in which case mutant cells accumulate a classic, multi-cisternae Golgi structure (42). Some years later, Chris Kaiser, a talented postdoctoral fellow with considerable experience in yeast genetics, revisited the *SEC* genes that govern traffic early in the pathway and uncovered a distinct smaller vesicle species that mediates traffic between the ER and the Golgi complex (43). He classified a set of *SEC* genes that governs vesicle formation and another set required for vesicle consumption, presumably by a process of membrane fusion at the Golgi complex. Importantly, he showed that the two sets of genes show extensive genetic interactions, with mutations in each group exacerbating the mutant phenotype of other members of that group but not between the two groups. This behavior, referred to as synthetic lethal interaction, suggested that the members of each group function together, possibly by physical interaction with one another. These results led to a picture of the secretory pathway in yeast that was essentially the same as Palade had shown for mammalian cells, but with the crucial bonus that each step in the elaborate chain of events was now defined by genes and thus proteins that would surely illuminate the molecular mechanisms of this pathway (Figs. 5, 6).

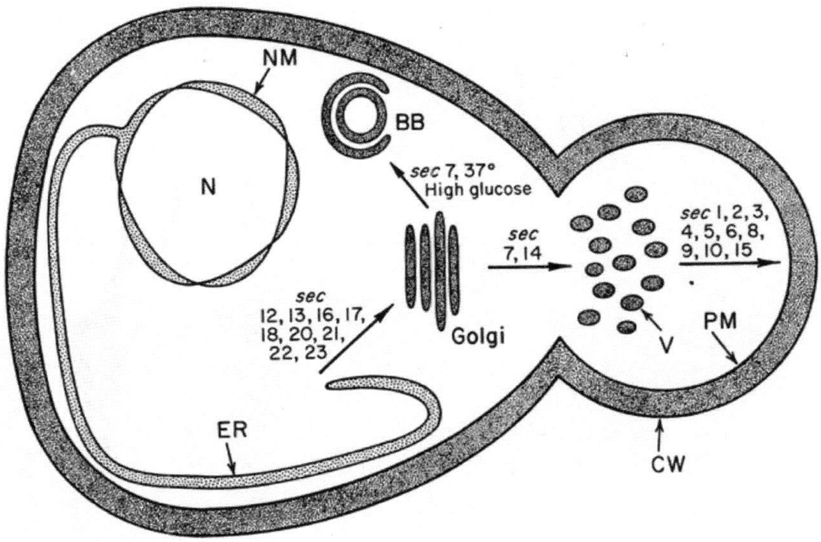

FIGURE 5. Yeast secretory pathway circa 1981. Reproduced from ref. #42.

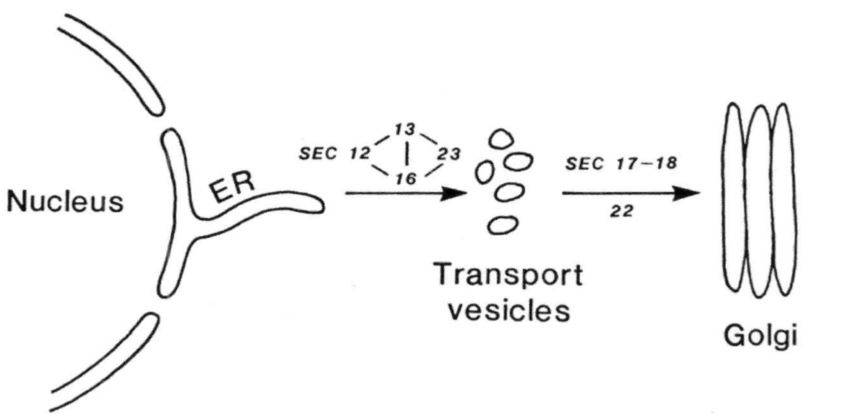

FIGURE 6. ER – Golgi vesicular traffic pathway circa 1990. Reproduced from ref. #43.

Two other studies added molecular detail to the emerging view of the secretory pathway in yeast. Brent Esmon, a graduate student in the lab, applied a histochemical stain for invertase on cell lysate samples that were electrophoretically resolved on a native polyacryamide gel. He discovered that the mutants defective in protein transport from the ER accumulate discrete forms of glycosylated invertase, distinct from invertase that progressed to the Golgi compartment and into secretory vesicles. Using antibodies that diagnose the "outer chain" carbohydrate epitopes of yeast glycoproteins, Brent learned that the division of labor between the ER and the Golgi complex in yeast with respect to *N*-glycan maturation is much the same as in mammalian cells (44). Tom Stevens, a postdoctoral fellow, studied the traffic of a protein to the yeast vacuole and found that it is diverted from the Golgi complex, similar to the traffic of lysosomal proteins in mammalian cells (45). Stevens and another postdoctoral fellow, Scott Emr, took this part of the pathway to their own labs at the University of Oregon and Cal Tech, respectively, to develop powerful genetic selections to uncover the genes that govern this sorting limb of the secretory pathway. The *VPS* genes continue to illuminate the process of sorting from the Golgi complex to the endosome and on to the vacuole or lysosome in all nucleated organisms.

Given our finding that the yeast and mammalian secretory pathways are fundamentally conserved, the biotech industry was quick to exploit the fermentation possibilities of yeast culture to engineer the expression of commercial quantities of important human secreted proteins. Chiron, near Berkeley in the San Francisco Bay Area was the first to succeed. Recombinant expression of the hepatitis B surface antigen in yeast resulted in the production of virus-like membrane particles that proved to be highly immunogenic and which were commercialized as a potent hepatitis vaccine, the sole source of that product in use today (46). As hepatitis B is the major cause of primary liver cancer, the successful introduction of this product of the yeast secretory pathway could, if fully implemented, dramatically reduce the incidence of liver cancer. Indeed this commercial product is considered the first anti-cancer vaccine. Chiron next engineered the expression and secretion of human insulin in yeast and that product, now marketed by Novo Nordisk, accounts for one-third of the world supply of human recombinant insulin.

I never patented any of our discoveries or thought to do work directed to commercial application in my laboratory because I was completely absorbed by the pursuit of fundamental knowledge. Nonetheless, as a consultant to Chiron I did benefit financially and was enormously gratified to see our work applied to such important practical goals. My view is that the work of drug discovery and practical application is best left to the private sector and that University scientists should focus on basic discovery.

IMPORTANT GENES UNCOVERED BY OTHER MEANS

Although the initial set of *SEC* genes revealed the broad outline of the secretory pathway, it became clear that key elements in the process were not reflected in the Novicks' mutants. We had hoped to find mutations that block the insertion of secretory polypeptides into the lumen of the ER and thus to define genes that constitute the translocation channel predicted by the classic work of Palade, Sabatini and Blobel. The key prediction was that mutations in a putative channel would accumulate unglycosylated secretory precursor polypeptides in the cytoplasm. No such defects were found in the initial set of *sec* mutations. Susan Ferro conducted a wider search for mutants using the density gradient technique and turned up two that accumulated unglycosylated forms of invertase (47). However, on closer inspection these mutations identified genes involved in the biosynthesis of glycans on secretory proteins rather than bona fide catalysts of translocation (48, 49). Clearly, a different, more directed approach was needed.

Studies in *E. coli* and in yeast showed that the N-terminal signal peptide is necessary and sufficient for the translocation of a secretory protein across the cytoplasmic membrane or ER membrane, respectively (50, 51). The recombinant expression of a chimeric protein constructed by the fusion of a signal peptide coding sequence and the *E. coli* β-galactosidase gene, encoding a soluble cytoplasmic enzyme, result in the membrane translocation of the hybrid protein. Beckwith and colleagues found the expression of such a hybrid protein in *E. coli* provided a selectable growth phenotype, which they used to isolate translocation defective *sec* mutations, defining the novel cytoplasmic proteins SecA and SecB (52). Using other genetic approaches, Silhavy, Ito and colleagues identified a gene encoding a membrane protein, PrlA/SecY, a candidate for the bacterial translocation channel (53, 54).

Ray Deshaies, an unusually creative and confident graduate student joined the lab in the mid 1980s and after an initial effort with the existing *sec* mutants, he decided to revisit the translocation problem. In three brilliant but entirely independent efforts, he succeeded in defining a number of genes required in the translocation process. Ray reasoned that if a signal peptide were appended to a cytoplasmic enzyme required for the production of an essential nutrient, the enzyme would be sequestered in the ER, removed from contact with its substrate. In this situation, cells would grow on the nutrient but not on its substrate unless a mutation was introduced that blocked the translocation of the hybrid protein into the ER. Of course, a mutation in an essential channel protein would likely kill the cell, so the quest was for mutations that crippled but did not destroy proteins required for the assembly process. Temperature-sensitive lethal mutations often exert a partial effect at a permissive temperature, thus the search was for mutations that grow at 30C on the substrate, in this case histidinol, the substrate of the enzyme histidinol dehydrogenase, the last step in the biosynthesis of histidine, but which fail to form colonies at 37C on rich growth medium. Ray's first mutant was called *sec61* and further searches using the same selection identified five other genes that encode additional functions essential for translocation, including other subunits of the channel complex and a subunit of the signal recognition particle (SRP) (55, 56). Subsequent cloning of these genes revealed that *SEC61* is homologous to the PrlA/SecyY gene of *E. coli* (57). Comparable genes are found in mammals, and biochemical analysis demonstrated that the Sec61 protein constitutes the core of the channel protein through which secretory and membrane proteins pass during assembly in the ER (58, 59).

Deshaies also tackled the question of how certain secretory proteins may be translocated post-translationally in yeast. In contrast to the classical rule of co-translational translocation discovered by Blobel, Peter Walter, a protégé of Blobel's, discovered that at least one substrate, the precursor of the yeast mating pheromone α-factor, could pass across the ER membrane after the completion of translation (60). The assumption was that something extrinsic or intrinsic to α-factor precursor held it in a form that could readily unfold during the translocation event.

In reading an influential review article by Hugh Pelham on the possible role of the heat shock protein family hsp70 in dispersing protein aggregates (61), Ray imagined that hsp70 might also serve to retain partially unfolded forms of post-translational substrates such as α-factor precursor. Fortunately, we were in a position to test this *in vivo* because Margaret Werner-Washburn and Elizabeth Craig had just constructed a yeast strain missing three members of the major hsp70 class of proteins and with a *ts* mutation in the remaining fourth gene such that the quadruple mutant was *ts* lethal. Ray established in short order that this mutant accumulated untranslocated α-factor precursor and as a bonus, he found that the β subunit of the mitochondrial F_1-ATPase, also post-translationally translocated into that organelle, accumulated in the cytoplasm. Ray and independently Chirico and Blobel showed that the requirement for Hsp70 could be reproduced in the cell-free reaction that reconstitutes the translocation of α-factor precursor into isolated yeast ER membranes (62, 63).

In a third example of Deshaies' creative instinct, he solved a problem that had bedeviled a postdoc, Peter Bohni, who had struggled for two years to devise a selection for a mutation in the yeast signal peptidase, the enzyme that Blobel demonstrated cleaves the signal on a secretory polypeptide as it emerges on the luminal side of the ER. Neither the enzyme nor the gene for the peptidase had been obtained, thus it was of interest to test the function of the protein, which at that time remained a candidate for a subunit of the translocation channel. We knew that a mutation at the yeast invertase signal peptide cleavage site delayed the secretion of active enzyme, which accumulates in a precursor form in the ER (64). Attempts to devise a selection for mutations in the peptidase based on that secretion delay proved futile. Ray suggested that some uncleaved cargo proteins might be delayed more seriously than others and that a peptidase mutant could be in our original collection of *sec* mutants and would have the unusual characteristic of blocking only a subset of cargo proteins. In Peter Novick's last effort as a graduate student, he had devised a cell surface chemical labeling procedure to assess the full range of major cargo proteins and how their cell surface appearance is affected in *sec* mutant cells incubated at 37C (65). Curiously, one mutant in the original collection, sec11, showed an anomalous effect with certain cargo proteins blocked and others less so. With this insight, Bohni immediately investigated the *sec11* mutant and found that it accumulated uncleaved invertase at a restrictive temperature (66). The *SEC11* gene was cloned and found to be the prototype of all eukaryotic signal peptidases (67).

CLONING GENES AS AN ADJUNCT TO FUNCTIONAL ANALYSIS OF SEC PROTEINS

With the advent of cloning yeast genes by complementation, pioneered by Hinnen and Fink in 1978 (68), we had the immediate prospect of a molecular description of the *SEC* genes and a possible alignment of these genes with comparable functions in simple metazoans and perhaps even mammals. I resisted the temptation to launch in this direction because it seemed unlikely that the *SEC* genes would look like anything else then known. After all, DNA sequencing was still in its infancy and genome databases were nonexistent. Almost from the outset of our characterization of the *sec* mutants, my focus was on attempting to develop a cell-free reaction that reproduced the function of Sec proteins. Most students and fellows who joined the lab resisted my entreaties or took up only half-hearted attempts. One initial effort in this direction yielded a feeble signal that seemed unlikely to prove useful (69). And yet, just miles away in his new lab at Stanford, Jim Rothman had succeeded in developing a reaction that appeared to measure a significant limb of the Golgi traffic pathway reconstituted in a lysate of mammalian cells (70). My own efforts remained on hold until I found a courageous student to take up the challenge.

SEC53 was the first *SEC* gene cloned and identified with a biochemical function. Although *sec53* was isolated and initially characterized as a mutant defective in translocation, the gene sequence predicted a soluble protein (71), which on closer inspection proved to be to the enzyme phosphomannomutase involved in the production of GDP-mannose, the precursor of *N*- and *O*-glycans in yeast (48). Other *SEC* genes were cloned but other than predicting that *SEC12* encoded an ER membrane protein and *SEC18* encoded a soluble cytoplasmic protein, no functional biochemical role could be seen in the sequences (72,73).

The first real breakthrough with respect to vesicular traffic came in 1987 when Novick, now in his own lab at Yale, cloned and sequenced *SEC4*, which he showed encoded a small GTP-binding protein of the RAS family (74). Novick's focus on *SEC4* was no accident. We had agreed that he could take charge of the group of *sec* mutants that block late in the pathway and accumulate mature secretory vesicles. Salminen and Novick found that *SEC4* overexpression suppressed the growth defect of several members of the group of late acting sec mutants, and that double mutants constructed among the members of this class displayed a synthetic lethal form of genetic interaction. As the genomes of other organisms were sequenced, it became clear that *SEC4* was a prototype of what are now called Rab proteins, each of which defines a unique destination for the fusion of vesicles to a target membrane. Continuing on the brilliant path he established right from the start of his graduate work, Novick has built a substantial body of highly original work that reveals detailed mechanisms associated with the production, migration and fusion of transport vesicles at the yeast cell surface. And given the fundamental conservation of the *SEC* gene sequences, it is no surprise that Novick's insights extend to all comparable vesicle targeting/fusion events in metazoans and mammals. Indeed, *SEC1* was found to be related to the unc-18 gene isolated in the original collection of uncoordinated mutants of *C. elegans* isolated by Sydney Brenner (75,76). And the Sec1 protein is known to play a universal role in the control of SNARE protein action in vesicle fusion.

Jim Rothman's pioneering initial effort to purify proteins required for vesicle fusion yielded the soluble ATPase, NSF (NEM-sensitive factor), which on cloning revealed a striking similarity to the yeast Sec18 protein, a gene that had been cloned by Scott Emr in his own lab at Cal Tech (73,77). At around the same time, Chris Kaiser in my lab had detected a vesicle intermediate between the ER and Golgi, whose consumption by fusion required the genetically interacting genes *SEC18*, *SEC17* and *SEC22* (43). In a joint paper, our labs showed that *SEC17* encodes the yeast equivalent of α-SNAP, a protein Rothman's lab discovered as the factor required for NSF to bind a membrane site, later defined as the SNARE protein (78). Later work showed that *SEC22* encodes one such yeast SNARE protein. These results made it clear that the two labs were working on fundamentally the same problem and forged a persuasive link between the mechanism of vesicle targeting/fusion in yeast and mammalian cells.

The mechanism of secretory vesicle budding was now accessible to molecular analysis. Palade had seen coated vesicles at the ER exit site in sections of pancreatic exocrine cells and the view was that the mechanism of budding would involve a coat similar to the classic clathrin coat first visualized as a coated pit engaged in yolk protein internalization in insect oocytes and characterized molecularly by Barbara Pearse with isolated bovine brain clathrin coated vesicles (79, 80). Rothman had evidence to suggest a role for clathrin in the transport of vesicular stomatitis virus G protein from the ER in cultured mammalian cells (81). Thus, clathrin or a similar coat protein was a candidate for one or more of the *SEC* genes required for traffic from the ER.

Greg Payne decided to assess the role of clathrin directly by cloning the gene for the heavy chain and characterizing the phenotype of a clathrin gene knockout in yeast. Given the expected role of clathrin in vesicular traffic, we assumed the gene would – like the *SEC* genes – be essential for cell viability. Yet, after disruption of the heavy chain gene in a diploid strain, Greg was shocked to see 2 disrupted spores in each tetrad growing after a several day lag phase. Clathrin deficient cells were sickly but continued to secrete even when the gene was knocked out in a number of different genetic backgrounds (82). Lemmon and Jones reported a strain in which the heavy chain gene was essential but it now seems likely this strain carried an additional mutation that exerted a synthetic lethal effect in the absence of clathrin (83). Further analysis showed that clathrin was required for the proper sorting/retention of a Golgi-localized dibasic peptidase essential for the proteolytic maturation of α-factor precursor (84). These results conformed nicely to the suggestion by Lelio Orci that clathrin coats mediate the retrieval of the proinsuln processing protease from condensing granules in pancreatic β cells (85). The search continued for a coat mechanism in the formation of secretory transport vesicles.

A YEAST CELL-FREE VESICULAR TRANSPORT REACTION

I knew that the full potential of the *sec* mutant collection awaited the development of a cell-free reaction to recapitulate at least a portion of the pathway *in vitro*. Finally, in 1985, I recruited a brilliant and creative graduate student, David Baker, who shared my vision and had the talent to make it happen. Up to that point we had relied on the accumulation of precursor glycoproteins in *sec* mutant cells arrested at 37C to serve as substrates in *in vitro* reactions. Immature glycoproteins become modified by specific outer chain glycan decorations *en route* through the Golgi complex when cells are returned to the permissive temperature, and we assumed the same would be true *in vitro*. This assumption proved wrong. The first hint of a problem came in the evaluation of *sec53* mutant phosphomannomutase, which proved to be inactive even in lysates of cells that were grown at a permissive temperature (48). But without such a block to accumulate substrates in the ER, the assay for traffic would have to rely on a low level of immature glycoproteins radiolabelled for a brief time during biosynthesis. Rothman had succeeded with just such an approach (71), but the transit time of glycoproteins in yeast is much quicker than in mammalian cells.

David had a fresh idea. Peter Walter's lab (as well as the labs of David Meyer and Blobel) had reconstituted the translocation of radiolabled α-factor precursor into ER membranes prepared by mechanical disruption of yeast spheroplasts (61). The product of this incubation was a core *N*-glycosylated species that migrated at a discrete position on SDS-PAGE separation. David guessed that membranes prepared by a more gentle lysis procedure, basically a quick freeze-thaw of yeast spheroplasts, might preserve membrane organization well enough to permit vesicular traffic of the core glycan modified synthetic α-factor precursor. Within a few weeks of starting, David observed the production of a heterogeneous spread of low electrophoretic mobility forms of the radioactive precursor, which importantly was precipitated by antibodies directed against mannose epitopes added to N-glycans in the yeast Golgi complex. The reaction required cytosol, ATP and incubation at a physiological temperature. The results were most promising and the assay was amenable to quantification and easy repetition with many samples.

The crucial test of Baker's reaction was to examine the effect of an ER-blocked *sec* mutant in the cell-free reaction. Linda Hicke, an ambitious and technically gifted graduate student had cloned *SEC23*, one of the four genes Kaiser found to interact in the formation of ER-derived transport vesicles. She collaborated with Baker to reproduce the α-factor precursor transport reaction in separate incubations containing membranes from wild type (wt) cells mixed with cytosol fractions from wild type (wt), mutant and mutant cells complemented with the wt gene. The results were stunning, with a clear *ts* defect in transport complemented by a wt copy of Sec23p supplied in the mutant cytosol fraction (86) (Fig. 7). Amazingly, Susan Ferro-Novick and her graduate student Hannele Ruohola, developed virtually the same methodology yielding similar results in their laboratory at Yale (87).

Baker and Hicke's results were precisely what I had dreamed of and the experimental design was modeled on my own graduate research, in which I used complementation of mutant lysates as an assay to purify functional DNA replication enzymes (19). With her assay, Linda was able to purify overexpressed recombinant Sec23p and then to show that it copurified with anther protein that was not represented in our original mutant collection but which proved to be encoded by another essential gene, which we then called *SEC24* (88).

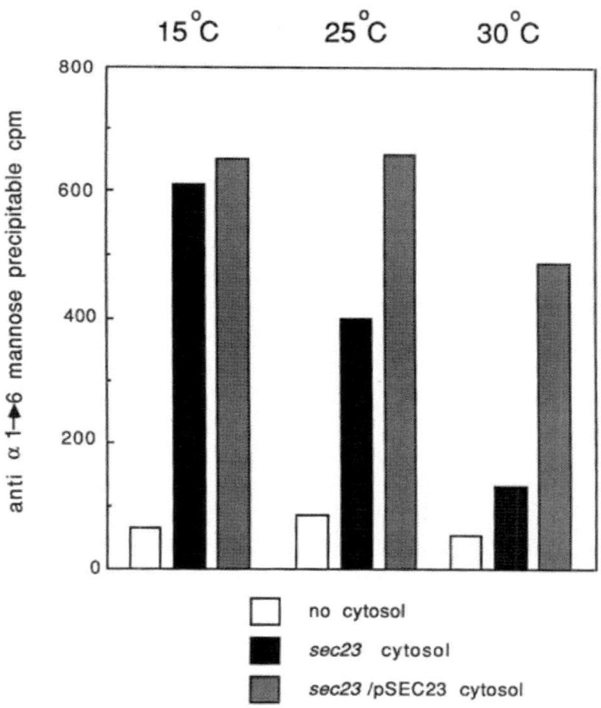

FIGURE 7. Temperature sensitive transport of α-factor precursor. Golgi glycan-modified precursor in incubations at 15C, 25C and 30C containing yeast membranes and no cytosol (open bar), sec23 mutant ytosol (dark bar) or cytosol from sec23 mutant strain complemented with SEC23.

By itself the purified heterodimer of functional Sec23/24p did not offer any clues to its role in ER vesicle budding. For this we required purified forms of the other cytosolic components necessary for budding of α-factor precursor. The next factor came by a circuitous route. Akihiko Nakano, the first of a series of outstanding postdoctoral fellows from Japan, had cloned the ER membrane protein Sec12 that we knew from Kaiser's genetic work was intimately connected to the set of soluble Sec proteins involved in vesicle budding (43, 59). We had in our collection a set of genes cloned by overexpression suppression of the *sec12* mutation. One clone suppressed *sec12 ts* growth even when its copy number was only two-fold of normal. Aki took this gene back to his lab in Japan and found that it encoded another small GTP binding protein, though of a class distinct from *SEC4*. This gene, which he called *SAR1*, also proved essential for secretion (89). Christophe D'Enfert, a postdoc from Paris, found that membranes isolated from a strain overexpressing *SEC12* were defective in the transport reaction unless the cytosol contained overexpressed Sar1p (90). This became the assay to purify functional Sar1 that we found could also be isolated by recombinant expression in *E. coli* (91).

As the proteins required for budding were being lined-up, it became clear that the requirements for the full transport reaction were quite complex and it seemed reasonable to devise a simpler assay to focus only on vesicle formation. Michael Rexach joined the lab as a graduate student and brought considerable skill and stubborn determination to this goal. Using a simple technique of differential centrifugation, Michael observed that ER membranes remained intact during the course of the cell-free incubation, as measured by the rapid sedimentation of ER marker proteins. In contrast, he found as the incubation proceeded that a substantial fraction of the core glycosylated α-factor precursor, which was initially contained within large ER envelopes, was transferred into a slowly-sedimenting vesicle species, which lacked translocation activity and other marker proteins of the ER membrane and lumen. Importantly, the formation of this vesicle species was blocked in the mutants that Kaiser showed to be defective in the production of the vesicle intermediate *in vivo* (*sec12* and *sec23*), but not in mutants blocked later (*sec18*) (92). Again, similar results were obtained in Ferro-Novick's lab (93). Rexach's work provided us with the essential tool we needed to complete the purification and functional analysis of the proteins required for vesicle budding from the ER.

Two other genes required for ER vesicle formation remained to be functionally identified: *SEC13* and *SEC16*. In his own lab at MIT, Kaiser cloned and characterized *SEC16* and learned that it encodes a 240kD peripheral membrane protein, not readily released into the cytosol (94). Nancy Pryer, a postdoc in our lab, cloned *SEC13* and found that it encodes a small cytosolic protein that contains a series of WD-40 repeats, very similar to the G protein β subunit (95). Members of this family have a 7-member β propeller structure common to proteins that engage in reversible multi-subunit protein interactions. Nina Salama, an effervescent graduate student in the lab, used Rexach's budding reaction to purify a functional form of Sec13p and found that it co-purifies with an additional subunit, which we cloned and characterized as a novel *SEC* gene, *SEC31* (96). With this last piece of the puzzle, we found that the budding reaction was sustained with isolated membranes and pure, recombinant Sar1p, Sec23/24p and Sec13/31p, with Sec16p presumably being supplied by the membrane fraction. A complete functional analysis of the mechanism of vesicle budding was now at hand.

COPII MEDIATES VESICLE BUDDING FROM THE ER

We had few clues as to the mechanism of vesicle budding mediated by the pure Sec proteins in our collection. Rothman's lab had identified and characterized a novel coat protein complex, coatomer, required for vesicle budding in transport within the Golgi complex (97). He suggested that this coat may also be required for vesicular traffic from the ER, but we found no evidence for subunits of the coatomer in our purified set of Sec proteins. In addition, we had cloned and characterized a different *SEC* gene, *SEC21*, that encodes a subunit of coatomer and although the *sec21* mutant is blocked in traffic from the ER, it did not fit neatly into one of Kaiser's mutant classes, and we attributed its effect on traffic from the ER to a backlog of cargo that accumulates when Golgi function is disrupted (98).

Several key insights developed in the1990s that consolidated our efforts. Two wonderful new postdocs in the lab, Charles Barlowe and Tohru Yoshihisa, discovered a cycle of GTP hydrolysis and exchange on Sar1p. Tohru found that the Sec23 subunit is a GTP hydrolysis catalyst (GAP) specific for Sar1p and Charlie found that the cytoplasmic domain of Sec12p catalyzes nucleotide exchange on Sar1p (99,100). Several years later Bruno Antonny, a tremendously skilled and perceptive biophysicist, discovered that the Sec31 subunit of the 13/31 heterotetramer complex accelerates the GAP activity of Sec23 10-fold (101). Clearly, a coordinated assembly event controlled by GTP binding and hydrolysis, served to frame the budding process. Given Rothman's discovery of a role for GTP binding in the control of coatomer assembly and vesicle budding on Golgi membranes, we were primed for the prospect of a novel coat complex (102).

Fate intervened again in the form of a phone call from the maestro of membrane morphology, Lelio Orci at the University of Geneva Medical School. Orci was instrumental in the effort to discover the morphologic stages in vesicle formation and fusion in the Golgi complex uncovered in the Rothman lab cell-free transport reaction. His skills were so extraordinary that I had attempted, unsuccessfully, to engage his interest when our work uncovered a role for clathrin in the retrieval of a Golgi enzyme similar to his discovery of the organization of clathrin and proinsulin processing in β-cells of the pancreas (85). His call in 1990 was prompted by our recent publication of Kaiser's analysis of the vesicle species that mediates traffic from the ER. Lelio took pity on us for the primitive standards of our thin section EM analysis and graciously offered his help in a collaboration to examine the organization of the Sec proteins involved in ER vesicle formation. His first success was in using our antibody against the yeast Sec23p to localize the mammalian homolog precisely at the ER exit site in sections of pancreatic tissue (103). But the greatest excitement came when he discovered a novel coat that surrounded the vesicles formed in a reaction with yeast membranes and our purified Sec proteins. Barlowe isolated these vesicles and we saw a hint of a coat in thin sections prepared by my skilled EM technician, Susan Hamamoto, but the images Orci produced were simply breathtaking (Fig. 8). We called this novel coat COPII and suggested that the Rothman/Orci coat be referred to as COPI (104). I count it as one of the great privileges of my career to have enjoyed over 20 years of continuous collaboration with Orci, a scholar and experimentalist of the highest distinction.

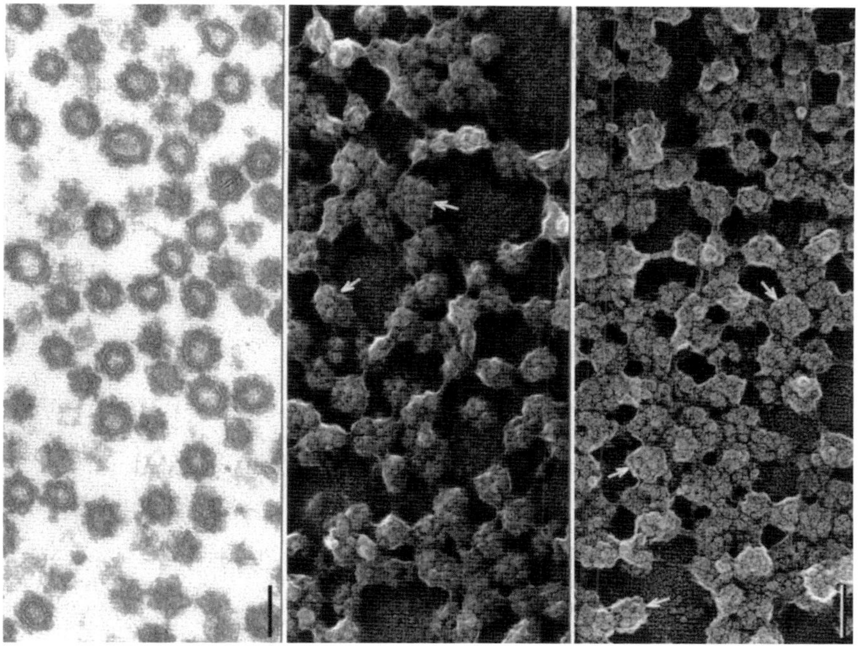

FIGURE 8. Thin section transmission and scanning EM images of COPII vesicles. Bar, 100nm. Courtesy of Lelio Orci, Univ. of Geneva.

In a crucial initial collaboration, Orci and a new postdoc in the lab, Sebastian Bednarek, defined the ER as the morphological site of COPII budding. Sebastian purified yeast nuclei as a source of pure ER membrane and with Orci showed that COPII proteins, and curiously also COPI, form buds and incorporate cargo molecules from the outer nuclear membrane. Using a sequential binding assay, Sebastian demonstrated that the COPII assembles in pieces with Sar1p and Sec23/24p binding first and constituting an inner layer of the coat with Sec13/31p forming the outer layer of the coat (105).

With a purified ensemble of cytosolic proteins in hand, we turned our attention to the contribution of membrane proteins and lipids in an effort to define the minimum requirements for vesicle budding.

Sec16p represented the most obvious part of the machinery not accounted for in our reconstituted reaction. Two successive postdoctoral fellows, Joe Campbell and Frantisek Supek, found conditions in which a role for Sec16p in the budding reaction could be observed (106, 107). Eugene Futai succeeded in purifying recombinant Sec16p and found conditions in which it controlled the GTPase cycle mediated by the interaction of the full set of COPII proteins and Sar1 (108). Yet even now, it is not clear if Sec16 participates actively in the cycle of vesicle budding or rather plays a regulatory role in organizing COPII proteins at the ER exit site.

We considered the possibility that coat assembly may be regulated by the availability of membrane cargo proteins. Tom Yeung, a graduate student in the lab, found that membranes isolated from cells treated with cycloheximide, and thus purged of newly-synthesized cargo, were perfectly active in budding COPII vesicles as assayed by the incorporation of a SNARE protein (109). Although biosynthetic cargo may not be essential for vesicle budding, we suggested that proteins cycling between the ER and Golgi might constitute an essential element of the membrane contribution to the formation of a COPII bud (110).

To test directly the role of membrane proteins and lipids in the budding event, Yeung initiated an effort to solubilize the membrane with detergents to see if membrane proteins and lipids could be reconstituted into liposomes capable of budding synthetic COPII vesicles. To our surprise, Yeung and a meticulous new postdoctoral fellow, Ken Matsuoka, systematically documented that synthetic COPII vesicles bud and could be isolated by density gradient sedimentation from reactions conducted with pure phospholipid liposomes of defined composition provided the reaction was conducted in the presence of a non-hydrolyzable analog of GTP (111). Bruno Antonny developed an elegant real time light scattering assay to monitor the stepwise assembly and disassembly of the coat in incubations containing GTP or a nonhydrolyzable analog (101). Eugene Futai then showed that GTP could replace a nonhydrolyzable analog to produce a stable COPII coated membrane provided the reaction was supplemented with the cytoplasmic domain of the Sar1p nucleotide exchange catalyst, Sec12p, presumably stabilizing the coat by repeated rounds of GTP nucleotide exchange. Curiously, these reactions arrested with buds on liposomes, but few if any completed COPII vesicles (112). More recently, Kirsten Bacia, another postdoctoral fellow, reconstituted the budding reaction on giant unilamellar vesicles where the process may be visualized in real time by light and fluorescence microscopy without potentially damaging manipulation, e.g. centrifugation. In these conditions, incubations containing the COPII proteins and nonhydrolyzable GTP produce long, multi-lobed, coated tubules with regular points of constriction but with little evidence of vesicle fission (113). The nature of the COPII fission reaction remains unresolved but appears to hinge on spatial regulation of GTP binding and hydrolysis at the vesicle bud neck.

The initial event that leads to a bud may begin when Sar1p acquires GTP through interaction with Sec12. Structural analysis showed that the soluble GDP-bound form of Sar1 shields an N-terminal amphipathic helix in a cleft of the folded protein (114). Nucleotide exchange displaces the N-terminus and renders activated Sar1p highly insoluble and prone to membrane insertion. Marcus Lee, an insightful postdoctoral fellow, reasoned that the embedment of the N-terminus in the bilayer may laterally displace phospholipids and create a local asymmetry in the surface area of the two leaflets, much as Sheetz and Singer had proposed decades earlier in the bilayer couple hypothesis (115). In a series of elegant experiments conducted in collaboration with Orci, Lee showed that Sar1p promotes the formation of membrane tubules from synthetic liposomes dependent on the insertion of the amphipathic N-terminal helix and that this insertion is required for COPII vesicle formation *in vitro* and protein transport *in vivo* (116).

Tremendous progress has been made on the structural analysis of the COPII coat, principally by the laboratories of Jonathan Goldberg and William Balch (117, 118, 119). We now have a detailed understanding of the mechanism of polymerization of the two layers of the coat and a key insight concerning the scaffold complex that forms the outer layer, a regular polyhedral lattice that Balch discovered in a self-assembly reaction with purified mammalian Sec13/31 heterotetramer. A former postdoctoral co-worker, Giulia Zanetti, using cryo-electron microscopy has now visualized the lattice network of COPII formed on the surface of a synthetic liposome (120). Although little evidence suggests any significant structural or functional differences between the yeast and mammalian COPII proteins, mammals have the capacity to regulate the size of the coat to accommodate large or irregularly-shaped cargo complexes such as lipoproteins and pro-collagen. A posttranslational modification, ubiquitylation of Sec31, may serve to regulate some aspect of coat assembly to create a more flexible carrier (121).

An unexpected connection developed between the structure and function of the two layers of the COPII coat in the discovery of a mutation in the human Sec23A subunit. Simeon Boyadjiev and Waffa Eyaid, a Saudi colleague, examined a Bedouin family in which children have a rare craniofacial disorder. The recessive mutation maps to an invariant phenylalanine residue corresponding to a position on the structure of yeast Sec23p facing away from the surface predicted to abut the cytoplasmic face of the ER, a residue not at that time known to have any particular role in coat function or assembly. Orci examined primary skin fibroblasts from one of the afflicted children and observed a profound distortion of the ER and an accumulation of procollagen consistent with a severe defect in secretion (122). Fortunately for us, Jinoh Kim, a courageous postdoc in the lab, had systematically perfected a COPII vesicle budding reaction using membranes isolated from cultured mammalian cells (123). Chris Fromme, another ambitious and skilled postdoctoral fellow, took up the effort to recapitulate the defect seen in the human F382L mutant Sec23A. Chris found conditions that reproduce a budding defect and showed that the defect could be suppressed by increasing the level of recombinant human Sec13/31 in a budding reaction. Further he showed, with all pure mammalian COPII proteins, that the F382L mutant Sec23A has trouble making contact with the Sec13/31 complex as reflected in reduced stimulation of Sar1p GTP hydrolysis (124). At the same time, Goldberg's lab had solved the structure of the yeast Sec23/24 heterodimer in complex with a fragment of yeast Sec31 that stimulates the GAP activity of Sec23p (125). The point of closest contact between Sec31and Sec23 was located within angstroms of the position corresponding to the human F382 residue. Thus, the structure of the yeast protein and the functional deficit resulting from mutation in humans could be perfectly reconciled.

THE COPII COAT GUIDES CARGO SELECTION IN YEAST AND IN MAMMALIAN CELLS AND TISSUES

In the early 90s the prevailing view was that sorting of secretory and ER resident proteins occurs after cargo exits the ER, mediated by retrieval receptors that return escaped resident proteins back to the ER. Powerful support for this model came with the discovery and characterization of a retrieval signal and a receptor for soluble resident ER proteins such as the luminal hsp70 chaperone, BiP (126). Measurements of the rate of traffic of certain artificial proteins introduced into the secretory pathway argue against the need for active sorting of secretory proteins *en route* through the pathway (127). Furthermore, two major proteins secreted in the liver appear not to be concentrated in buds that form at the ER exit site, but instead later at the point of COPI-mediated resident protein retrieval (128). Although this issue continues to be the subject of considerable disagreement (129), the results of our vesicle budding reaction where resident proteins are largely excluded from COPII vesicles formed *in vitro* support an alternative view that active protein sorting accompanies the budding reaction and that resident protein retrieval mediated by sorting receptors in the Golgi membrane may represent a back up mechanism to reinforce the primary event in the ER (92,104). Substantial evidence developed over the past 15 years documents a role for ER-localized secretory cargo receptors and one particular subunit of the COPII coat, Sec24p, in the concentrative sorting of membrane and soluble luminal cargo proteins into COPII transport vesicles (130).

If secretory proteins are actively sorted into COPII vesicles, it should be possible to define a sorting signal by the isolation of point mutant forms that produce properly folded precursors that persist in the ER lumen. In practice this has proved difficult because of the uncertainly that a mutant protein may be subject to the quality control retention of misfolded proteins in the ER. Irene Schauer, one of the early graduate students in my lab, isolated just such a mutant of invertase that accumulates in the ER in what appears to be a perfectly active, properly assembled and fully soluble enzyme, but which is secreted from the ER 4–5 fold more slowly than normal (65).

With respect to membrane cargo proteins, early evidence supported a direct interaction with the inner subunits of the COPII coat, Sar1p and Sec23/24p, prior to the complete formation of the coated vesicle. Meta Kuehn, a postdoc in the lab, detected an interaction of plasma membrane permease and SNARE proteins but not luminal ER resident proteins with the inner COPII subunits dependent on incubation of membranes in the presence of a non-hydrolyzable analog of GTP (131). Bill Balch's lab observed a similar interaction of mammalian Sec23/24 with a transit intermediate of the VSV G protein, and discovered the interaction depends on a C-terminal sorting sequence, ..DxE., in the G-protein (132). Sebastian Springer reinforced this idea with the observation of a stable and selective complex of Sar1p, Sec23/24p and pure recombinant forms of the cytosolic domain of two ER SNARE proteins, Bet1p and Bos1p (133).

For secretory proteins, the best evidence for selective sorting comes from the discovery of ER sorting receptors. David Ginsburg's laboratory identified the genes involved in a rare, combined hemophilia in which two blood-clotting factors, V and VIII, are delayed in the ER. One gene encodes a lectin-binding membrane protein, ERGIC53 (or LMAN1) (134), that cycles between the ER and Golgi and which is actively packaged into COPII vesicles in a cell-free budding reaction prepared from permeabilized cultured mammalian cells (previous ref). The heavily glycosylated protein domains of factors V and VIII are suggested to interact with the luminal lectin-binding domain of ERGIC 53 to promote their exit from the ER (135). An appreciation of the exact role of ERGIC53 as a sorting receptor awaits the development of an approach to measure the incorporation of a blood-clotting factor into transport vesicles.

A breakthrough in yeast came with the discovery by Charles Barlowe, now in his own laboratory at Dartmouth, of the sorting receptor necessary for the transport of α-factor precursor. In a survey of membrane proteins in isolated COPII vesicles, Barlowe characterized Erv29p, a protein that had not turned up in any genetic screen (136). Deletion of *ERV29* produced a viable strain with a pronounced defect in the secretion of α-factor, the mature species produced by proteolytic processing of the precursor in the trans Golgi (137). Unfortunately, *ERV29* had evaded detection in classic selections for pheromone deficient yeast mutants because even the 30-fold delay in secretion of α-factor seen in the *erv29* deletion strain is inadequate to reduce the steady state level of secreted pheromone below that necessary to produce an infertile strain of yeast. Other work showed that ERV29 speeds the transport of a vacuolar protease from the ER and likely several other secreted proteins, though notably not invertase (138). Barlowe went on to demonstrate that Erv29p is required to package α-factor precursor into COPII vesicles *in vitro* and to map the residues responsible for Erv29p interaction with the precursor (137).

One could argue that ERGIC53 and Erv29p serve primarily as species-specific folding chaperones that accompany cargo molecules into the cis Golgi and then are recycled for reuse in the ER and that in their absence the cognate cargo molecules remain subtly unfolded and subject to quality control retention. Such appears to be the case for a large number of species-specific ER membrane chaperones, e.g. Shr3p required for the transport of amino acid permeases in yeast, which remain in the ER and do not accompany cargo into COPII vesicles (139). However, Per Malkus, a graduate student in my lab, showed that α-factor precursor is chemically concentrated 3-fold with respect to a soluble bulk flow marker, a glycotripeptide, within COPII vesicles produced in a budding reaction. This result favors a model of active sorting as opposed to bulk flow in the capture of cargo proteins into COPII vesicles (140).

A complementary line of evidence demonstrates that the COPII coat, specifically the Sec24p subunit, directs the selection of cargo molecules during the budding event. Yeast has three paralogs of Sec24, mammals have four, and genetic and biochemical evidence shows that several are responsible for the capture of particular subsets of cargo membrane proteins. Chris Kaiser's lab at MIT was the first to recognize the important role of the *SEC24* paralog he called *LSTI* in the transport of the major plasma membrane ATPase, Pma1p (141). Although deletion of *LST1* is not a lethal event, cells are sickly and deficient in the surface presentation of the ATPase, which instead accumulates in the ER. Kaiser suggested that Lst1p might form an alternate complex with Sec23p to favor the packaging of Pma1p and that in its absence, the normal Sec24p may not properly sort Pma1p into COPII vesicles. Yuval Shimoni, a postdoc in my lab, proved that directly using a Pma1p budding reaction programmed with either Sec23/ Sec24p or Sec23/Lst1p. Lst1p dramatically promoted the packaging of Pma1p into COPII vesicles *in vitro* (142).

Liz Miller, a wonderfully enthusiastic and talented postdoc, joined the lab to explore the details of cargo sorting mediated by COPII. Following Shimoni's isolation of functional Sec23/Lst1p, Liz found a remarkably different spectrum of membrane proteins packaged into vesicles produced by the alternative heterodimer, including a defect in the incorporation of α-factor precursor, presumably because Lst1p is not required to recognize most membrane cargo or sorting receptor proteins, including Erv29p (143). Liz then undertook a detailed mutagenesis study designed to identify the residues of Sec24p devoted to the sorting of particular cargo proteins (144). She found mutant alleles that were synthetically lethal when one or both of the other *SEC24* paralogs was deleted. One mutation mapped to a binding pocket Jonathan Goldberg had defined structurally on a lateral surface of Sec24p that interacts with the ..DXE.. sorting signal Bill Balch had discovered as important for the traffic of mammalian VSV G protein from the ER (132, 145). Using the budding reaction, Liz showed that Sec24p mutations in this binding site were fully capable of budding certain cargo but not those dependent on the ..DXE.. sorting motif. Per Malkus had identified a ..DXD.. motif in the C-terminal cytoplasmic domain of the yeast amino acid permeases which Liz showed was recognized perfectly adequately by a Sec24p mutant that failed to recognize the ..DXE.. motif (140). These and many results since then have built up a picture of a Sec24p coat subunit with multiple independent cargo binding sites which combined with the two Sec24p paralogs, helps to explain how the diverse repertoire of cargo molecules may be deciphered by a combinatorial code.

An even greater range of cargo proteins is encountered in the mammalian ER. Two striking examples of cargo specificity in sorting mediated by mammalian *SEC24* paralogs have been reported. Chain terminating mutations in the mouse SEC24B gene cause an extreme form of neural tube closure defect referred to as craniorachiscisis (146, 147). The same arrest is seen in deletions of the neural forms of such signaling receptors as Frizzled and Vangl, two neural epithelium surface proteins that are assembled on the distal and proximal plasma membranes of neural epithelial cells, respectively (148). Using permeabilized cultured mammalian cells, Devon Jensen, a graduate student in my lab collaborating with the laboratory of David Ginty, found that the Sec24B protein stimulated the packaging specifically of Vangl2 protein into COPII vesicles, again consistent with the sequence or structure-selective sorting of membrane proteins at the ER (146). Mutant alleles of human SEC24B may appear in children afflicted with a genetic form of spina bifida. Xiaowei Chen in David Ginsburg's lab found a striking cargo preference mediated by another paralog,

SEC24A. Deletion of SEC24A in the mouse leads to a striking decrease in cholesterol levels in the blood that Chen was able to attribute to a defect in ER transport and secretion of a soluble serum protein, PCSK9, which controls the itinerary of the LDL receptor (149). Lower levels of PCSK9 allow the LDL receptor to cycle efficiently and control cholesterol biosynthesis, thus explaining the low cholesterol in animals deficient in PCSK9 secretion. Chen's results argue that the export of PCSK9 from the ER is mediated by a sorting receptor that is recognized and packaged into COPII vesicles by SEC24A. The nature of this receptor and its role in sorting of other cargo molecules remain to be discovered. It seems likely that many other such sorting receptors in the ER will be found, adding to the picture of an active process of cargo selection by the COPII coat, and by extension, by other coats involved in the intracellular traffic of membrane and soluble proteins.

LESSONS LEARNED AND CREDIT GIVEN

Summarizing almost 40 years of work is a daunting experience, but if I may, three key conclusions follow from the work I have described:

1. Secretion and plasma membrane assembly are physically and functionally linked through a series of obligate organelle intermediates.
2. The polypeptide translocation and vesicular traffic machinery has been conserved over a billion years of evolution.
3. The COPII coat sorts cargo molecules by the recognition of transport signals and physically deforms the ER membrane to create budded vesicles.

Limitations of space and time have made it impossible to acknowledge all the many contributions of the nearly 200 students, fellows and colleagues with whom it has been my privilege to collaborate over the years. Although I end this story here, the work continues in my lab in spite of the many distractions that the call from Stockholm has brought to my life. I am grateful to the present members of my lab for their patience with me this year but even more importantly for the enthusiasm and dedication they bring to the work at hand. None of this would have been possible without the steadfast love and support of my family and friends, and the wise investment that the U.S. and California made in building educational and research opportunities second to none.

The subject of membrane assembly and vesicular traffic is rich with opportunity and remains an area with great potential for molecular and even atomic resolution in the years ahead. The connections between basic discovery and practical, medical application are certainly more tangible now than when I began my independent work in 1976. However, I trust the pursuit of basic discovery unconnected to any practical application will continue to motivate young scholars and that the agencies, government and private, that made discovery an adventure for me will continue to do so for as long as we thirst for knowledge of the natural world.

REFERENCES

1. Palade, G. (1975). "Intracellular aspects of protein secretion." *Science* **189**: 347–358.
2. Kornberg, A., Lehman, I. R., Bessman, M. J. & Simms, E. S. "Enzymatic synthesis of desoxyribonucleic acid." *Biochim. Biophys. Acta* **21**: 197–198 (1956).
3. De Lucia, P. and Cairns, J. (1969). "Isolation of an *E. coli* Strain with a Mutation affecting DNA Polymerase." *Nature* **224**: 1164–1166.
4. Josse, J., Kaiser, A.D. and Arthur Kornberg (1961). "Enzymatic Synthesis of Deoxyribonucleic Acid: VIII. Frequencies of the nearest neighbor base sequences in deoxyribonucleic acid." *J. Biol. Chem.* **236**: 864–875.
5. Goulian, M. and Kornberg, A. (1967). "Enzymatic synthesis of DNA, XXIII, Synthesis of circular replicative form phage φX174 DNA." *Proc. Natl. Acad. Sci. USA* **58**: 1723–1730
6. Goulian, M., Kornberg, A. and Sinsheimer, R.L. (1967). "Enzymatic synthesis of DNA, XXIV. Synthesis of infectious phage φX174 DNA." *Proc. Natl. Acad. Sci. USA* **58**(6): 2321– 2328.
7. Kelly, R., Atkinson, M., Huberman, J., and Kornberg, A. (1969). "Excision of Thymine Dimers and Other Mismatched Sequences by DNA Polymerase of *Escherichia coli*." *Nature* **224**: 495–501.
8. De Waard, A., Paul, A., and Lehman, I.R. (1965). "The structural gene for deoxyribonucleic acid polymerase in bacteriophages T4 and T5." *Proc. Natl. Acad. Sci. USA* **54**: 1241–1248.
9. Hirota, Y., Ryter, A., and Jacob F. (1968). "Thermosensitive mutants of *E. coli* affected in the processes of DNA synthesis and cellular division." *Cold Spring Harb Symp Quant Biol.* **33**: 677–693.
10. Fangman, W. and Novick, A. (1968). "Characterization of two bacterial mutants with temperature-sensitive synthesis of DNA." *Genetics* **60**: 1–17.
11. Kornberg, T. & Gefter, M. L. "DNA synthesis in cell-free extracts of a DNA polymerase-defective mutant." *Biochem. Biophys. Res. Commun.* **40**: 1348–1355 (1970).
12. Gefter, M., Hirota, Y., Kornber, T., Wechsler, J. and Barnoux, C. (1971). "Analysis of DNA polymerases II and III in mutants of *Escherichia coli* thermosensitive for DNA Synthesis." *Proc. Natl. Acad. Sci. USA* **68**: 3150–3153.
13. Watson, J.D. (1966). *The Molecular Biology of the Gene* (W.A. Benjamin, New York).
14. Epstein, R., Bolle, A., Steinberg, C., Kellenberger, E., Boy de la Tour, E., Chevalley, R., Edgard, R., Susman, M., Denhardt, G., and Leilausis, A. (1963). "Physiological

Studies of Conditional Lethal Mutants of Bacteriophage T4D." *Cold Spring Harbor Symposia on Quantitative Biology* **28**: 375–394.
15. Benzer, S. (1957). *The elementary units of heredity. In a symposium on the chemical basis of heredity*, edited by W.D. McElroy and B. Glass. Baltimore: The Johns Hopkins Press, p. 70–133.
16. Edgar, R. and Wood, W., (1966). "Morphogenesis of bacteriophage T4 in extracts of mutant-infected cells." *Proc. Natl. Acad. Sci. USA* **55**: 498–505.
17. Brutlag, D., Schekman, R. W., and Kornberg, A. (1971). "A possible role for RNA polymerase in the initiation of M13 DNA synthesis." *Proc. Natl. Acad. Sci. USA* **68**: 2826.
18. Wickner, W., Brutlag, D., Schekman, R., and Kornberg, A. (1972). "RNA synthesis initiates *in vitro* conversion of M13 DNA to its replicative form." *Proc. Natl. Acad. Sci. USA* **69**: 965.
19. Schekman, R. W., Wickner, W., Westergaard, O., Brutlag, D., Geider, K., Bertsch, L. L., and Kornberg, A. (1972). "Initiation of DNA synthesis: synthesis of ϕX174 replicative form requires RNA synthesis resistant to rifampicin." *Proc. Natl. Acad. Sci. USA* **69**: 2691.
20. Olivera, B. and Bonhoeffer, F. (1972). "Replication of φX174 DNA by *polA*- in vitro." *Proc. Natl. Acad. Sci. USA* 69: 25–29.
21. Barry, J. and Alberts, B. (1972). "In vitro complementation as an assay for new proteins required for bacteriophage T4 DNA replication: Purification of the complex specified by T4 genes 44 and 62." *Proc. Natl. Acad. Sci. USA* **69**: 2717–2721.
22. Schekman, R., Weiner, A., and Kornberg, A. (1974). "Multienzyme systems of DNA replication." *Science* **186:** 987.
23. Hartwell, L., Mortimer, R., Culotti, J., and Culotti, M. (1973). "Genetic control of cell division cycle in yeast: Genetic analysis of *cdc* mutants." *Genetics* **74**: 267–286.
24. Redman, C., Siekevitz, P., and Palade, G. (1966). "Synthesis and Transfer of Amylase in Pigeon Pancreatic Microsomes." *J. Biol. Chem.* **241**: 1150–1158.
25. Redman, C. and Sabatini, D. (1966). "Vectorial discharge of peptides released by puromycin from attached ribosomes." *Proc. Natl. Acad. Sci. USA* **56**: 608–615.
26. Singer, S.J. and Nicholson, G. (1972). "The fluid mosaic model of membrane structure." *Science* **175**(4023): 720–31.
27. Tokuyasu, K. (1973). "A technique for ultracryotomy of cell suspensions and tissues." *J. Cell Biol.* **57**: 551–565.
28. Hirano, H., Parkhouse, B, Nicholson, G., Lennox, E., and Singer, S.J. (1972). "Distribution of saccharide residues on membrane fragments from a melanoma cell homogenate: Its implications for membrane biogenesis." *Proc. Natl. Acad. Sci. USA* **69**: 2945–2949.
29. Schekman, R. and Singer, S. J. (1976). "Clustering and endocytosis of membrane receptors can be induced in mature erythrocytes of neonatal humans but not adults." *Proc. Natl. Acad. Sci. USA* **73**: 4075.
30. Blobel, G. and Dobberstein B. (1975a). "Transfer of proteins across membranes. I. Presence of proteolytically processed and unprocessed nascent immunoglobulin light chains on membrane-bound ribosomes of murine myeloma." *J. Cell Biol.* **67**: 835–51.

31. Blobel G. and Dobberstein B. (1975b). "Transfer of proteins across membranes. II. Reconstitution of functional rough microsomes from heterologous components." *J. Cell Biol.* **67**: 852–862.
32. Byers, B. and Goetsch, L. (1976). "A highly ordered ring of membrane-associated filaments in budding yeast." *J. Cell Biol.* **69**: 7171–721.
33. Cabib, E. and Bowers, B. (1971). "Chitin and yeast budding." *J. Biol Chem.* **246**: 152–159.
34. Byers, B. and Goetsch, L. (1974). "Duplication of spindle plaques and integration of the yeast cell cycle." *Cold Spring Harb Symp Quant Biol.* **38**: 123–131.
35. Boer, P., Van Rijn, H.J., Reinking, A., Seryn-Parvé, E.P. (1975). "Biosynthesis of acid phosphatase of baker's yeast. Characterization of a protoplast-bound fraction containing precursors of the exo-enzyme." *Biochim. Biophys. Acta*, Feb 19; **377**(2): 331–342.
36. Scott, J. H. and Schekman, R. (1980). "Lyticase: Endoglucanase and protease activities that act together in yeast cell lysis." *J. Bact.* **142**: 414.
37. Novick, P. and Botstein, D. (1985). "Phenotypic analysis of temperature-sensitive yeast actin mutants." *Cell* **40**(2): 405–16.
38. Schekman, R. and Brawley, V. (1979). "Localized deposition of chitin on the yeast cell surface in response to mating pheromone." *Proc. Natl. Acad. Sci. USA* **76**: 645.
39. Henry, S., Atkinson, K., Kolat, A., and Culbertson, M. (1977). "Growth and metabolism of inositol-starved *Saccharomyces cerevisia.*" *J. Bact.* **130**: 472–484.
40. Novick, P. and Schekman, R. (1979). "Secretion and cell surface growth are blocked in a temperature sensitive mutant of *Saccharomyces cerevisiae.*" *Proc. Natl. Acad. Sci. USA* **76**: 1858–1862.
41. Novick, P., Field, C., and Schekman, R. (1980). "The identification of 23 complementation groups required for post-translational events in the yeast secretory pathway." *Cell* **21**: 205–215.
42. Novick, P., Ferro, S., and Schekman, R. (1981). "Order of events in the yeast secretory pathway." *Cell* **25**: 461–469.
43. Kaiser, C. A. and Schekman, R. (1990). "Distinct sets of *SEC* genes govern transport vesicle formation and fusion early in the secretory pathway." *Cell* **61**: 723–733.
44. Esmon, B., Novick, P., and Schekman, R. (1981). "Compartmentalized assembly of oligosaccharides on exported glycoproteins." *Cell* **25**: 451–460.
45. Stevens, T., Esmon, B., and Schekman, R. (1982). "Early stages in the yeast secretory pathway are required for transport of carboxypeptidase Y to the vacuole." *Cell* **30**: 439–448.
46. Valenzuela, P., Medina, M., Rutter, W., Ammerer, G., and Hall, B. (1982). "Synthesis and assembly of hepatitis B surface antigen particles in yeast." *Nature* **298**: 347–350.
47. Ferro-Novick, S., Novick, P., Field, C., and Schekman, R. (1984). "Yeast secretory mutants that block the formation of active cell surface enzymes." *J. Cell Biol.* **98**: 35–43.
48. Kepes, F. and Schekman, R. (1988). "The yeast *SEC53* gene encodes phosphomannomutase." *J. Biol. Chem.* **263**: 9155–9161.

49. Bernstein, M., Kepes, F., and Schekman, R. (1989). "*SEC59* encodes a membrane protein required for core glycosylation in yeast." *Mol. Cell. Biol.* **9**: 1191–1199.
50. Silhavy, T.J., Casadaban, M.J., Shuman, H.A., and Beckwith, J.R. "Conversion of beta-galactosidase to a membrane-bound state by gene fusion." *Proc. Natl. Acad. Sci. USA* 1976 Oct; **73**(10): 3423–3427.
51. Emr, S. D., Schauer, I., Hansen, W., Esmon, P., and Schekman, R. (1984). "Invertase β-galactosidase hybrid proteins fail to be transported from the endoplasmic reticulum in yeast." *Mol. Cell Biol.* **4**: 2347–2356.
52. Oliver, D.B. and Beckwith, J. (1981). "*E. coli* mutant pleiotropically defective in the export of secreted proteins." *Cell* Sep; **25**(3): 765–72.
53. Emr, S.D. and Silhavy, T.J. (1980). "Mutations affecting localization of an *Escherichia coli* outer membrane protein, the bacteriophage lambda receptor." *J. Mol. Biol.* **141**: 63–90.
54. Shiba, K., Ito, K., Yura, T., and Cerretti, D.P. "A defined mutation in the protein export gene within the spc ribosomal protein operon of Escherichia coli: isolation and characterization of a new temperature-sensitive secY mutant." *EMBO J.* 1984 Mar; **3**(3): 631–635.
55. Deshaies, R. and Schekman, R. (1987). "A yeast mutant defective at an early stage in import of secretory protein precursors into the endoplasmic reticulum." *J. Cell Biol.* **105**: 633–645.
56. Rothblatt, J. A., Deshaies, R. J., Sanders, S., Daum, G., and Schekman, R. (1989). "Multiple genes are required for proper insertion of secretory proteins into the endoplasmic reticulum in yeast." *J. Cell Biol.* **109**: 2641–2652.
57. Stirling, C. A., Rothblatt, J., Hosobuchi, M., Deshaies, R., and Schekman, R. (1992). "Protein translocation mutants defective in the insertion of integral membrane proteins into the endoplasmic reticulum." *Mol. Biol. Cell* **3**: 129–142.
58. Gorlich, D., Prehn, S., Hartmann, E., Kalies, K-U., and Rapoport, T. (1992). "A mammalian homolog of SEC61p and SECYp is associated with ribosomes and nascent polypeptides during translocation." *Cell* **71**: 489–503
59. Nakano, A., Brada, D., and Schekman, R. (1988). "A membrane glycoprotein, Sec12p, required for protein transport from the endoplasmic reticulum to the Golgi apparatus in yeast." *J. Cell Biol.* **107**: 851–863.
60. Gorlich, D. and Rapoport, T. (1993). "Protein translocation into proteoliposomes reconstituted from purified components of the endoplasmic reticulum membrane." *Cell* **75**: 615–630.
61. Hansen, W., Garcia, P., and Walter, P. (1986). "In vitro protein translocation across the yeast endoplasmic reticulum: ATP-dependent posttranslational translocation of the prepro-alpha-factor." *Cell* **45**: 397–406.
62. Pelham, H. (1986). "Speculations on the functions of the major heat shock and glucose-regulated proteins." *Cell* **46**: 959–961.
63. Deshaies, R. J., Koch, B. D., Werner-Washburne, M., Craig, E. A., and Schekman, R. (1988). "A subfamily of stress proteins facilitates translocation of secretory and mitochondrial precursor polypeptides." *Nature* **332**: 800–805.
64. Chirico, W. J., Waters, M. G., and Blobel, G. (1988). "70K heat shock related proteins stimulate protein translocation into microsomes." *Nature* **332**: 805–810.

65. Schauer, I., Emr, S., Gross, C., and Schekman, R. (1985). "Invertase signal and mature sequence substitutions that delay intercompartmental transport of active enzyme." *J. Cell Biol.* **100**: 1664–1675.
66. Novick, P. and Schekman, R. (1983). "Export of major cell surface proteins is blocked in yeast secretory mutants." *J. Cell Biol.* **96**: 541–547.
67. Böhni, P. C., Deshaies, R. J., and Schekman, R. W. (1988). "*SEC11* is required for signal peptide processing and yeast cell growth." *J. Cell Biol.* **106**: 1035–1042.
68. Greenberg, G., Shelness, G and Blobel, G. (1989). "A subunit of the mammalian signal peptidase is homologous to the yeast SEC11 protein." *J. Biol. Chem.* **264**: 15762–5.
69. Hinnen, A., Hicks, J., and Fink, G. (1978). "Transformation of yeast." *Proc. Natl. Acad. Sci. USA* **75**: 1929–1933.
70. Haselbeck, A. and Schekman, R. (1986). "Interorganelle transfer and glycosylation of yeast invertase in vitro." *Proc. Natl. Acad. Sci. USA* **83**: 2017–2021.
71. Fries, E. and Rothman, J.E. (1980). "Transport of vesicular stomatitis virus glycoprotein in a cell-free extract." *Proc. Natl. Acad. Sci. USA* **77**: 3870–3874.
72. Bernstein, M., Hoffmann, W., Ammerer, G., and Schekman, R. (1985). "Characterization of a gene product (Sec53p) required for protein assembly in the yeast endoplasmic reticulum." *J. Cell Biol.* **101**: 2374–2382.
73. Eakle, K., Bernstein, M., and Emr, S. (1988). "Characterization of a component of the yeast secretion machinery: identification of the SEC18 gene product." *Mol. Cell Biol.* **8**: 4098– 4109.
74. Salminen, A. and Novick, P.J. (1987). "A ras-like protein is required for a post-Golgi event in yeast secretion." *Cell* **49**: 527–538.
75. Gengyo-Ando, K., Kamiya, Y., Yamanaka, A., Kodaira, I. K., Nishiwaki, K., Miwa, J., Hori, I., and Hosono R. (1993). "The *C. elegans unc-18* gene encodes a protein expressed in motor neurons." *Neuron* **11**: 703–711.
76. Brenner, S. (1974). "The genetics of *Caenorhabditis elegans*." *Genetics* **77**: 71–94.
77. Wilson, D.W., Wilcox, C.A., Flynn, G.C., Chen, E., Kuang, W.J., Henzel, W.J., Block, M.R., Ullrich, A., and Rothman, J.E. (1989). "A fusion protein required for vesicle-mediated transport in both mammalian cells and yeast." *Nature* **339**: 355–359.
78. Griff, I. C., Schekman, R., Rothman, J. E., and Kaiser, C. A. (1992). "The yeast *SEC17* gene product is functionally equivalent to mammalian α-SNAP protein." *J. Biol. Chem.* **267**: 12106–12115.
79. Roth, T. and Porter, K., (1964). "Yolk protein uptake in the oocyte of the mosquito *Aedes aegypti*." *J. Cell Biol.* **20**: 313–331.
80. Pearse, B. (1976). "Clathrin: a unique protein associated with intracellular transfer of membrane by coated vesicles." *Proc. Natl. Acad. Sci. USA* **73**: 1255–1259.
81. Rothman, J. and Fine, R. (1980). "Coated vesicles transport newly-synthesized membrane glycoproteins to plasma membrane in two successive stages." *Proc. Natl. Acad. Sci. USA* **77**: 280–284.
82. Payne, G. S. and Schekman, R. (1985). "A test of clathrin function in protein secretion and cell growth." *Science* **230**: 1009–1014.

83. Lemmon, S. and Jones, E. (1987). "Clathrin requirement for normal growth of yeast." *Science* **238**: 504–509.
84. Payne, G. S., and Schekman, R. (1989). "Clathrin: A role in the intracellular retention of a Golgi membrane protein." *Science* **245**: 1358–1365.
85. Orci, L., Ravazzola, M., Storch, M-J., Anderson, R., Vassalli, J-D., and Perrelet, A. (1987). "Proteolytic maturation of insulin is a post-Golgi event which occurs in acidifying clathrin-coated secretory vesicles." *Cell* **49**: 865–868.
86. Baker, D., Hicke, L., Rexach, M., Schleyer, M., and Schekman, R. (1988). "Reconstitution of *Sec* gene product-dependent intercompartmental protein transport." *Cell* **54**: 335–344.
87. Ruohola, H., Kabcenell, A., and Ferro-Novick, S. (1988). "Reconstitution of protein transport from the endoplasmic reticulum to the Golgi complex in yeast: The acceptor Golgi compartment is defective in the *sec23* mutant." *J. Cell Bio.* **107**: 1465–76.
88. Hicke, L., Yoshihisa, T., and Schekman, R. (1992). "Sec23p and a novel 105 kD protein function as a multimeric complex to promote vesicle budding and protein transport from the ER." *Mol. Biol. Cell* **3**: 667–676.
89. Nakano, A. and Muramatsu, M. (1989). "A novel GTP-binding protein, Sar1p, is involved in transport from the endoplasmic reticulum to the Golgi apparatus." *J. Cell Biol.* **109**: 2677– 2691.
90. d'Enfert, C., Wuestehube, L. J., Lila, T., and Schekman, R. (1991). "Sec12p-dependent membrane binding of the small GTP-binding protein Sar1p promotes formation of transport vesicles from the ER." *J. Cell Biol.* **114**: 663–670.
91. Barlowe, C., d'Enfert, C., and Schekman, R. (1993). "Purification and characterization of SAR1p, a small GTP-binding protein required for transport vesicle formation from the endoplasmic reticulum." *J. Biol. Chem.* **268**: 873–879.
92. Rexach, M. and Schekman, R. (1991). "Distinct biochemical requirements for the budding, targeting, and fusion of ER-derived transport vesicles." *J. Cell Biology* **114**: 219–229.
93. Groesch, M., Ruohola, H., Bacon, R., Rossi, G., and Ferro-Novick, S. (1990). "Isolation of a functional vesicle intermediate that mediates ER-Golgi transport in yeast." *J. Cell Biol.* **111**: 45–53.
94. Espenshade P., Gimeno R. E., Holzmacher E., Teung P., and Kaiser C. A., (1995). "Yeast SEC16 gene encodes a multidomain vesicle coat protein that interacts with Sec23p." *J. Cell Biol.* **131**: 311–324.
95. Pryer, N. K., Salama, N. R., Schekman, R., and Kaiser, C. A. (1993). "Cytosolic Sec13p complex is required for vesicle formation from the endoplasmic reticulum *in vitro*." *J. Cell Biol.* **120**: 865–875.
96. Salama, N. R., Yeung, T., and Schekman, R. (1993). "The Sec13p complex and reconstitution of vesicle budding from the ER with purified cytosolic proteins." *EMBO J.* **12**: 4073–4082.
97. Malhotra, V., Serafini, T., Orci, L., Shepherd, J.C., and Rothman, J.E. (1989). "Purification of a novel class of coated vesicles mediating biosynthetic protein transport through the Golgi stack." *Cell* **58**: 329–336

98. Hosobuchi, M., Kreis, T., and Schekman, R. (1992). "*SEC21* is a gene required for ER to Golgi protein transport that encodes a subunit of a yeast coatomer." *Nature* **360**: 603–605.
99. Yoshihisa, T., Barlowe, C., and Schekman, R. (1993). "Requirement for a GTPase-activating protein in vesicle budding from the endoplasmic reticulum." *Science* **259**: 1466–1468.
100. Barlowe, C. and Schekman, R. (1993). "*SEC12* encodes a guanine nucleotide exchange factor essential for transport vesicle formation from the ER." *Nature* **365**: 347–349.
101. Antonny, B., Madden, D., Hamamoto, S., Orci, L., and Schekman, R. (2001). "Dynamics of the COPII coat with GTP and stable analogues." *Nature Cell Biol.* **3**: 531–537.
102. Melancon, P., Glick, B.S., Malhotra, V., Weidman, P.J., Serafini, T., Gleason, M.L., Orci, L., and Rothman, J.E. (1987). "Involvement of GTP-binding "G" proteins in transport through the Golgi stack." *Cell* **51**: 1053–1062.
103. Orci, L., Ravazzola, M., Meda, P., Holcomb, C., Moore, H-P., Hicke, L., and Schekman, R. (1991). "Mammalian Sec23p homologue is restricted to the endoplasmic reticulum transitional cytoplasm." *Proc. Natl. Acad. Sci. USA* **88**: 8611–8615.
104. Barlowe, C., Orci, L.,Yeung, T., Hosobuchi, M., Hamamoto, S., Salama, N., Rexach, M. F., Ravazzola, M., Amherdt, M., and Schekman, R. (1994). "COPII: A membrane coat formed by Sec proteins that drive vesicle budding from the endoplasmic reticulum." *Cell* **77**: 895– 907.
105. Bednarek, S. Y., Ravazzola, M., Hosobuchi, M., Amherdt, M., Perrelet, A., Schekman, R., and Orci, L. (1995). "COPI- and COPII-coated vesicles bud directly from the endoplasmic reticulum in yeast." *Cell* **83**: 1183–1196.
106. Campbell, J. L. and Schekman, R. (1997). "Selective packaging of cargo molecules into endoplasmic reticulum-derived COPII vesicles." *Proc. Natl. Acad. Sci. USA* **94**: 837–842.
107. Supek, F., Madden, D. T., Hamamoto, S., Orci, L., and Schekman, R. (2002). "Sec16p potentiates the action of COPII proteins to bud transport vesicles." *J. Cell Biol.* **158**: 1029–1038.
108. Kung, L. F., Pagant, S., Futai, E., D'Arcangelo, J. G., Buchanan, R., Dittmar, J. C., Reid, R. J. D., Rothstein, R., Hamamoto, S., Snapp, S., Schekman, R., and Miller, E. A. (2011). "Sec24p and Sec16p cooperate to regulate the GTP cycle of the COPII coat." *EMBO J.* **31**: 1014–1027.
109. Yeung, T., Barlowe, C., and Schekman, R. (1995). "Uncoupled packaging of targeting and cargo molecules during transport vesicle budding from the endoplasmic reticulum." *J. Biol. Chem.* **270**: 30567–30570.
110. Springer, S., Spang, A., and Schekman, R. (1999). "A primer on vesicle budding." *Cell* **97**: 145–148.
111. Matsuoka, K., Orci, L., Amherdt, M., Bednarek, S.Y., Hamamoto, S., Schekman, R., and Yeung, T. (1998). "COPII-Coated vesicle formation reconstituted with purified coat proteins and chemically defined liposomes." *Cell* **93**: 263–275.

112. Futai, E., Hamamoto, S., Orci, L., and Schekman, R. (2004). "GTP/GDP exchange by Sec12p enables COPII vesicle bud formation on synthetic liposomes." *EMBO J.* 4146–4155.
113. Bacia, K., Kutai, E., Prinz, D., Meister, A., Daum, S., Glatte, D., Briggs, J.A.G., and Schekman, R. (2011). "Multibudded tubules formed by COPII on artificial liposomes." *Scientific Reports* **1**: 17.
114. Huang, M., Weissman, J., Beraud, S., Luan, P., Wang, C., Chen, W., Aridor, M., Wilson, I., and Balch, W. (2001). "Crystal structure of Sar1-GDP at 1.7 Å." *J. Cell Biol.* **155**: 937–948.
115. Sheetz, M. and Singer, S.J. (1974). "Biological membranes as bilayer couples. A mechanism of drug-erythrocyte interactions." *Proc. Natl. Acad. Sci. USA* **71**: 4457–4461.
116. Lee, M. C, Orci, L., Hamamoto, S., Futai, E., Ravazzola, M., and Schekman, R. (2005). "Sar1p N-terminal helix initiates membrane curvature and completes the fission of a COPII vesicle." *Cell* Aug 26; **122**(4): 605–17.
117. Bi, X., Corpina, R., and Goldberg, J. (2002). "Structure of the Sec23/24-Sar1 pre-budding complex of the COPII coat." *Nature* **419**: 271–277.
118. Stagg, S. M., Gürkan, C., Fowler, D. M., LaPointe, P., Foss, T. R., Potter, C.S., Carragher, B., and Balch, W.E. (2006). "Structure of the Sec13/31 COPII coat cage." *Nature* **439**: 234–238.
119. Fath, S., Mancias, J. D., Bi, X., and Goldberg, J. (2007). "Structure and organization of coat proteins in the COPII cage." *Cell* **129**: 1325–1336.
120. Zanetti, G., Prinz, S., Daum, S., Meister, A., Schekman, R., Bacia, K., and Briggs, J.A.G. (2013). "The structure of the COPII coat assembled on membranes." *eLife* **2**: e00951.
121. Jin, L., Pahuja, K. B., Wickliffe, K. E., Gorur, A., Baumgartel, C., Schekman, R., and Rape, M. (2012). "biquitin-dependent regulation of COPII coat size and function." *Nature* **482**: 495–500.
122. Boyadjiev, S. A., Fromme, J. C., Ben, J., Chong, S. S., Nauta, C., Hur, D. J., Zhang, G., Hamamoto, S., Schekman, R., Ravazzola, M., Orci, L., and Eyaid, W. (2006). "Cranio-lenticulo-sutural dysplasia is caused by a SEC23A mutation leading to abnormal endoplasmic-reticulum-to-Golgi trafficking." *Nature Gen.* **38**: 1192–1197.
123. Kim, J., Hamamoto, S., Ravazzola, M., Orci, L.,, and Schekman, R. (2004). "Uncoupled packaging of amyloid precursor protein and presenilin 1 into COPII vesicles." *J. Biol. Chem.*, published online, December 2004, 10.1074.
124. Fromme, J. C., Ravazzola, M., Hamamoto, S., Al-Balwi, M., Eyaid, W., Boyadjiev, S. A., Cosson, R., Schekman, R., and Orci, L. (2007). "The genetic basis of a craniofacial disease provides insight into COPII coat assembly." *Developmental Cell* **13**: 623–634.
125. Bi, X. et al. (2007). "Insights into COPII coat nucleation from the structure of Sec23–Sar1 complexed with the active fragment of Sec31." *Dev. Cell* **13**: 635–645.
126. Semenza, J., Hardwick, K., Dean, N. and Pelham, H. (1990). "ERD2, a yeast gene required for the receptor-mediated retrieval of ER luminal proteins from the secretory pathway." *Cell* **61**: 1349–1357.

127. Wieland, F., Gleason, M., Serafini, T., and Rothman, J. (1987). "The rate of bulk flow from the endoplasmic reticulum to the cell surface." *Cell* **50**: 289–300.
128. Martinez-Menarguez, J., Geuze, H., Slot, J., and Klumpermann, J., (1999). "Vesicular tubular clusters between the ER and Golgi mediate concentration of soluble secretory proteins by exclusion from COPI-coated vesicles." *J. Cell Biol.* **98**: 81–90.
129. Thor, F., Gautschi, M., Geiger, R. and Helenius, A. (2009). "Bulk flow revisited: Transport of a soluble protein in the secretory pathway. *Traffic* **10**: 1819–1830.
130. Zanetti, G., Pahuja, K. B, Studer, S., Shim, S., and Schekman, R. (2011). "COPII and the regulation of protein sorting in mammals." *Nature Cell Biol.* **14**: 20–28.
131. Kuehn, M. T., Herrmann, J. M., and Schekman, R. (1998). "COPII-cargo interactions direct protein sorting into ER-derived transport vesicles." *Nature* **391**: 187–190.
132. Nishimura, N. and Balch, W. (1997). "A di-acidic signal required for selective export from the endoplasmic reticulum." *Science* **277**: 556–558.
133. Springer, S. and Schekman, R. (1998). "Nucleation of COPII vesicular coat complex by ER to Golgi v-SNAREs." *Science* **281**: 698–700.
134. Nichols, W.C., Seligsohn, U., Zivelin, A., Terry, V.H., Hertel, C.E., Wheatley, M.A., Moussalli, M.J., Hauri, H.P., Ciavarella, N., Kaufman, R.J., and Ginsburg, D. (1998). "Mutations in the ER-Golgi intermediate compartment protein ERGIC-53 cause combined deficiency of coagulation factors V and VIII." *Cell* **93**: 61–70.
135. Moussalli, M., Pipe, S.W., Hauri, H.P., Nichols, W.C., Ginsburg, D., and Kaufman, R.J. (1999). "Mannose-dependent endoplasmic reticulum (ER)-Golgi intermediate compartment-53-mediated ER to Golgi trafficking of coagulation factors V and VIII." *J. Biol. Chem.* **12**: 32539–42.
136. Belden, W.J. and Barlowe, C. (1996). "Erv25p, a component of COPII-coated vesicles, forms a complex with Emp24 that is required for efficient endoplasmic reticulum to Golgi transport." *J. Biol. Chem.* **271**: 26939–26946.
137. Belden, W. J. and Barlowe, C. (2001). "Role of Erv29p in collecting soluble secretory proteins into ER-derived transport vesicles." *Science* **294**: 1528–1531.
138. Caldwell, S., Hill, K., and Cooper, A. (2001). "Degradation of ER quality control substrates requires transport between the ER and Golgi." *J. Biol. Chem.* **276**: 23296–23303.
139. Kuehn, M., Schekman, R., and Ljungdahl, P. (1996). "Amino acid permeases require COPII components and the ER resident membrane protein in Shr3p for packaging into transport vesicles *in vitro*." *J. Cell Biol.* **135**: 585–595
140. Malkus, P., Jiang, F., and Schekman, R. (2002). "Concentrative sorting of secretory cargo proteins into COPII-coated vesicles." *J. Cell Biol.* **159**, 915–921.
141. Roberg, K., Crotwell, P., Espenshade, R., Gimeno, C., and Kaiser, C. (1999). "LST1 is a SEC24 homologue used for selective export of the plasma membrane ATPase from the endoplasmic reticulum." *J. Cell Biol.* **145**: 659–672.
142. Shimoni, Y., Kurihara, T., Ravazzola, M., Amherdt, M., Orci, L., and Schekman, R. (2000). "Lst1p and Sec24p cooperate in sorting of the plasma membrane ATPase into COPII vesicles in *Saccharomyces cerevisiae*." *J. Cell Biol.* **151**: 973–984.

143. Miller, E., Antonny, B., Hamamoto, S., and Schekman, R. (2002). "Cargo selection into COPII vesicles is driven by the Sec24p subunit." *EMBO J.* **21**: 6105–6113.
144. Miller, E., Beilharz, T. H., Malkus, P. N., Lee, M.C.S., Hamamoto, S., Orci, L., and Schekman, R. (2003). "Multiple cargo binding sites on the COPII subunit Sec24p ensure capture of diverse membrane proteins into transport vesicles." *Cell* **114**: 1–20.
145. Mosseseva, E., Bickford, L.C., and Goldberg, J., (2003). "SNARE selectivity of the COPII coat." *Cell* **114**: 483–495.
146. Merte, J., Jensen, D., Wright, K., Sarsfield, S., Wang, Y., Schekman, R., and Ginty, D. D. (2010). "Sec24b selectively sorts Vangl2 to regulate planar cell polarity during neural tube closure." *Nature Cell Biol.* **12**: 4–46.
147. Wansleeben, C., Feitsma, H., Montcouquiol, M., Kroon, C., Cuppen, E., and Meljlink, F. (2010). "Planar cell polarity defects and defective Vangl2 trfficking in mutants for the COPII gene Sec24b." *Development* **137**: 1067–1073.
148. Wu, J. and Mlodzik, M. (2009). "A quest for the mechanism regulating global planar cell polarity." *Trends in Cell Biology* **19**: 295–305.
149. Chen, X.-Y,E., Baines, E., Yu, G., Sartor, M.A., Zhang, B., Yi, Z., Lin, J., Young, S. G., Schekman, R., and Ginsburg, D. (2013). "SEC24A Deficiency Lowers Plasma Cholesterol through Reduced PCSK9 Secretion." *eLife*, April 9; 2:e00444.doi:10.7554/eLife.00444.

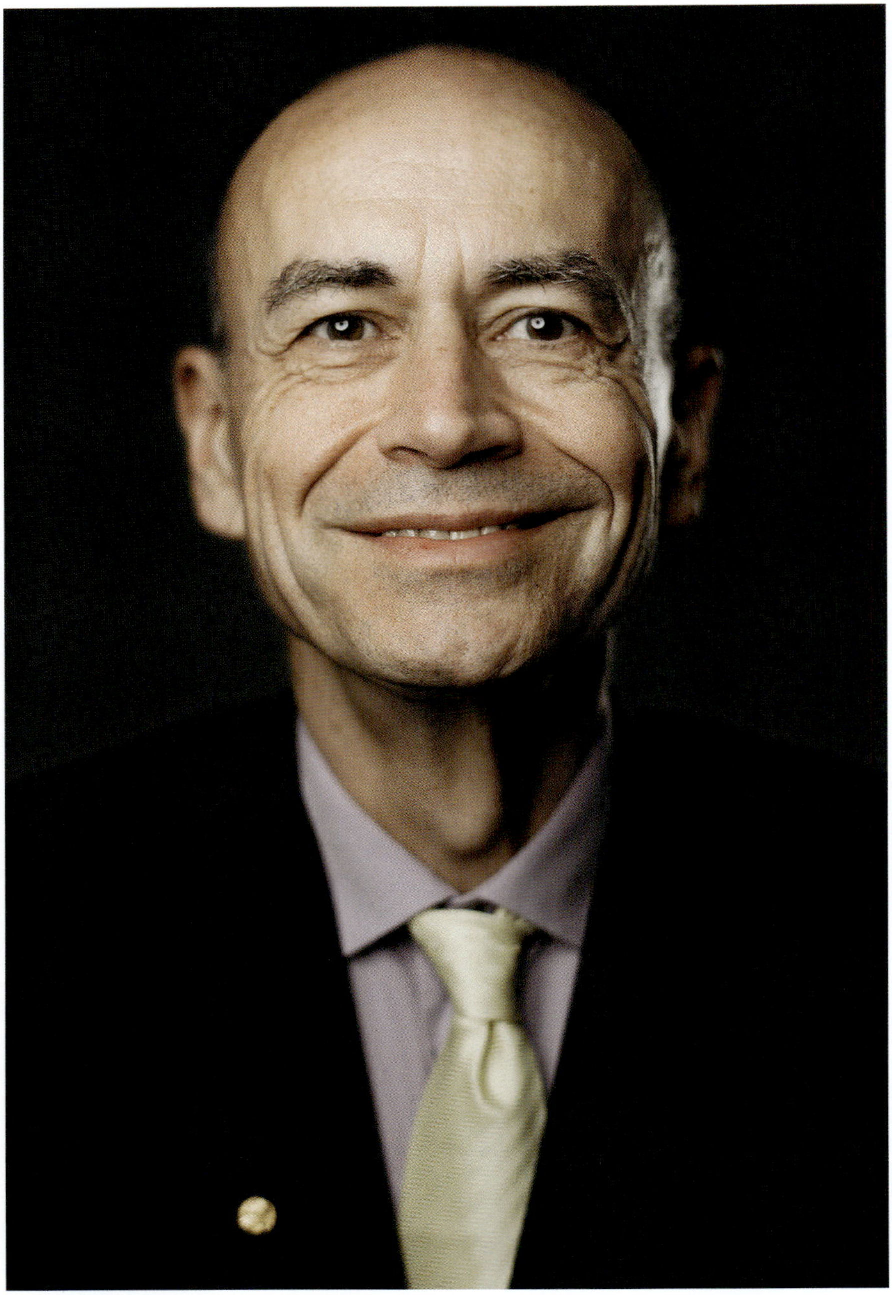

Thomas C. Südhof. © Nobel Media AB. Photo: A. Mahmoud

Thomas C. Südhof

UPBRINGING

I was born in Göttingen on December 22, 1955. At that time, the aftermaths of the Second World War were still reverberating. Mine was an anthroposophical family; my maternal grandparents had been early followers of Rudolf Steiner's teaching, and worked for Waldorf schools when Hitler assumed power and banned the anthrophosophical movement. Waldorf schools were forced to close, and my grandfather was conscripted to work in a chemical munitions factory—it was a miracle he survived the war. My uncle was drafted into the army out of school, and when I was born, he had just returned from the Soviet Union after 10 years as a prisoner of war. I was the second of four children. My parents were physicians, with my father pursuing a career in academic medicine, while my mother cared for our growing family. My father's training led him to the United States during the time I was born; as a result, he learned of my arrival by telegram as he was learning biochemical methods in San Francisco, close to where—by a twist of fate—I now live.

I spent my childhood in Göttingen and Hannover, and graduated from the Hannover Waldorf School—resurrected after the war—in 1975. My strongest childhood memories were those of my maternal grandmother telling me stories about the time during the war, how she was reading Dostoyevski while trying to escape the bombs in underground shelters and hoping that my grandfather would survive. She imbued me with the importance of Goethe and detested Kant, whom I learned to love. I learned from my grandmother how important an intellectual life is under any circumstance, and that values are spiritual even if you are an atheist.

My father was a successful doctor who managed an entire hospital district and wrote countless books on general internal medicine; he worked very hard, and was continuously frustrated by what he felt were the inadequacies of the medical care system and the academic world. However, when I was in high

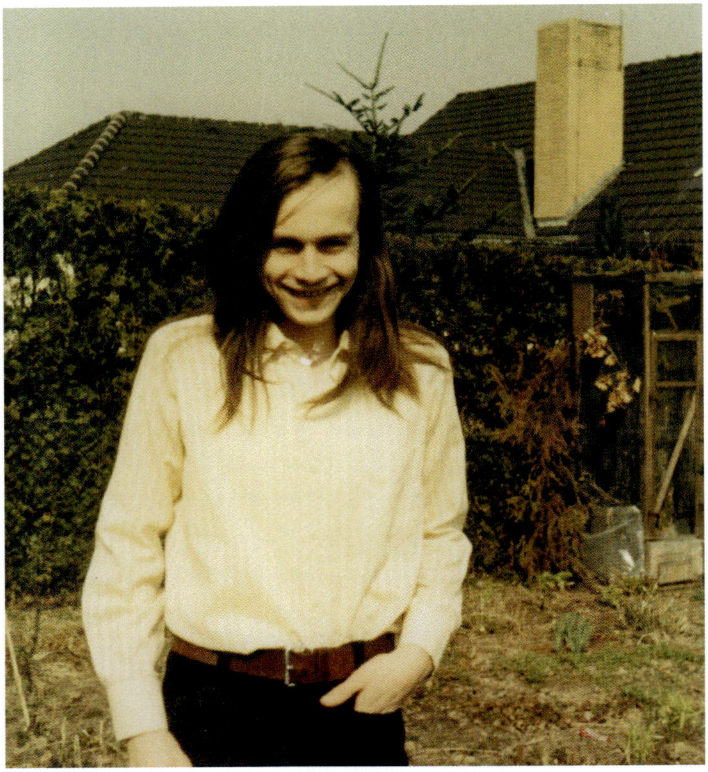

FIGURE 1. Thomas Südhof at age 16 in the garden of his parents' home in Gehrden near Hannover.

school, my father died of a heart attack, brought about by inattention to his health, and my mother had to cope with life alone with four children—a difficult and sad but an also partially liberating experience for her, as she explained to me later. Her strength was an example to me, her ability to accept what happened without giving up, and to concentrate on what was important to her.

I had been interested in many different subjects in high school, in fact all subjects except for sports which I found primitive—now ironic to me as I have become addicted to regular exercise. Early on, I became fascinated by classical music. After unsuccessful attempts at playing the violin, I gave this instrument up to the delight of everyone around me who had to listen to me trying. However, I then decided to learn to play bassoon, which I pursued with a vengeance, motivated by a wonderful teacher (Herbert Tauscher) who was the solo-bassoonist at the local opera house, and who probably taught me more about life than most of my other teachers. I credit my musical education with my dual appreciation for discipline and hard work on the one hand, and for creativity on the other. I think trying to be marginally successful in learning how to be a musician taught me how to be a scientist: there is no creativity if one does not master the subject and pay exquisite attention to the details, but there is also no creativity if one cannot transcend the details and the common interpretation of such details, and use one's mastery of the subject like an instrument to develop new ideas.

I did not know what to do with my life after school, except that I was determined not to serve in the military. More by default than by vocation, I decided to enter medical school, which kept all avenues open for a possible career in science or as a practitioner of something useful—as a physician—and allowed me to defer my military service. I thought that music, philosophy, or history were more interesting subjects than medicine, but I did not feel confident that I had sufficient talent to succeed in these difficult areas, whereas I thought that almost anybody can become a reasonably good medical doctor.

FIRST EXPERIMENTS

I studied first in Aachen, the beautiful former capital of Charles the Great, and then transferred to Göttingen, the former scientific center of the Weimar republic, in order to have better access to laboratory training since I became more and more interested in science.

Soon after arriving in Göttingen, I decided to join the Dept. of Neurochemistry of Prof. Victor P. Whittaker at the Max-Planck-Institut für biophysikalische Chemie as a 'Hilfswissenschaftler' (literally an 'assisting scientist', but more accurately a kind of 'sub-scientist'). I was attracted to Whittaker's department because it focused on biochemical approaches to probe the function of the brain, following up on Whittaker's development of purification methods for synaptosomes and synaptic vesicles in the two preceding decades. Moreover, when I entered his lab, Whittaker had become increasingly interested in the cell biology of synaptic vesicle exo- and endocytosis, which I thought were fascinating. However, I never got a chance to work on the brain or synaptic vesicles when I was in Whittaker's lab. As a lowly 'Hilfswissenschaftler', I was assigned to the task of examining the biophysical structure of chromaffin granules, which are the secretory vesicles of the adrenal medulla that store catecholamines. Although my project developed well, I started exploring other questions in parallel as I became more and more familiar with doing experiments, while simultaneously studying medicine at the university. A helpful factor was that my supposed supervisor, a senior US scientist who worked with Whittaker, departed soon after I started in Whittaker's lab, leaving me completely alone in my experiments since

Whittaker was not really interested in that work. I am infinitely grateful to Victor Whittaker for giving me complete freedom in his department in pursuing whatever I thought was interesting. I continued working in his department after my graduation from medical school in 1982 until I moved to the US a year later in 1983.

Among the work I performed during my time in Whittaker's department in Göttingen, the most significant is probably the isolation and characterization of a new family of calcium-binding proteins that we called 'calelectrins' because we had initially purified them from the electric organ of Torpedo marmorata, although we also identified them in bovine liver and brain. 'Calelectrins' were among the first identified members of an enigmatic and evolutionarily ancient family of calcium-binding proteins now called annexins. Annexins were at the same time discovered in several other laboratories, and I am proud of the fact that we contributed to the first description of this intriguing protein family, although to this date their function remains unknown.

POSTDOCTORAL TRAINING

After finishing medical school, I decided to become an academic physician, along the mold of my deceased father. Although my time in Whittaker's laboratory had taught me to love doing science, I wanted to do something more practical, exciting, and immediately useful than what I had seen in the Max-Planck-Institut in Göttingen. The standard career for an academic physician in Germany was to go abroad for a couple of years to acquire more clinically oriented scientific training before starting her/his clinical specialty training. Upon surveying the scientific landscape, I decided to join the laboratory of Mike Brown and Joe Goldstein at the University of Texas Southwestern Medical School in Dallas for postdoctoral training. Brown and Goldstein were already famous for their brilliant cell-biological studies when I made this decision. They were equally renowned for using cutting-edge scientific tools to address a central question in medicine, namely how cholesterol in blood is regulated. When I announced my decision to go to Dallas instead of the more conventional Boston or San Francisco, my friends and family were disappointed, but it was the best professional decision I ever made.

While in Joe Goldstein's and Mike Brown's laboratory, I cloned the gene encoding the LDL receptor, which taught me molecular biology, revealed to me the beauty of sequences and protein organizations, and opened up genetic analyses of this gene in human patients suffering from atherosclerosis. I also became interested in how expression of the LDL receptor is regulated by cholesterol, and identified a sequence element in the LDL receptor gene called 'SRE' for sterol-regulatory element that mediates the regulation of the LDL receptor expression by cholesterol. During my time in their laboratory, Joe Goldstein and Mike Brown were awarded the Nobel Prize (in 1985), which I still consider one of the best Nobel Prizes given. After I left, discovery of the SRE led to the identification of the SRE-binding protein in Brown and Goldstein's laboratory, which in turn identified new mechanisms of transcriptional regulation effected by intramembrane proteolysis.

The contrast between Göttingen and Dallas could not have been bigger. When I arrived in Dallas, Texas was not yet the extremely conservative bastion of religious fundamentalism that it is now, but a vast state with an optimistic 'can-do' culture that was very different from the culture to which I had been exposed in Göttingen. The difference in scientific environment was even more extreme. In Dallas, scientific life was teeming with enthusiasm and energy, work was a pleasure, and excitement was pulsating through every experiment because the importance of the goals was self-evident. In Göttingen, as I realized when I

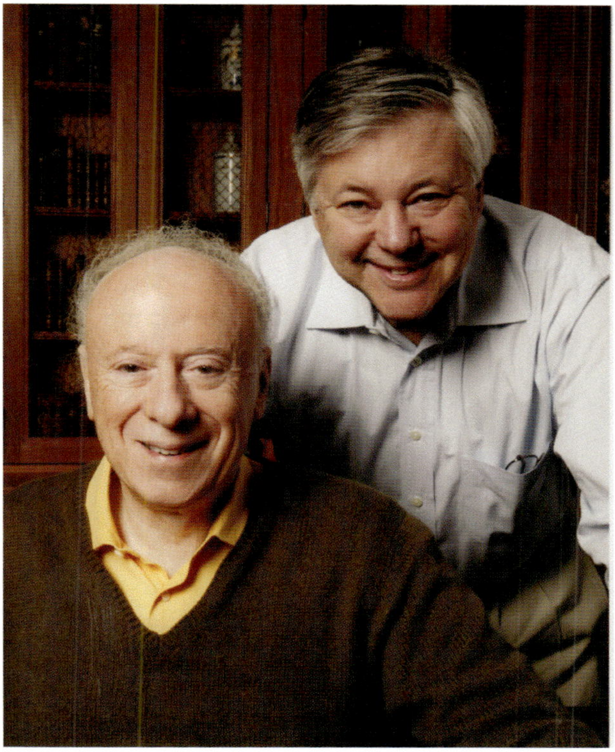

FIGURE 2. Joseph L. Goldstein and Michael S. Brown (picture taken 2008 in Dallas, TX; gift of Drs. Goldstein and Brown).

was in Dallas, although the approach was very scholarly in the sense of pursuing knowledge, much of that pursuit was without regard to the importance of the subject. As a result, people often asked uninteresting questions, and possibly even wasted their time. To this date, I find it one of the hardest challenges in science to achieve the right balance between trusting my own judgment and listening to others. If I only rely on my own judgment, there is no corrective for mistakes, no adjustment of unreasonable impressions. However, if I listen only to the 'world', I will only follow fashions, will always be behind, and often will be just as wrong. Among the many things I credit Brown and Goldstein with for teaching me, the realization of this challenge and their example of how to deal with this challenge is among the most important. This challenge resembles that of composing music in which pure harmony is boring and meaningless, but pure dissonance is unbearable, and it is really the back and forth between these extremes that creates meaning.

EARLY YEARS OF THE SÜDHOF LAB

In 1986, at the end of my postdoctoral training, I faced the choice of resuming my clinical training, or of establishing my own laboratory. Probably the best advice Brown and Goldstein gave me was now: they suggested I forego further clinical training and do 'only' science, and they backed up this advice by providing me with the opportunity to start my own laboratory at Dallas. This I did, and ended up staying for another 22 years, interrupted only by a short guest appearance as a Max-Planck Director in Göttingen (see below).

When I started my laboratory at Dallas in 1986, I decided to attack a question that was raised by Whittaker's work, but neglected since: what are synaptic vesicles composed of, and how do they undergo exo- and endocytosis, i.e., what is the mechanism of neurotransmitter release that underlies all synaptic transmission? We had learned from Whittaker's work that synaptic vesicles could be biochemically purified, but nothing was known about the molecular mechanisms guiding synaptic vesicle exo- and endocytosis. Our initial approach, performed in close collaboration with Reinhard Jahn, whose laboratory at that time had just been set up in Munich, was simple: We set out to purify and clone every protein that might conceivably be involved, and worry about their functions later. This approach was initially criticized for being too descriptive, but turned out to be more fruitful than I could have hoped for, and has arguably led to a plausible understanding of neurotransmitter release.

In the nearly three decades since I started my laboratory, our work, together with that of others, led to the identification of the key proteins that are involved

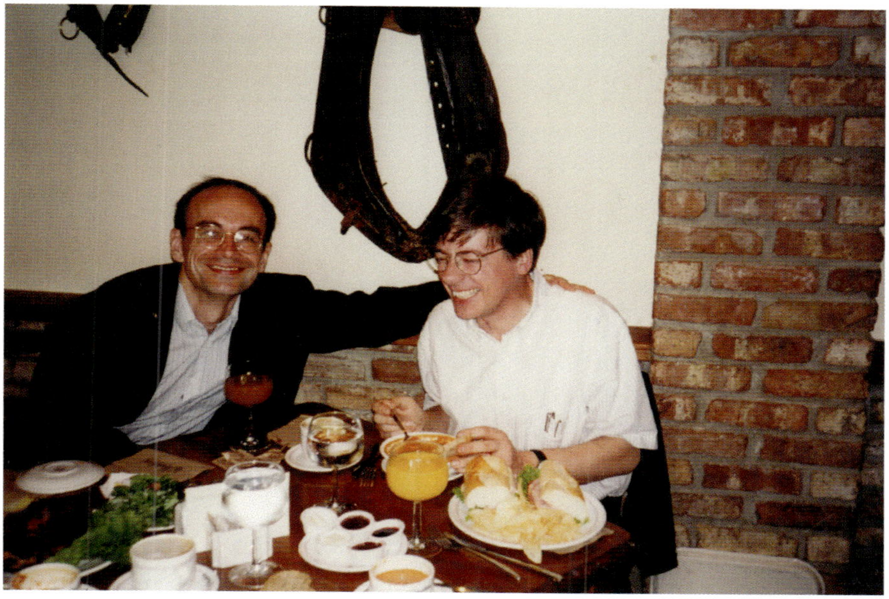

FIGURE 3. Thomas Südhof together with Reinhard Jahn at a Dallas restaurant (around 1992).

in synaptic vesicle exocytosis. In particular, this work shed light on the molecular mechanisms underlying membrane fusion during synaptic vesicle exocytosis, explained how calcium signals control these mechanisms, and described the molecular organization of the presynaptic terminal that allows fast coupling of an action potential and the ensuing calcium influx to neurotransmitter release. Some of the proteins whose function we identified are now scientific household names and have general roles in eukaryotic membrane fusion that go beyond a synaptic function, while other proteins are specific to synapses and in part account for the exquisite precision and plasticity of synapses as elementary computational elements in brain. I feel fortunate to have stumbled onto this overarching neuroscience question at a time when it was ready to be addressed, and it has been tremendous fun to work our way through the various synaptic proteins and their properties that shape the functions of these proteins.

It is important to note, however, that the nature of our studies was not revolutionary. In my career, no single major discovery changed the field all at once. Instead, our work progressed in incremental steps over two decades. I think this is a general property of scientific progress in understanding how something works—a single experiment rarely explains a major question, but usually a body of work is required. In contrast, scientific progress in developing tools normally advances in spurts, and often a single flash of genius creates a completely new method (e.g., see monoclonal antibodies, patch clamping, PCR, or shRNAs, to name a few).

The closest our work came to inducing a radical change in the field was probably the identification of synaptotagmins as calcium-sensors for fusion, and of Sec1/Munc18-like proteins (SM-proteins) as membrane fusion proteins, but both hypotheses took decades to develop and to become accepted by the field—in fact, the SM-protein hypothesis was only recently adopted by others, 20 years after we proposed it, and is still in flux. Thus, our work in parallel with that of others (Reinhard Jahn, James Rothman, Jose Rizo, Randy Scheckman, Richard Scheller, Cesare Montecucco, and Axel Brunger come to mind) produced a steady incremental advance that resulted a better understanding of how membranes fuse, one step at a time. As a result of this combined effort, we now know that SNAREs are the fusion catalysts at the synapse, first shown when SNAREs were shown to be the substrates of clostridial neurotoxins, that SM-proteins in general and Munc18-1 in particular are essential contributors to all membrane fusion events, that a synaptotagmin-based mechanism assisted by complexin underlies nearly all regulated exocytosis, and that synaptic exocytosis

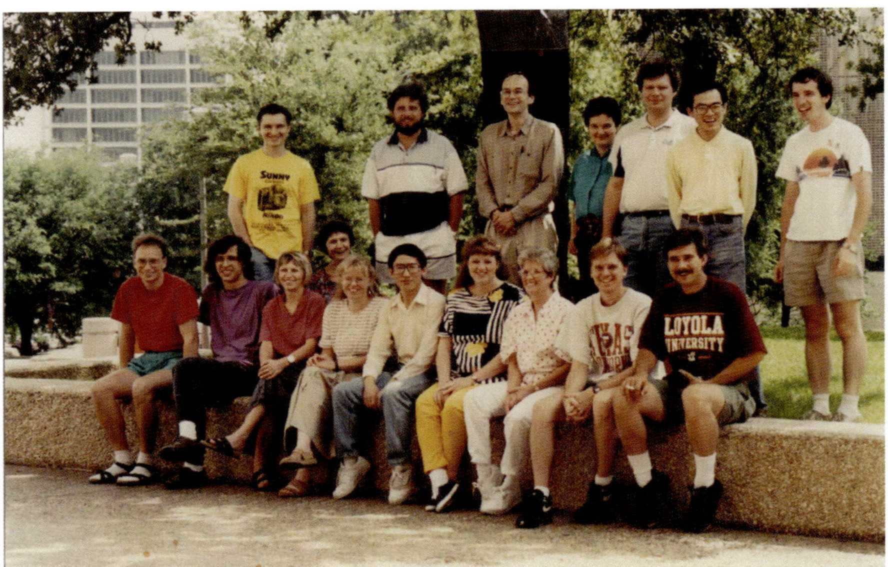

FIGURE 4. The Südhof laboratory in Dallas in 1995. Sitting in the first row left to right: Thomas Rosahl, Martin Geppert, Ewa Borowicz, Izabella Kornblum [sitting behind the row], Else Fykse, Cai Li, Andrea Roth, Shirley Clement, Christopher Newton, and Greg Mignery. Standing left to right: Konstantin Ichtechenko, Alexander Petrenko, Thomas Südhof, Beate Ullrich, Andrei Khokhlatchev, Yutaka Hata, and Harvey McMahon.

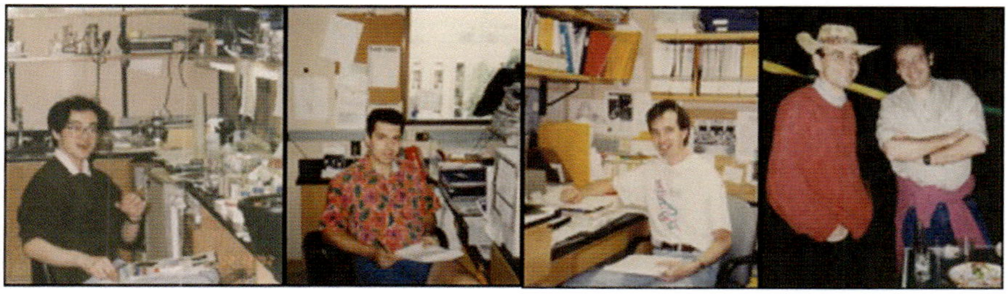

FIGURE 5. Work in the Südhof laboratory in Dallas in the 1990s. Left, Yutaka Hata at his bench; middle right, Nils Brose at his desk; middle right, Harvey McMahon getting ready to think; right, Thomas Südhof and Rafael Fernandez-Chacon after work.

is organized in time and space by an active zone protein scaffold containing RIM and Munc13 proteins as central elements.

The work in my lab would have been impossible without the contributions of many brilliant postdoctoral fellows who have now gone on to successful careers on their own. Ever since I started my laboratory, I have found the pleasure of working with others the best part of my life. The continuing friendship of my former trainees has been one of the major satisfactions of my career. Among these were Mark Perin with whom I cloned synaptotagmin, Yutaka Hata who discovered Munc18, Martin Geppert who performed the initial mouse genetics experiments in my lab, Nils Brose who identified Munc13, Harvey McMahon who identified complexins, Yun Wang who isolated RIM, and many others who made essential contributions. Complementing these great co-workers, I had the best collaborators I could possibly wish for. Besides Reinhard Jahn (who had moved to Yale after Munich, and then on to Göttingen), the most important of these collaborators were Jose Rizo in Dallas with whom we worked out the atomic structures of many of the proteins we studied, Bob Hammer in Dallas who helped us with the mouse genetics, and Chuck Stevens at the Salk Institute who introduced us to the beauty of electrophysiological analyses.

MY GERMAN INTERMEZZO

Ten years after I started my laboratory, while the work described above was progressing, I was offered the opportunity to return to Germany and to organize a Department of Neuroscience at the Max-Planck-Institut für experimentelle Medizin in Göttingen, my home town. I enthusiastically took on the challenge, planned and oversaw the building of a new animal facility, hired scientists, and organized the renovations and equipment of a suite of laboratories. However, after a few years the leadership of the Max-Planck-Society changed. It soon became clear that the Max-Planck-Society's new president, Prof. Hubert Markl, developed doubts about my recruitment, and wanted to rebuild the institute that I was recruited into in directions that were quite different from what I had been promised. In a personal discussion, Prof. Markl suggested I resign my position at the Max-Planck-Institut and look for a future in the U.S., which I did.

I have never regretted my work for the Max-Planck-Institut in Göttingen, which laid the foundation for much of what happened there subsequently, including the subsequent recruitment of one of my postdoctoral fellows (Nils Brose) as a new director who has done a much better job than I could have done. However, I have also never regretted following Prof. Markl's suggestion and returning to the U.S., where the breadth and tolerance of the system allowed me to operate in a manner that was more suitable for my somewhat iconoclastic temperament. Overall, my work as a director at the Max-Planck-Institut in Göttingen was a very positive experience that shaped my thinking when I subsequently had the opportunity to help build the Department of Neuroscience at the University of Texas Southwestern Medical Center in Dallas.

MATURITY

Soon after I returned full-time to UT Southwestern at Dallas in 1998, I accepted the position of director of the Center for Basic Neuroscience, which was later transformed into the Department of Neuroscience. Building a Center and Department of Neuroscience partly occupied the following ten years, and was a lot of fun. Southwestern had a free-flowing and unbureaucratic environment that was extremely supportive. It was a pleasure to hire young people and see them develop, and I greatly appreciated the support of my colleagues in every respect.

Scientifically the 10 years between 1998 and 2008 were even more important. The flurry of discoveries of the 1990s created the impression that everything was already solved in membrane fusion and neurotransmitter release, but nothing could have been farther from the truth. I decided to continue to work on these questions, and believe that some of the most important observations in the field came out of our work during that time period.

For example, it was well established in 2000 that SNAREs 'do' fusion and that they 'do so' by pulling membranes together, but it was unknown whether SNAREs were just nanomachines that acted as force-generators in approximating membranes, or whether they actually catalyze the fusion process, possibly by their transmembrane regions. Similarly, although we found that the SM-protein Munc18-1 was absolutely essential for fusion, Munc 18-1 appeared to bind to a form of the SNARE protein syntaxin-1 that was 'closed' and was thought to block fusion, whereas the yeast homolog Sec1p, as shown in elegant work by

Peter Novick, bound to assembled SNARE complexes. How could the same protein be essential for fusion and inhibit SNARE-complex formation? Comparably puzzling questions surrounded the role of synaptotagmin as a calcium sensor in neurotransmitter release. Furthermore, a major question in understanding synapses had never been addressed, namely how the presynaptic machinery is organized in a manner that allows tight coupling of calcium-influx to the calcium-triggering of release. The significance of this latter question is often underestimated outside of the esoteric realm of neurophysiologists, but this tight coupling is the most important prerequisite for the speed and brevity of neurotransmitter release—in essence this coupling is what makes a synapse precise.

In the years after 1998, my lab and the labs of others, foremost those of my former postdoctoral fellows Nils Brose, Harvey McMahon, and Matthijs Verhage, of Christian Rosenmund, of Peter Novick, and of Jim Rothman, established several key points that address these questions. The most important was the demonstration that synaptotagmin is truly the calcium-sensor for release by showing that point mutations in synaptotagmin that change its calcium-affinity change release accordingly. Maybe equally important was the finding that Munc18 acts by binding to SNARE complexes after assembly, not by binding to one SNARE protein before assembly. Other significant findings of these years included the demonstration of the priming function of Munc13, the discovery that complexin acts as a 'sidekick' to support synaptotagmin function and that both synaptotagmin and complexin clamp minis in addition to the major action as activators of release, and that multiple synaptotagmins generally function as calcium-sensors in release. Moreover, in these years we identified specific chaperones that support the proper folding of SNAREs, opening up a new perspective on how SNARE function is maintained in neurons, an important issue because the loss of these chaperone activities were found to cause neurodegeneration. These were very productive years that did more than complete the stories we had begun in the 90s—they extended these stories into new directions, including an explanation of at least some forms of neurodegeneration. The one major issue that remained unresolved was how calcium-channels are recruited to the active zone, a question that was really only resolved after I moved to Stanford in 2008.

NEW AND OLD DIRECTIONS

The currently final chapter in my career began when I moved my laboratory from UT Southwestern to Stanford University in 2008. After 10 years as a chair of a Neuroscience Center and then Department in Dallas, I felt that I wanted to devote more of my time to pure science, and to embark on a new professional direction, with an environment that was focused on academics. Moreover, I decided to redirect a large part of my efforts towards a major problem in neuroscience that appeared to be unexplored: how synapses are formed. Thus, in this currently last chapter of my work, I am probing the mechanisms that allow circuits to form in brain, and to form with often nearly magical properties dictated by the specific features of particular synapses at highly specific positions. I am fascinated by the complexity of this process, which far surpasses the numerical size of the genome, and interested in how disturbances in this process contribute to neuropsychiatric diseases such as autism and schizophrenia. This is what I would like to address in the next few years, hoping for at least some interesting insights.

As early as 1992, my laboratory had identified a family of cell-surface proteins called neurexins whose properties suggested that they may be involved in synapse formation. Neurexins were discovered because they are presynaptic receptors for the black widow spider venom component α-latrotoxin which paralyses small prey by causing excessive neurotransmitter release. However, the importance of neurexins and their ligands—such as the neuroligins, cerebellins, and neurexophilins which we and others identified—only became apparent in recent years when we started to analyze mouse mutants of these proteins.

Apart from these new directions, at Stanford we followed up on two 'old' questions about release: how calcium-channels are recruited to active zones, and what mediates the calcium-triggered release that remains in synapses which lack fast synaptotagmin calcium-sensor isoforms. Both questions had haunted me for decades—I was convinced of their importance but could not solve them. Only in the last few years did we develop answers to these questions in identifying the scaffolding proteins RIMs and RIM-BPs as the organizers of calcium-channels in the presynaptic active zone, and another synaptotagmin isoform (synaptotagmin-7) as a calcium-sensor for the remaining release in synaptotagmin-1 deficient forebrain neurons. Fittingly, this last observation was submitted a few weeks before the announcement of the Nobel Prize, and published coincidently with the award ceremony!

LIFE LESSONS

After nearly 60 years of life and nearly 40 years as a scientist, I would like to draw the following personal conclusions, none of them very original. First, being a scientist, although socially a privilege and luxury, is not socially rewarding—for personal happiness, this profession is only worth it if a person obtains individual satisfaction in doing science. A scientist has to have the attitude of an adherent to Philip Spener's pietism in Lutheran Germany in the 18th century—what counts are not outward successes, money, and social decorations, but the conviction of truth obtained from personal inspection of the evidence. After a glorious period of ascendance in Western Europe from Bacon's England over Courvoisier's France to Boltzmann's Germany, the scientific method is now increasingly being challenged based on ideological grounds. In the most powerful country of the world, the United States, the majority of the governing elite at present feels free to dismiss some established scientific facts as fantasy, even suspecting evolution or climate science as communist conspiracies at a time when there is no communism left anywhere. At this stage—different from previous centuries—the only reason to pursue a career in science is an enormous curiosity to know what is really true.

Second, I at least have learned most from personal contacts, not from reading the literature or listening to talks. Although reading books or papers provided me with an indispensable background of facts, I learned how to think, how to assess a subject, and how to value a perspective from insightful comments of others. Thus, for a scientific career the most important elements are good teachers and mentors, and a great environment—not only during early years as student and postdoc, but throughout the entire career of a scientist. Now at an arguably rather advanced stage of my career, I need mentors and teachers more than ever—I need people who know better than I to tell me when I am wrong, and to make me aware of my mistakes! As an immediate consequence of this realization, I would advise everybody to make career choices primarily based on the people involved, not on the geographic location of a place or the fashionableness of the subject or the techniques. I believe this is true for all stages of a career.

Third, once a scientist has the opportunity to choose what to work on (increasingly a rarity in our world where political prescriptions of what scientists are supposed to discover are becoming more and more prevalent), he/she should make sure that whatever the choice of subject is, it is both important and tractable. I am personally often amazed about the choice of subject by some of my colleagues, possibly because I simply fail to recognize the importance of the subject. However, if one looks at the history of science over the last 50 years or so, I think one can argue that some approaches and goals have proved to be highly productive whereas others have not. For example, investments into bacterial and bacteriophage genetics early on eventually led to the golden age of molecular biology that all of science, but particularly cellular neuroscience, has benefitted from, whereas the parallel large investments into systems neuroscience has only recently started to bear some fruit after the tools developed by molecular and cellular neurobiology were beginning to be applied.

Finally, quantity doesn't matter very much, nor does the place one publishes—in the end what counts is discovery which is often not immediately apparent. Most articles in "high-impact journals," although highly cited initially, are soon forgotten. Especially in our time, when it is basically the editor of a journal and not the reviewers who decides what gets published—an editor who often has limited knowledge of the subject but knows what is 'exciting'—the major journals publish many papers that are composed of true data with contrived interpretations and very little long-term import. As scientists, we have to intellectually dissociate ourselves from fashion and journals, and focus on what is the actual content of a study, what the data really say (not what the abstract says!). We can then take pride and pleasure in work that reports an actual advance—I feel that this is the most important ability I tried to learn from my mentors, and I am trying to teach my students.

THANK YOU

Throughout my career, I have been generously supported by the Howard Hughes Medical Institute and the National Institute of Mental Health. I am grateful to both for their unflinching support. I have received several recognitions, all of them unexpected, among which I particularly cherish the Alden Spencer Award from Columbia University in 1993, the von Euler Lectureship from the Karolinska Institutet in 2004, the Kavli Award in 2010, the Lasker~deBakey Award in 2013, and—of course—the Nobel Prize. I am not sure I deserve any of these awards, as conceptual advances in science always represent incremental progress to which many minds contribute, but I immensely appreciate receiving them. Finally, I feel indebted beyond words to my family, my wife Lu Chen and my children Saskia, Alexander, Leanna, Sören, Roland, and Moritz, without whom I would be barren and rudderless, and who have been more considerate of me than I deserve, and finally to my ex-wife Annette Südhof who greatly supported me in earlier stages of my life, and to my brothers Markus and Donat Südhof and my sister Gudrun Südhof-Müller whom I appreciate more the older I get.

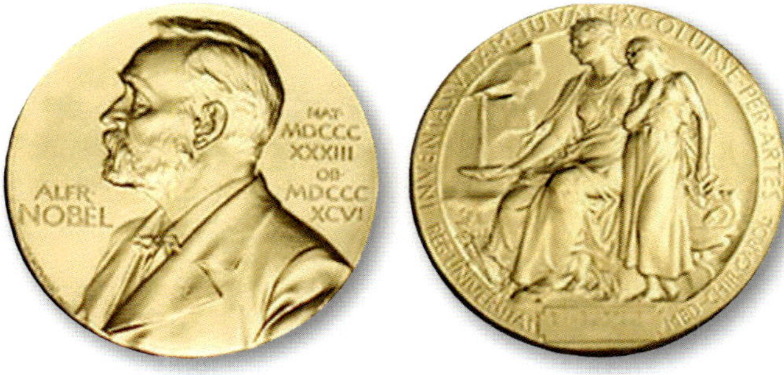

The Molecular Machinery of Neurotransmitter Release

Nobel Lecture, 7 December 2013

by Thomas C. Südhof
Dept. of Molecular and Cellular Physiology, and Howard Hughes Medical Institute, Stanford University, USA.

1. THE NEUROTRANSMITTER RELEASE ENIGMA

Synapses have a long history in science. Synapses were first functionally demonstrated by Emil duBois-Reymond (1818–1896), were morphologically identified by classical neuroanatomists such as Rudolf von Kölliker (1817–1905) and Santiago Ramon y Cajal (1852–1934), and named in 1897 by Michael Foster (1836–1907). Although the chemical nature of synaptic transmission was already suggested by duBois-Reymond, it was long disputed because of its incredible speed. Over time, however, overwhelming evidence established that most synapses use chemical messengers called neurotransmitters, most notably with the pioneering contributions by Otto Loewi (1873–1961), Henry Dale (1875–1968), Ulf von Euler (1905–1983), and Julius Axelrod (1912–2004). In parallel, arguably the most important advance to understanding how synapses work was provided by Bernard Katz (1911–2003), who elucidated the principal mechanism of synaptic transmission (Katz, 1969). Most initial studies on synapses were carried out on the neuromuscular junction, and central synapses have only come to the fore in recent decades. Here, major contributions by many scientists, including George Palade, Rodolfo Llinas, Chuck Stevens, Bert Sakmann, Eric Kandel, and Victor Whittaker, to name just a few, not only confirmed the principal results obtained in the neuromuscular junction by Katz, but also revealed that synapses exhibit an enormous diversity of properties as well as an unexpected capacity for plasticity.

Arguably, the most important property of synaptic transmission is its speed. At most synapses, synaptic transmission lasts for only a few milliseconds. This amazing speed is crucial for the overall workings of the brain—how else could a goalkeeper react to a shot in less than a second, or a ballerina pirouette without crashing to the floor? Synapses differ dramatically from each other in properties such as strength and plasticity, but always operate by the same canonical principle to achieve this speed, as first elucidated by Bernard Katz. When an action potential travels down an axon, it depolarizes the nerve terminals and opens presynaptic Ca^{2+}-channels. The in-flowing Ca^{2+} then triggers neurotransmitter release in less than a millisecond, with a delay of possibly less than 100 microseconds (Sabatini and Regehr, 1996). Amazingly given this speed, presynaptic neurotransmitter release is mediated by membrane traffic. Presynaptic terminals are chock-full with synaptic vesicles—uniformly small organelles with a 35 nm diameter—that contain high concentrations of neurotransmitters. Release is triggered when Ca^{2+} induces the rapid fusion of these vesicles with the presynaptic plasma membrane at a specialized region, the so-called active zone. The active zone is located exactly opposite the postsynaptic density containing the neurotransmitter receptors; as a result, neurotransmitters are released directly onto their receptors (Fig. 1).

The active zone is the organizing principle that ensures the speed and precision of synaptic transmission. The active zone recruits and docks synaptic vesicles at the release sites, transforms synaptic vesicles into a fusion-competent 'primed' state that is responsive to Ca^{2+}-triggering of release, and tethers Ca^{2+}-channels next to the docking sites (Südhof, 2012). By co-localizing Ca^{2+}-channels and primed vesicles at the synaptic cleft, the active zone enables the tight coupling of neurotransmitter release to an action potential and directs neurotransmitter release to the synaptic cleft. After exocytosis, synaptic vesicles recycle by different pathways, including fast endocytic mechanisms that are sometimes referred to as 'kiss-and-run' (Ceccarelli et al., 1973), as well as slower endocytic mechanisms involving clathrin-coated pits (Heuser and Reese, 1973; Fig. 1).

Compared to presynaptic neurotransmitter release, postsynaptic neurotransmitter reception is conceptually more straightforward since it is largely mediated by transmitter binding to ligand-gated ion channels. Postsynaptic ionotropic receptors are highly developed molecular machines that are clustered opposite to the presynaptic active zone, and quickly convert an extracellular neurotransmitter signal into an intracellular ionic signal (Fig. 1). The apparent simplicity of postsynaptic mechanisms, however, is deceptive because

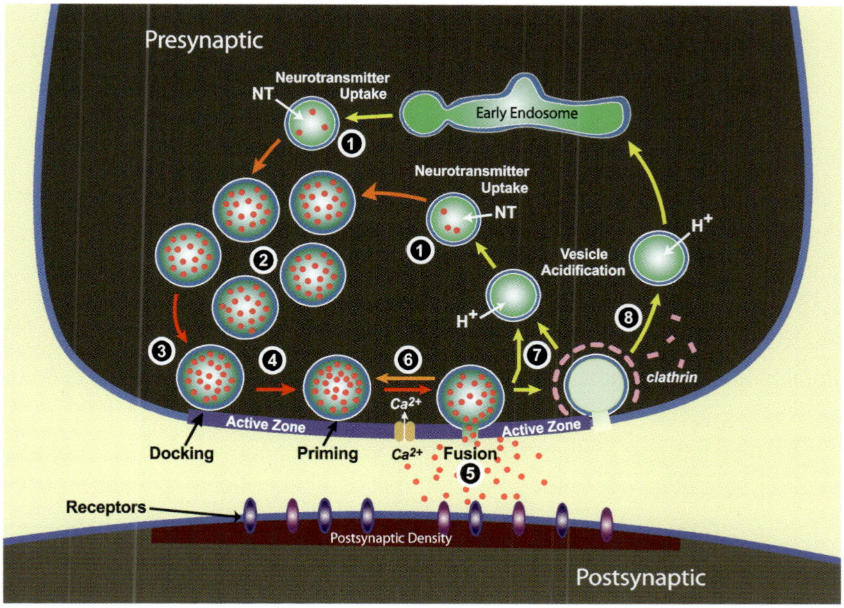

FIGURE 1. *The synaptic vesicle cycle.* Synaptic vesicles undergo a membrane trafficking cycle in presynaptic terminals that mediates neurotransmitter release. Step *1*, vesicles are replenished from endosomes or by recycling after exo- and endocytosis, and are filled with neurotransmitters (NT); Step *2*, vesicles are transported to the active zone of the presynaptic plasma membrane, where they reside in a cluster ready to be recruited for exocytosis; Step *3*, vesicles are tethered to the presynaptic active zone in a 'docking' reaction that depends on the synaptic vesicle proteins Rab3/27 and the active zone protein RIM (see Fig. 14); Step *4*, vesicles are 'primed' to render them competent for Ca^{2+}-triggered fusion; Step *5*, Ca^{2+} triggers fusion-pore opening, releasing the neurotransmitters; Steps *6–8*, vesicles recycle locally immediately after fusion-pore opening (6, 'kiss-and-stay'), by endocytosis via a rapid pathway that is likely clathrin-independent (7, 'kiss-and-run'), or by a clathrin-dependent pathway that involves an endosomal intermediate (8). Note that most of the recycling pathways were worked out in classical studies by Heuser and Reese (1973), Ceccarelli et al. (1973), and Zimmermann and Whittaker (1977). Drawing was adapted from Südhof and Jahn (1991) and Südhof (2004).

postsynaptic neurotransmitter receptors are subject to complex regulatory processes, including vesicular trafficking, that are incompletely understood. Moreover, postsynaptic signal-transduction pathways are organized in a sophisticated and compartmentalized manner that differs between various types of synapses. Considering the simple yet complex canonical design of a chemical synapse, one cannot but marvel at the ingenuity of this design that enables the requisite speed and plasticity of synaptic transmission using specialized pre- and postsynaptic machineries.

When I started my laboratory in 1986, neurotransmitter release had been described in exquisite physiological detail. However, there was no mechanistic understanding, not even a hypothesis, of how synaptic vesicles might fuse, how Ca^{2+} could possibly trigger such fusion so rapidly, and how the release machinery is organized by the presynaptic active zone. No molecular component of the release machinery had been characterized, and no conceptual framework was available to explain the extraordinary plasticity and precision of Ca^{2+}-triggered release. I focused on these questions, as opposed to studying postsynaptic neurotransmitter reception, because I was mesmerized by the apparent incomprehensibility of the speed of Ca^{2+}-triggered release, and intrigued by the general implications of understanding release for other membrane-trafficking reactions, such as hormone secretion.

In the following, I will provide a brief personal overview of what we found. I will present our work in the context of that of others which was indispensable for our progress, but given space constraints I will not be able to do justice to the many important contributions made by others. We performed our studies as part of a larger scientific community working on this problem, and I will try to provide as balanced an account of the field as I can within my space allowance.

2. MOLECULAR ANATOMY OF THE PRESYNAPTIC TERMINAL

When we started, we chose a simple approach to the understanding of neurotransmitter release: to isolate and clone all major proteins of presynaptic terminals. Largely in collaboration with Reinhard Jahn, we first focused on synaptic vesicles because they could be obtained at high yield and purity (Whittaker and Sheridan, 1965; Südhof and Jahn, 1991). Later on, we expanded this approach to the presynaptic active zone. With these initial experiments, we aimed to assemble a molecular catalogue of presynaptic proteins as a starting point for a functional dissection of release.

The first synaptic vesicle proteins we purified and cloned were synaptophysin (Südhof et al., 1987), cytochrome b561 (Perin et al., 1988), synapsins (Südhof et al., 1989a), synaptobrevins (Südhof et al., 1989b; also independently cloned by R.H. Scheller and named vesicle-associated membrane protein [VAMP]; Trimble et al., 1988), proton pump components (Südhof et al., 1989c; Perin et al., 1991), and synaptotagmins (Perin et al., 1990; Geppert et al., 1991; Li et al., 1995). In addition, we found that Rab3 proteins, the brain's most abundant GTP-binding proteins originally identified as ras-homologous sequences (Touchot et al., 1987), are associated with synaptic vesicles (von Mollard et al.,

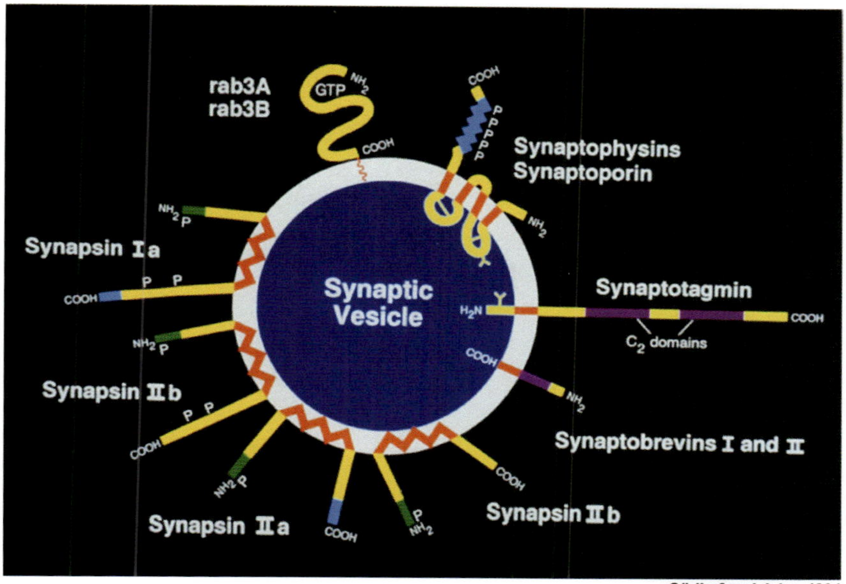

FIGURE 2. *Diagram of synaptic vesicle proteins involved in neurotransmitter release as seen in 1991.* At the beginning of the effort to map the molecular anatomy of synaptic vesicles, five major classes of synaptic vesicle proteins were identified: the synapsins that were at that time thought to be major candidates for regulating neurotransmitter release (Südhof et al., 1989a), Rab3 proteins (von Mollard et al., 1990), synaptophysins (Südhof et al., 1987), synaptotagmins (Perin et al., 1990), and synaptobrevins/VAMPs (Südhof et al., 1989b). Of these proteins, three classes (Rab3, synaptotagmins, and synaptobrevins) turned out to be crucial for release in subsequent studies (reproduced from Südhof and Jahn, 1991).

1990), and that Rab3 proteins cycle on and off synaptic vesicles during exocytosis (von Mollard et al., 1991).

Thus, in the beginning of the 1990s a fairly comprehensive characterization of the synaptic vesicle as an organelle had emerged (Südhof and Jahn, 1991; Fig. 2). Subsequently, we and others cloned a series of additional vesicle proteins, including SVOP (Janz et al., 1998) and SCAMPs (Fernandez-Chacon et al., 2000). Furthermore, we expanded our attempts to molecularly characterize the release machinery to the active zone, and identified Munc18s (Hata et al., 1993), complexins (McMahon et al., 1995), Munc13s (Brose et al., 1995), CASK (Hata et al., 1996), RIMs (Wang et al., 1997), RIM-BPs (Wang et al., 2000), and ELKS (Wang et al., 2002; independently described by Ohtsuka et al., 2002). These studies were complemented by those of others identifying as active-zone proteins α-liprins

(Zhen and Jin, 1999), bassoon (tom Diek et al., 1998) and piccolo (Wang et al., 1999; Fenster et al., 2000).

After having elucidated the primary structures of a growing number of synaptic proteins, we faced the challenge of determining their functions. We decided to examine these molecules broadly in an un-biased manner as systematically as possible, and used a combination of methods ranging from biochemistry and cell biology to structural biology, mouse genetics, and electrophysiology.

As I will describe in the following account, these studies enabled a new understanding of neurotransmitter release. However, not all efforts were productive, and not all abundant and conserved synaptic proteins were found to be important. For example, prominent proteins such as synapsins and synaptophysins turned out to have only ancillary roles in the synaptic vesicle cycle that may be important for the overall organism, but are not essential for the basic process of synaptic vesicle exo- and endocytosis (e.g., Rosahl et al., 1993 and 1995; Janz et al., 1999).

In the following description, I will divide neurotransmitter release into three processes, membrane fusion as the basic mechanism that mediates release by synaptic vesicle exocytosis, Ca^{2+}-triggering as the key event that enables fast synaptic transmission, and the spatial organization of the release machinery by the active zone that allows precise coupling of a presynaptic action potential to a postsynaptic response.

3. MECHANISM OF SYNAPTIC MEMBRANE FUSION

SNARE Proteins in Fusion

The first insights into how synaptic vesicles fuse with the presynaptic plasma membrane during neurotransmitter release came from studies of tetanus and botulinum toxins. These neurotoxins, which as disease agents cause tetanus and botulism but also have great therapeutic value, are among the most powerful neurotoxins known (Grumelli et al., 2005). Tetanus and botulinum toxins are metalloproteases that block neurotransmitter release at nanomolar concentrations by arresting the fusion of synaptic vesicles with the presynaptic plasma membrane.

In 1992, studies in Cesare Montecucco's, Heiner Niemann's, and Reinhard Jahn's laboratories—to which we contributed—showed that tetanus toxin and botulinum B toxin block synaptic vesicle fusion by proteolytic cleavage of Synaptobrevin-2/VAMPs (Link et al., 1992; Schiavo et al., 1992). In the following year, the same laboratories showed that other types of botulinum toxins cleave two other presynaptic membrane proteins, SNAP-25 and Syntaxin-1 (Blasi et al., 1993a and 1993b; Schiavo et al., 1993). Moreover, we demonstrated that a ubiquitously distributed synaptobrevin isoform (Cellubrevin) is also a tetanus toxin substrate, suggesting that the inhibition of vesicle fusion by tetanus toxin-dependent cleavage of Synaptobrevin-2 reflects a general function of synaptobrevin-like molecules in membrane fusion (McMahon et al., 1993). Together, these findings provided the first, and arguably still most compelling evidence that Synaptobrevin-2, SNAP-25, and Syntaxin-1 are essential components of the presynaptic membrane fusion machinery. As we will see now, evidence about how these proteins, later named SNARE proteins (for 'soluble NSF-attachment protein receptors'), might work came from parallel studies in James Rothman's laboratory.

Rothman had been studying membrane fusion by biochemically reconstituting vesicular traffic between compartments of the Golgi apparatus (Balch et al., 1984). Using this assay, Rothman isolated an N-ethyl maleimide-sensitive factor (referred to as NSF) and NSF-adaptor proteins that attach NSF to membranes (referred to as SNAPs, an unfortunate coincidence of acronyms with SNAP-25). Both NSF and SNAPs were essential for *in vitro* fusion in Rothman's assay, and were found to be homologous to yeast genes involved in secretion, suggesting a fundamental function in membrane traffic (Wilson et al., 1989; Clary et al., 1990). In a crucial study, Rothman's laboratory then used immobilized NSF and SNAPs as an affinity matrix to purify SNAP 'receptors' (i.e., SNAREs) from brain because brain was the richest source of such receptors. He isolated Synaptobrevin-2, Syntaxin-1 and SNAP-25, just as these proteins were revealed to be tetanus and botulinum toxin substrates (Söllner et al., 1993a). Subsequently, Rothman went on to show in collaboration with Richard Scheller that Synaptobrevin-2, Syntaxin-1, and SNAP-25 formed a complex with each other, and that this complex is dissociated by NSF which acts as an ATPase (Söllner et al., 1993b). This brilliant experiment provided an explanation for how these proteins might work in fusion, although it took many more years to formulate a compelling mechanism for their fusion function. Collaborating with Heiner Niemann, we found that SNARE complexes are SDS-resistant and extremely tight, and that only the SNARE complex but not individual SNARE proteins binds to SNAPs and NSF, while only free SNARE proteins but not SNARE proteins in the complex are substrates for botulinum and tetanus toxins (Hayashi et al., 1994; McMahon et al., 1995a).

Viewed together, these studies suggested to us that formation of SNARE complexes between the synaptic vesicle and presynaptic plasma membranes may mediate fusion, but the mechanism of fusion was unclear. One hypothesis was that NSF and SNAPs are the actual fusion proteins, and that SNARE proteins ensure the specificity of the fusion reaction mediated by NSF and SNAPs by acting as their receptors after SNARE complexes have assembled (Söllner et al., 1993a and 1993b). An alternative idea that we favored was motivated by the botulinum and tetanus toxin data, and stated that SNARE proteins, especially synaptobrevin, are actually directly involved in fusion, although we did not know by what mechanism (Südhof et al., 1993).

Two subsequent key experiments clarified the question whether NSF/SNAPs or SNAREs are the actual membrane-fusion proteins. First, Bill Wickner's laboratory elegantly showed in yeast vacuole fusion assays that yeast NSF does not function in fusion, but is only required to activate SNARE proteins for fusion and to recycle the SNARE machinery after fusion (Mayer et al., 1996). Second, in a seminal experiment Reinhard Jahn and John Heuser demonstrated that SNARE complexes assemble in a parallel manner, such that SNARE-complex assembly forces the C-terminal transmembrane regions of SNARE proteins into close proximity (Hanson et al., 1997). This key observation by Heuser and Jahn provided an immediate model for how SNARE proteins may mediate fusion, namely by zippering up in an N- to C-terminal direction, thereby forcing membranes that contain their C-terminal transmembrane regions into close proximity. This model was quickly confirmed using biophysical studies and crystallography (Lin and Scheller, 1997; Poirier et al., 1998, Sutton et al., 1998), and further elaborated by Rothman and others using *in vitro* reconstitution experiments with liposomes (Weber et al., 1998). It is now the standard model of the field.

SM proteins are obligatory SNARE partners in membrane fusion

In 1993, just at the time at which SNARE proteins were being discovered as membrane fusion proteins, we searched for other components of the fusion machinery using affinity chromatography on immobilized Syntaxin-1 (Hata et al., 1993). We isolated a 65 kDa protein that we named Munc18-1 because of its sequence homology to the C. elegans *unc18* gene (Fig. 3A). Sidney Brenner had isolated *unc18*-mutants because the mutant worms did not move properly (were '*unc*oordinated'), but the function of the *unc18* gene was unknown (Brenner, 1974). However, because Munc18 bound to the SNARE membrane-fusion machinery and because C. elegans *unc18* was essential for movement, we hypothesized that Munc18-1 was an intrinsic component of the fusion machinery, and co-operates with SNARE proteins in fusion (Fig. 3A).

Further analyses revealed that Munc18-1 was also homologous to *sec1*, which was the first gene isolated by Peter Novick and Randy Schekman in screens for secretory yeast mutants, but whose function, like that of the previously described *unc18*, was unknown (Novick and Schekman, 1979). In fact, this homology led some investigators to refer to Munc18-1 as n-sec1 or rb-sec1 (Garcia et al., 1994, Pevsner et al., 1994). Multiple additional homologs of Sec1p and Munc18 were subsequently described, and the whole gene family is now referred to as Sec1/*M*unc18-like proteins (*SM* proteins; Rizo and Südhof, 2012).

After the discovery of Munc18-1, considerable confusion reigned about its function, fueled by paradoxical observations. On the one hand, in yeast *sec1* mutations blocked fusion (Novick and Schekman, 1979), in Drosophila deletion of the Munc18-1 gene (*rop*) abolished synaptic transmission (Harrison et al., 1994), and in mice knockout of Munc18-1 ablated neurotransmitter release (Verhage et al., 2000; Fig. 3B). These results suggested an essential role for Munc18-1 in fusion itself, a hypothesis that was further supported by Novick's elegant studies demonstrating that yeast Sec1p binds to assembled SNARE complexes (Carr et al., 1999), and acts downstream of SNARE-complex assembly (Grote et al., 2000). On the other hand, we found that outside of the SNARE complex, Syntaxin-1 assumes a 'closed' conformation in which its N-terminal Habc-domain folds back on its SNARE-motif, and that Munc18-1 specifically binds to this closed conformation of Syntaxin-1 (Dulubova et al., 1999). Habc-domains are a conserved feature of syntaxins, and account for half of their sequences, while the SNARE motifs of synaxins form SNARE complexes by assembling with similar SNARE motifs in synaptobrevins and SNAP-25 or their homologs into a four-helical bundle (Fig. 3C; Fernandez et al., 1998; Sutton et al., 1998). As a result, the intramolecular interaction in the closed Syntaxin-1 conformation of the N-terminal Habc-domain with the SNARE motif prevents Syntaxin-1 from assembling into SNARE complexes, suggesting that Munc18-1 may be a negative regulator of SNARE-complex assembly. Thus, paradoxically at this junction Munc18-1 seemed to be at the same time essential for fusion itself and preventing fusion by blocking SNARE-complex assembly.

We found a resolution to this apparent contradiction when we observed in collaboration with Josep Rizo that both in vertebrates and in yeast, the SM protein involved in vesicular transport from the endoplasmic reticulum to the Golgi apparatus (Sly1) binds to its cognate syntaxins (Syntaxin-5 and -18 in vertebrates, and Sed5p and Ufe1p in yeast) via a short, conserved N-terminal peptide (the 'N-peptide'; Yamaguchi et al., 2002; Figs. 3C and 3D). We also found that the same mechanism applies to another SM protein—Vps45—that

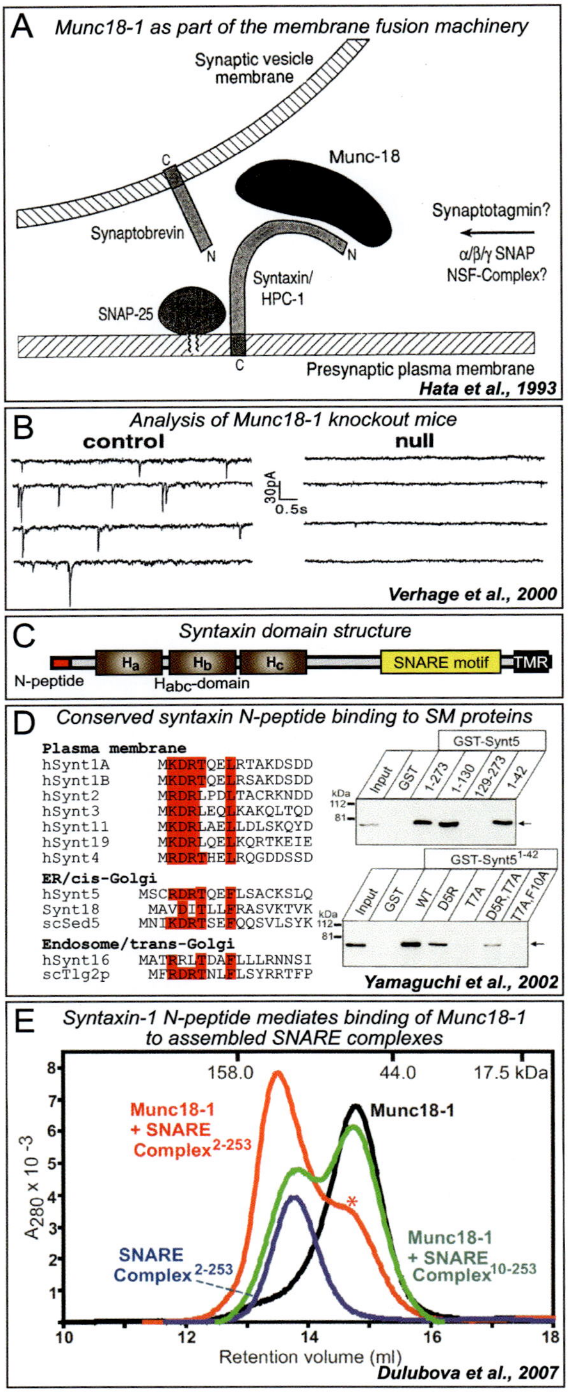
A
Munc18-1 as part of the membrane fusion machinery
Synaptic vesicle membrane
Munc-18
C
Synaptotagmin?
Synaptobrevin
N
N
α/β/γ SNAP
NSF-Complex?
Syntaxin/
HPC-1
SNAP-25
C
Presynaptic plasma membrane
Hata et al., 1993
B
Analysis of Munc18-1 knockout mice
control
null
30pA
0.5s
Verhage et al., 2000
C
Syntaxin domain structure
Ha
Hb
Hc
SNARE motif
TMR
N-peptide
Habc-domain
D
Conserved syntaxin N-peptide binding to SM proteins
Plasma membrane
hSynt1A MKDRTQELRTAKDSDD
hSynt1B MKDRTQELRSAKDSDD
hSynt2 MRDRLPDLTACRKNDD
hSynt3 MKDRLEQLKAKQLTQD
hSynt11 MKDRLAELLDLSKQYD
hSynt19 MKDRLQELKQRTKEIE
hSynt4 MRDRTHELRQGDDSSD
ER/cis-Golgi
hSynt5 MSCRDRTQEFLSACKSLQ
Synt18 MAVDITLLFRASVKTVK
scSed5 MNIKDRTSEFQQSVLSYK
Endosome/trans-Golgi
hSynt16 MATRRLTDAFLLLRNNSI
scTlg2p MFRDRTNLFLSYRRTFP
GST-Synt5
Input
GST
1-273
1-130
129-273
1-42
kDa
112
81
GST-Synt5 1-42
Input
GST
WT
D5R
T7A
D5R,T7A
T7A,F10A
kDa
112
81
Yamaguchi et al., 2002
E
Syntaxin-1 N-peptide mediates binding of Munc18-1 to assembled SNARE complexes
158.0
44.0
17.5 kDa
Munc18-1 + SNARE Complex 2-253
Munc18-1
SNARE Complex 2-253
Munc18-1 + SNARE Complex 10-253
A280 x 10 -3
Retention volume (ml)
Dulubova et al., 2007

is involved in endosome and trans-Golgi fusion, and that binds to its cognate Syntaxin-16 (Tlg2p in yeast) again via a very similar N-peptide sequence (Dulubova et al., 2002). Owing to this binding mechanism, these SM proteins could remain associated with their cognate syntaxins throughout SNARE-complex assembly, consistent with Novick's studies on Sec1p (Grote et al., 2000; note, however, that the details of Sec1p binding in yeast to the SNARE complex may differ). We observed that the vertebrate plasma membrane syntaxins contain an extremely similar conserved N-terminal sequence (Fig. 3D), prompting us to search for a similar binding mode of Munc18-1 to Syntaxin-1.

FIGURE 3. *(opposite) Definition of the interactions of Sec1/Munc18-like ('SM') proteins with syntaxins and the SNARE complex during synaptic vesicle fusion.*

A. Diagram of the Munc18-1/SNARE interactions proposed in the description of Munc18-1 (originally referred to as 'Munc-18') as a Syntaxin-1 binding protein that contributes to the fusion machinery (reproduced from Hata et al., 1993).

B. Demonstration that Munc18-1 is essential for vesicle fusion and does not primarily function as a negative regulator of fusion. Images show synaptic activity recorded from the cortex of newborn littermate wild-type (control) and Munc18-1 knockout mice (null), demonstrating complete electrical silence in the absence of Munc18-1 (reproduced from Verhage et al., 2000).

C. Domain structure of syntaxins composed of a conserved N-terminal sequence (N-peptide), an autonomously folded Habc-domain comprising three α-helices (Fernandez et al., 1998), the SNARE motif that associates into a SNARE complex with the homologous sequences present in synaptobrevins and SNAP-25 or their homologs, and a C-terminal transmembrane region (TMR). Outside of the SNARE complex, syntaxins spontaneously form a 'closed' conformation in which the N-terminal Habc-domain folds back onto the SNARE motif, thereby occluding this motif and hindering SNARE-complex assembly (Dulubova et al., 1999).

D. Discovery of a conserved N-terminal sequence motif of syntaxins that mediates binding of most SM proteins to their cognate syntaxins. An alignment of the N-terminal syntaxin sequences is shown on the left (red, conserved residues involved in SM-protein binding), and immunoblots of the initial binding experiments demonstrating that the N-terminus of the ER/Golgi syntaxin-5 binds to the SM protein Sly1 in a manner dependent on the conserved N-terminal Syntaxin-5 sequence motif are shown on the right (reproduced from Yamaguchi et al., 2002).

E. Demonstration by gel-filtration of a stable complex containing Munc18-1 bound to fully assembled SNARE complexes. Munc18-1 or synaptic SNARE complexes containing the full N-terminal sequence of Syntaxin-1 were analyzed alone (black and blue traces, respectively), or Munc18-1 was analyzed together with SNARE complexes containing either the full N-terminal Syntaxin-1 sequence (red trace) or N-terminally truncated Syntaxin-1 lacking 8 residues (green trace). Note that in the presence of SNARE complexes containing full-length Syntaxin-1, most Munc18-1 co-elutes with SNARE complexes, whereas in the presence of SNARE complexes containing N-terminally truncated Syntaxin-1, no Munc18-1 co-elutes with the SNARE complexes (reproduced from Dulubova et al., 2007).

Indeed, we found that Munc18-1 bound tightly to assembled SNARE complexes in a manner that depended on the Syntaxin-1 N-peptide (Fig. 3E; Dulubova et al., 2007). The Munc18-1/SNARE-complex assembly was stable during size-exclusion chromatography, but disrupted by deletion of the N-peptide from Syntaxin-1 (Fig. 3E; note that James Rothman's laboratory simultaneously made similar observations [Shen et al., 2007]). Fusing as little as a Myc-epitope to the N-peptide of Syntaxin-1 impaired this binding mode, whereas binding of Munc18-1 to the monomeric closed conformation of Syntaxin-1 did not require the Syntaxin-1 N-peptide.

Viewed together, these results showed that Munc18-1 binds to Syntaxin-1 in two sequential modes that involve different Syntaxin-1 conformations (Fig. 4): an exocytosis-specific binding mode in which Munc18-1 binds to 'closed' Syntaxin-1 independent of the N-peptide (Dulubova et al., 1999), and a general

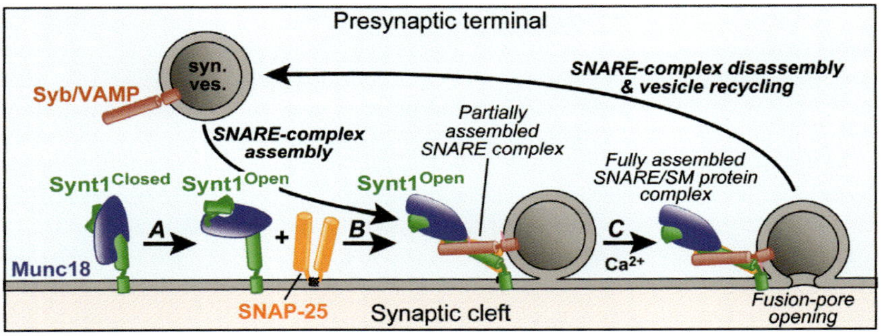

FIGURE 4. *Conformational changes of SNARE and SM proteins mediating synaptic vesicle fusion.* Prior to fusion, Syntaxin-1 assumes a default 'closed' conformation that binds Munc18-1 via an interaction which does not require the Syntaxin-1 N-peptide (Dulubova et al., 1999). In Reaction *A*, Syntaxin-1 is 'opened' (probably by Munc13-mediated catalysis; Ma et al., 2011) to initiate synaptic vesicle priming. In Reaction *B*, SNARE complexes partially assemble via N- to C-terminal zippering (Hanson et al., 1997), while Munc18-1 stays associated with Syntaxin-1 during SNARE-complex assembly via its binding to the Syntaxin-1 N-peptide (Khvotchev et al., 2007). In Reaction *C*, Ca^{2+}-triggers fusion-pore opening by stimulating the completion of SNARE-complex assembly; Munc18-1 contributes to this process and is required for fusion-pore opening during this step because the continuing association of Munc18-1 with SNARE-complexes is essential for fusion-pore opening (Zhou et al., 2013a). After fusion, vesicles are endocytosed (see Fig. 1), and SNARE complexes are disassembled by the NSF ATPase and its SNAP protein adaptor (no relation to the SNARE protein SNAP-25). Munc18-1 remains associated with Syntaxin-1, and reverts to the heterodimeric interaction with 'closed' Syntaxin-1. Thus, there are two major conformational transitions during exocytotic membrane fusion: opening of Syntaxin-1 with rearrangement of the mode of Munc18-1 binding, and folding of SNARE proteins into SNARE complexes.

binding mode shared with some other SM protein/SNARE complex interactions in which Munc18-1 binds to 'open' Syntaxin-1 assembled into SNARE complexes via the Syntaxin-1 N-peptide, and additionally interacts with other parts of the SNARE complex (Dulubova et al., 2007).

What are the functions of the two Munc18-1 binding modes to SNARE proteins, and which of the two modes is more important for fusion? Initial peptide competition experiments in the calyx-of-Held synapse showed that displacing the Syntaxin-1 N-terminus from Munc18-1 impairs synaptic vesicle fusion (Khvotchev et al., 2007). Further studies described that mutations in Munc18-1 which decrease Munc18-1 binding to the Syntaxin-1 N-terminal sequences also decrease fusion (Deak et al., 2009). It should be noted that in a later study in which this result was disputed using similar but weaker mutations (Meijer et al., 2012), the Munc18-1 mutations caused only a partial decrease in binding to the Syntaxin-1 N-peptide. In these studies, all physiology was performed with a high degree of overexpression, which could have easily compensated for the decrease in binding affinity. Furthermore, elegant experiments in C. elegans revealed that the Syntaxin-1 N-peptide was essential for fusion, but that it did not actually need to be on Syntaxin-1 in order to function, as long as it was positioned close to SNARE complexes (Rathore et al., 2010). Finally, we showed that in mammalian synapses, the Syntaxin-1 N-peptide was also required for fusion under physiological conditions (Zhou et al., 2013b).

These experiments show that binding of Munc18-1 to 'open' Syntaxin-1 within the SNARE complex is essential for fusion, and validate the function of Munc18-1—analogous to that of Sec1p—as an intrinsic component of the fusion machine. What then is the role of Munc18-1 binding to 'closed' Syntaxin-1? To test this role, we created knock-in mice in which Syntaxin-1 was rendered constitutively 'open' (Syntaxin-1^{Open}), and thus binding of Munc18-1 to 'closed' Syntaxin-1 was suppressed (Gerber et al., 2008). In these mice, both Munc18-1 and Syntaxin-1 were destabilized and decreased in levels, consistent with other evidence suggesting that the complex of Munc18-1 with the closed conformation of Syntaxin-1 stabilizes both proteins (Verhage et al., 2000). The decreased levels of Syntaxin-1 and Munc18-1 in Syntaxin-1^{Open} synapses resulted in decreased vesicle priming, presumably because fewer slots for vesicle fusion were available (Gerber et al., 2008; Acuna et al., 2014).

Nevertheless, the probability of Ca^{2+}-triggered neurotransmitter release was dramatically enhanced in Syntaxin-1^{Open} synapses, and fusion was accelerated. Even the fusion of individual vesicles, as judged by the kinetics of single miniature release ('mini') events, was faster in Syntaxin-1^{Open} than in wild-type synapses (Acuna et al., 2014). These data, together with the finding that the

Habc-domain of Syntaxin-1, different from its N-peptide, is not essential for fusion (Zhou et al., 2013a) demonstrate that Munc18-1 binding to the closed conformation of Syntaxin-1 is not required for fusion, whereas binding to 'open' Syntaxin-1 in the SNARE complex is essential for fusion. Binding of Munc18-1 to closed Syntaxin-1 appears to serve two other functions that are not directly part of fusion itself: to stabilize both proteins in the complex, and to 'gate' SNARE-complex assembly mediating fusion, i.e., to regulate the rate of fusion.

How do SNARE and SM proteins mediate fusion?

In principle, SNARE proteins act in fusion via a simple mechanism: SNARE proteins are attached to both membranes destined to fuse, and form a trans-complex that involves a progressive zippering of the four-helical SNARE-complex bundle in an N- to C-terminal direction, forcing the fusing membranes into close proximity and destabilizing their surfaces. This opens a fusion pore, whose expansion then converts the initial 'trans'-SNARE complexes into 'cis'-SNARE complexes which are subsequently dissociated by the NSF and SNAP adapter proteins, thereby allowing a recycling of the vesicles and the SNARE proteins for another round of fusion (Fig. 4).

However, at least two major questions arise at this point. First, do SNARE proteins primarily act as force-generators to pull membranes together (which may be sufficient for inducing *in vitro* fusion), or do SNARE proteins actually open the fusion pore? Second, what is the precise function of SM proteins in fusion—why are they required?

In vitro, the transmembrane regions of synaptobrevin and Syntaxin-1 interact with each other in the plane of the membrane. The SNARE motifs of these proteins form a continuous, rigid a-helix with their transmembrane regions, suggesting that the SNARE protein transmembrane regions may actively contribute to the fusion pore (Stein et al., 2009). However, in recent experiments we found that Synaptobrevin-2 and Syntaxin-1 still mediate fusion when both are attached to their resident membranes via lipid anchors, not transmembrane regions, demonstrating that SNARE transmembrane regions are not essential components of the fusion machine (Zhou et al., 2013b). These results support the notion that SNARE proteins act as force generators, and that their transmembrane regions do not act as fusion catalysts.

What then do SM proteins do in fusion? The fact that SM proteins are required continuously during SNARE-complex assembly argues for a role either in organizing proper SNARE-complex assembly and in preventing dead-end inappropriate SNARE complexes, or in catalyzing lipid mixing during fusion. At present, no conclusive data argue one way or the other, and this question will clearly keep many of us busy for years to come.

SNARE chaperones are essential for maintaining the integrity of the presynaptic terminal

Neurons fire action potentials often in bursts or trains, with high frequencies, sometimes exceeding 100 Hz. Each neurotransmitter release event involves the folding and unfolding of reactive SNARE proteins, exposing the presynaptic cytosol to potentially deleterious misfolding of SNARE proteins and formation of inappropriate complexes by reactive SNARE motifs. It is thus not surprising that neurons express specialized chaperones which help proper folding of SNARE proteins, and that deletion of these chaperones leads to neurodegeneration.

We identified two classes of such chaperones, CSPα (for cysteine-string protein-α, so named because it contains an eponymous string of cysteine residues that are palmitoylated to attach CSPα to the synaptic vesicle membrane; Gundersen et al., 1994), and synucleins (so named because it was initially thought that these presynaptic proteins may also be in the nucleus; Maroteaux et al., 1988).

Our discovery that these proteins function as SNARE chaperones was pure serendipity. We found that deletion of CSPα in mice leads to massive neurodegeneration that kills affected mice in 3-4 months and is caused by an impairment in SNARE-complex formation (Fernandez-Chacon et al., 2004). Surprisingly, this neurodegeneration was suppressed by modest overexpression of α-synuclein (Chandra et al., 2005). Following up on these observations, we showed that CSPα—which contains a DNA-J domain and forms a catalytically active, ATP-dependent chaperone complex with Hsc70 and the tetratricopeptide-repeat protein SGT (Tobaben et al., 2000)—catalyzes the proper folding of SNAP-25, rendering SNAP-25 competent for SNARE-complex assembly (Sharma et al., 2011a, 2011b, and 2012). In CSPα KO mice, misfolding of SNAP-25 impaired SNARE-complex assembly which then caused neurodegeneration. α-Synuclein rescued this neurodegeneration by independently promoting SNARE-complex assembly via a non-classical, ATP-independent chaperone activity (Burre et al., 2010).

Although these observations uncovered a potentially interesting facet of SNARE protein biology, we do not yet understand how the physiological activities of α-synuclein relate to its neurotoxic role in Parkinson's disease. One attractive hypothesis is that α-synuclein aggregation in Parkinson's disease may deplete neurons of all available functional α-synuclein, and thus cause SNARE protein misfolding that is then deleterious, but alternative hypotheses, such as a direct neurotoxic non-physiological activity of α-synuclein oligomers, are equally plausible.

4. CA^{2+}-TRIGGERING OF FUSION: SYNAPTOTAGMINS AND MORE

At the same time as our work on synaptic membrane fusion was progressing, we were studying a related question: how is neurotransmitter release by synaptic membrane fusion triggered by Ca^{2+}? Ever since I was a graduate student in Victor Whittaker's laboratory in Göttingen, I had been fascinated by this question. The central importance of Ca^{2+}-triggered neurotransmitter release for brain function intrigued me, its improbable speed and plasticity puzzled me, and the similarity of Ca^{2+}-induced synaptic vesicle exocytosis to other types of Ca^{2+}-induced exocytosis, such as those underlying hormone secretion, mast cell degranulation, or fertilization, suggested to me that understanding Ca^{2+}-triggered neurotransmitter release may be generally relevant for cellular signaling processes. Although some key discoveries about synaptotagmins were made at the same time as those about SNARE and SM proteins, the work on synaptotagmins extended over a longer time period to satisfy even the most stringent critics, and some of the most important observations are quite recent.

Discovery of Synaptotagmin-1: identification of C2-domains as versatile Ca^{2+}-binding domains

During our studies of the molecular anatomy of synaptic vesicles, we searched for a candidate Ca^{2+}-sensor that might mediate Ca^{2+}-triggering of synaptic vesicle exocytosis. When we purified and cloned Synaptotagmin-1 (Syt1)—which had been described earlier as a synaptic vesicle protein using a monoclonal antibody raised against synaptosomes (Matthew et al., 1981)—we were intrigued by its primary structure because Syt1 included two C_2-domains that were anchored on the vesicle membrane by a transmembrane region (Perin et al., 1990; Figs. 2 and 5A). At that time, nothing was known about C_2-domains except that they represented the "2nd constant sequence" in classical protein-kinase C (PKC) isozymes (Coussens et al., 1986). Since classical PKC isozymes are Ca^{2+}-regulated and interact with phospholipids, we speculated that the synaptotagmin C2-domains may represent Ca^{2+}-binding modules that interact with phospholipids, and that Syt1 may be a Ca^{2+}-sensor for neurotransmitter release (Perin et al., 1990). In pursuing this hypothesis over two decades, we showed that Ca^{2+}-triggering of neurotransmitter release is mediated by Ca^{2+}-binding to Syt1 and other synaptotagmins, and that different synaptotagmin isoforms additionally perform similar Ca^{2+}-sensor functions in other types of Ca^{2+}-dependent exocytosis in neuronal and non-neuronal cells.

The first challenge after describing Syt1 was to test whether the Syt1 C2-domains were indeed a novel type of Ca^{2+}/phospholipid-binding domain. We found that the Syt1 C2-domains bound to phospholipids (Perin et al., 1990), that such binding was mediated by purified brain Syt1 in a Ca^{2+}-dependent manner (Brose et al., 1992), and that a single C_2-domain of Syt1—the first 'C2A-domain—constituted an autonomously folded domain that bound Ca^{2+} and phospholipids in a ternary complex (Davletov and Südhof, 1993 and 1994; Fig. 5B). In addition, we and others observed that the Syt1 C_2-domains also bind to Syntaxin-1 and to SNARE-complexes as a function of Ca^{2+} (Li et al., 1995a and 1995b; Chapman et al., 1995). In collaboration with Steven Sprang and Josep Rizo, we obtained atomic structures of the C2-domains of Syt1, and defined the architecture of their Ca^{2+}-binding sites (Sutton et al., 1995; Shao et al., 1996 and 1997; Ubach et 1998 and 2001; Fernandez et al., 2001; Fig. 5A). Our structural studies demonstrated that the Syt1 C2-domains are composed of stable β-sandwiches with flexible loops emerging from the top and bottom, and that Ca^{2+} exclusively binds to the top loops of the C2-domains with incomplete coordination spheres (Figs. 5A and 5C). As a result, intrinsic Ca^{2+}-binding to Syt1 C2-domains exhibited low affinity, but was dramatically enhanced by binding of phospholipids which complete the Ca^{2+}-coordination spheres (Davletov and Südhof, 1993 and 1994; Ubach et al., 1998 ; Fernandez et al., 2001).

The biochemical and structural definition of the Syt1 C2A-domain as an autonomously folded Ca^{2+}-binding module – the first for any C2-domain—proved paradigmatic for all C2-domains, which are now known to represent a common Ca^{2+}-binding motif found in many proteins (Rizo and Südhof, 1998; Corbalan-Garcia and Gómez-Fernández, 2014). However, not all C2-domains bind Ca^{2+}. Some C2-domains are Ca^{2+}-independent phospholipid-binding modules (e.g., the PTEN C2-domain; Lee et al., 1999), while others are Ca^{2+}-independent protein interaction domains (e.g., the N-terminal C2-domain of Munc13 that binds to RIMs as discussed below; Dulubova et al., 2005; Lu et al., 2006). Even C2-domains that bind Ca^{2+} are functionally diverse. For example, different from Syt1 C2-domains, some C2-domains exhibit a high intrinsic Ca^{2+}-affinity also in the absence of phospholipids (e.g., the central C2-domain of Munc13-2; Shin et al., 2010). Thus, C2-domains are versatile protein modules that most often are Ca^{2+}/phospholipid-binding domains but can adopt multifarious other functions.

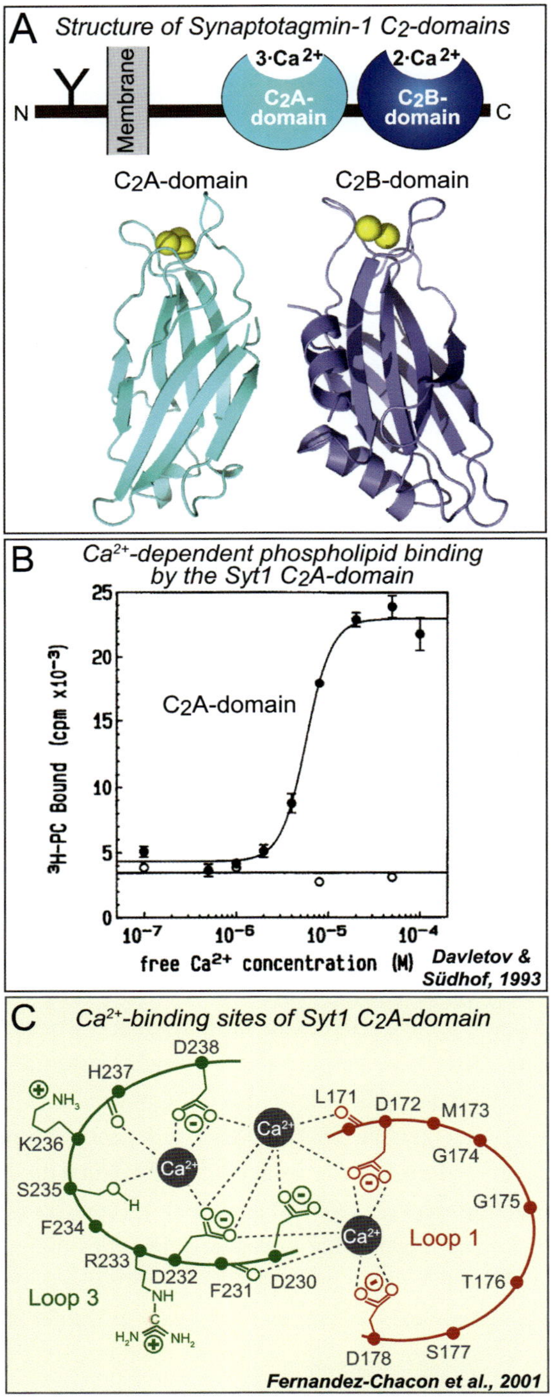
A Structure of Synaptotagmin-1 C2-domains
3·Ca2+
2·Ca2+
N
Membrane
C2A-domain
C2B-domain
C
C2A-domain
C2B-domain
B Ca2+-dependent phospholipid binding by the Syt1 C2A-domain
3H-PC Bound (cpm x10−3)
C2A-domain
free Ca2+ concentration (M)
Davletov & Südhof, 1993
C Ca2+-binding sites of Syt1 C2A-domain
D238
H237
K236
S235
F234
R233
D232
F231
D230
L171
D172
M173
G174
G175
T176
S177
D178
Loop 1
Loop 3
Ca2+
Fernandez-Chacon et al., 2001

Demonstration that Syt1 is a Ca^{2+}-sensor for exocytosis

After the biochemical studies had established that Syt1 binds Ca^{2+}, the next challenge was to show whether Syt1 constitutes Katz's long-sought Ca^{2+}-sensor for neurotransmitter release. Initial experiments in C. elegans and Drosophila disappointingly indicated that at least some neurotransmitter release remained after deletion of Syt1, even though release was significantly reduced (Littleton et al., 1993; DiAntonio et al., 1993; Nonet et al., 1993). Our electrophysiological analyses of Syt1 knockout mice in which higher resolution measurements of release were possible then revealed that Syt1 is selectively and absolutely required for fast synchronous synaptic fusion in forebrain neurons, whereas it is dispensable for other, slower forms of Ca^{2+}-induced release (Fig. 6; Geppert et al., 1994; Maximov and Südhof, 2005). These experiments, carried out in collaboration with Chuck Stevens at the Salk Institute, accounted for the Drosophila and C. elegans phenotypes, and established that Syt1 is essential for fast Ca^{2+}-triggered release, but is not required for fusion as such—is not even necessary for all Ca^{2+}-triggered fusion. Moreover, deletion of Syt1 increased spontaneous 'mini' release in some synapses, suggesting that Syt1 normally contributes to clamping spontaneous synaptic vesicle exocytosis (Maximov and Südhof, 2005; Xu et al., 2009).

The Syt1 knockout analyses thus supported the 'synaptotagmin Ca^{2+}-sensor hypothesis', but did not exclude the possibility that Syt1 positions vesicles next to voltage-gated Ca^{2+}-channels (a function now known to be mediated by RIMs and RIM-BPs [Kaeser et al., 2011]). Such a 'positioning function' would enable another 'real' Ca^{2+}-sensor to do the actual Ca^{2+}-triggering, consistent with the remaining Ca^{2+}-induced release in Syt1 knockout synapses—an alternative hypothesis that was widely discussed (Penner and Neher, 1994), but could not account for why Syt1 itself binds Ca^{2+}.

FIGURE 5. *(opposite) Domain structure and Ca^{2+}-binding of Synaptotagmin-1*

A. Domain structure of Synaptotagmin-1 (Syt1) and structure of the Syt1 C2-domains (courtesy of J. Rizo; Shao et al., 1998; Fernandez et al., 2001).

B. Demonstration that the C2A-domain of Syt1, and by extension other C2-domains, are autonomously folding Ca^{2+}-binding domains. The data illustrate high-affinity and highly cooperative Ca^{2+}-regulation of phospholipid binding by the purified recombinant Syt1 C2A-domain (reproduced from Davletov and Südhof, 1993).

C. Architecture of the Syt1 C2A-domain Ca^{2+}-binding sites as determined by NMR-spectroscopy (modified from Fernandez-Chacon et al., 2001). Note that multiple Ca^{2+}-ions are ligated in incomplete coordination spheres by multiple overlapping aspartate residues.

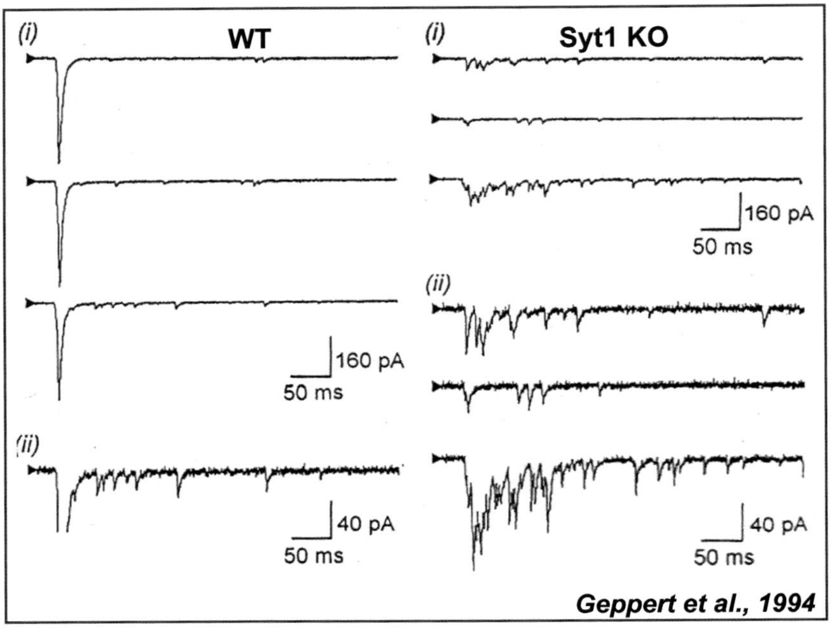

FIGURE 6. *Synaptotagmin-1 (Syt1) knockout selectively ablates fast synchronous neurotransmitter release.* Traces of evoked synaptic responses recorded from hippocampal neurons cultured from newborn littermate wild-type (WT, left) and Syt1 knockout mice (right). Synaptic responses were induced by isolated action potentials; two different scales are shown under (i) and (ii) as indicated by the calibration bars. Note that the Syt1 knockout completely ablates fast synchronous response, but not slow asynchronous responses (reproduced from Geppert et al., 1994a).

To directly test whether Ca^{2+}-binding to Syt1 actually triggers neurotransmitter release, we introduced into the endogenous mouse Syt1 gene a point mutation (R233Q) that decreased the Syt1 Ca^{2+}-binding affinity during phospholipid binding ~2-fold, but had no detectable effect on Ca^{2+}-dependent Syntaxin-1 binding (Figs. 7A and 7B; Fernandez-Chacon et al., 2001). Electrophysiological recordings, carried out in collaboration with Christian Rosenmund, revealed that the R233Q mutation converted synaptic depression during stimulus trains into synaptic facilitation, consistent with a decrease in release probability (Fig. 7C). Importantly, this decrease in release probability was revealed to be caused by a ~2-fold decrease in the apparent Ca^{2+}-affinity of neurotransmitter release, formally proving that Syt1 is the Ca^{2+}-sensor for release (Fig. 7D).

In subsequent studies, we extended this analysis, and introduced into knock-in mice other point mutations, including a mutation (D232N) that increased the Ca^{2+}-dependent interaction of Syt1 with SNARE proteins (Fig. 7E; Pang et al., 2006a). We found that this mutation increased neurotransmitter release accordingly. We showed in a detailed comparison of the R233Q and D232N point mutations, which decrease or increase the apparent Ca^{2+}-affinity of Syt1, respectively, that they have corresponding opposite effects on the apparent Ca^{2+}-affinity of release (Figs. 7F and 7G). Moreover, in parallel experiments in chromaffin cells performed in collaboration with Erwin Neher, we found that Syt1 also functions as a Ca^{2+}-sensor for endocrine granule exocytosis (Voets et al., 2001; Sorensen et al., 2002), although here the Syt1 deletion causes only a very small impairment in Ca^{2+}-triggered exocytosis because Syt1 function is largely redundant with that of Syt7 in chromaffin cells (Schonn et al., 2008; see discussion below).

Together, these studies proved that Syt1 functions as a Ca^{2+}-sensor in synaptic vesicle exocytosis. We next wondered whether Ca^{2+}-binding to both of the C2-domains of Syt1 contributes to triggering release. Initial studies in Drosophila demonstrated that the C2B-domain Ca^{2+}-binding sites of Syt1 are essential for release (Mackler and Reist, 2001). A similar study suggested that the C2A-domain Ca^{2+}-binding sites are dispensable (Robinson et al., 2002), but the signal-to-noise ratio of this study was too low to rule out a significant contribution of the C2A-domain. Using systematic rescue experiments to perform a direct quantitative comparison of the Ca^{2+}-triggering activities of Syt1 mutants lacking either C2A- or C2B-domain Ca^{2+}-binding sites, we found that in addition to the C2B-domain Ca^{2+}-binding sites, the C2A-domain Ca^{2+}-binding sites significantly contribute to release (Shin et al., 2009). Moreover, we observed that in the absence of the C2A-domain Ca^{2+}-binding sites, Ca^{2+}-triggered release exhibited a significantly decreased apparent Ca^{2+}-cooperativity, documenting that Ca^{2+}-binding to the C2A-domain of Synaptotagmin-1 directly participates in the Ca^{2+}-triggering of fast release.

Diversity of synaptotagmins in fast Ca^{2+}-triggered neurotransmitter release

Mammalian genomes encode 16 synaptotagmins (defined as double C2-domain proteins with an N-terminal transmembrane region). The C2-domains of 8 synaptotagmins (Syt1-Syt3, Syt5-Syt7, Syt9, and Syt10) bind Ca^{2+}, whereas those of the other 8 synaptotagmins do not. The 8 Ca^{2+}-binding synaptotagmins comprise two classes which lack (Syt1, Syt2, Syt7, and Syt9) or contain N-terminal disulfide bond that covalently dimerizes the respective synaptotagmins (Syt3, Syt5, Syt6, and Syt10).

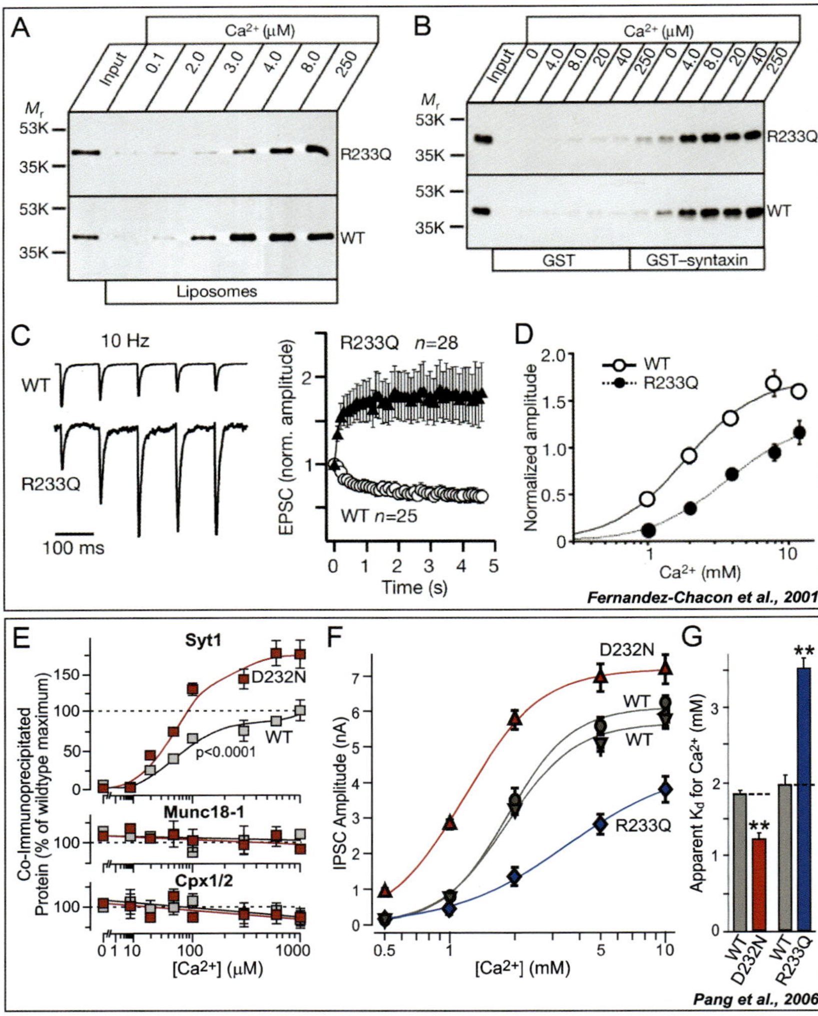

FIGURE 7. *Demonstration that Ca^{2+}-binding to Synaptotagmin-1 (Syt1) triggers neurotransmitter release using knock-in mice containing mutant Syt1 with altered Ca^{2+}-affinities*

A & B. A single amino-acid substitution in the Syt1 C2A-domain (R233Q) decreases the apparent Ca^{2+}-affinity of Syt1 during phospholipid but not during Syntaxin-1 binding. Data show measurements of Ca^{2+}-dependent binding of the entire cytoplasmic fragment of endogenous wild-type and R233Q-mutant mutant Syt1 obtained from littermate knock-in mice to liposomes (A) or immobilized GST-Syntaxin-1 (B).

C. The R233Q amino-acid substitution decreases the probability of neurotransmitter release as evidenced by a conversion of synaptic depression in wild-type synapses into synaptic facilitation in R233Q-mutant synapses. Synaptic responses during a 10 Hz stimulus train are measured (left, representative traces; right, normalized responses).

(continues)

When the diversity of synaptotagmins emerged (e.g., see Geppert et al., 1991; Li et al., 1995), it was surprising that the Syt1 knockout produced a dramatic phenotype because at least some of these other synaptotagmins are co-expressed with Syt1. However, using systematic rescue experiments we found that only three of the eight Ca^{2+}-binding synaptotagmins—Syt1, Syt2 and Syt9—mediate fast synaptic vesicle exocytosis (Xu et al., 2007). These synaptotagmins exhibit distinct kinetics, with Syt2 triggering release faster, and Syt9 slower than Syt1. Most forebrain neurons express only Syt1, accounting for the dramatic Syt1 knockout phenotype. Syt2 is the Ca^{2+}-sensor of fast synapses in the brainstem and the neuromuscular junction (Pang et al., 2006b; Sun et al., 2007; Figs. 8A and 8B), while Syt9 is primarily present in the limbic system (Xu et al., 2007). Thus, the kinetic properties of Syt1, Syt2, and Syt9 correspond to the functional needs of the synapses containing them.

In the initial Syt1 KO studies (Geppert et al., 1994), we observed that although fast release was ablated in Syt1-deficient synapses, a slower form of Ca^{2+}-triggered release remained (Fig. 6). We thus sought to biophysically define the

---

D. The R233Q-mutation decreases the apparent Ca^{2+}-affinity of neurotransmitter release approximately 2-fold similar to its effect on the apparent Ca^{2+}-affinity of phospholipid binding (see A), which accounts for the decrease in release probability in C. Data show normalized amplitudes of synaptic responses as a function of extracellular Ca^{2+}-concentration.

E. Another single amino-acid substitution in the Syt1 C2A-domain (D232N) has a distinct effect on the Ca^{2+}-binding properties of Syt1: it increases Ca^{2+}-dependent binding of Syt1 to SNARE complexes. Data show measurements of Ca^{2+}-dependent binding of wild-type and D232N-mutant endogenous Syt1 to SNARE complexes in brain homogenates from knock-in mice solubilized with Triton X-100. SNARE complexes were immunoprecipated at the indicated concentrations of free Ca^{2+}, and immunoprecipiates were analyzed by quantitative immunoblotting for Syt1 (top graph), Munc18-1, and and complexins (bottom graphs). Note that Munc18-1 and complexin constitutively co-immunoprecipitate with SNARE complexes whereas the co-IP of Syt1 is dramatically enhanced at increasing Ca^{2+}-concentrations.

F & G. Direct comparisons of the effects of D232N- and R233Q-knock-in mutations in Syt1 demonstrate that these two mutations that have opposite effects on the Ca^{2+}-binding properties of Syt1 produce opposite shifts in the apparent Ca^{2+}-affinity of release. F. Measurements of the absolute amplitude of evoked inhibitory postsynaptic currents as a function of extracellular Ca^{2+} in neurons cultured from littermate D232N- or R233Q-mutant knock-in mice and their wild-type (WT) littermates; each mutant has its own wild-type control. Synaptic amplitudes are fit to a Hill function. G. Apparent Ca^{2+}-affinity for release calculated by Hill function fits of the data in F comparing wild-type controls to D232N- or R233Q-mutant synapses.

Panels A–D were reproduced from Fernandez-Chacon et al. (2001); and panels E–G from Pang et al. (2006) and Xu et al. (2009).

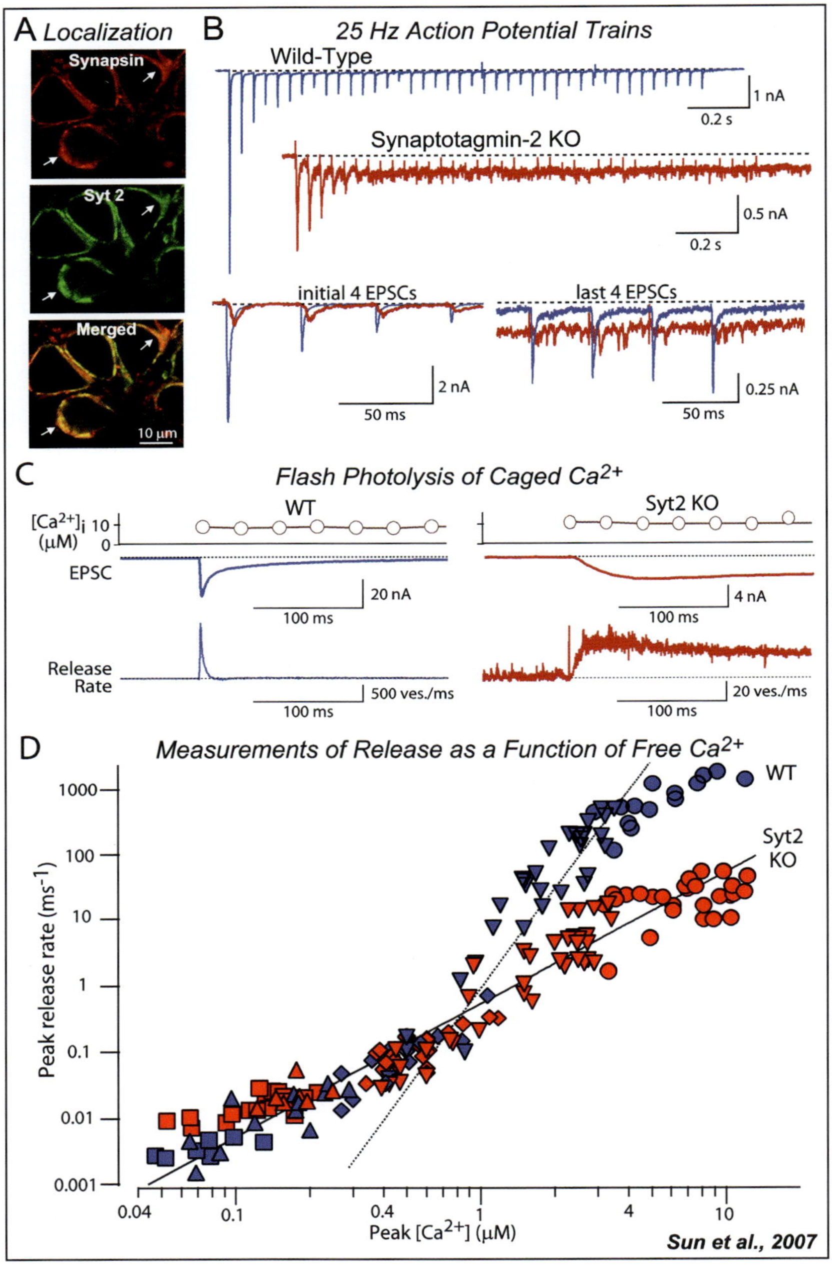

FIGURE 8. *Deletion of Synaptotagmin-2 (Syt2) the fast Ca^{2+}-sensor for release in the Calyx of Held synapse, uncovers a slower form of Ca^{2+}-triggered release that is controlled by a secondary Ca^{2+}-sensor with a much lower Ca^{2+}-cooperativity than Syt2.*

(continues)

contribution of the 'fast' synaptotagmin-dependent form of release, and to describe the properties of the slower remaining form. To do so, we used the calyx-of-Held synapse as a model system because it allows simultaneous patching of pre- and postsynaptic compartments, providing an unparalleled resolution of electrophysiological measurements (Forsythe, 1994; Borst and Sakmann, 1996). The calyx-of-Held synapse expresses only Syt2 among the 'fast' synaptotagmins (Fig. 8A; Sun et al., 2007). Knockout of Syt2 ablated all fast Ca^{2+}-triggered neurotransmitter release; only a slower form of release remained (Fig. 8B). In the Syt2 KO calyx synapse, this remaining Ca^{2+}-triggered release did not facilitate during high-frequency stimulus trains, different from what we observed in Syt1 KO synapses in hippocampal and cortical neurons (see Maximov and Südhof, 2005, and Fig. 9 below). As a result, the Syt2 KO blocked the vast majority of

---

A. Localization of Syt2 by immunocytochemistry of Calyx synapses demonstrates abundant expression in presynaptic terminals.

B. Knockout (KO) of Syt2 in calyx synapses ablates most fast synchronous neurotransmitter release induced by a high-frequency action potential train (40 stimuli at 25 Hz). Representative traces of synaptic responses (EPSCs) recorded during the overall train are shown on top (note that wild-type and mutant traces are shown with different scales), and expansions of the initial and the final 4 EPSCs at the bottom (note that here wild-type and mutant traces have the same scales, but scales differ for the first and last 4 EPSCs). The baseline shift in the Syt2 KO traces reflects unclamping of unsynchronous release that is not observed in wild-type synapses.

C. KO of Syt2 severely impairs neurotransmitter release triggered by high concentrations of Ca^{2+} in the calyx of Held synapse. Presynaptic terminals were filled via a patch pipette with caged Ca^{2+} and a Ca^{2+}-indicator dye, and release was triggered by Ca^{2+} released by flash photolysis. The amount of release was measured postsynaptically by monitoring the EPSC and then calculating the number of vesicles released at a given time (release rate). Simultaneously, the presynaptic Ca^{2+}-concentration was measured by microfluorometry.

D. Ca^{2+}-triggered neurotransmitter release exhibits a biphasic Ca^{2+}-concentration dependence in wild-type (WT) calyx synapses with a low apparent Ca^{2+}-cooperativity of release (~2 Ca^{2+}-ions) at low Ca^{2+}-concentrations, and a high apparent Ca^{2+}-cooperativity at high Ca^{2+}-concentrations (~5 Ca^{2+}-ions). KO of Syt2 selectively ablates the high Ca^{2+}-cooperativity release phase, decreasing the release rates at physiological Ca^{2+}-concentrations nearly 100-fold without significantly affecting Ca^{2+}-triggered release at low Ca^{2+}-concentrations. Data show summary graph of EPSC peak release rates as a function of different free Ca^{2+}-concentrations in the presynaptic terminal. The dashed line represents a fit of a 5th power function to the data from wild-type terminals at >1 μM free Ca^{2+}; the solid line a 2nd power function to the data from mutant terminals at all Ca^{2+}-concentrations. Note that the solid line also fits the wild-type responses at low Ca^{2+}-concentrations.

All data were adapted from Sun et al. (2007).

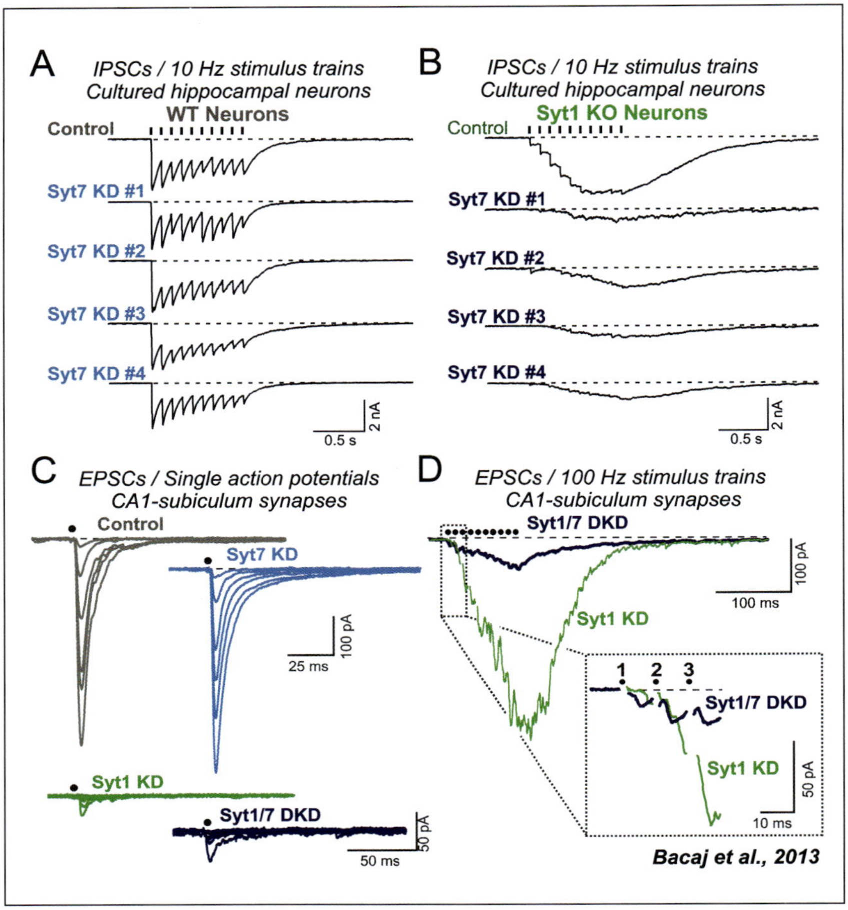

FIGURE 9. *Synaptotagmin-7 (Syt7) knockdown impairs the slow release remaining in Synaptotagmin-1 (Syt1) knockout neurons*

A & B. In cultured hippocampal neurons, suppression of Syt7 expression by knockdown (KD) has no major effect on neurotransmitter release evoked by a high-frequency stimulus train in wild-type synapses (A). However, suppressing Syt7 expression in Syt1-deficient neurons (Syt1 KO) impairs most of the slow and facilitating Ca^{2+}-triggered release that remains after the Syt1 KO (B). Data show representative traces of IPSCs evoked by a 10 Hz stimulus train obtained in control neurons and neurons expressing four different Syt7 shRNAs to assure reproducibility. Note that in hippocampal neurons, the high-frequency stimulus train induces in Syt1 KO neurons a strongly facilitating form of asynchronous release, such that the amount of total release during the train is similar in Syt1 KO and wild-type neurons. By contrast, in Syt2 KO calyx synapses no such facilitation of the residual release is observed (see Fig. 8B).

C & D. In acute slices, suppression of Syt7 expression by itself also has no significant effect on release, but here again suppression of Syt1 expression ablates only the initial fast phase of release but retains a strongly facilitating asynchronous form of release that is severely

(continues)

Ca^{2+}-triggered release in this synapse independent of the stimulation frequency (Sun et al., 2007).

We then analyzed the Ca^{2+}-dependence of neurotransmitter release in calyx synapses from wild-type and littermate Syt2 KO mice using flash-photolysis of caged-Ca^{2+}. We performed simultaneous measurements of the postsynaptic response (which allows precise calculations of synaptic vesicle exocytosis) and of presynaptic Ca^{2+}-levels by microfluorometry, an approach that had been pioneered by the Sackmann, Schneggenburger, and Neher laboratories (Bollmann et al., 2000; Schneggenburger and Neher, 2000). We found that as described previously (Bollmann and Sakmann, 2000), release triggered by physiological Ca^{2+}-concentrations exhibited an apparent Ca^{2+}-cooperativity of 5, similar to the number of Ca^{2+}-ions bound to synaptotagmins (Figs. 8C and 8D). However, the small amount of remaining Ca^{2+}-triggered release in Syt2 KO calyx synapses exhibited an apparent Ca^{2+}-cooperativity of only 2, suggesting that this release was mediated by a different Ca^{2+}-sensor that at least in the calyx of Held synapse has properties distinct from those of Syt1, Syt2, and Syt9 (Sun et al., 2007).

Testing the function of Synaptotagmin-7 in slow Ca^{2+}-triggered release

Which Ca^{2+}-sensor induces the remaining release in Syt1 and Syt2 KO synapses, and could this release be mediated by one of the other 5 Ca^{2+}-binding synaptotagmins? The remaining release in Syt1 KO neurons exhibits distinct, synapse-dependent properties. Whereas in Syt2-deficient calyx-of-Held synapses the remaining release remains small and constant even at high stimulation frequencies (Fig. 8B), in Syt1-deficient hippocampal and cortical synapses the remaining 'asynchronous' release is massively facilitating at high stimulation frequencies (Fig. 9A). As a result, in the latter synapses the total amount of Ca^{2+}-triggered release induced by high-frequency stimulus trains is similar in wild-type and Syt1-deficient synapses, even though the initial rate of fast release differs more than 10-fold (Maximov and Südhof, 2005; Xu et al., 2012).

impaired by additional suppression of Syt7 expression. Data show measurements of EPSCs elicited by isolated stimuli applied with increasing strength (C) or by a 100 Hz, 0.1 sec stimulus train (D; representative traces with an expansion of the initial response below). Measurements were performed in acute hippocampal slices from mice whose CA1 region had been injected with viruses encoding shRNAs for knockdown of the indicated synaptotagmins two weeks prior to the experiments. EPSCs were measured in postsynaptic subiculum neurons after presynaptic stimulation of axons emanating from CA1 region neurons.

All data were adapted from Bacaj et al. (2013).

To define the Ca^{2+}-sensor for the remaining release in Syt1-deficient hippocampal neurons, we focused on Syt7. We had found earlier that Syt7, similarly to Syt1, functions as a Ca^{2+}-sensor for exocytosis in chromaffin and other neuroendocrine and endocrine cells (Sugita et al., 2001; Gustavsson et al., 2008 and 2009; Schonn et al., 2009), and Paul Brehm had observed a role for Syt7 in release at the neuromuscular junction (Wen et al., 2010). We found that although Syt7 loss-of-function did not produce a major change in neurotransmitter release in Syt1-containing wild-type neurons (Maximov et al., 2008), it impaired most of the remaining slow Ca^{2+}-triggered release in Syt1 knockout neurons (Bacaj et al., 2013; Fig. 9). The Syt7 loss-of-function phenotype in Syt1-deficient neurons could be rescued only by Syt7 containing functional Ca^{2+}-binding sites, suggesting that Syt7 functions as a Ca^{2+}-sensor. Different from Syt1 in which the C2B-domain Ca^{2+}-binding sites were more important than the C2A-domain Ca^{2+}-binding sites, blocking the Syt7 C2B-domain Ca^{2+}-binding sites of Syt7 had no effect on rescue. However, blocking the Syt7 C2A-domain Ca^{2+}-binding sites abolished its rescue activity (Bacaj et al., 2013). This result indicates that the mechanisms of action of Syt1 and Syt7 partly differ from each other.

Viewed together, these observations suggest that Syt7—like the other synaptotagmins of its class (Syt1, Syt2, and Syt9)—functions as a Ca^{2+}-sensor for exocytosis, but exhibits a slower kinetics than Syt1, Syt2, and Syt9. The relatively slow action of Syt7 normally occludes its function in many wild-type synapses in which the faster Syt1 or Syt2 probably outcompetes the slower Syt7. Although the function of Syt7 was not immediately apparent at most normal synapses (Fig. 9), paired recordings showed that Syt7 does contribute physiologically to release during stimulus trains even in the presence of Syt1 (Bacaj et al., 2013). Therefore four synaptotagmins (Syt1, Syt2, Syt7, and Syt9) together account for nearly all neurotransmitter release at a synapse. The different speed of action of Syt1 and Syt7 may be related to their localizations because Syt7 has been consistently found to be absent from synaptic vesicles (Sugita et al., 2002; Maximov et al., 2008), even though it is present on endocrine granules, suggesting that it is slow because it is not as close to the site of Ca^{2+}-triggered fusion as Syt1.

Complexins support synaptotagmin-dependent Ca^{2+}-triggering of fusion

We identified complexins as small proteins bound to SNARE complexes but not to individual SNARE proteins (McMahon et al., 1995; also later independently identified by Ishizuka et al., 1995). The crystal structure of complexin bound to the SNARE complex, obtained in collaboration with Josep Rizo, revealed that complexin contains a central α-helix that nestles in an antiparallel orientation into the groove formed by the Syntaxin-1 and Synaptobrevin-2 SNARE motifs (Chen et al., 2002). The central α-helix of complexin is N-terminally preceded by an accessory α-helix and a short unstructured sequence, and C-terminally followed by a longer unstructured sequence. Analysis of complexin-deficient neurons showed that complexin represents a co-factor for synaptotagmin that functions physiologically both as a clamp and as an activator of Ca^{2+}-triggered fusion (Reim et al., 2001; Tang et al., 2006; Huntwork and Littleton, 2007; Maximov et al., 2009; Yang et al., 2010). Complexin-deficient neurons exhibited a milder phenocopy of Syt1-deficient neurons, with a partial suppression of fast synchronous exocytosis and an increase in spontaneous exocytosis, suggesting that complexins and synaptotagmins are functionally interdependent.

Some confusion developed regarding complexin function because *in vitro* fusion assays suggested that complexins act only as a clamp of fusion (Giraudo et al., 2006), whereas in analyses of synaptic transmission in autapses (in which isolated neurons form synapses with themselves for want of a better partner), complexins acted only as an activator of Ca^{2+}-triggered fusion (Reim et al., 2001). Subsequent studies in cultures of dissociated neurons readily uncovered both complexin activities in that the loss-of-function of complexin produced a large increase in spontaneous 'mini' release (interpreted as unclamping) and a major impairment in evoked release (interpreted as a lack of activation; Fig. 10 [Maximov et al., 2009]).

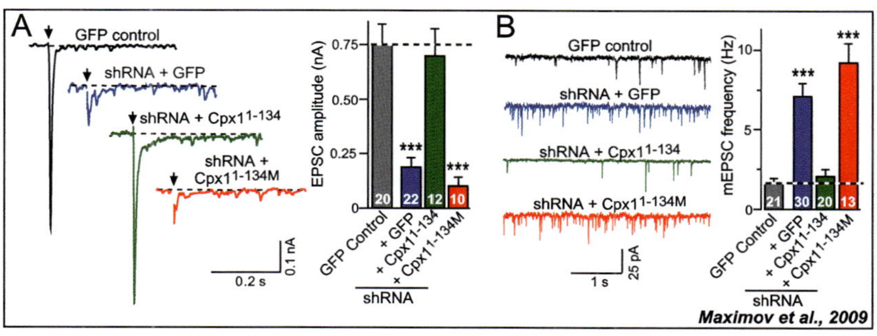

FIGURE 10. *Complexin functions both as an activator and as a clamp of synaptic vesicle fusion*

A & B. Excitatory postsynaptic currents (EPSCs) elicited by isolated action potentials (A) and spontaneous miniature EPSCs (mESPCs; B) monitored in control neurons and complexin knockdown neurons without or with expression of complexin rescue constructs (wild-type complexin-1 [$Cpx^{1\text{-}134}$] and mutant complexin-1 unable to bind to SNARE complexes [$Cpx^{1\text{-}134M}$]). Representative traces are shown on the left, and summary graphs on the right to illustrate the dual nature of complexin action as an activator of Ca^{2+}-triggered exocytosis (A) and as a clamp of spontaneous mini release (B). Data are adapted from Maximov et al. (2009).

How does a small molecule like complexin, composed of only ~130 residues, act to activate and clamp synaptic vesicles for synaptotagmin action? The central complexin α-helix that is bound to the SNARE complex is essential for all complexin function (Fig. 10; Maximov et al., 2009). The accessory α-helix is required only for the clamping but not the activating function of complexin, demonstrating that clamping is not a prerequisite for the activation function of complexin (Yang et al., 2010). The flexible N-terminal sequence of complexin, conversely, mediates only the activating but not the clamping function of complexin (Xue et al., 2007; Maximov et al., 2009). Recent results indicate that the activating function of complexin is unexpectedly complex (no pun intended) in that complexin also contributes to the priming of synaptic vesicles, but that for this facet of its activating function the C-terminal sequence is required (Yang et al., 2010; Kaeser-Woo et al., 2012).

Based on these studies, our current model posits that complexin binding to SNAREs activates the SNARE/SM protein complex, and that at least part of complexin competes with synaptotagmin for SNARE-complex binding and clamps the complex to prevent its complete assembly (Tang et al., 2006). Ca^{2+}-activated synaptotagmin displaces this part of complexin, thereby enabling fusion-pore opening (Fig. 11). However, it is likely that the clamping function of complexin is relatively less important than its activation function. Even though a 10-fold increase in the rate of spontaneous mini release induced by loss of complexin function is significant, it is very small on a per synapse basis. If one considers that each neuron receives thousands of synaptic inputs, the increased mini rate still translates into only one release event or less per synapse and per minute (Yang et al., 2013). Moreover, some complexin isoforms that are generally expressed at low levels (complexin-3 and -4) do not exhibit a clamping function (Kaeser-Woo et al., 2012), and the function of complexin in Ca^{2+}-triggered exocytosis of IGF-1 containing vesicles (see below) does not involve clamping (Cao et al., 2013). Thus, it is likely that complexin primarily functions as an activator of exocytosis, and that its clamping function is either an epiphenomenon, or a more minor fine-tuning activity in synaptic transmission.

An approximation of how SNARE and SM proteins collaborate with synaptotagmins and complexins in Ca^{2+}-triggered fusion

The convergence of biochemical and biophysical studies on the neurotransmitter release machinery lead us to a preliminary model of how Ca^{2+}-triggered neurotransmitter release proceeds (Fig. 11).

Sketching the atomic structures of SNARE proteins, complexin and synaptotagmin into the context of a docked and primed synaptic vesicle in an in-scale drawing reveals a crowded space in which all partners are placed into close proximity, allowing for rapid interactions (Fig. 11A). When we consider how sequential interactions of SNARE and SM proteins with complexin and synaptotagmin may mediate Ca^{2+}-triggered fusion, the most plausible model is that complexin and synaptotagmin act on top of the two sequential major conformational changes involved in SNARE/SM protein complex assembly (Fig. 11B; see also Fig. 4). Specifically, after docked and tethered vesicles are primed for fusion by opening up the closed conformation of Syntaxin-1 and by partial trans-SNARE-complex assembly (Priming I, Fig. 11B), complexin binds to the partially assembled trans-SNARE complex to 'superprime' it and to energize the vesicles for Ca^{2+}-triggered fusion (Priming II). Synaptotagmins probably also constitutively bind to assembling SNARE complexes independent of Ca^{2+}, and the complexin- and synaptotagmin-binding may contribute to 'freeze' the partly assembled SNARE complex and thus 'clamp' it. Ca^{2+} then triggers fusion-pore opening by binding to synaptotagmin, which in turn binds to phospholipids and changes its interaction with the trans-SNARE complex to partly displace complexin. It is likely that synaptotagmin and complexin constitutively interact with the SNARE/SM protein complex in a Ca^{2+}-independent manner to form a single prefusion complex, and that Ca^{2+} does not cause an all-or-none binding of synaptotagmin to the SNARE complex as it does for binding of synaptotagmin to phospholipids, but instead causes a rearrangement of the prefusion complex (e.g., see Shin et al., 2003).

The simplest mechanism by which Ca^{2+}-binding to synaptotagmin could open the fusion pore would be by pulling on the SNARE/SM protein complex, a pulling action that could be induced by Ca^{2+}-triggered binding of synaptotagmin to phospholipids. After fusion-pore opening, the pore expands, and NSF and SNAPs are recruited to the assembled cis-SNARE complex. NSF then dissociates the cis-SNARE complex, the Munc18-1/SNARE complex assembly is transformed into the heteromeric Munc18-1/Syntaxin-1 complex, and synaptic vesicles recycle via one of several forms of endocytosis (see Fig. 1).

Parallel synaptotagmin-mediated pathways of Ca^{2+}-triggered exocytosis

The 4 synaptotagmins that lack N-terminal disulfide bonds (Syt1, Syt2, Syt7, and Syt9) function in synaptic vesicle and neuroendocrine exocytosis, but what about the other 4 Ca^{2+}-binding synaptotagmins that are disulfide-bonded

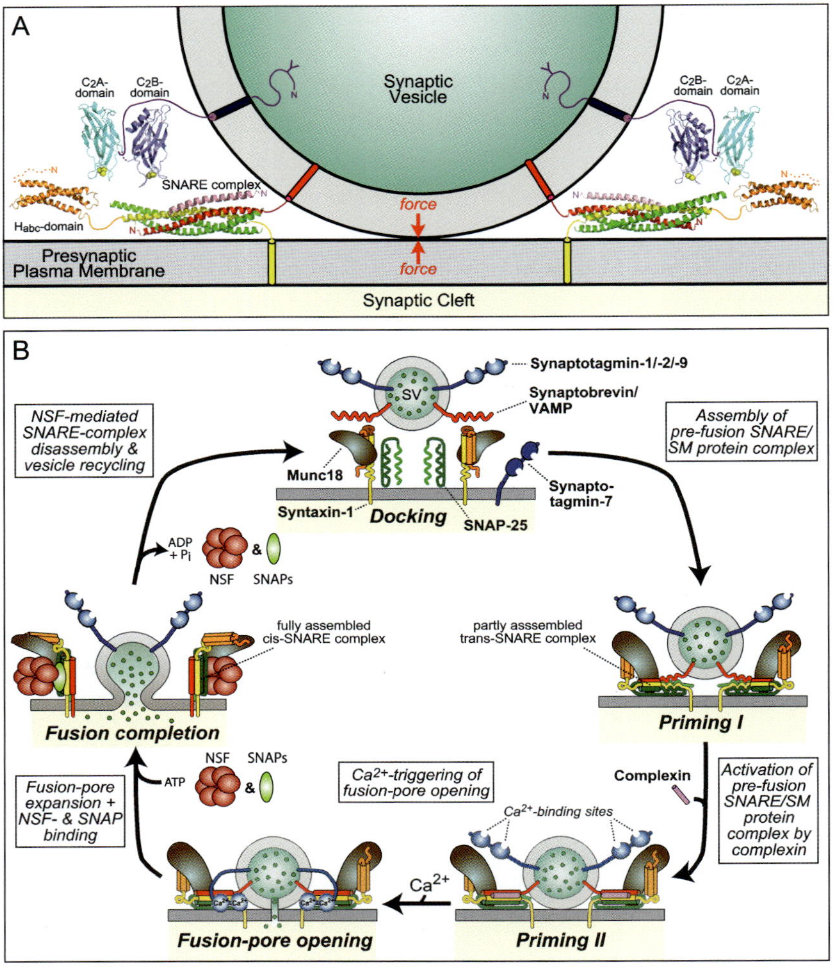

FIGURE 11. *Modeling how SNARE and SM proteins collaborate with synaptotagmins and complexins in Ca^{2+}-triggered neurotransmitter release*

A. Atomic structures of SNARE proteins, complexin, and Syt1 during synaptic vesicle fusion. The illustration summarizes atomic structures obtained in collaboration with Josep Rizo (UT Southwestern) of the Syt1 C2-domains (Shao et al., 1998; Fernandez et al., 2001), the Syntaxin-1 Habc-domain (Ferndandez et al., 1997), and the assembled SNARE complex containing bound complexin (pink; Chen et al., 2002). Transmembrane regions are depicted as cylinders, and linker sequences as lines. All structures are in scale relative to the synaptic vesicle, illustrating the space constraints of the collaboration between Syt1 and the SNARE complex/complexin assembly. Munc18-1 is also bound to the SNARE complex at the same time (see Figs. 3D and 4) but is not shown since no structure of Munc18-1 bound to the SNARE complex is available. The direction of the force produced by SNARE complex assembly that destabilizes the phospholipid membrane surfaces is indicated.

(continues)

dimers? Recent studies revealed that one of these synaptotagmins, Syt10, also acts as a Ca^{2+}-sensor in exocytosis, but in a form of exocytosis that differs from synaptic vesicle and neuroendocrine granule exocytosis. Specifically, we found that Syt10 functions in olfactory neurons as a Ca^{2+}-sensor for specialized vesicles containing IGF-1 (Cao et al., 2011). These vesicles differ from neuropeptide-containing vesicles present in the same neurons (which are more like neuroendocrine granules and contain Syt1; Cao et al., 2013). Among others, these experiments demonstrated that even in a single neuron, different synaptotagmins act as Ca^{2+}-sensors for distinct Ca^{2+}-triggered fusion reactions (Fig. 12). Moreover, these observations indicated that Ca^{2+}-triggered exocytosis generally depends on synaptotagmin Ca^{2+}-sensors, and that different synaptotagmins contribute to the specificity and differential properties of distinct exocytosis pathways.

Interestingly, complexin not only supports synaptotagmins acting in neurotransmitter release, but also Syt10-dependent IGF1 secretion, despite the different covalent structures of Syt1 and Syt10 (Cao et al., 2013). Thus, complexin likely is a general co-factor for all synaptotagmins in regulated exocytosis. This hypothesis is supported by the fact that complexin is ubiquitously present in all cells (McMahon et al., 1995), and is also central for the postsynaptic insertion of AMPA-type glutamate receptors during LTP (Ahmad et al., 2012), suggesting that complexins are general cofactors for regulated exocytosis.

B. Schematic diagram of the action of synaptotagmins and complexins in the SNARE/SM protein cycle. The SNARE/SM protein cycle is composed of the assembly of the SNARE proteins Synaptobrevin/VAMP, SNAP-25, and Syntaxin-1 into complexes whose full formation forces fusion-pore opening; the SM protein Munc18-1 remains associated with Syntaxin-1 throughout the cycle and is essential for fusion-pore opening. After fusion, the chaperone ATPase NSF and its SNAP adaptors catalyze SNARE-complex dissociation. Complexin binds to partially assemble SNARE complexes during priming, and serves as an essential adaptor that enables synaptotagmin to act as a Ca^{2+}-sensor in triggering fusion-pore opening (bottom limb of the cycle). Note that synaptotagmin likely constitutively interacts with the SNARE/SM protein complex in a Ca^{2+}-independent manner to form a single prefusion complex prior to Ca^{2+}-triggering of exocytosis, and that Ca^{2+} does not cause an all-or-none binding of synaptotagmin to the SNARE complex as it does for binding of synaptotagmin to phospholipids, but instead causes a rearrangement of the prefusion complex. However, this is not shown in the diagram due to difficulties of representing these multifarious three-dimensional interactions in a two-dimensional format. Both synaptotagmins and complexins additionally clamp spontaneous release, probably via their Ca^{2+}-independent constitutive binding to partly assembled SNARE complexes. Three vesicular synaptotagmins act as Ca^{2+}-sensors for fast exocytosis (Syt1, Syt2, and Syt9); in addition, Syt7 that is not present on synaptic vesicles but probably localizes to the presynaptic plasma membrane (Sugita et al., 2001) mediates slower forms of Ca^{2+}-triggered exocytosis (Syt7 is only shown in the top overview for simplicity). Drawing was modified from Südhof (2013).

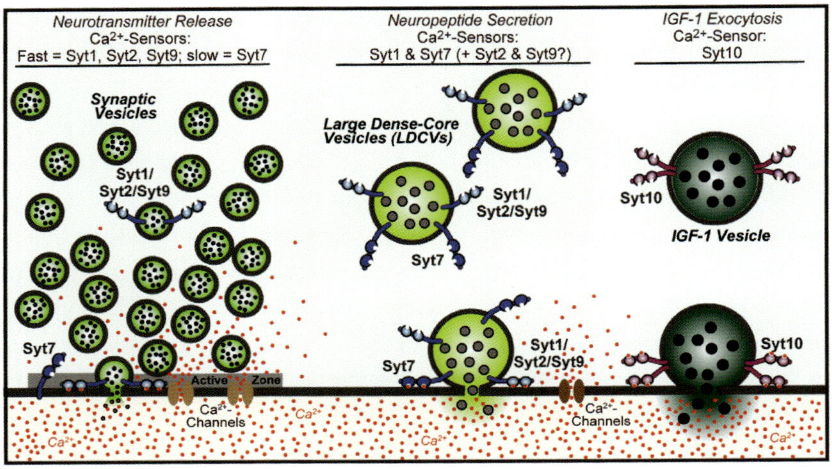

FIGURE 12. *Overlapping and non-overlapping functions of different synaptotagmins in Ca^{2+}-triggering of various types of exocytosis in a single neuron.* Three types of Ca^{2+}-triggered exocytosis are illustrated: Left, synaptic vesicle exocytosis mediating neurotransmitter release that uses Syt1, Syt2, and/or Syt9 as fast Ca^{2+}-sensors (Xu et al., 2007), and Syt7 as a slow Ca^{2+}-sensor (Bacaj et al., 2013). Center, large dense-core vesicle (LDCV) exocytosis that uses the same Ca^{2+}-sensors as synaptic vesicle exocytosis (Syt1 and Syt7 based on work in chromaffin cells [Sugita et al., 2001; Schonn et al., 2007], and probably also Syt2 and Syt9). Right, exocytosis of a separate class of peptidergic vesicles that are larger than LDCVs and utilize Syt10 as a Ca^{2+}-sensor (Cao et al., 2011 and 2013). Note that although Syt7 has been shown to operate in both synaptic vesicle and LDCV exocytosis, it is absent from synaptic vesicles but present on LDCVs, and is thought that act more slowly in neurotransmitter release because of its different localization. Diagram was modified from Cao et al. (2011).

5. ORGANIZING THE RELEASE MACHINERY AT THE ACTIVE ZONE

In a presynaptic terminal, synaptic vesicles dock and fuse at the active zone of the presynaptic plasma membrane. The active zone is a specialized area that appears dense in electron microscopy pictures of fixed tissue and is localized precisely opposite postsynaptic receptor clusters (Fig. 1). The first specific active zone protein we identified was Munc13-1 (Brose et al., 1995). Munc 13-1 was named like Munc18-1 (no relation!) after a homologous gene in C. elegans (*unc13*) that is essential for coordinated worm movements but whose function was unknown (Brenner, 1974). Based on this homology, the 'uncoordinated' worm phenotype, and its localization to the active zone, we speculated that Munc13-1 may be a component of the neurotransmitter release machinery (Brose et al., 1995).

This supposition was confirmed when we analyzed knockout synapses lacking Munc13-1, which exhibited a dramatic loss of synaptic vesicle priming (Augustin et al., 1999).

Quickly after Munc13-1, we identified a series of additional active zone proteins such as CASK (Hata et al., 1996), RIMs (for Rab3-interacting molecules; Wang et al., 1997), RIM-BPs (Wang et al., 2000), and ELKS (Wang et al., 2002; see also Ohtsuka et al., 2002), while others identified additional active zone proteins such as α-liprins (Zhen and Jin, 1999), bassoon (tom Dieck et al., 1998), and piccolo (Wang et al., 1999; Fenster et al., 2000). Interestingly, most of these proteins directly or indirectly bind to each other, forming a protein network at the active zone (Südhof, 2012). Specifically, RIMs bind to Munc13-1, to RIM-BPs, to ELKS (although it is not clear whether this binding is physiologically important) and to α-liprins, suggesting that RIMs are the central hub of this network, while additional interactions connect some of the other proteins with each other (Wang et al., 2000 and 2003; Betz et al., 2001; Schoch et al., 2002). Clearly, many questions about the active zone are still unanswered, most importantly what mechanisms position the active zone precisely opposite a postsynaptic specialization. Nevertheless, we now have a plausible view of how the active zone performs its three main functions, namely the tethering ('docking') of synaptic vesicles at the plasma membrane, the priming of such vesicles for fusion, and the recruitment of Ca^{2+}-channels next to docked and primed vesicles.

Tethering ('docking') of synaptic vesicles to the active zone

As in other membrane-trafficking processes, synaptic vesicle tethering involves Rab proteins, small GTPases that are distantly related to ras proteins. The central role of Rab proteins in membrane traffic was discovered in Novick's studies on Sec4p (Salminen and Novick, 1987). Following up on Novick's work, we observed in 1992 in collaboration with Reinhard Jahn that Rab3, the most abundant Rab protein in brain, is highly enriched on synaptic vesicles at rest but dissociates from the vesicles during exocytosis, suggesting a role in neurotransmitter release (von Mollard et al., 1990 and 1991). Subsequent mouse genetic analyses of the four different Rab3 isoforms (Rab3A, 3B, 3C, and 3D) confirmed that Rab3 plays a central role in neurotransmitter release (Geppert et al., 1994b; Schlüter et al., 2004 and 2006). Moreover, single Rab3 isoforms did perform essential functions on their own in that deletions of Rab3A or Rab3B caused major but distinct changes in short- and long-term forms of presynaptic plasticity (Geppert et al., 1994b; Schlüter et al., 2004 and 2006; Tsetsenis et al., 2011).

In our search for a mechanism of action for Rab3s, we initially tested the functional role of rabphilin, the first putative Rab3-effector identified by Yoshimi Takai (Shirataki et al., 1993). However, rabphilin deletions produced only minor changes in release, suggesting that is it not a major player (Schlüter et al., 1999; Deak et al., 2006).

We then searched for additional Rab3-effector proteins, defined by the GTP-dependent binding to Rab3 but not other major Rabs. We identified RIMs (for 'Rab3-interacting molecules'), a family of large multi-domain active zone proteins that are evolutionarily conserved (Wang et al., 1997 and 2000). In mammals, four RIM-related genes are expressed, of which only two (*RIMS1* and *RIMS2*) produce proteins that contain the Rab3-binding domain (Wang et al., 2000 and 2002). The RIMS1 and RIMS2 genes, however, include multiple independent promoters, resulting in five principal forms (RIM1α, RIM1β, RIM2α, RIM2β, and RIM2γ) that are further diversified by extensive alternative splicing.

Subsequent studies extending over 15 years revealed that RIMs perform multiple functions in the active zone which extend far beyond their role as Rab3-effectors. As we will see below, RIMs are critical not only for tethering/docking synaptic vesicles, but also for recruiting Ca^{2+}-channels to the active zone, for mediating short- and long-term presynaptic plasticity, and for activating the priming function of Munc13 proteins. As regards the tethering/docking function of RIMs that was suggested by their active zone localization and Rab3-binding, this function was first validated in C. elegans, which contains only a single RIM gene (referred to as *unc10*; Koushika et al., 2001; Gracheva et al., 2008). However, in mice deletions of single RIM isoforms, including that of the predominant RIM1α, did not detectably alter vesicle docking as analyzed by conventional electron microscopy (Schoch et al., 2002), but double conditional knockouts that deleted all isoforms produced by the *RIMS1* and *RIMS2* genes exhibited a dramatic decrease in vesicle docking (Kaeser et al., 2011; Han et al., 2011). Based on these studies, it is plausible that synaptic vesicles are tethered ('docked') to active zones via a GTP-dependent binding of active zone RIM proteins to synaptic vesicle Rab3/27 proteins.

It should be noted that no other proteins besides RIMs were found to be essential for synaptic vesicle docking when such docking was analyzed in electron micrographs of chemically fixed and traditionally stained sections. However, a completely different picture emerges when electron microscopy is performed on unfixed, rapidly frozen tissue—now, a large number of additional genes were found to be essential for 'docking'. In such preparations, even the single RIM1α

knockout exhibits a docking phenotype. However, it is implausible that so many proteins tether vesicles without redundancy, and these phenotypes may more closely reflect priming than docking. Thus, although multiple molecules can contribute to the stable attachment of synaptic vesicles to the active zone, only RIMs appear to be truly required for docking. It should also be noted that 'docking' of secretory granules in chromaffin cells behaves differently from docking of synaptic vesicles at the active zone. For example, the Syt1 KO blocks secretory granule docking (de Wit et al., 2009) but not synaptic vesicle docking (Geppert et al., 1994). However, the Syt1 KO has only a small effect on Ca^{2+}-triggered exocytosis in chromaffin cells in contrast to its large effect on synaptic exocytosis, probably because Syt1 is fully redundant with Syt7 in chromaffin exocytosis but not in synaptic exocytosis (Xu et al., 2007; Schonn et al., 2008). This discrepancy between docking and exocytosis suggests that different from synapses, docking may not even be essential for exocytosis in chromaffin cells.

Priming vesicles for fusion

Priming is thought to transfer vesicles into a readily-releasable pool (RRP) of vesicles that are then competent for Ca^{2+}-triggered fusion. A large number of proteins have been implicated in priming. In addition to those proteins that are involved in fusion itself (e.g., SNARE and SM proteins) and to complexin, the most important priming factors are probably Munc13 and RIMs that bind to each other.

Analyses largely carried out in Nils Brose's and Josep Rizo's laboratories revealed that Munc13 is essential for vesicle priming, probably because it catalyzes SNARE-complex assembly via its MUN domain (Augustin et al., 1999; Varoqueaux et al., 2002). The purified MUN domain can facilitate the opening of 'closed' Syntaxin-1 for subsequent SNARE-complex assembly, providing a mechanism for the phenotypes observed in mutant mice (Ma et al., 2011). A striking observation is that Munc13 function is tightly regulated by multiple signaling pathways. Among others, neuronal Munc13 isoforms contain a C1-domain N-terminal to the central Ca^{2+}-binding C2-domain. The Munc13 C1-domain binds diacylglycerol physiologically, and is activated pharmacologically by phorbol esters (Betz et al., 1998). Diacylglycerol binding to the Munc13 C1-domain regulates synaptic function since mouse mutants lacking phorbol ester binding to Munc13-1 exhibit a dramatic impairment in priming and short-term plasticity (Rhee et al., 2002). The Ca^{2+}-binding C2-domain of Munc13s is equally important since it also significantly contributes to short-term plasticity of synapses (Shin et al., 2010). Finally, Munc13s bind to calmodulin which additionally modulates its function (Lipstein et al., 2013).

Deletions of RIMs also cause a major impairment in priming (Schoch et al., 2002; Koushika et al., 2001). The mechanism of this impairment, however, seems to be indirect because RIMs bind to Munc13s and activate Munc13 function (Deng et al., 2011). Specifically, the N-terminal sequence of RIMs includes a zinc-finger motif that avidly binds to the N-terminal Ca^{2+}-independent C2-domain of Munc13 (Dulubova et al., 2005; Lu et al., 2006). Without such binding, the Munc13-1 C2-domain forms a constitutive homodimer; upon RIM zinc-finger binding, the homodimer is converted into a RIM-Munc13 heterodimer. Strikingly, we found that the priming impairment in RIM-deficient synapses can be at least partly suppressed by overexpression of an N-terminally truncated Munc13-1 mutant that lacks the N-terminal C2-domain and no longer homodimerizes, whereas overexpression of wild-type Munc13-1 has no effect (Deng et al., 2011). These observations portray at least one mechanism by which RIMs regulate the priming function of Munc13, consistent with an overall central function of RIMs in all active zone activities.

Recruiting Ca^{2+}-channels to the active zone

In order to achieve fast synchronous neurotransmitter release that is precisely coupled to an action potential, the most important requirement is that Ca^{2+}-channels are localized at the active zone adjacent to docked and primed synaptic vesicles. Only such an arrangement produces the short Ca^{2+}-diffusion pathways required for the requisite speed of a synapse, and only a short Ca^{2+}-diffusion path can explain how the extremely brief presynaptic Ca^{2+}-transient triggers release—after all, the Ca^{2+}-sensors for neurotransmitter release and neuroendocrine exocytosis are the same, even though the latter are much slower than the former.

A molecular mechanism that explains how synapses achieve the required arrangement of Ca^{2+}-channels and synaptic vesicles emerged with the demonstration that RIMs collaborate with their binding partners RIM-BPs to recruit Ca^{2+}-channels to release sites (Kaeser et al., 2011; Fig. 13). Since RIMs are also the tethering agents for synaptic vesicles and contribute crucially to vesicle priming, RIMs are thus the central elements in the organization of the active zone that enable the amazing properties of neurotransmitter release. This simple architecture of the active zone, whereby a single protein is the central agent in assembling all components at one location, is at the same time parsimonious and effective (Fig. 14).

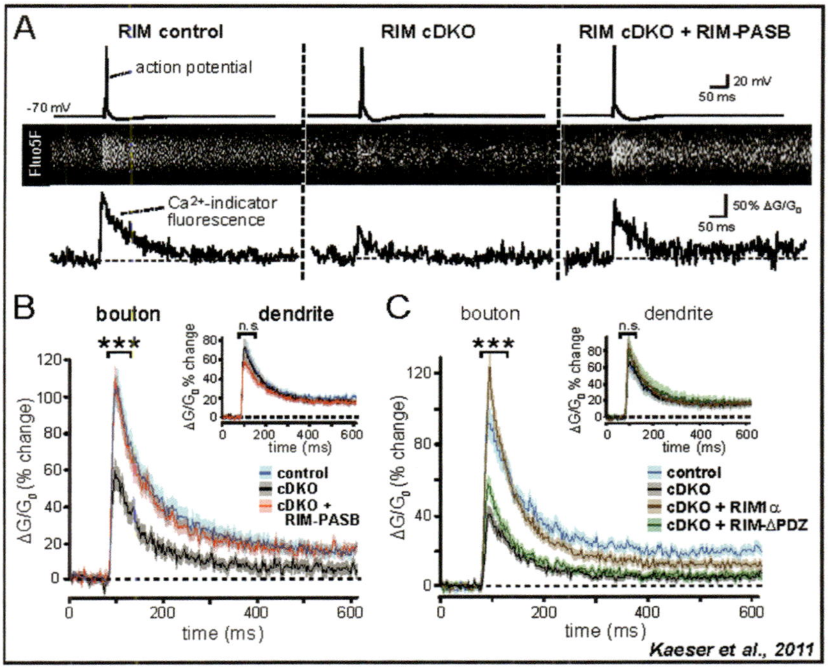

FIGURE 13. *RIM deletion decreases presynaptic Ca^{2+}-transients*

A. Isolated action potentials cause a rise in presynaptic Ca^{2+}-concentrations that is impaired by deletion of RIM proteins (RIM cDKO) but can be rescued by expression of a RIM1 fragment which binds to Ca^{2+}-channels (RIM-PASB). Data show representative traces of action potentials (top); line scans of Ca^{2+}-transients in presynaptic boutons induced by these action potentials, and monitored by fluorescence of the Ca^{2+}-indicator Fluo5F (middle); and quantitations of Ca^{2+}-transients (bottom).

B. Summary plots of the time course of the intracellular Ca^{2+}-concentration in presynaptic terminals and in dendrites (inset) during an action potential. Data show average Ca^{2+}-concentrations monitored as shown in A in multiple independent experiments in control neurons, neurons lacking RIM proteins (cDKO), and RIM-deficient neurons that express a RIM fragment binding to Ca^{2+}-channels (cDKO + RIM-PASB).

C. Same as B, except that rescue of impaired Ca^{2+}-transients in RIM-deficient synapses was tested for full-length wild-type RIM1α or for full-length RIM1α lacking the PDZ-domain.

All images are from Kaeser et al. (2011).

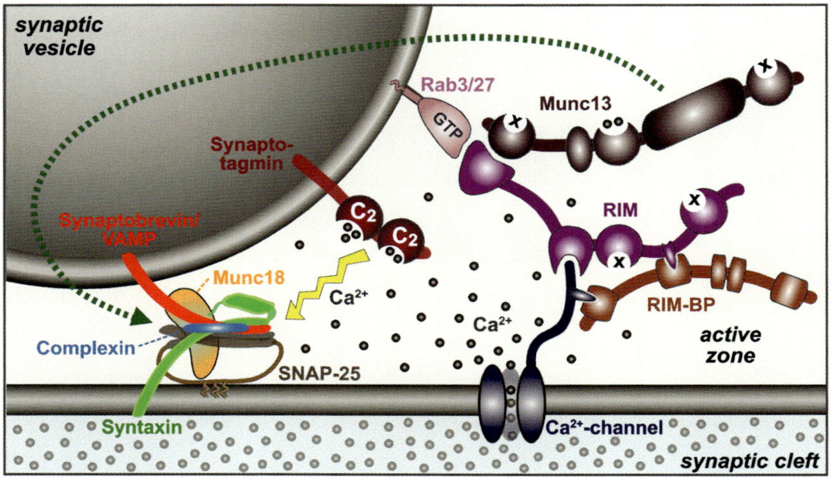

FIGURE 14. *Schematic diagram of the RIM, RIM-BP, and Munc13 protein complex that binds simultaneously to Rab3/27 on the synaptic vesicle and to Ca^{2+}-channels on the plasma membrane, thereby mediating the tethering ('docking') of vesicles at release sites, the priming of vesicles for release (arrow with dotted line), and the recruitment of Ca^{2+}-channels adjacent to tethered vesicles.* RIM, RIM-BP, and Munc13 are multidomain proteins that form a tight complex which mediates three essential functions of active zones: recruitment of Ca^{2+}-channels to enable tight coupling of action potentials to release by localizing Ca^{2+}-influx next to the Ca^{2+}-sensor synaptotagmin; docking of vesicles at the release site; and Munc13-dependent priming of the fusion machinery composed of the SNARE syntaxin, SNAP-25, synaptobrevin/VAMP, and Munc18-1. Spheres denote Ca^{2+}-ions; of the domains shown, only C2-domains are specifically labeled. Other active zone proteins bind to the RIM/Munc13/RIM-BP complex such as α-liprins and ELKS, and contribute to release but are not shown. Modified from Kaeser et al. (2011) and Südhof (2012).

We found that RIMs directly and selectively bind to Ca^{2+}-channels expressed in presynaptic active zones. Similar to the identification of the role of RIMs in vesicle tethering/docking, however, identification of the role of RIMs in recruiting Ca^{2+}-channels to the active zone only became possible when we deleted all RIM isoforms from presynaptic terminals (Kaeser et al., 2011). We found that deletion of RIMs causes a decrease of presynaptic Ca^{2+}-influx, a loss of presynaptic Ca^{2+}-channels, and a loss of the tight coupling of a presynaptic action potential to release (Fig. 13; Han et al., 2011; Kaeser et al., 2011 and 2012). RIMs perform their functions by forming a large complex with the Ca^{2+}-channels, with other active zone proteins such as RIM-BPs (which in turn also bind to Ca^{2+}-channels) and Munc13-1, and with synaptic vesicles. The role of RIMs and RIM-BPs in recruiting Ca^{2+}-channels and docking vesicles to active zones is evolutionarily conserved (Liu et al., 2011; Graf et al., 2012), and represents a fundamental mechanism underlying synaptic transmission.

6. PUTTING IT ALL TOGETHER

The three levels of release that we have been studying—membrane fusion, Ca^{2+}-triggering of fusion, and the organization of the Ca^{2+}-controlled fusion machinery at the active zone—form a hierarchy of interdependent processes. Like a Russian doll, these three levels are nestled into each other, with membrane fusion as the inner core, and the scaffolding organizing the various components into a single machine as the outer layer. Our work, together with that of others, uncovered a plausible mechanism explaining how the synaptic vesicle membrane and the plasma membrane undergo rapid fusion during neurotransmitter release, how such fusion is triggered by Ca^{2+}, and how those processes are spatially organized in the presynaptic terminal, such that opening of Ca^{2+}-channels by an action potential allows rapid translation of the entering Ca^{2+} signal into a fusion event.

Together, the neurotransmitter release machinery that we uncovered accounts for the astounding speed and precision of Ca^{2+}-triggered release. Moreover, the overall design of this machinery and the identification of regulatory domains in it suggest mechanisms to explain the dramatic short- and long-term plasticity of release that plays a central role in determining circuit properties. Nevertheless, many crucial questions remain. For example, what are the physicochemical mechanisms underlying membrane fusion, how precisely do SNARE and SM proteins work, what is the role of the fusion machine as outlined here in disorders like Parkinson's disease, how do presynaptic terminals undergo long-term structural changes during plasticity, and what is the role of plasticity in long-term memory? Moreover, what mechanisms render various types of synapses different from each other—why do inhibitory synapses for example often exhibit a higher release probability than excitatory synapses, and what mechanisms confer distinct forms of plasticity onto different types of synapses? How is the presynaptic active zone precisely aligned with the postsynaptic density, and how is the size of a synapse regulated? Much remains to be done, and I hope to see at least some of these intriguing questions addressed in my lifetime!

ACKNOWLEDGEMENTS

I thank my life-long mentors in science M.S. Brown, V.P. Whittaker, and J.L. Goldstein for continuous advice, and my co-workers and collaborators for invaluable guidance and support, in particular Reinhard Jahn, Robert E. Hammer, Nils Brose, Rafael Fernandez-Chacon, Zhiping Pang, Irina Dulubova, Jianyuan Sun, Axel Brunger, Christian Rosenmund, and Josep Rizo. I am grateful to the Howard Hughes Medical Institute, the NIMH, and NINDS for financial support for almost 30 years.

REFERENCES

Acuna C, Guo Q, Burre J, Sharma M, Sun J, and Südhof TC (2014). "Microsecond Dissection of Neurotransmitter Release: SNARE-Complex Assembly Dictates Speed and Ca^{2+}-Sensitivity." *Neuron* **82**,1088–1100.

Ahmad M et al. (2012). "Postsynaptic Complexin Controls AMPA Receptor Exocytosis During LTP." *Neuron* **73**, 260–267.

Augustin I, Rosenmund C, Südhof TC, Brose N (1999). "Munc-13 is essential for fusion competence of glutamatergic synaptic vesicles." *Nature* **400**, 457–461.

Bacaj T et al. (2013). "Synaptotagmin-1 and -7 Trigger Synchronous and Asynchronous Phases of Neurotransmitter Release." *Neuron* **80**, 947–959.

Balch WE, Dunphy WG, Braell WA and Rothman JE (1984). "Reconstitution of the transport of protein between successive compartments of the Golgi measured by the coupled incorporation of N-acetylglucosamine." *Cell* **39**:405–416.

Betz A et al. (1998). "Munc13-1 is a presynaptic phorbol ester receptor that enhances neurotransmitter release." *Neuron* **21**:123–36.

Betz A et al. (2001). "Functional interaction of the active zone proteins Munc13-1 and RIM1 in synaptic vesicle priming." *Neuron* **30**:183–196.

Bollmann JH, Sakmann B and Borst JG (2000). "Calcium sensitivity of glutamate release in a calyx-type terminal." *Science* **289**:953–957.

Borst JG and Sakmann B (1996). "Calcium influx and transmitter release in a fast CNS synapse." *Nature* **383**:431–434.

Brenner S (1974). "The genetics of Caenorhabditis elegans." *Genetics* **77**:71–94.

Brose N, Petrenko AG, Südhof TC and Jahn R (1992). "Synaptotagmin: A Ca^{2+}-sensor on the synaptic vesicle surface." *Science* **256**:1021–1025.

Burré J et al. (2010). "α-Synuclein Promotes SNARE-Complex Assembly in Vivo and in Vitro." *Science* **329**:1664–1668.

Cao P, Maximov A and Südhof TC (2011). "Activity-Dependent IGF-1 Exocytosis is Controlled by the Ca^{2+}-Sensor Synaptotagmin-10." *Cell* **145**:300–311.

Cao P, Yang X and Südhof TC (2013). "Complexin Activates Exocytosis of Distinct Secretory Vesicles Controlled by Different Synaptotagmins." *J. Neurosci.* **33**:1714–1727.

Carr CM et al. (1999). "Sec1p binds to SNARE complexes and concentrates at sites of secretion." *J. Cell Biol.* **146**:333–344.

Ceccarelli B, Hurlbut WP and Mauro A (1973). "Turnover of transmitter and synaptic vesicles at the frog neuromuscular junction." *J. Cell Biol.* **57**:499–524

Chandra S et al. (2005). "α-Synuclein Cooperates with CSPα in Preventing Neurodegeneration." *Cell* **123**, 383–396.

Chapman ER, Hanson PI, An S and Jahn R (1995). "Ca^{2+} regulates the interaction between synaptotagmin and syntaxin 1." *J. Biol. Chem.* **270**:23667–23671.

Chen X et al. (2002). "Three-dimensional structure of the complexin/SNARE complex." *Neuron* **33**:397–409.

Clary DO, Griff IC and Rothman JE (1990). "SNAPs, a family of NSF attachment proteins involved in intracellular membrane fusion in animals and yeast." *Cell* **61**:709–721.

Coussens L et al. (1986). "Multiple, distinct forms of bovine and human protein kinase C suggest diversity in cellular signaling pathways." *Science* **233**:859–66.

Corbalan-Garcia S and Gómez-Fernández JC (2014). "Signaling through C2 domains: More than one lipid target." *Biochim Biophys Acta* **1838**:1536–1547.

Davletov BA and Südhof TC (1993). "A single C2-domain from synaptotagmin I is sufficient for high affinity Ca^{2+}/phospholipid-binding." *J. Biol. Chem.* **268**:26386–26390.

Davletov BA and Südhof TC (1994). "Ca^{2+}-dependent conformational change in synaptotagmin I." *J. Biol. Chem.* **269**:28547–28550.

Deák F et al. (2006). "Rabphilin Regulates SNARE-Dependent Re-Priming of Synaptic Vesicles for Fusion." *EMBO J.* **25**:2856–2866.

de Wit H et al. (2009). "Synaptotagmin-1 docks secretory vesicles to Syntaxin-1/SNAP-25 acceptor complexes." *Cell* **138**:935–946.

Deng L, Kaeser PS, Xu W and Südhof TC (2011). "RIM Proteins Activate Vesicle Priming by Reversing Auto-Inhibitory Homodimerization of Munc13." *Neuron* **69**:317–331.

DiAntonio A, Parfitt KD and Schwarz TL (1993). "Synaptic transmission persists in synaptotagmin mutants of Drosophila." *Cell* **73**:1281–1290.

Dulubova I, et al. (1999). "A conformational switch in syntaxin during exocytosis." *EMBO J.* **18**:4372–4382.

Dulubova I et al. (2002). "How Tlg2p/syntaxin16 'snares' Vps45." *EMBO J.* **21**:3620–3631.

Dulubova I et al. (2005). "A Munc13/RIM/Rab3 Tripartite Complex: From Priming to Plasticity?" *EMBO J.* **24**:2839–2850.

Dulubova I, Khvotchev M, Südhof TC and Rizo J (2007). "Munc18-1 Binds Directly to the Neuronal SNARE Complex." *Proc. Natl. Acad. Sci. U.S.A.* **104**: 2697–2702.

Fenster SD et al. (2000). "Piccolo, a presynaptic zinc finger protein structurally related to bassoon." *Neuron* **25**:203–214.

Fernandez I et al. (1998). "Three-dimensional structure of an evolutionarily conserved N-terminal domain of syntaxin 1A." *Cell* **94**:841–849.

Fernandez I et al. (2001). "Three-dimensional structure of the synaptotagmin 1 C2B-domain: Synaptotagmin 1 as a phospholipid binding machine." *Neuron* **32**:1057–1069.

Fernández-Chacón R et al. (2001). "Synaptotagmin I functions as a Ca^{2+}-regulator of release probability." *Nature* **410**:41–49.

Fernandez-Chacon R and Südhof TC (2000). "Novel SCAMPs lacking NPF repeats: ubiquitous and synaptic vesicle-specific forms implicate SCAMPs in multiple membrane-trafficking functions." *J. Neurosci.* **20**:7941–7950.

Fernandez-Chacon et al. (2004). "The synaptic vesicle protein CSPα prevents presynaptic degeneration." *Neuron* **42**:237–251.

Forsythe ID (1994). "Direct patch recording from identified presynaptic terminals mediating glutamatergic EPSCs in the rat CNS, in vitro." *J. Physiol.* **479** (Pt 3):381–387.

Garcia EP et al. (1994). "A rat brain Sec1 homologue related to Rop and UNC18 interacts with syntaxin." *Proc. Natl. Acad. Sci. U.S.A.* **91**:2003–2007.

Geppert M, Archer BT III and Südhof TC (1991). "Synaptotagmin II: a novel differentially distributed form of synaptotagmin." *J. Biol. Chem.* **266**:13548–13552

Geppert M et al. (1994a). "Synaptotagmin I: A major Ca^{2+}-sensor for transmitter release at a central synapse." *Cell* **79**:717–727.

Geppert M et al. (1994b). "The role of Rab3A in neurotransmitter release." *Nature* **369**:493–497.

Gerber SH et al. (2008). "Conformational Switch of Syntaxin-1 Controls Synaptic Vesicle Fusion." *Science* **321**:1507–1510.

Giraudo CG, Eng WS, Melia TJ and Rothman JE (2006). "A clamping mechanism involved in SNARE-dependent exocytosis." *Science* **313**:676–80.

Gracheva EO, Hadwiger G, Nonet ML and Richmond JE (2008). "Direct interactions between C. elegans RAB-3 and Rim provide a mechanism to target vesicles to the presynaptic density." *Neurosci Lett.* **444**:137–142.

Graf ER et al. (2012). "RIM promotes calcium channel accumulation at active zones of the Drosophila neuromuscular junction." *J. Neurosci.* **32**:16586–16596.

Grote E, Carr CM and Novick PJ (2000). "Ordering the final events in yeast exocytosis." *J. Cell Biol.* **151**:439–452.

Grumelli C et al. (2005). "Internalization and mechanism of action of clostridial toxins in neurons." *Neurotoxicology* **26**:761–767.

Gundersen CB, Mastrogiacomo A, Faull K and Umbach JA (1994). "Extensive lipidation of a Torpedo cysteine string protein." *J. Biol Chem.* **269**:19197–19199.

Gustavsson N et al. (2008). "Impaired insulin secretion and glucose intolerance in Synaptotagmin-7 null mutant mice." *Proc. Natl. Acad. Sci. U.S.A.* **105**:3992–3997.

Gustavsson N et al. (2009). "Synaptotagmin-7 is a principal Ca^{2+} sensor for Ca^{2+}-induced glucagon exocytosis in pancreas." *J. Physiol.* **587**:1169–1178

Han Y, Kaeser PS, Südhof TC and Schneggenburger R (2011). "RIM determines Ca^{2+}-channel density and vesicle docking at the presynaptic active zone." *Neuron* **69**:304–316.

Hanson PI et al. (1997). "Structure and conformational changes in NSF and its membrane receptor complexes visualized by quick-freeze/deep-etch electron microscopy." *Cell* **90**:523–35.

Harrison SD, Broadie K, van de Goor J and Rubin GM (1994). "Mutations in the Drosophila Rop gene suggest a function in general secretion and synaptic transmission." *Neuron* **13**:555–66.

Hata Y, Slaughter CA and Südhof TC (1993). "Synaptic vesicle fusion complex contains unc-18 homologue bound to syntaxin." *Nature* **366**:347–351.

Hayashi T et al. (1994). "Synaptic vesicle membrane fusion complex: Action of clostridial neurotoxins on assembly." *EMBO J.* **13**:5051–5061.

Heuser JE and Reese TS (1973). "Evidence for recycling of synaptic vesicle membrane during transmitter release at the frog neuromuscular junction." *J. Cell Biol.* **57**:315–344.

Huntwork S and Littleton JT (2007). "A complexin fusion clamp regulates spontaneous neurotransmitter release and synaptic growth." *Nat. Neurosci.* **10**:1235–1237.

Ishizuka T, Saisu H, Odani S and Abe T (1995). "Synaphin: a protein associated with the docking/fusion complex in presynaptic terminals." *Biochem. Biophys. Res. Commun.* **213**:1107–1114.

Janz R, Hofmann K and Südhof TC (1998). "SVOP, an evolutionarily conserved synaptic vesicle protein, suggests novel transport functions of synaptic vesicles." *J. Neurosci.* **18**:9269–9281.

Janz, R et al. (1999). "Essential roles in synaptic plasticity for synaptogyrin I and synaptophysin I." *Neuron* **24**:687–700.

Katz B (1969). "The Release of Neural Transmitter Substances." *Liverpool: Liverpool Univ. Press.*

Kaeser PS et al. (2011). "RIM proteins tether Ca^{2+}-channels to presynaptic active zones via a direct PDZ-domain interaction." *Cell* **144**:282–295.

Kaeser PS, Deng L, Fan M and Südhof TC (2012). "RIM Genes Differentially Contribute to Organizing Presynaptic Release Sites." *Proc. Natl. Acad. Sci. U.S.A.* **109**:11830–11835.

Kaeser-Woo YJ, Yang X and Südhof TC (2012). "C-terminal Complexin Sequence is Selectively Required for Clamping and Priming but Not for Ca^{2+}-Triggering of Synaptic Exocytosis." *J. Neurosci.* **32**:2877–2885.

Khvotchev M et al. (2007). "Dual Modes of Munc18-1/SNARE Interactions Are Coupled by Functionally Critical Binding to Syntaxin-1 N-terminus." *J. Neurosci.* **27**:12147–12155.

Koushika SP et al. (2001). "A post-docking role for active zone protein Rim." *Nat. Neurosci.* **4**:997–1005.

Lee JO et al. (1999). "Crystal structure of the PTEN tumor suppressor: implications for its phosphoinositide phosphatase activity and membrane association." *Cell* **99**:323–34.

Li C et al. (1995). "Ca^{2+}-dependent and Ca^{2+}-independent activities of neural and non-neural synaptotagmins." *Nature* **375**:594–599.

Li C, Davletov BA and Südhof TC (1995). "Distinct Ca^{2+}- and Sr^{2+}-binding properties of synaptotagmins: definition of candidate Ca^{2+}-sensors for the fast and slow components of neurotransmitter release." *J. Biol. Chem.* **270**:24898–24902.

Lin RC and Scheller RH (1997). "Structural organization of the synaptic exocytosis core complex." *Neuron* **19**:1087–94.

Link E, et al. (1992). "Tetanus toxin action: Inhibition of neurotransmitter release linked to synaptobrevin poteolysis." *Biochem. Biophys. Res. Comm.* **189**:1017–1023.

Lipstein N et al. (2013). "Dynamic control of synaptic vesicle replenishment and short-term plasticity by Ca^{2+}-calmodulin-Munc13-1 signaling." *Neuron* **79**:82–96.

Littleton JT et al. (1993). "Mutational analysis of Drosophila synaptotagmin demonstrates its essential role in Ca^{2+}-activated neurotransmitter release." *Cell* **74**:1125–1134.

Liu KS et al. (2011). "RIM-binding protein, a central part of the active zone, is essential for neurotransmitter release." *Science* **334**:1565–1569.

Lu J et al. (2006). "Structural Basis for a Munc13-1 Homodimer-Munc13-1/RIM Heterodimer Switch: C2-domains as Versatile Protein-Protein Interaction Modules." *PLOS Biology* 4:e192.

Ma C, Li W, Xu Y and Rizo J (2011). "Munc13 mediates the transition from the closed syntaxin-Munc18 complex to the SNARE complex." *Nat. Struct. Mol. Biol.* **18**:542–549.

Mackler JM and Reist NE (2001). "Mutations in the second C2 domain of synaptotagmin disrupt synaptic transmission at Drosophila neuromuscular junctions." *J. Comp. Neurol.* **436**:4–16.

Maroteaux L, Campanelli JT and Scheller RH (1988). "Synuclein: a neuron-specific protein localized to the nucleus and presynaptic nerve terminal." *J. Neurosci.* **8**:2804–15.

Matthew WD, Tsavaler L and Reichardt LF (1981). "Identification of a synaptic vesicle-specific membrane protein with a wide distribution in neuronal and neurosecretory tissue." *J. Cell Biol.* **91**:257–69.

Maximov A and Südhof TC (2005). "Autonomous Function of Synaptotagmin 1 in Triggering Synchronous Release Independent of Asynchronous Release." *Neuron* **48**:547–554.

Maximov A et al. (2008). "Genetic analysis of Synaptotagmin-7 function in synaptic vesicle exocytosis." *Proc. Natl. Acad. Sci. U.S.A.* **105**:3986–3991.

Maximov A et al. (2009). "Complexin Controls the Force Transfer from SNARE complexes to membranes in Fusion." *Science* **323**:516–521.

Mayer A, Wickner W and Haas A (1996). "Sec18p (NSF)-driven release of Sec17p (alpha-SNAP) can precede docking and fusion of yeast vacuoles." *Cell* **85**:83–94.

McMahon H et al. (1993). "Cellubrevin: A ubiquitous tetanus-toxin substrate homologous to a putative synaptic vesicle fusion protein." *Nature* **364**:346–349.

McMahon HT and Südhof TC (1995). "Synaptic core complex of synaptobrevin, syntaxin, and SNAPS forms high affinity α-SNAP binding site." *J. Biol. Chem.* **270**:2213–2217.

McMahon HT, Missler M, Li C and Südhof TC (1995). "Complexins: cytosolic proteins that regulate SNAP-receptor function." *Cell* **83**:111–119.

Meijer M et al. (2012). "Munc18-1 mutations that strongly impair SNARE-complex binding support normal synaptic transmission." *EMBO J.* **31**:2156–2168.

Nonet ML, Grundahl K, Meyer BJ and Rand JB (1993). "Synaptic function is impaired but not eliminated in C. elegans mutants lacking synaptotagmin." *Cell* **73**:1291–1305.

Novick P and Schekman R (1979). "Secretion and cell-surface growth are blocked in a temperature-sensitive mutant of Saccharomyces cerevisiae." *Proc. Natl. Acad. Sci. U.S.A.* **76**:1858–1862.

Ohtsuka T et al. (2002). "Cast: a novel protein of the cytomatrix at the active zone of synapses that forms a ternary complex with RIM1 and munc13-1." *J. Cell Biol.* **158**:577–590.

Pang ZP et al. (2006a). "A gain-of-function mutation in Synaptotagmin-1 reveals a critical role of Ca^{2+}-dependent SNARE-complex binding in synaptic exocytosis." *J. Neurosci.* **26**, 12556–12565.

Pang ZP et al. (2006b). "Genetic Analysis of Synaptotagmin 2 in Spontaneous and Ca^{2+}-Triggered Neurotransmitter Release." *EMBO J.* **25**:2039–2050.

Pang ZP et al. (2007). "Synaptotagmin-2 is Essential for Survival and Contributes to Ca^{2+}-Triggering of Neurotransmitter Release in Central and Neuromuscular Synapses." *J. Neurosci.* **26**:13493–13504.

Perin MS, Fried VA, Slaughter CA and Südhof TC (1988). "The structure of cytochrome b561, a secretory vesicle-specific electron transport protein." *EMBO J.* **7**:2697–2703.

Perin MS et al. (1990). "Phospholipid binding by a synaptic vesicle protein homologous to the regulatory region of protein kinase C." *Nature* **345**:260–263.

Perin MS et al. (1991). "Structure of the 116 kDa polypeptide of the clathrin-coated vesicle/synaptic vesicle proton pump." *J. Biol. Chem.* **266**:3877–3881.

Perin MS et al. (1991). "Structural and functional conservation of synaptotagmin (p65) in Drosophila and humans." *J. Biol. Chem.* **266**:615–622.

Pevsner J, Hsu SC and Scheller RH (1994). "n-Sec1: a neural-specific syntaxin-binding protein." *Proc. Natl. Acad. Sci. U.S.A.* **91**:1445–1449.

Poirier MA et al. (1998). "The synaptic SNARE complex is a parallel four-stranded helical bundle." *Nat Struct Biol.* **5**:765–769.

Rathore SS et al. (2010). "Syntaxin N-terminal peptide motif is an initiation factor for the assembly of the SNARE-Sec1/Munc18 membrane fusion complex." *Proc. Natl. Acad. Sci. U.S.A.* **107**:22399–22406.

Regehr WG (2012). "Short-term presynaptic plasticity." *Cold Spring Harb Perspect Biol.* **4**:a005702.

Reim K et al. (2001). "Complexins regulate the Ca^{2+}-sensitivity of the synaptic neurotransmitter release machinery." *Cell* **104**:71–81.

Rhee JS et al. (2002). "Beta phorbol ester- and diacylglycerol-induced augmentation of transmitter release is mediated by Munc13s and not by PKCs." *Cell* **108**:121–133.

Rizo J and Südhof TC (1998). "C2-domains, structure of a universal Ca^{2+}-binding domain." *J. Biol. Chem.* **273**:15879–15882.

Rizo J and Südhof TC (2012). "The Membrane Fusion Enigma: SNAREs, SM Sec1/Munc18 Proteins, and Their Accomplices—Guilty as Charged?" *Annu. Rev. Cell Dev. Biol.* **28**: 279–308.

Robinson IM, Ranjan R and Schwarz TL (2002). "Synaptotagmin I and IV promote transmitter release independently of Ca^{2+} binding in the C2A domain." *Nature* **418**:336–340.

Rosahl TW et al. (1993). "Short term synaptic plasticity is altered in mice lacking synapsin I." *Cell* **75**:661–670.

Sabatini BL and Regehr WG (1996). "Timing of neurotransmission at fast synapses in the mammalian brain." *Nature* **384**:170–172.

Salminen A and Novick PJ (1987). "A ras-like protein is required for a post-Golgi event in yeast secretion." *Cell* **49**:527–538.

Schiavo G et al. (1992). "Tetanus and botulinum-B neurotoxins block neurotransmitter release by proteolytic cleavage of synaptobrevin." *Nature* **359**:832–835.

Schiavo G et al. (1993). "Identification of the nerve terminal targets of botulinum neurotoxin serotypes A, D, and E." *J. Biol. Chem.* **268**:23784–23787.

Schlüter OM et al. (1999). "Rabphilin knock-out mice reveal rat rabphilin is not required for rab3 function in regulating neurotransmitter release." *J. Neurosci.* **19**:5834–5846.

Schlüter OM et al. (2004). "A complete genetic analysis of neuronal Rab3 function." *J. Neurosci.* **24**:6629–6637.

Schlüter OM, Südhof TC and Rosenmund C (2006). "Rab3 Superprimes Synaptic Vesicles for Release: Implications for Short Term Synaptic Plasticity." *J. Neurosci.* **26**:1239–1246.

Schoch S et al. (2002). "RIM1α forms a protein scaffold for regulating neurotransmitter release at the active zone." *Nature* **415**:321–326.

Schonn J et al. (2008). "Synaptotagmin-1 and -7 are functionally overlapping Ca^{2+} sensors for exocytosis in adrenal chromaffin cells." *Proc. Natl. Acad. Sci. U.S.A.* **105**: 3998–4003.

Schoch S et al. (2002) RIM1α forms a protein scaffold for regulating neurotransmitter release at the active zone." *Nature* **415**:321–326.

Shao X et al. (1996). "Bipartite Ca^{2+}-binding motif in C2 domains of synaptotagmin and protein kinase C." *Science* **273**:248–251.

Shao X et al. (1997). "Synaptotagmin-syntaxin interaction: the C2-domain as a Ca^{2+}-dependent electrostatic switch." *Neuron* **18**:133–142.

Shao X, Fernandez I, Südhof TC and Rizo J (1998). "Solution structures of the Ca^{2+}-free and Ca^{2+}-bound C2A domain of synaptotagmin I: does Ca^{2+} induce a conformational change? *Biochemistry* **37**:16106–16115.

Sharma M et al. (2011a). "CSPα Knockout Causes Neurodegeneration by Impairing SNAP-25 Function." *EMBO J.* **31**:829–841.

Sharma M, Burré J and Südhof TC (2011b). "CSPα Promotes SNARE-Complex Assembly by Chaperoning SNAP-25 during Synaptic Activity." *Nature Cell Biol.* **13**:30–39.

Sharma M, Burré J and Südhof TC (2012). "Proteasome Inhibition Alleviates SNARE-Dependent Neurodegeneration in CSPα Knockout Mice." *Science Transl. Medicine* **4**: 147ra113.

Shen J et al. (2007). "Selective activation of cognate SNAREpins by Sec1/Munc18 proteins." *Cell* **128**:183–95.

Shirataki H et al. (1993). "Rabphilin-3A, a putative target protein for smg p25A/rab3A p25 small GTP-binding protein related to synaptotagmin." *Mol. Cell Biol.* **13**:2061–8.

Shin O-H et al. (2003). "Sr^{2+}-Binding to the Ca^{2+}-Binding Site of the Synaptotagmin 1 C2B-Domain Triggers Fast Exocytosis Without Stimulating SNARE Interactions." *Neuron* **37**:99–108.

Shin O-H, Xu J, Rizo J and Südhof TC (2009). "Differential but convergent functions of Ca^{2+}-binding to Synaptotagmin-1 C2-domains mediate neurotransmitter release." *Proc. Natl. Acad. Sci. U.S.A.* **106**:16469–16474.

Shin O-H et al. (2010). "Munc13 C2B-domain—an activity-dependent Ca^{2+}-regulator of synaptic exocytosis." *Nature Struct. Mol. Biol.* **17**:280–288.

Schneggenburger R and Neher E (2000). "Intracellular calcium dependence of transmitter release rates at a fast central synapse." *Nature* **406**:889–893.

Söllner T et al. (1993). "SNAP receptors implicated in vesicle targeting and fusion." *Nature* **362**:318–324.

Söllner T, Bennett MK, Whiteheart SW, Scheller RH and Rothman JE (1993). "A protein assembly-disassembly pathway in vitro that may correspond to sequential steps of synaptic vesicle docking, activation, and fusion." *Cell* **75**:409–418.

Sørensen JB, Fernandez-Chacon R, Südhof TC and Neher E (2003). "Examining synaptotagmin 1 function in dense core vesicle exocytosis under direct control of Ca^{2+}." *J. Gen. Physiol.* **122**:265–276.

Stein A, Weber G, Wahl MC and Jahn R (2009). "Helical extension of the neuronal SNARE complex into the membrane." *Nature* **460**:525–8.

Südhof TC (2004). "The synaptic vesicle cycle." *Annu. Rev. Neurosci.* **27**:509–547.

Südhof TC (2012). "The presynaptic active zone." *Neuron* **75**:11–25.

Südhof TC (2013). "A molecular machine for neurotransmitter release: Synaptotagmin and beyond." *Nature Medicine* **19**:1227–1231.

Südhof TC (2013). "Neurotransmitter release: The last millisecond in the life of a synaptic vesicle." *Neuron* **80**:675–690.

Südhof TC et al. (1987). "Synaptophysin: A synaptic vesicle protein with four transmembrane regions and a novel cytoplasmic domain." *Science* **238**:1142–1144.

Südhof TC et al. (1989a). "Synapsins: mosaics of shared and individual domains in a family of synaptic vesicle phosphoproteins." *Science* **245**:1474–1480

Südhof TC, Baumert M, Perin MS and Jahn R (1989b). "A synaptic vesicle membrane protein is conserved from mammals to Drosophila." *Neuron* **2**:1475–1481.

Südhof TC et al. (1989c). "Human endomembrane H+-pump strongly resembles the ATP-synthetase of archaebacteria." *Proc. Natl. Acad. Sci. U.S.A.* **86**:6067–6071.

Südhof TC and Jahn R (1991). "Proteins of synaptic vesicles involved in exocytosis and membrane recycling." *Neuron* **6**:665–677.

Südhof TC, DeCamilli P, Niemann H and Jahn R (1993). "Membrane fusion machinery: Insights from synaptic proteins." *Cell* **75**:1–4.

Südhof TC and Rothman JE (2009). "Membrane Fusion: Grappling with SNARE and SM Proteins." *Science* **323**:474–477.

Sugita S, Hata Y and Südhof TC. (1996). "Distinct Ca^{2+} dependent properties of the first and second C2-domains of synaptotagmin I." *J. Biol. Chem.* **271**:1262–1265

Sugita S et al. (2001). "Synaptotagmin VII as a plasma membrane Ca^{2+}-sensor in exocytosis." *Neuron* **30**:459–473

Sugita S et al. (2002). "Synaptotagmins form a hierarchy of exocytotic Ca^{2+}-sensors with distinct Ca^{2+}-affinities." *EMBO J.* **21**:270–280

Sun J et al. (2007). "A Dual Ca^{2+}-Sensor Model for Neuro-transmitter Release in a Central Synapse." *Nature* **450**:676–682.

Sutton RB et al. (1995). "Structure of the first C2-domain of synaptotagmin I: A novel Ca^{2+}/phospholipid binding fold." *Cell* **80**:929–938.

Sutton RB, Fasshauer D, Jahn R and Brunger AT (1998). "Crystal structure of a SNARE complex involved in synaptic exocytosis at 2.4 A resolution." *Nature* **395**:347–353.

Tang J et al. (2006). "A Complexin/Synaptotagmin-1 Switch Controls Fast Synaptic Vesicle Exocytosis." *Cell* **126**:1175–1187.

tom Dieck S et al. (1998). "Bassoon, a novel zinc-finger CAG/glutamine-repeat protein selectively localized at the active zone of presynaptic nerve terminals." *J. Cell Biol.* **142**:499–509.

Tobaben S et al. (2001). "A trimeric protein complex functions as a synaptic chaperone machine." *Neuron* **31**:987–999.

Touchot N, Chardin P and Tavitian A (1987). "Four additional members of the ras gene superfamily isolated by an oligonucleotide strategy: molecular cloning of YPT-related cDNAs from a rat brain library." *Proc. Natl. Acad. Sci. U.S.A.* **84**:8210–8214.

Tsetsenis T et al. (2011). "Rab3B protein is required for long-term depression of hippocampal inhibitory synapses and for normal reversal learning." *Proc. Natl. Acad. Sci. U.S.A.* **108**:14300–14305.

Varoqueaux F et al. (2002). "Total arrest of spontaneous and evoked synaptic transmission but normal synaptogenesis in the absence of Munc13-mediated vesicle priming." *Proc. Natl. Acad. Sci. U.S.A.* **99**:9037–9042.

Verhage M et al. (2000). "Synaptic assembly of the brain in the absence of neurotransmitter secretion." *Science* **287**:864–869.

Voets T et al. (2001). "Intracellular calcium dependence of large dense-core vesicle exocytosis in the absence of synaptotagmin I." *Proc. Natl. Acad. Sci. U.S.A.* **98**:11680–11685.

von Mollard GF et al. (1990). "Rab3 is a small GTP-binding protein exclusively localized to synaptic vesicles." *Proc. Natl. Acad. Sci. U.S.A.* **87**:1988–1992.

von Mollard GF, Südhof TC and Jahn R (1991). "A small GTP-binding protein (rab3A) dissociates from synaptic vesicles during exocytosis." *Nature* **349**:79–81.

Wang Y et al. (1997). "RIM: A putative Rab3-effector in regulating synaptic vesicle fusion." *Nature* **388**:593–598.

Wang X et al. (1999). "Aczonin, a 550-kD putative scaffolding protein of presynaptic active zones, shares homology regions with Rim and Bassoon and binds profilin." *J. Cell Biol.* **147**:151–162.

Wang Y, Sugita S and Südhof TC (2000). "The RIM/NIM family of neuronal SH3-domain proteins: interactions with Rab3 and a new class of neuronal SH3-domain proteins." *J. Biol. Chem.* **275**:20033–20044.

Wang Y, Liu X, Biederer T and Südhof TC. (2002). "A family of RIM-binding proteins regulated by alternative splicing: Implications for the genesis of synaptic active zones." *Proc. Natl. Acad. Sci. U.S.A.* **99**:14464–14469.

Weber T et al. (1998). "SNAREpins: minimal machinery for membrane fusion." *Cell* **92**: 759–772.

Wen H et al. (2010). "Distinct roles for two synaptotagmin isoforms in synchronous and asynchronous transmitter release at zebrafish neuromuscular junction." *Proc. Natl. Acad. Sci. U.S.A.* **107**:13906–13911.

Whittaker VP and Sheridan MN (1965). "The morphology and acetylcholine content of isolated cerebral cortical synaptic vesicles." *J. Neurochem.* **12**:363–372

Wilson DW et al. (1989). "A fusion protein required for vesicle-mediated transport in both mammalian cells and yeast." *Nature* **339**:355–359.

Xu J, Mashimo T and Südhof TC (2007). "Synaptotagmin-1, -2, and -9: Ca^{2+}-sensors for fast release that specify distinct presynaptic properties in subsets of neurons." *Neuron* **54**: 801–812.

Xu J, Pang ZP, Shin OH and Südhof TC (2009). "Synaptotagmin-1 functions as a Ca^{2+} sensor for spontaneous release." *Nature Neurosci.* **12**, 759–766.

Xue M et al. (2007). "Distinct domains of complexin I differentially regulate neurotransmitter release." *Nat. Struct. Mol. Biol.* **14**:949–958.

Yamaguchi T et al. (2002). "Sly1 binds to Golgi and ER syntaxins via a conserved N-terminal peptide motif." *Developmental Cell* **2**:295–305.

Yang X et al. (2010). "Complexin Clamps Asynchronous Release by Blocking a Secondary Ca^{2+}-Sensor via its Accessory a-Helix." *Neuron* **68**:907–920.

Yang X, Cao P and Südhof TC (2013). "Deconstructing complexin function in activating and clamping Ca^{2+}-triggered exocytosis by comparing knockout and knockdown phenotypes." *Proc. Natl. Acad. Sci. U.S.A.* **110**:20777–20782.

Zhen M and Jin Y (1999). "The liprin protein SYD-2 regulates the differentiation of presynaptic termini in C. elegans." *Nature* **401**:371–375.

Zhou P et al. (2013). "Syntaxin-1 N-Peptide and Habc-Domain Perform Distinct Essential Functions in Synaptic Vesicle Fusion." *EMBO J.* **32**:159–171.

Zhou P et al. (2013b). "Lipid-Anchored SNARE Lacking Transmembrane Regions Support Membrane Fusion During Neurotransmitter Release." *Neuron* **80**:470–483.

Zimmermann H and Whittaker VP (1997). "Morphological and biochemical heterogeneity of cholinergic synaptic vesicles." *Nature* **267**:633–635.

Physiology or Medicine 2014

John O'Keefe, May-Britt Moser and Edvard I. Moser

"for their discoveries of cells that constitute a positioning system in the brain"

The Nobel Prize in Physiology or Medicine

Speech by Professor Ole Kiehn of the Nobel Assembly at Karolinska Institutet.

Your Majesties, Your Royal Highnesses, Esteemed Laureates, Ladies and Gentlemen,

We do it every day. Many times a day. You did it when you came to this Nobel Prize Ceremony: you found your way! And when you entered the room and sat down, you immediately knew where you were and got a sense of the place. Should you come here again, you will know that this is the Stockholm Concert Hall and not any other concert hall in the world. The ability to orient in space, to find our way, and to remember places that we have visited is necessary to survive, both for animals and human beings. For this to happen, we need our brain and our "inner GPS".

But where in the brain is the positioning system, the inner GPS, located? And how can nerve cells code such abstract mental activities? The work of this year's Nobel Laureates in Physiology or Medicine has given us answers to these fundamental questions, which are among the greatest in neuroscience.

In the late 1960s, John O'Keefe performed experiments in rats that were moving freely around. While they were doing that, he recorded from nerve cells in a structure deep inside the brain, called the hippocampus. Here he discovered cells that were active only when the rat was in a specific location in the environment. When it moved to other places, new cells were active. He called these cells "place cells". The place cells report the position of the rat and build up an inner map that represents a mental picture of the environment. O'Keefe suggested that memory of a place may be stored as a specific combination of place cell activities. By these groundbreaking experiments, O'Keefe showed how specialised nerve cells encode an awareness of space, so that familiar, as well as unfamiliar environments may be recognised.

More than thirty years after O'Keefe's discovery, May-Britt Moser and Edvard Moser discovered an amazing pattern of nerve cell activity in a brain region near the hippocampus, called the entorhinal cortex. Here certain cells, which they named "grid cells", were active when the rat was at several places. When a grid cell was active, its activity formed a hexagonal grid pattern in the environment. The Mosers showed that this hexagonal pattern was not imported from the environment but generated entirely by activity in the brain. The activity of many grid cells provides the brain with a coordinate system that divides the environment into longitudes and latitudes and allows us to keep track of how far we are from a starting point as we navigate our environment. The Mosers groundbreaking discovery showed that the brain holds a mental representation of a coordinate system that can be used to find the way in the external world.

Continued research showed that grid cells, together with other types of cells of the entorhinal cortex, form a circuitry with place cells in the hippocampus. Together, this nerve cell circuitry constitutes a positioning system in the brain, an inner GPS.

Today we know that humans also have place cells and grid cells similar to the ones found in rats. Your place cells and grid cells may have made it possible for you to find your way here tonight, to have an awareness of where you are in this magnificent Hall, and recognise it should you come back. Without these cells you could easily get lost in space.

Professors John O'Keefe, May-Britt Moser and Edvard Moser,

The discovery of the place and grid cells, key elements in the brain's positioning system, is a paradigm shift in our understanding of how groups of specialised nerve cells work together to execute higher brain functions. Through brilliant experiments, you have given us new insight into one of the greatest mysteries of life: how the brain creates behaviour and provides us with fascinating mental proficiencies.

On behalf of the Nobel Assembly at Karolinska Institutet, I wish to convey to you our warmest congratulations. May I now ask you to step forward to receive the Nobel Prize from the hands of His Majesty the King.

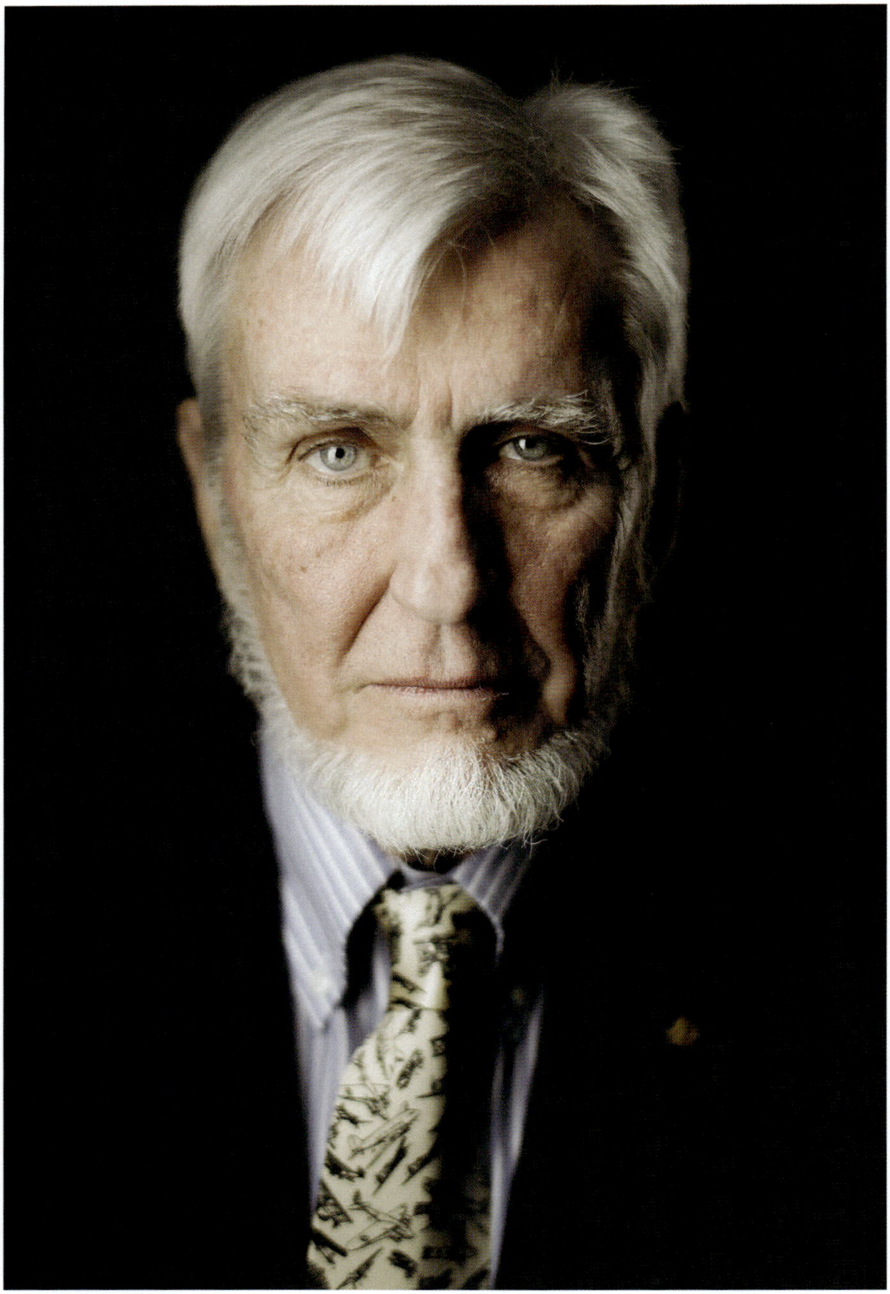

John O'Keefe. © Nobel Media AB. Photo: A. Mahmoud

John O'Keefe

EARLY YEARS

I was born in November 1939 in Harlem, New York to Irish immigrant parents and grew up in the South Bronx. My parents had landed in New York on the eve of the depression; my father's hope was that I would never have to live through one myself. My mother's passage was funded by an uncle and redeemed by seven years' indentured labour. Neither had completed elementary school in Ireland but my father studied in the evening in New York and attained a high school degree. His dream to become an aircraft mechanic was thwarted by a shipyard accident during the war. Most of his life was spent as a nightshift mechanic on the New York bus system where he repaired the buses which became inoperative during the daytime and which couldn't be fixed by the daytime mechanics. My mother worked as a welder in the Newark shipyards during the war, which reinforced her strong sense of confidence and mastery. Following elementary education at my local Catholic school, I won a scholarship to Regis, the academically ambitious Jesuit high school in Manhattan, while my best friends went to local Bronx schools. My time at Regis was unsuccessful. I felt like an outsider and never got to grips with Latin and Greek. Four years of poor grades and low test marks left me demoralised and prevented me from getting any help with college fees, which even then were unaffordable. So I went out to work: an entry-level clerical job in a stock brokerage house on Wall Street was followed swiftly by a bookkeeping job in the engineering department of an insurance company. I did not see this as my long-term future and decided to have another crack at the academic world. It was the era of Sputnik, aeronautical engineering was a glamorous profession, and I wanted to put as much distance between myself and the classics as I could. I spent three years studying aeronautical engineering at New York University in the evening while working in the daytime. After the first year I was lucky to attend a talk by one of the project engineers at Grumman Aircraft

Corporation on Long Island who encouraged me to apply for a job there, which I duly got. I worked on several different aeroplanes, spending considerable time on the shop floor as well as at the drafting board. In the end, however, the gruelling schedule involving over 100 miles commuting a day in rush hour traffic and 12–16 hours of evening lectures per week in addition to a full-time job took its toll and I pined for the freedom of a full-time college student. It was also during this time that I became interested in philosophy through some of my non-engineering courses and decided that many of the perennial problems in philosophy might be solvable through brain research.

CITY COLLEGE OF NEW YORK AND MCGILL UNIVERSITY

So in 1960 I give up my job and went back to college full-time. This was a particularly difficult decision since Grumman's response was to offer me a substantial raise and a role in the development of the Lunar Expedition Module component of the Apollo spacecraft programme, which they were preparing to tender for and eventually were awarded. A path not taken . . . I was fortunate to be accepted for full-time study at City College of New York, a part of the City University of New York and one of the few tuition-free colleges in the United States. At CCNY, I took courses across a wide range of subjects, paying scant attention to faculty or discipline boundaries. I studied filmmaking, advanced English literature, physics and a wide range of psychology and philosophy courses. I met my wife Eileen in an advanced philosophy course on ethics. There were of course no neuroscience courses in those days but I was fortunate to take courses in physiological psychology (as it was then called) with Daniel Lehrman, one of the early neuroethologists, and Philip Ziegler, a young enthusiastic researcher just starting his own laboratory. Phil allowed me to join his team working on the effects of lesions of the wulst on pigeon exploratory behaviour. I got a first-hand taste for experimental brain research and was hooked. During this period I supported myself working in the library, showing classic European films for various courses, and driving a taxi cab in the evening. I loved every minute of it and had no thought for the future. Eventually I was summoned to the office of an irate Dean who pointed out that I had accumulated enough credits to receive several degrees and would I please choose one and get out. I opted to major in psychology and minor in philosophy and graduated in 1963. Faced with the unthinkable prospect of working for a living again, I took the advice of one of my professors and applied for graduate school. Again I was lucky and was accepted to study in the McGill University Psychology Department, where Donald Hebb was still active and influential. Hebb was one of the founders of physiological psychology who, in his landmark book *The Organisation of Behaviour*, provided the theoretical framework which enabled us to think about the neural network basis of cognitive representations. McGill at that time was the Mecca for the study of physiological psychology. In addition to Hebb, the faculty included Peter Milner, who had discovered rewarding electrical self-stimulation of the brain with Jim Olds, Brenda Milner, whose investigations of the famous patient HM had identified the memory functions of the hippocampus, Wilder Penfield and Herbert Jasper at the Montréal Neurological Institute, who had pioneered electrical stimulation of the brain of conscious patients undergoing surgery for epilepsy, and Ronald Melzack an expert in pain who became my PhD advisor. McGill provided a wonderful environment where students were encouraged to think hard about the brain and creatively about experiments but where resources were initially extremely limited. Fortunately just after I arrived Melzack received a large grant to study alternative techniques for monitoring brain activity and generously allowed myself and Ken Casey, a postdoctoral fellow who went on to become Head of Neurology at the University of Michigan, to build a state-of-the-art electrophysiological recording laboratory. Ken also taught me the fundamentals of electrophysiology during experiments in which we looked for the midbrain targets of the ascending somatosensory projections. During my final year there I learned a considerable amount of experimental technique from Dr Herman Bouma, who had originally come to work with Hebb on vision but joined me in my amygdala project. On his return to Holland, Herman became the head of the Perceptual Research Laboratory at Phillips, Einthoven where he subsequently had a successful career discovering important principles governing reading.

During my PhD thesis work I developed techniques for recording from chronic animals and concentrated on the amygdala. Jim Olds, although he had left McGill before I got there, was revered there as the co-discoverer of self-stimulation with Peter Milner. In 1966, I learned from Ken Casey, who had visited Olds' laboratory at Michigan as part of a job interview, that he was successfully recording from single units in awake rats using implanted microwires. I purchased the minimum order of 50,000 feet of coated nichrome microwire, set up a poor man's version of Olds' gold-plated lab and improved on his techniques in three ways. Firstly, I used differential recording between adjacent electrodes, which eliminated much of the movement and muscle artefact. Secondly, I introduced the use of preamplifiers made from miniature field effect transistors (which had just become available in 1965) on the animal's head which greatly improved the signal-to-noise ratio and allowed us to move away from the thick and cumbersome microdot noise reduction cables to lightweight flexible hearing aid wires, greatly improving the animal's mobility. Finally, I started playing with head-mounted microdrives, first at McGill but then more extensively when I went to London. Many of our early microdrives had four independently movable electrodes and it was only when Caroline Harley came to London on sabbatical and asked for a simpler single drive electrode that I developed the "poor lady's" single-screw microdrive that we still use extensively and which is now sold by Axona. For the amygdala work, I had recorded from several silent cells for long periods (in some cases days and weeks) before discovering the specific ethological stimulus which caused them to first become active: cells there responded to highly specific stimuli approximating to the classical much-maligned grandmother cells of Jerry Lettvin. I found mouse detectors, specific food detectors, and bird song detectors. In contrast, the more active cells were sensitive to a broader range of stimuli, for example responding to pure tones of a wide spectrum of audio frequencies. On this basis I formulated my first law of the nervous system, which is that the silent cells are the important ones. I was intellectually and methodologically prepared to tackle the hippocampus and in particular its silent cells. But not quite yet.

POSTDOC AT UNIVERSITY COLLEGE LONDON

After McGill, Eileen and I decided we wanted to go to Europe and in particular to England. I originally went to University College London in 1967 as a US-NIMH postdoctoral fellow to work on somatosensation with Patrick Wall. We immediately fell in love with Britain. Our first son was born soon after we arrived and, in contrast to our experience in Québec where agencies found us insufficiently religious, the adoption of our second son proceeded smoothly a few years later. British institutions such as the National Health Service, the Ordnance Survey Map with its well-marked walking trails, and the BBC offered a cultural and social landscape that meshed with our lifestyle. University College London also proved the ideal location for me to carry out single unit recording in the freely moving animal. After my NIH Fellowship ran out, I applied for and obtained several grants from the Wellcome Trust and various British research councils which paid my salary as well as providing monies to carry out experiments. This high-risk strategy of funding my own salary as well as my research allowed me to minimise my teaching and administrative duties and maximise research time, and I carried on doing this for my entire career. I got used to letters from the University Human Resources Department advising me to prepare to exit the lab and UCL if my next grant wasn't funded. Thankfully the emphasis now given to high-impact translational research and rapid, frequent publication had not yet gained ascendancy in those days, allowing for the funding of the risky time-consuming basic research that is my addiction.

I first began recording single units in the hippocampus following an experiment which went astray. The time was 1970 and my project was to record from the dorsal column nuclei during various behaviours in the behaving rat to see whether the descending afferents from the neocortex would modify the excitability of these first-order sensory cells. This was an extremely difficult project, since the juncture of the foramen magnum and the C1 spinal vertebra is designed to be maximally flexible and obtaining decent stable recordings was well-nigh impossible. After two years, the project was clearly not going anywhere. A much easier task would be to record from somatosensory thalamus and neocortex and that's what I did in my spare time. During one of these experiments I tried to implant a microelectrode in the somatosensory thalamus, but the coordinates I used were too lateral and it strayed into the hippocampus. The first hippocampal cell I recorded was an interneuronal "theta" cell and I was immediately struck by the strong correlation of its activity with the hippocampal sinusoidal 8–10 Hz local field potential theta pattern on one hand and the animal's motor behaviour on the other. I had previously made LFP recordings from the hippocampus at McGill and was aware of Case Vanderwolf's claim that theta activity in the rat was correlated with voluntary movements. And here, at the single unit level, was striking confirmation of his claim. I decided then and there to leave the somatosensory system and begin research on the hippocampus. I was intrigued by the apparent conflict between the motor correlates of the cells at single cell level and the widely accepted memory function which had been ascribed to the hippocampus by Brenda Milner on the basis of her research with HM and which I had completely accepted. Brenda had been one of my teachers at the McGill Psychology department and I and many of the other graduate students routinely traipsed across the frozen campus to attend her lectures at the Montréal Neurological Institute.

In addition to the theta unit it was clear that there were other cells in the hippocampus which were mostly silent except for the occasional action potential to announce their presence. Again I was hooked. My amygdala-inspired first law of the nervous system was that silent cells are the important ones and here was a brain region chock-a-block full of them.

I will always be grateful to Pat Wall for allowing me to make this shift to a part of the brain which was outside his immediate field of interest. In addition to his support he signed off on grant applications and provided space for many of the early years of our hippocampal research, turning a deaf ear to the many naysayers who considered the whole approach a waste of time.

DISCOVERY OF THE PLACE CELLS

Around this time Jonathan Dostrovsky, an MSc student, joined the laboratory. We recorded single units while the animal was engaged in a wide variety of tasks including basic everyday behaviours such as eating, drinking, grooming, exploring novel environments, searching for foods as well as during simple learned tasks such as lever pressing and approaching different stimuli for food. We noticed two things almost immediately. First, there were two types of cells distinguishable on the basis of strictly physiological properties: spike amplitude and width, and baseline firing rates. As I had originally observed, many of the cells with large amplitude action potentials were silent most of the time, only occasionally showing a burst of spikes when the animal sat quietly or during slow-wave sleep. These bursts occurred on large sharp wave spikes in the extracellular hippocampal LFP accompanied by a high frequency waveform which we originally called "wiggles" but quickly changed to the more euphoneous term "ripples." When we mapped the distribution of these two potentials we found that the ripples were largest in the centre of the CA1 pyramidal cell layer but that the associated sharp wave peaked several hundred microns below in the apical dendrites of the pyramidal cells. More recently, Gyuri Buzsaki, Matt Wilson and Bruce McNaughton have suggested that ripples represent a form of replay of immediately previous spatial learning and might be involved in consolidation of recent memory traces.

It was also immediately obvious that the correlate of the second cell type, which had a much higher resting firing rate and showed a clear phase locking to the ongoing LFP theta oscillations, was a tight coupling to some aspect of movement as I had noticed on my first foray into the hippocampus. This movement correlate was not related to any single limb movement or any specific behaviour but was associated with some higher aspect of the movement such as the vigour or speed with which the movement was executed. Movements which changed the animal's location seemed to be particularly important. It took much longer for us to identify the correlate of the major cell type, the low firing-rate pyramidal cell. Over a period of months, I began to suspect that their activity didn't depend so much on what the animal was doing or why it was doing it but had something to do with where it was doing it. And then on one electrifying day I realised with a flash of insight that the cells were responding to the animal's location or place in the environment. We quickly verified that changing many aspects of the environment one at a time had little effect on the locational response of the cell but if major alterations were made, e.g. by removal of the curtains surrounding the platform, the cell activity altered abruptly. In thinking about these results over the next day I was assailed by a montage of ideas about the potential significance of this finding: the first was that it might mean that the hippocampus was the neural site of Tolman's cognitive map, a vague hypothetical construct that he had used to explain some aspects of rodent maze behaviour but which had never gained much acceptance in the animal learning field and which was little discussed in the 1960s. It was clear he had given little thought to the neural basis of this 'map', much less envisaged that it would be localised in a particular brain structure. This spatial map idea provided a clear function for the movement-related hippocampal cells and the LFP theta activity, since a map would need information about higher order aspects of an animal's behaviour such as speed in order to calculate the distance it had travelled. I decided subsequently to christen these movement-related cells "displace cells" to reflect this idea. It also dawned on me that the difficulties that animals with hippocampal damage had in experiments such as those of the Blanchards might be in identifying places in the environment as opposed to objects as the source of threat. The Blanchards had shown that hippocampal-damaged animals could learn to avoid specific threatening objects but were less good at identifying less specific threats such as electric shocks delivered through the floor. Perhaps the hippocampus in rodents was a specialised type of memory system, a memory system for places which, when elaborated, might provide the basis for the more general episodic memory system of the human. Finally, I realised that if the hippocampus were involved in spatial representation we could draw on several millennia of mathematical, philosophical, and geographical thought to help us understand its functions. One of my philosopher heroes had been Immanuel Kant, who had suggested that our sense of space was a special property of the brain which provided a framework for the representation of other aspects of the world such as objects and which existed prior to experience with those objects. Had we found the neural basis for Kant's a priori spatial faculty of sensibility? Would the hippocampus provide brain researchers with a neural Rosetta Stone, a portal into the mysterious world of cortical brain function? Throughout the day, I experienced a prolonged euphoria of the classical Archimedean type.

I decided to write a short paper on our findings and also to announce the idea that the hippocampus was Tolman's cognitive map. The paper was originally rejected by *Brain Research* but after minor modifications finally accepted. I confidently sat back and waited for the chorus of approval from the hippocampal community. Instead there was a deafening silence, with the exception of a small number of isolated voices (see below).

Unbeknownst to me, Jim Ranck at the University of Michigan and subsequently Downstate Medical Center in Brooklyn was carrying out similar recording experiments in the rat hippocampus and finding similar behavioural correlates. His 'theta' cells were identical to our displace neurons and his approach-consummate and approach-consummate mismatch cells might be place cells since they consistently fired when the animal approached a reward location on a particular trajectory, i.e., passing through the same place. Ranck did not explore this possibility but on a subsequent sabbatical visit to our laboratory agreed that the animal's location might be the primary correlate. In subsequent work with Phil Best he confirmed our findings and supported our interpretation. Importantly, he went on to discover the head-direction cells, providing strong support for the cognitive map theory (see below).

THE HIPPOCAMPUS AS A COGNITIVE MAP

Around this time Lynn Nadel joined the UCL Anatomy Department to work on the visual system. He quickly became interested in place cells and the cognitive map idea and we decided to write a short review article fleshing out some of the ideas and showing how they applied to the literature on the effects of hippocampal lesions on behaviour. Pat Wall was strongly supportive of the idea, but I'm sure he had no idea how extensive and ambitious the project would become. Our first draft ran to several hundred pages and it was clear that we had a book rather than a review article on our hands. In 1972, we sent the first draft to 50 colleagues and asked for their opinion, and I am still grateful to all those who replied and gave us such constructive comments. However, Oxford University Press, which had agreed to publish the book, also sent the manuscript to reviewers, one of whom was the foremost expert on animal behaviour. He gave it a long, detailed blisteringly negative review, making it clear that we knew little about animal behaviour and that the book suffered badly from this lack of expertise. We could either scrap the project or become experts in animal learning theory and totally rewrite it. We chose to do the latter and found to our amazement that many of the ideas we were expressing about the role of hippocampus in behaviour made a lot of sense within the context of animal learning theory. In total it took us six years to write the book and since many copies of the 1972 version had found their way into the hands and minds of a large number of physiological psychologists, a degree of scepticism developed about whether the book would ever be published at all.

The Hippocampus as a Cognitive Map (HCM) was an ambitious book in conception, daunting to write, and an unavoidably demanding read. The modest

OUP run of a few thousand protected many from the effort. It remained cited by many but read by few, until around 2005 when I had it laboriously scanned and made available on the web where it has been and still is free to download (www.cognitivemap.net/).

During the writing of the book, I continued to work on place cells and explore their properties, leading to a more extensive publication in 1976. I reported that in addition to the standard place cell there were other types of spatial cells in the hippocampus including *misplace* cells which fired maximally when the animal went to a familiar location and found a new object there or failed to find an expected object, and *displace* cells which Jim Ranck called theta cells because of their close relationship to the ongoing LFP theta and which I characterised as being related to the same aspects of movement as Vanderwolf had attributed to the LFP. In the discussion section of the paper, I speculated that there were two independent ways in which a place cell could be activated. The first was by direct activation from the environmental sensory inputs which impinged upon the animal in a particular location and the second was through a path integration mechanism internal to the hippocampus itself, which used abstract measures of the animal's behaviour such as its direction and distance of movement since the previous known location to update the representation. This idea has received considerable support since, most recently from work in our lab by Guifen Chen showing that, in a virtual reality environment, 25% of place cells are influenced primarily by the visual inputs while most of the rest receive a significant path integration input as well, i.e. receive a combination of both.

EXPERIMENTAL TEST AND SUPPORT: LESION STUDIES

Nadel and I were joined in our analysis of the lesion literature by Abe Black from McMaster University, who came to London every summer and worked with us on ideas about the application of the theory to the normal animal learning literature and the lesion literature. Abe was a world leader in the field of animal learning theory, with a particular interest in avoidance learning, and the three of us published a paper on this in 1975. To our great regret Abe was diagnosed with stomach cancer and died in 1978 at the very young age of 49. I sometimes wonder what the hippocampal field would look like today if he had survived.

What was lacking however was a spatial memory task specifically designed to depend on the capabilities we had attributed to the cognitive map. In the mid-1970s, a newly graduated animal learning theorist, Richard Morris, came to visit Lynn Nadel and myself announcing that he had experienced a Pauline conversion and would like to work on the cognitive map idea. The theory made the strong prediction that hippocampal damage would lead to deficits in allocentric spatial navigation. Lynn and I had tried to develop a land-based navigation task which would be a sensitive test of this hypothesis. The basic idea was that the animal would be started from several locations and had to find a safe location in the environment despite having to move in different directions on each trial to get there. We failed to come up with a workable task, but Richard succeeded. His important idea was to require the animal to go a hidden platform in a swimming pool where there were no local cues to guide it. Together with Nick Rawlins, we subsequently tested rats with hippocampal lesions and found they had pronounced deficits: the Morris water maze was a superb test of hippocampal function and is still the best and most widely used behavioural assay available.

EXPERIMENTAL TEST AND SUPPORT: SINGLE UNIT STUDIES

The Cognitive Map theory also made strong predictions about the existence of other types of spatial information in the hippocampal formation, for example predicting the existence of cells representing distance and direction which would bind together the place representations into a map-like structure. Cells signalling the animal's heading direction were found by Ranck, Taube, Muller and colleagues in the presubiculum in the 1980s; grid cells in the entorhinal cortex which may be signaling distance travelled in a particular direction have recently been described by the Mosers and their colleagues in 2005 (see below). In the early '80s I was lucky enough to attract Bruce McNaughton and Carol Barnes to spend a year as postdocs in my laboratory. They were already experts in intracellular recording, long-term potential studies and behavioural studies. It was during an earlier visit to Graham Goddard's (another McGill graduate) lab in Dalhousie that I first met them. Using a minicomputer and an overhead camera head tracking system to record unit activity on an 8-arm maze, we carried out the first quantitative measurement of place fields. We showed for the first time that the firing rate of place cells was dependent on the animal's speed. Surprisingly, unlike on open platforms where the rat was free to move in all directions, on the behaviourally constraining narrow arms of the radial maze almost all of the cells had unidirectional fields, firing as the animal moved in one direction but not the other. We also implemented an idea of Bruce's that two electrodes looking at the same cells might enable us to separate action potentials from anatomically close cells by giving us a stereoscopic view. The stereotrode was born to be followed in a short time by the tetrode, a 4 electrode version which is now in wide use (see below).

Over the next few years, our group showed that place cells could learn to distinguish between square and circular enclosures (Colin Lever) and under certain circumstances could do so in an all-or-nothing manner reflective of attractor dynamics (Tom Wills). A particularly revealing experiment during this period was one in which Neil Burgess and I showed that the firing fields of place cells stretched as the enclosure was stretched from a square shape to a rectangle. This led to the idea that one set of inputs to the place cells reflected the distance to one or more walls of the enclosure in particular allocentric directions. As the box was stretched, these inputs maintained their relationship to the opposing walls resulting in expanded fields. The predicted *boundary* cells were subsequently found in the subiculum by Colin Lever in our lab and in the medial entorhinal cortex by Trygve Solstad in the Moser lab.

PHASE PRECESSION

For many years, I struggled with the functional role of the hippocampal sinusoidal LFP theta and tried unsuccessfully to integrate it into the cognitive map theory. I knew from my own unpublished work in the late '70s that at any given time different hippocampal place cells could have different theta phase correlates and even that the same place cell could have different phase correlates at different times. Every so often I would run into Gyuri Buzsaki, who has had a lifetime interest in theta and other hippocampal oscillations and he would ask me what was the relationship of theta to pyramidal cell activity. Given my experience I told him that unlike hippocampal interneurons, they didn't have a fixed phase of firing relative to theta. I had also been troubled by the possibility that the dentate granule cells might fire like interneurons (it appeared that there were just too many theta cells in the granule layer for them all to be interneurons) and was trying to understand how the interactions between several high-rate dentate granule cells might be translated into low-rate CA3 place cell activity. This got me thinking about interference patterns and led indirectly to my 1985 philosophy paper which suggested that the hippocampus might store and manipulate theta-frequency holograms and that theta was the neural substrate of consciousness (O'Keefe, J. (1985), "Is consciousness the gateway to the hippocampal cognitive map? A speculative essay on the neural basis of mind," in D.A. Oakley (ed), *Brain and Mind*, 59–98, Methuen, London.). Around this time I also began exploring the relationship between hippocampal theta sinusoids and vectors. In particular, I pursued the phasor coding idea from engineering in which sinusoids are represented by rotating vectors, but inverted it so that the sinusoids were used to represent vectors and not vice versa. In this version, the length of the vector is represented by the amplitude of the sinusoid and the angle relative to some reference direction is represented by the phase shift relative to a reference sinusoid. This would enable the hippocampus to do vector algebra using sinusoids to represent the locations of environmental landmarks in a polar co-ordinate system (see my paper O'Keefe, J. (1991) "The hippocampal cognitive map and navigational strategies," in, J. Paillard (ed)., *Brain and Space*. Oxford University Press, 273–295).

So with all of these ideas in mind, I thought I should have another go at trying to make sense of the relationship between place cells and theta. I went back and looked carefully at the data from one particular place cell from a spatial memory experiment on a +-shaped maze with narrow arms that Andrew Speakman and I had published in 1987. We had also recorded the slow-wave theta LFP from the same electrodes. I quickly confirmed that the phase relationship between the firing of this cell changed from one wave to the next. But how? Was there some systematic relationship between the two? Over several days I looked at run after run on the maze over and over again but couldn't make any sense of the pattern until one day I found one run on which the spikes fired on every wave and realised that they were systematically moving to earlier phases on each successive wave as the animal ran straight through the field on the narrow track. I also noticed that quite often the phase would continue to precess in the second half of the field despite the fact that the firing rate was falling. This suggested that a simple depolarisation model might not be adequate to explain the effect. Harking back to my thinking about interference patterns, I realised that the wavelet produced by the interference pattern between two waves of slightly different frequencies would produce the required effect. The number of spikes on each theta burst would increase towards the centre of the field and then decrease while the peak of the interference wavelet would continue to progress relative to extracellular theta LFP. I guessed that the phase might correlate with the animal's location in the field rather than with time or some other variable and this proved to be the case. Following rejection from several journals, the paper by Michael Recce and myself was eventually published in *Hippocampus*. This was also the first published paper in which tetrodes were used. We considered the possibility that there was a second higher frequency wave in one of the inputs to the hippocampus, so Kate Jeffery looked for it in the entorhinal cortex and Charles King looked for it in the medial septal. Neither found it and we were forced to conclude that if it existed it was located in the dendrites of the pyramidal cells themselves.

GRID CELLS

I first met Edvard and May Britt Moser, my Nobel co-laureates, when they were graduate students in the lab of Per Andersen in Oslo. They were clearly very bright and ambitious and I was more than happy subsequently to agree to their spending some time in my UCL lab to learn the techniques of single unit recording in free-moving animals. Following a string of high-profile important papers on place cells in journals such as *Science* and *Nature*, they and their students Torkil Hafting and Marianne Fynn produced their monumental 2005 paper announcing the existence of grid cells in the entorhinal cortex. The grid cells looked like they might provide the metric for the map, completing the spatial information necessary for creating the hippocampal cognitive map. Although others including ourselves had looked in the entorhinal cortex for spatial cells we had all missed the grid cells. I have no doubt that this discovery together with the findings on the spatial role of the human hippocampus (see below) have had a major impact on the neuroscientific community's acceptance of the cognitive map theory. But how were the grid cells constructed? Neil Burgess, Caswell Barry and I suggested that a generalised two-dimensional version of the oscillatory interference model using interference patterns between several theta-like oscillations might provide a good model for the generation of grid cells. And how universal is the grid pattern? Recently Julia Krupic and Marius Bauza in our group have shown that the walls of the environment have a much greater influence on the structure of the grids then had previously been realised, even to the point of destroying the grid pattern in highly structured asymmetrical environments such as trapezoids. We still have a lot to learn about the function of the grids and how these remarkable cells are created by the brain.

HUMAN HIPPOCAMPUS

One of the major obstacles to the acceptance of the cognitive map theory was the belief that the human hippocampus had a broader function than the spatial one proposed for the rodent hippocampus. The strongest contestant here was the declarative memory theory championed by Larry Squire. Declarative memory theory held that the deficit following hippocampal damage included both factual memories as well as episodic memories for events of the past. The cognitive map extension to the human disagreed with this, predicting that the global memory deficit was limited to episodic memories comprised of memories for what happened in a particular place at a particular time. The idea was that episodes were built upon the basic spatial framework through the addition of a linear sense of time amongst other higher-order cognitive capacities.

One problem in studying the role of the human hippocampus in spatial memory was that most of the tasks had usually been presented on a tabletop or as video displays which, could also be solved by non-hippocampal strategies in particular egocentric ones in which objects were located relative to axes fixed to the eyes, head or trunk as well as by hippocampal-dependent allocentric ones. What was needed was a large-scale environment comparable to the mazes in which rodent spatial navigation was tested. Better still if navigation could be carried out by participants whose heads were immobile, so that their brains could be scanned using the rapidly developing imaging technology. The solution was to use one of the newly developed first-person shoot-em-up virtual reality games which were just becoming available in the '90s and were all the rage with teenagers. Importantly, some came with editors which allowed the games to be modified and components added or deleted. Neil Burgess, with help from Jim Donnett removed all of the monsters, guns etc. from the game Duke Nukem, which provided an excellent complex 70 x 70 m virtual environment with multiple rooms and pathways, and the layout of which participants could explore and learn to navigate around in a reasonable amount of time. Eleanor Maguire and Neil carried out an imaging experiment in which healthy volunteers had their brains scanned while they navigated between locations using either a cognitive map strategy or a route-finding one in which they followed a series of marked paths, a non-hippocampal strategy. To our delight, the hippocampus and surrounding parahippocampal gyrus become active during map-based way-finding in virtual reality environments. Importantly there was a good correlation between the accuracy of navigation and the amount of blood flow in the right hippocampus. Subsequently, we used fMRI to study the role of the hippocampus in episodic memory within a virtual reality context and showed that the left hippocampus is more involved than the right. We also studied the spatial and episodic memories of patients with bilateral and unilateral mesial temporal lobe damage in virtual environments and corroborated the imaging work, with the left temporal patients displaying selective recognition deficits in episodic memory and the right showing deficits in spatial memory, object recognition and navigation. The bilateral hippocampal patient showed deficits in both episodic and spatial recognition memory but interestingly not in object recognition memory, suggesting that this deficit in the right temporal-lobectomised patients was due to the additional damage to other areas of the temporal lobe outside the hippocampus. Eleanor Maguire went on to develop these ideas to include the notion that the human hippocampus is involved in the construction of spatial scenes and the prediction of future events. She also showed that the posterior hippocampus of expert and highly practised human navigators

(London taxicab drivers) was larger than in the rest of us, including bus drivers who extensively travel the streets of London but along fixed routes.

Another obstacle to the acceptance of the cognitive map theory was the evidence that the left human hippocampus was involved in memory for language and narrative. The problem here was that many psychologists believed that visual-spatial processing was at the opposite end of the cognitive spectrum from language processing, the former held to be represented in a two-dimensional static space while the latter being based on serial processing along a single dimension. How could language be processed and stored in a two- or three-dimensional spatial structure? Nadel and I had suggested that one clue might come from spatial language, which might be easier to store in a spatial structure and, if adequately modelled, might form the basis for much of non-spatial language by metaphorical extension. In follow-up articles, I have explored the use of a specific model of hippocampal spatial function to create a mathematical model underlying the meanings of the spatial prepositions in English, prepositions being one important way in which location and movement are captured. Spatial prepositions are part of the closed class elements of language, are usually limited to around 20 in most languages, and are more or less consistent across languages although not necessarily appearing as independent words in the surface structure. This 'vector grammar model' was based on the idea that place fields can be located in an environment on the basis of the distance of the animal's head from a landmark (usually a wall or boundary of the environment) in a specific allocentric direction (for example the wall of the room between the window and the door) generated by Neil Burgess, Tom Hartley and myself (see above). The vector grammar model postulated that almost all of the prepositions had a primary spatial meaning and these identified the underlying places, objects and vectors connecting them. For example in the phrase "to go from London to New York," "from" would be represented as the origin or tail of a vector at the place "London" with its head at the place "New York." The meanings of most prepositions can be described in a similar vector-based fashion.

TRANSLATIONAL POSSIBILITIES

We are optimistic that our understanding of hippocampus function at the network level will allow us to address the neural basis of neurodegenerative and psychiatric brain diseases. There is evidence that some of the earliest neuropathological manifestations of neurodegenerative diseases such as Alzheimer's occur in the entorhinal/hippocampal formation. One approach is to create mouse models of some aspects of AD and ask how place cells and other aspects of hippocampal physiology become dysfunctional during disease progression. We already know from work with Francesca Cacucci and Tom Wills that place cells are less able to identify the animal's current location in these mice and this functional loss correlates with the animals' inability on spatial memory tasks and its increased amyloid plaque burden. In another related approach, Neil Burgess and Dennis Chan are developing sensitive allocentric spatial tasks as diagnostic tests to look for changes in spatial memory during the early stages of dementia.

THE FUTURE

Having spent most of my career as a bench experimenter with a small lab, I have recently accepted the position as Inaugural Director of the Sainsbury Wellcome Centre for Neural Circuits and Behaviour at UCL. As the name implies, the SWC will provide a framework for the study of the neural correlates of perception, emotion, memory and behaviour using the latest techniques in optical and electrophysiological recording to identify the underline neural patterns and optogenetic manipulation of cell activity to control those patterns in a causal manner. It is a thrilling time to be taking on this job, given the numerous possibilities opening up for behavioural and systems neuroscience by these new technologies. So now back to the bench . . .

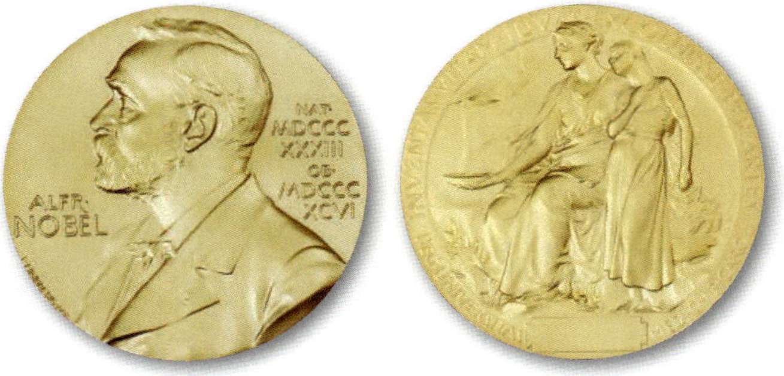

Spatial Cells in the Hippocampal Formation

Nobel Lecture, 7 December 2014

by John O'Keefe
University College London, United Kingdom.

INTRODUCTION

When I first started working on the hippocampus in 1970, the most important clue we had to its function had come from the work of Brenda Milner (Figure 1B) on the patient Henry Molaison (Figure 1A) (Scoville and Milner, 1957). Henry had undergone extensive removal of both medial temporal lobes including the hippocampus as well as surrounding structures for the relief of severe temporal lobe epilepsy (Figure 1C, 2A). While the epileptic seizures were ameliorated, the most dramatic result of the operation was a profound anterograde and retrograde amnesia. He not only failed to lay down new memories of his day-to-day experiences but was unable to recall ones previously stored. He suffered a profound episodic memory deficit. In the words of Sue Corkin (Figure 1D), one of Brenda's students who studied him extensively over the years

> He . . . cannot recall anything that relied on personal experience, such as a specific Christmas gift his father had given him. He retained only the gist of personally experienced events, plain facts but no recollection of specific episodes (Corkin, 2013, p. 219).

In the late 1960s, I had been recording somatosensory cells in the thalamus of the rat using our newly developed techniques for recording from single units in freely moving animals and on one occasion had inadvertently positioned electrodes more laterally in the hippocampus. There I found a cell which had a beautiful phase relationship to the 7–10 Hz local field potential theta activity

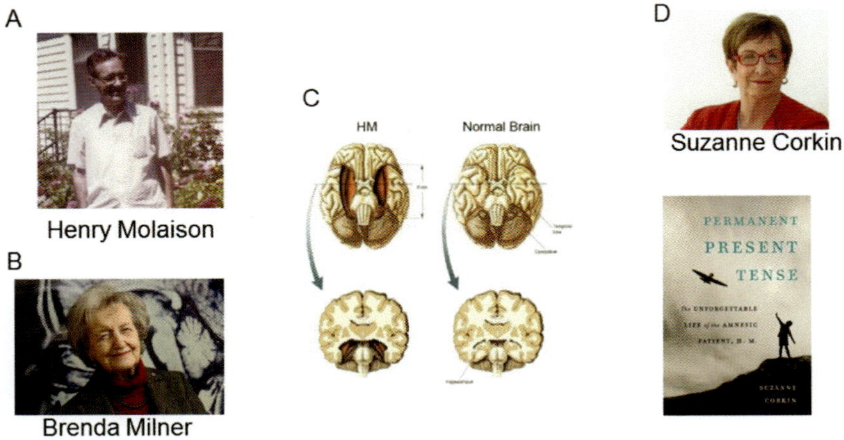

FIGURE 1. Henry Molaison (HM) (A) lost his episodic memory following medial temporal lobectomy (C). His amnesia was initially reported and studied by Brenda Milner (B) and more recently by Suzanne Corkin (D) as reported in her recent book "Permanent Present Tense."

and which clearly was activated by some higher-order aspect of the animal's movement such as speed of movement of the head. This behavioural correlate intrigued me since, on the face of it, it seemed very far removed from the type of cell you might expect to find in a memory system. I immediately decided to abandon the somatosensory system and move to the study of the hippocampus in an attempt to see what memories looked like at the single cell level. The hippocampus in the rat has very much the same anatomical structure (Figure 2B) as in the human and I reasoned that we might be able to gain considerable insight into how memories are stored and retrieved. Around this time I was joined in the lab by Jonathan Dostrovsky, an MSc student, and we decided to record from electrodes in the CA1 field (Figure 2B) as the animal performed simple memory tasks and otherwise went about its daily business. I have to say that at this stage we were very catholic in our approach and expectations and were prepared to see that the cells fire to all types of situations and all types of memories. What we found instead was unexpected and very exciting.

Over the course of several months of watching the animals behave while simultaneously listening to and monitoring hippocampal cell activity it became clear that there were two types of cells, the first similar to the one I had originally seen which had as its major correlate some non-specific higher-order aspect of movements, and the second a much more silent type which only sprang into activity at irregular intervals and whose correlate was much more difficult to

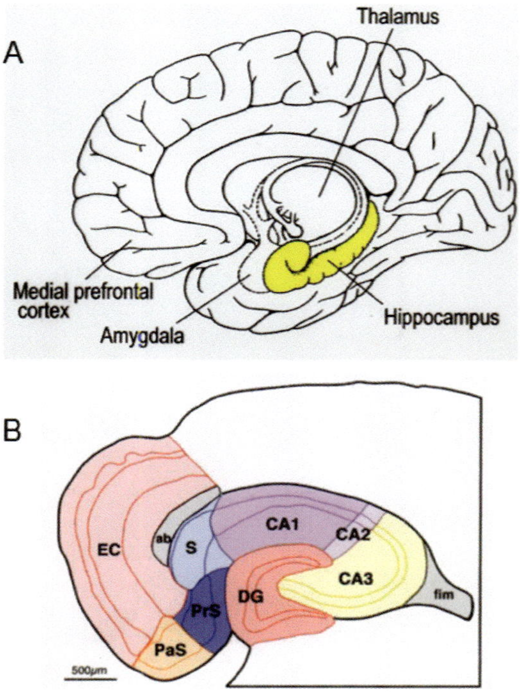

FIGURE 2. The human hippocampus is located in the medial temporal lobes (A). The rodent hippocampal formation (B) is composed of the hippocampus proper (CA fields and the dentate gyrus DG), the subicular region (subiculum S, pre-subiculum PrS, and para-subiculum PaS) and the entorhinal cortex EC.

identify. Looking back at the notes from this period it is clear that there were hints that the animal's location was important but it was only on a particular day when we were recording from a very clear well isolated cell with a clear correlate that it dawned on me that these cells weren't particularly interested in what the animal was doing or why it was doing it but rather they were interested in where it was in the environment at the time (Figure 3). The cells were coding for the animal's location! In the short three page paper (O'Keefe and Dostrovsky, 1971) that we wrote to summarise our initial findings, we said

> These findings suggest that the hippocampus provides the rest of the brain with a spatial reference map. Deprived of this map . . . it could not learn to go from where it happened to be in the environment to a particular place independently of any particular route (as in Tolman's experiments) . . . (pp. 174–5)

EC Tolman had been one of the doyens of American behavioural psychology who believed that animals found their way around environments by creating internal representations, which were more complicated and interesting than the simple associations between stimuli and responses beloved of the behaviourists of the Hullian persuasion. Tolman wrote:

> We believe that in the course of learning, something like a field map of the environment gets established in the rat's brain . . . The stimuli . . . are usually worked over . . . into a tentative, cognitive-like map of the environment. And it is this tentative map, indicating routes and paths and environmental relationships, which finally determines what responses, if any, the animal will finally release. (Tolman, 1948, p. 192).

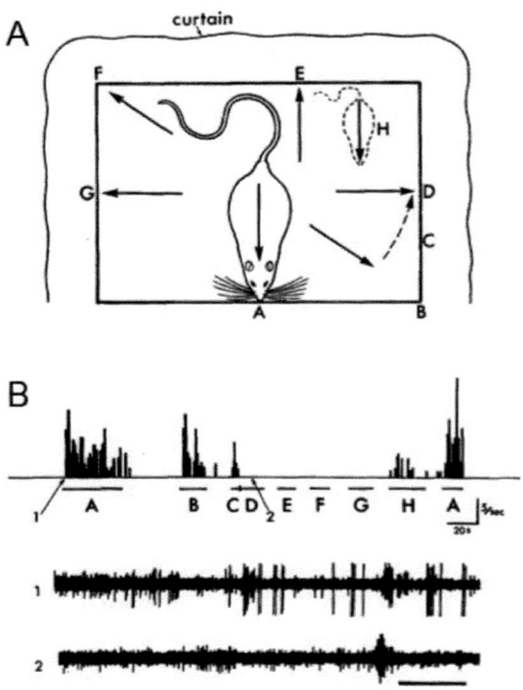

FIGURE 3. The first report of a place cell in the hippocampus of the freely moving rat. The animal went to different locations and faced in different directions on a rectangular platform surrounded on three sides by curtains (A). The cell fired when the animal was in locations A and B but not elsewhere. After O'Keefe and Dostrovsky (1971).

He never specified in any detail what this map would look like or consist of, and it is highly unlikely that he thought it would be localised in one brain system rather than being distributed throughout the whole brain. He also expected it to be involved in much more than spatial and navigational functions. This together with the absence of any techniques for identifying the cognitive map and its components led the idea to fall into disuse and the argument to be won by the Hullian behaviourists. But here Dostrovsky and I were recording from cells that looked like one important component of such a map, representing as they did different places in a familiar environment. Possessing such a map would surely furnish an animal with a very handy cognitive device enabling it to move around environments in a creative, flexible way rather than being reduced to the simple rigid stimulus-response routes envisaged by the behaviourists. This thinking led naturally to the prediction that damage to the hippocampus in rodents would result in a specific set of deficits in spatial location and spatial navigation as embodied in the quote from the 1971 paper. It also dawned on me that maps were rather sophisticated devices and needed more spatial information than that embodied by just a set of place representations. For one thing, it seemed likely that a place could be identified in at least two independent ways. In addition to a computation based on the sensory stimuli impinging on the animal when it found itself in that place it might be possible to compute that the animal had arrived at the same location on the basis of an updating of its position using information from its own movements, a technique not dissimilar to that used in the navigation systems of aeroplanes. In the subsequent paper in which I described the properties of place and misplace cells more extensively, I speculated that

> Each place cell receives two different inputs, one conveying information about a large number of environmental stimuli or events, and the other from a navigational system which calculates where an animal is in an environment independently of the stimuli impinging on it at that moment . . . When an animal had located itself in an environment (using environmental stimuli) the hippocampus could calculate subsequent positions in that environment on the basis of how far and in what direction the animal had moved in the interim . . . (O'Keefe, 1976)

And in a summary of the contents of a book "Hippocampus as a Cognitive Map"

> A small number of stimuli (two or three) occurring with a unique spatial configuration when an animal is in a particular part of an environment are sufficient to identify a place in the map. At any given point in an environment there are usually a large number of such sets of stimuli and therefore the identification of a place in an environment does not depend on any particular cue or group of cues. The distance and direction vectors which connect the places in the map of an environment are derived from the animal's movements in that environment. (O'Keefe and Nadel, 1979, p. 489).

An idea of what we had in mind in these quotes is shown in Figure 4 taken from a subsequent paper (O'Keefe, 1996) in which the place representations A, B and C are connected by vectors representing the distance between them in a certain direction. This type of representation would be useful in two ways: Firstly, if an animal found itself at location A in a familiar environment and wanted to go to location B (perhaps because it was hungry and had a representation that there was food there) then the system would generate the vector AB and send it to the motor system causing the animal to travel in a specific direction for a specific distance. The flexibility in the system arises from the fact that under circumstances in which the direct route AB is blocked, the system can generate a detour using the fact that the sum of vectors AC and CB equal AB. A second use of the system is in predictive mode. If the animal finds itself travelling along vector AB from location A, the mapping system will predict that it will end up at location B and furthermore what it should experience there. This ability of the internal navigation system to generate predictions about what will be experienced at particular locations forms the basis of learning in the cognitive map. If there is a mismatch between what the system predicts at B and what the animal experiences at B, a mismatch signal is generated which initiates

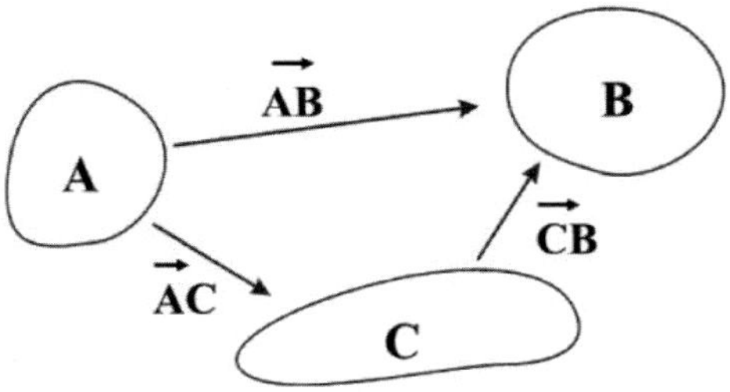

FIGURE 4. Schematic representation of a cognitive map of three places (A, B, C) and the vectors connecting them (AB, AC, CB). After O'Keefe (1996).

exploration behaviour designed to initially build maps of an unknown environment or to update existing maps where they are no longer veridical, perhaps due to small changes in the actual environment. In the 1976 paper, I reported the existence of a subset of place cells which I called misplace cells and which fired maximally when the animal went to a familiar place and found an unexpected novel object there or failed to find an expected familiar object. The ability of the mapping system to identify locations on the basis of subsets of environmental cues, to predict the sensory cues which would be found in particular locations, and flexible navigation involving the generation of both shortcuts and "umwegs" (detours) provide a powerful cognitive mechanism for learning about and representing an environment, and flexibly navigating through it.

Around this time, I was joined by Lynn Nadel in the Anatomy Department at UCL (Figure 5 right) and we decided to write a review paper showing how hippocampal anatomy and physiology could underpin the predicated mapping system and how the loss of such a map could explain the behavioural deficits following hippocampal damage. The review paper grew into a sizeable book and after a long gestation period was eventually published in 1978 by Oxford University press under the title "The Hippocampus as a Cognitive Map" (Figure 5 left). In it we covered the extant literature on the hippocampus, but in addition we tried to set our ideas in their historical context by covering the philosophical and psychological literature on space and spatial representation. We were deeply impressed by how important to many different behaviours such a spatial system might be and waxed lyrically about the role of space as shown in the poetic language with which we introduced the book.

THE
HIPPOCAMPUS
AS A COGNITIVE MAP

JOHN O'KEEFE
AND
LYNN NADEL

1478
1978

CLARENDON PRESS · OXFORD

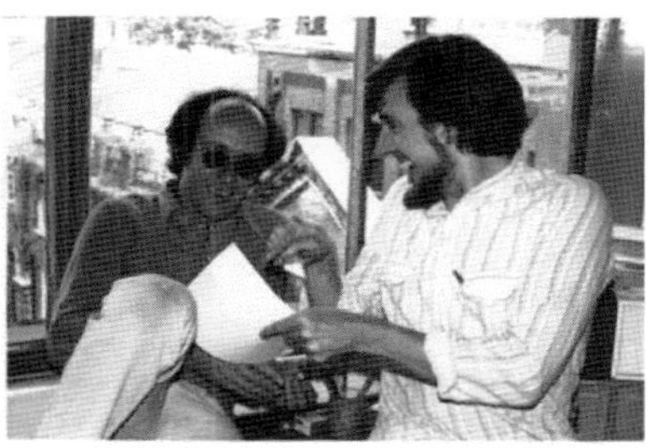

Lynn Nadel

FIGURE 5. Lynn Nadel and John O'Keefe kibitzing during the writing of the Hippocampus as a Cognitive Map.

SPACE
plays a role in all our behaviour.

We live in it, move through it, explore it, defend it.
We find it easy enough to point to bits of it:

the room,
the mantle of the heavens,
the gap between two fingers,
the place left behind when the piano
finally gets moved.

(O'Keefe and Nadel, 1978, p. 5).

Theories make predictions which go beyond the extant data. We predicted the existence of hippocampal signals coding for direction, distance and speed of movement and showed how the known effects of hippocampal lesions could be explained by impaired place learning, navigation, and exploration. Having reviewed the lesion literature, we also suggested that most existing behavioural tasks used to test hippocampal function were inadequate since they did not isolate the spatial components of the task sufficiently well to demonstrate that they were the crucial components. Further they did not adequately rule out alternative strategies based on remaining brain systems so that e.g., the animals couldn't learn using stimulus/response route-based strategies. The book had a limited production run and was not readily available for many years. To rectify this situation, some years ago I scanned the original book and placed the scanned version on the Internet (www.cognitivemap.net) to make it more accessible.

Well, if you make predictions and are lucky enough to have colleagues who take them seriously, they will set out to test them. One of the first persons to test a prediction of the theory was Richard Morris (Figure 6A). Inspired by the cognitive map idea, Richard who was then at St Andrews University devised a simple but powerful spatial navigation task which required the animal to approach a location defined by distal environmental cues when started from any one of several different start positions thus forcing it to approach the goal from different directions on different trials. The "Morris water maze," as it came to be known, consisted of a tub of opaque water within which was placed a hidden sunken escape platform effectively eliminating local cues (Figure 6B). Richard did all the important groundwork showing how normal animals performed on the maze and controlling for the influence of all but spatial information (Morris,

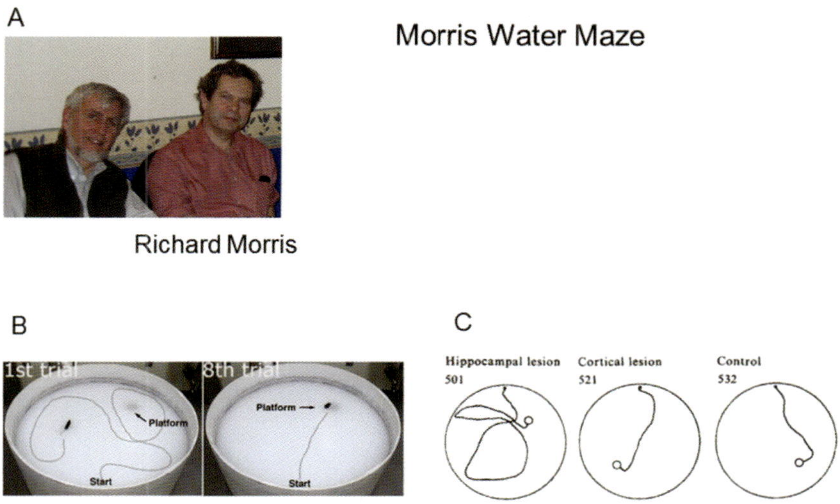

FIGURE 6. The Morris water maze was developed by Richard Morris (A) in order to test predictions of the cognitive map theory. The animal is placed in a tank filled with opaque water containing a hidden platform which it must locate on the basis of extramaze room cues (B). Control animals and those with neocortical lesions readily learn to do this but animals with damage to the hippocampus find it much more difficult (C).

1981). Subsequently Richard Morris, Nick Rawlins from Oxford and ourselves tested animals with hippocampal lesions on the task and showed that, unlike control animals and those with lesions of the overlying neocortex, these animals were severely deficient in learning to find the hidden platform (Figure 6C). The water maze has proved an invaluable test of hippocampal function and is now one of the most widely used behavioural testing apparatuses in neuroscience.

In the late 70s I was lucky enough to attract Bruce McNaughton and Carol Barnes to spend a year as postdocs in my laboratory (Figure 7 right). They were already experts in intracellular recording, long-term potentiation and behavioural studies. We had just introduced a minicomputer and an overhead camera head tracking system to the lab and Bruce, Carol and I carried out the first quantitative measurement of place fields albeit on the one-dimensional arms of an 8-arm maze (McNaughton et al., 1983). We also showed quantitatively for the first time that the firing rate of place cells was dependent on the animal's speed (Figure 7A). It was an important prediction of the cognitive map theory that the animal's speed would be represented in the hippocampus because this speed signal was needed to translate movements through the environment at different speeds into shifts of the same displacement within the map representation. Subsequently we were able to find a small number of pure speed cells in

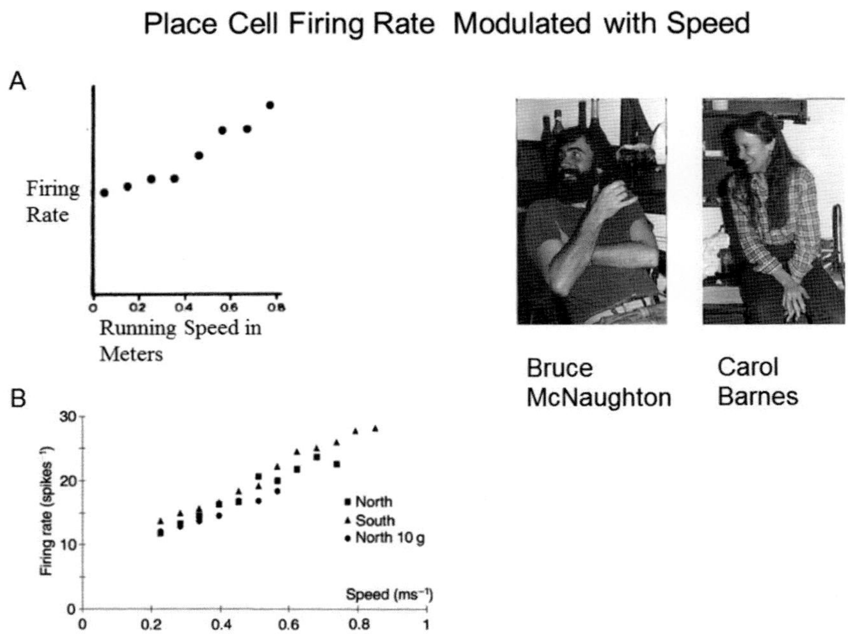

FIGURE 7. Place cell firing rate is modulated by the animal's speed of running. Bruce McNaughton and Carol Barnes (upper right) showed a good correlation between the two measures (A). Subsequently a small number of pure speed cells have been found in the hippocampus itself (B). Firing in these cells is not dependent on direction of movement or on the amount of exertion or force required to carry out the movement. After McNaughton et al. (1983) and O'Keefe et al. (1998).

the hippocampus which fired irrespective of the animal's location or direction of movement and which did not change markedly if the animal was pulling a 10 gram weight, ruling out a role for muscular effort (O'Keefe et al., 1998) (Figure 7B).

WHAT ABOUT THE OTHER CELL TYPES REQUIRED BY THE THEORY?

We now know that all the cell types required by the cognitive map theory exist in the greater hippocampal formation (Figure 8): place cells in the hippocampus proper which tell the animal where it is in a familiar environment (A), head direction cells in the presubiculum and entorhinal cortex which tell the animal which direction it is pointing in (D), boundary cells in the subiculum and entorhinal cortex which tell how close it is to a boundary in a particular direction (B), and last but not least, grid cells in the entorhinal cortex which appeared to

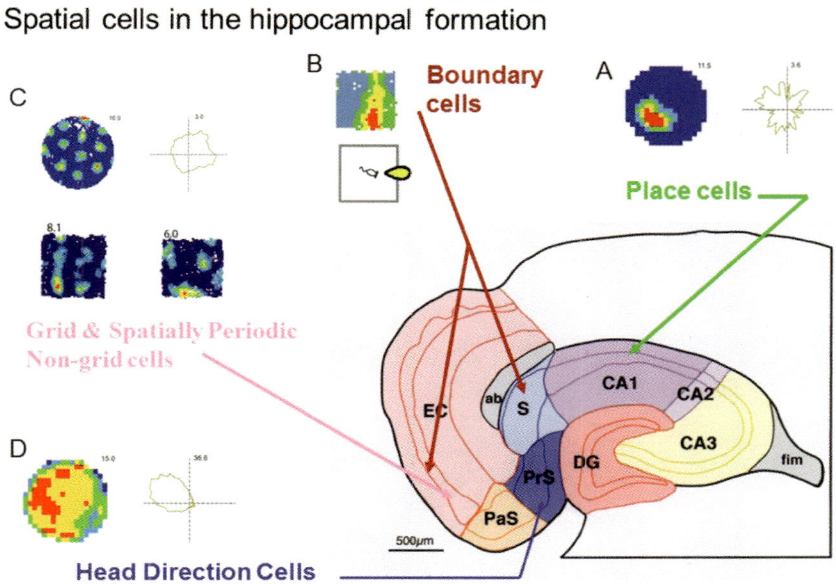

FIGURE 8. Spatial cells in the hippocampal formation include (A) place cells of the hippocampus proper which fire in localised parts of the environment (firing rate map, left) and in open fields irrespective of the animal's heading direction (polar plot, right), (B) boundary cells of the subiculum which fire when the animal is located a distance from a boundary in an allocentric direction, (C) grid and other spatially periodic cells of the medial entorhinal cortex which fire in multiple locations across an environment in a symmetrical hexagonal pattern (grids) or in other symmetrical but non-hexagonal patterns (spatially periodic non-grid cells), and (D) head direction cells of the pre-subiculum which fire when the animal's head is pointing in an allocentric direction (polar plot, right) irrespective of location in the environment (firing rate map, left). Boundary cells are also found in the entorhinal cortex where they are called border cells and head direction cells are also found in the entorhinal cortex. After Lever et al. (2009) & Krupic et al. (2012).

provide the metric for the map at least in some environments (C). In addition to the grid cells there are several other cell types in the entorhinal cortex including spatially periodic non-grid cells which fire in repeated regular patterns without the hexagonal symmetry of the grid cells and which may carry out some of the same functions as the grids (Krupic et al., 2012). In this review I can't possibly attempt to summarise all we know about these different cell types but will point out a few important aspects of each in the next few sections.

Place cells are typically recorded in boxes with square or circular walls (Figure 9A) where the animal is free to move in all directions except when it is close to the walls. In these environments, the place cells typically have one localised

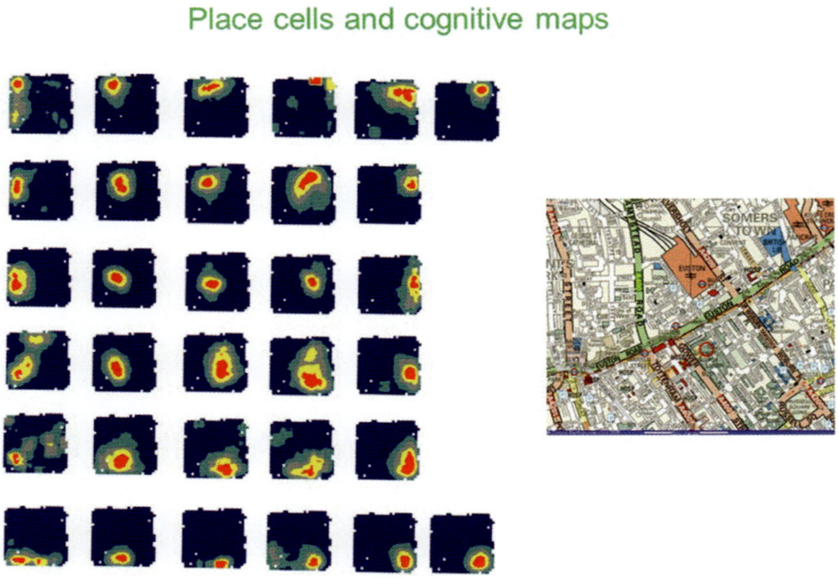

FIGURE 9. Different place cells have different firing fields and 32 simultaneously-recorded place fields taken together cover the surface of an environment. Firing rates are arranged to correspond to field locations in the environment and not to anatomical location in the hippocampus.

firing field within which it is happy to fire independently of the animal's direction of facing or movement. In environments in which the animal's movements are constrained to move in one or two directions (such as linear tracks, see Figure 12), the place cells typically have a preferred direction and fire much less or not at all in the opposite direction (McNaughton et al., 1983; O'Keefe and Recce, 1993). When a group of cells are recorded at the same time, each has its own firing field and, taken together, the firing fields of even a small group of cells tend to cover the entire surface of the environment (Figure 9). Place cells recorded in two familiar discriminable environments such as a square and a circle clearly discriminate between the two environments (Figure 10). Some fire in the square but not the circle (top row), others fire in the reverse pattern (second row), and still others fire in both boxes but not in the same locations (third row), and finally (bottom row) a small group fire in the same location in both boxes probably because the boxes were located in the same place in the laboratory and the cells were firing in the laboratory frame. Place cells recorded in three-dimensional environments have three-dimensional fields. The best demonstration of this is in bats, where the fields tend to be spherical and also cover the volume

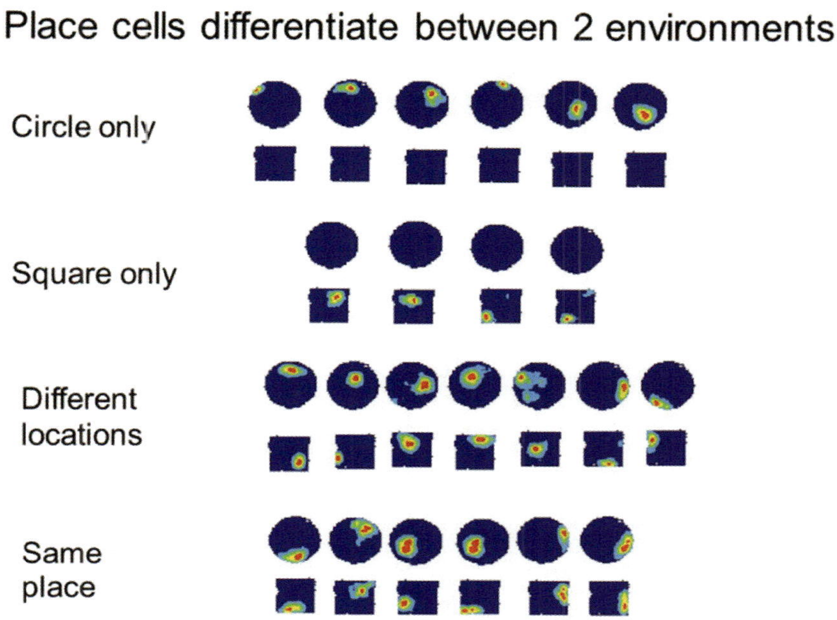

FIGURE 10. Place cells differentiate between 2 familiar environments, a circle and a square, either by firing only in the circle (top) or the square (2nd row), firing in both but in different locations (3+ row). A small number of cells fire in the same place in both boxes (bottom) probably because the boxes were set in the same location relative to the experimental room and the cells were responding to the absolute location in the room.

of space in the same way as two-dimensional place cells in the rat (Figure 11) (Yartsev and Ulanovsky, 2013).

Temporal coding in place cells allows place cells to identify locations in an environment with a much finer precision than if only firing rates are used (Figure 12). To know when an action potential has occurred, you need some sort of clock against which to measure time. The way the place cells do this is by using the population activity of the hippocampus as represented by the sinusoidal local field potential (LFP) called theta. The local field potential recorded from an electrode in the hippocampus shows a striking rhythmical oscillation called the theta rhythm which typically varies in frequency from 6 to 10 Hz (Figure 12A). When this oscillatory activity was first described, many thought it was an artefact since it didn't really seem likely that the brain was creating sine waves. In fact many years of experimentation have shown that theta is not only real but also a very important aspect of hippocampal function. Furthermore there is a nice behavioural correlate of theta as originally shown by Case Vanderwolf

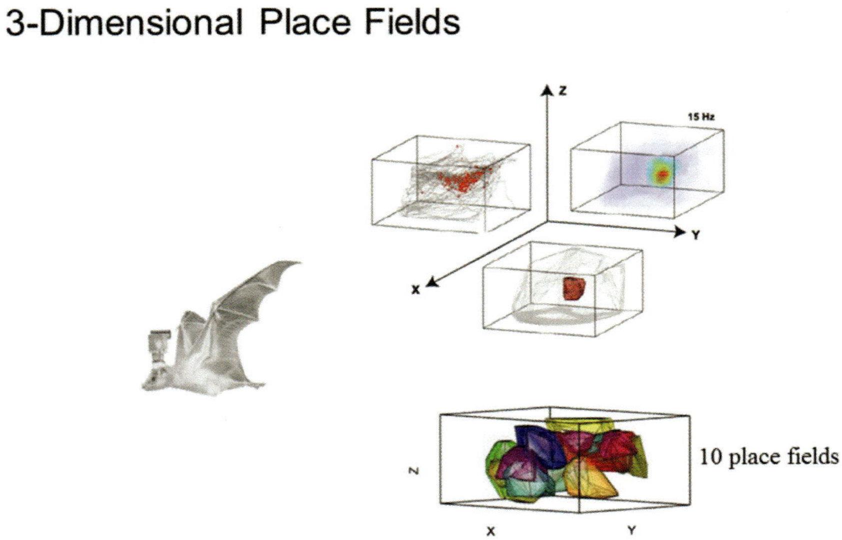

FIGURE 11. Three-dimensional place fields are found in the hippocampus of flying bats. The spherical fields of 10 place cells fill up the volume in which the animal is navigating. After Yartsev et al. (2013).

(Vanderwolf, 1969). It occurs primarily when the rat runs around an environment engaging in behaviours which translate its location relative to the environment (Figure 12A). In contrast when the animal sits still during drinking or eating, the rhythm typically disappears to be replaced by a less organised pattern with a broader range of frequencies. Over the years, Gyuri Buzsaki (Figure 12 upper left), who has studied hippocampal theta activity more than anyone else, would occasionally ask me about the relationship between the firing pattern of place cells and theta waves. We both knew from the earliest recording experiments that the interneuronal theta cells tended to have a fixed phase relationship to a particular part of the theta wave. In contrast I had not been able to identify any such fixed phase relationships between place cell firing and theta in earlier informal recordings and told him so more than once. Thinking about this around 1990, it seemed improbable that there would be no relationship whatsoever, so I decided to look more closely at the relationship on an individual run-by-run basis. I used a dataset that had been collected by Andrew Speakman and myself in a memory experiment carried out on a 4-armed plus-shaped maze with controlled environmental cues. The study was originally designed to monitor the firing of place cells when the animal was allowed to located itself relative to the environmental cues but then asked to navigate to a goal after these cues

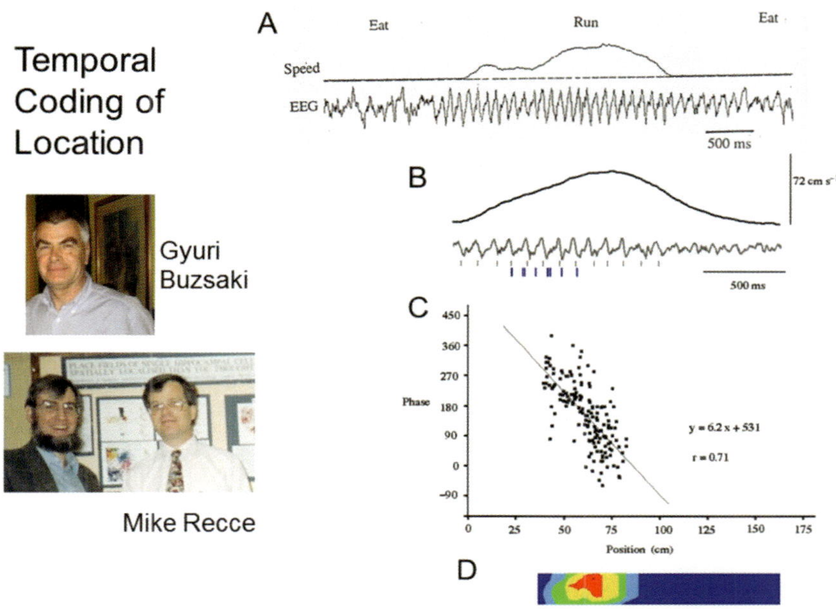

FIGURE 12. The timing of place cell firing as well as rate is used to code spatial information. Hippocampal local field potential shows 8–10 Hz theta oscillations as the animal runs in a linear track but a less organised irregular pattern as the animal sits at the end of the track eating (A). When the animal runs through the field of a place cell (D), the place cell emits a series of action potentials (B, blue) whose frequency is slightly higher than the simultaneously recorded LFP theta (B, black ticks). The result is that the spikes precess relative to the theta waves occurring at earlier phases each successive burst. The phase of place cell firing is highly correlated with the position of the animal (C). After O'Keefe and Recce (1993).

had been removed (O'Keefe and Speakman, 1987). I concentrated on the relationship between a well-isolated familiar place cell and the ongoing theta activity. After several days of pondering over what seemed at first to be a random relationship in which the spikes could fire at any phase of the theta wave, I realised that the relationship was not random but systematic: as the animal ran through the field each successive burst of spikes moved earlier and earlier relative to the theta wave. The spikes were precessing in a systematic way relative to the theta wave (Figure 12B). Notice how the blue spike moves earlier and earlier relative to the black ticks marking the + to –0° crossing of the theta wave as the animal runs through the place field. It seemed possible that this temporal code was carrying information. To study this more quantitatively, Michael Recce (Figure 12 lower left) and I recorded the place cells and theta waves as rats ran back and forth between the two ends of a linear track for a food reward. A typical instance of what we saw is shown in Figure 12C. When we plotted the phase of firing of the cell against the animal's location on the linear track we found a striking correlation suggesting that position is coded not only by the rate of firing of the cell but also by the exact timing of spikes relative to this wave. To this day, this phase coding for location is one of the best examples of a temporal code in the nervous system. More generally, temporal coding may be a very important property of cells in the cortex. In subsequent work with Neil Burgess and John Huxter (Huxter et al., 2003), we showed that the rate and temporal codes were relatively independent, opening up the possibility that the two variables might code for different aspects of the animal's behaviour or location. This might be one solution to the binding problem: how does the nervous system know that two different variables go together? Perhaps they are represented by different aspects of the same train of action potentials in a single cell.

Boundary cells may be part of the mechanism for identifying places in the environment on the basis of sensory information impinging on the animal at particular locations. The first clue to the existence of these cells came from an experiment that Neil Burgess (Figure 13 right) and I carried out on place cells in the mid-1990s. Bob Muller and his colleagues have reported that the size of place fields could be modified by increasing the size of the box in which they were recorded but that this scaling was not proportional to the increased area of the box. We wanted to understand this effect in greater detail. In order to do

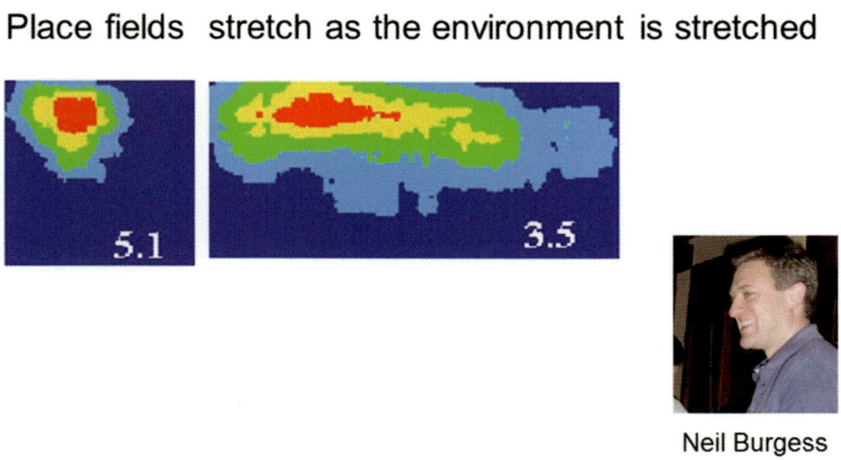

FIGURE 13. Place field stretches along the long dimension when the square is transformed into a rectangle. Number in white is peak firing rate marked by red. After O'Keefe and Burgess (1996).

so, we recorded from place cells in four boxes all placed in the same part of the room but differing in the ratio between the two adjacent sizes of the box. There was a small square, a large square with sides double those of the small square, and two rectangles with adjacent sides equal to the dimensions of the large and small square. The rectangles were essentially small squares stretched out along one dimension. The results show that quite often place fields were stretched along the same dimension as the boxes but were not affected in the orthogonal dimension (Figure 13). Thinking about this effect, Neil and I realised that the simplest model to explain it would be if the inputs to the place cells came from cells which were coding for the distance from a large environmental landmark such as the wall of the box in a particular direction. Cells which stretched along a particular dimension would be attached to the 2 opposing walls. With Tom Hartley, we modelled the firing fields of these cells (Figure 14A) and found that inputs from two or more of these boundary cells when added together followed by thresholding would produce realistic place fields in different environments

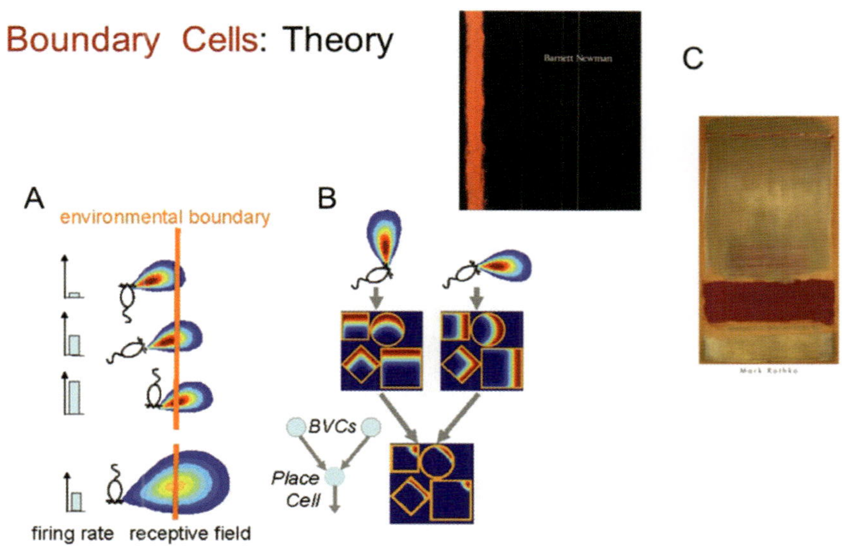

FIGURE 14. Properties of putative boundary cells providing inputs to the place cells to account for the stretching of place fields in the square to rectangle experiment. (A) Firing rate of boundary cells was predicted to increase as the animal got closer to the target distance from the environmental boundaries such as a wall of the box (red line). For some cells the preferred distance from the boundary was shorter (top) than for others (bottom). The fields of boundary cells recorded in different shaped environments were expected to look like the stripes in the paintings of Barnett Newman or Mark Rothko (C). Adding the inputs from 2 or more boundary cells together followed by a thresholding operation would produce place fields. After Hartley et al. (2000).

(B)(Hartley et al., 2000). The putative fields of these boundary cells looked very much like the bold stripes in the paintings of Barnett Newman and Mark Rothko delineating a small part of the two-dimensional space of the painting at a fixed distance from one of the walls (Figure 14C). Boundary cells with the predicted Rothko-like striped fields were subsequently looked for and found (Figure 15A & B) by Colin Lever in our lab (Figure 15 lower right) not in the hippocampus proper but in the neighbouring subiculum (D) (Lever et al., 2009). As predicted by the model, adding the inputs from these recorded two boundary cells followed by thresholding produces a respectable place field (C). Around the same time, similar cells with similar properties were found in the entorhinal cortex in the Moser lab (Solstad et al., 2008). They emphasised the closeness of the fields of many of their cells to the walls of the environment and called them border cells. It is still not clear whether these are the same cell types or the border cells are a subset of the boundary cells.

Head direction cells convey information about the direction in which the animal's head is pointing within the environmental frame (Figure 16A). They were originally identified by Jim Ranck about 1984 in an area called the presubiculum (PrS) nestled between the hippocampus and entorhinal cortex and

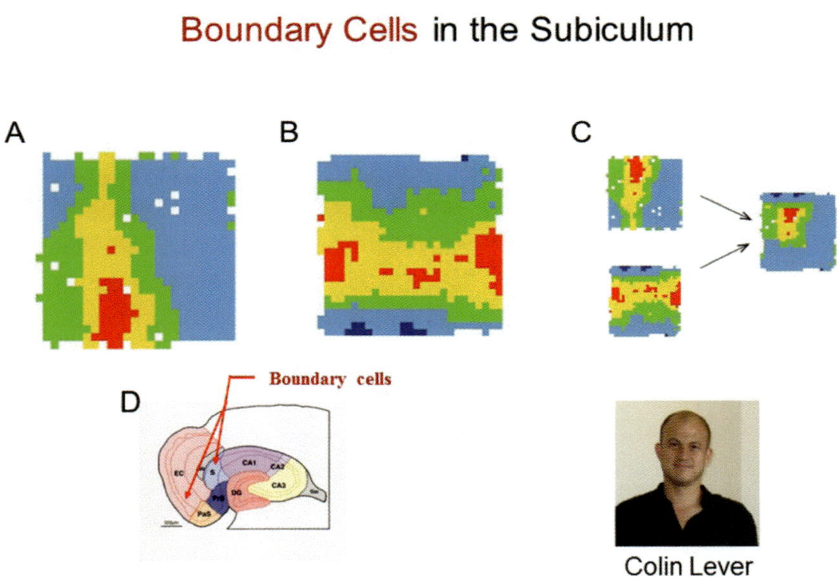

FIGURE 15. Boundary cells were found experimentally in the subiculum (D) by Colin Lever (lower right). Although many had fields close to the walls of the box, a number (A and B) fired away from the boundary and would be expected to produce place-like fields when combined (C). After Lever et al. (2009).

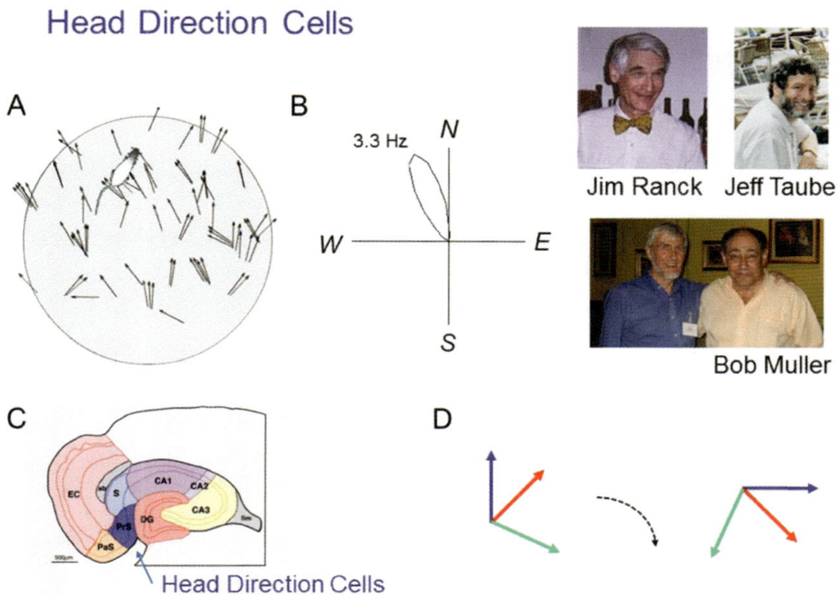

FIGURE 16. Head direction cells fire on the animal's head is pointing in the preferred heading direction (B) irrespective of the animal's location (A). They are found in many parts of the hippocampal circuit including the pre-subiculum (C) where they were discovered by Jim Ranck and studied extensively by Jeff Taube and Bob Muller (upper right). They appear to be wired together (D) such that rotation (dotted arrow) of the preferred direction of one (e.g., blue arrow) is accompanied by an equal rotation of the others (red and green arrows).

were subsequently studied extensively by Jim and his colleagues, Jeff Taube and Bob Muller. Bob Muller, who recently died, had one of the most incisive, original minds of anyone I have had the pleasure to discuss the brain with. The hippocampal spatial field is poorer for his loss. The firing fields of head direction cells are usually represented in a polar coordinate plot as shown in Figure 16B. The cell represented typically fired whenever the animal's head pointed in the North Northwest direction, irrespective of the animal's location in the environment (Figure 16A). An interesting property of these cells is that they seem to be wired together such that their preferred heading directions maintain a constant relationship with each other despite the fact that they can vary in their absolute relationship to the environment. For example, if the animal is briefly disoriented by spinning, the heading direction of a cell which originally pointed in the northward direction might be altered to point in the eastward direction (Figure 16 D, blue arrow); other head direction cells will alter their preferred directions (red and green arrows) in a concomitant fashion to maintain the internal angles constant. The constellation of cells appears to form a compass-like polar coordinate system upon which the rest of the spatial mapping system is built. As we shall see shortly, head direction cells appear earliest in development, at around the time that the infant rat is leaving the nest and opening its eyes and well before the place and grid components of the map. In addition to inputs about the animal's heading direction, a map needs a distance metric and the question arises as to whether this distance is represented by a one-dimension caliper-like signal in the manner suggested by William Blake's picture of Newton (Figure 17 B) or whether is it something more complicated as shown by the Lichtenstein painting Yellow Cliffs (Figure 17A)? In the latter a grid of dots is laid across the landscape and distance in two directions can be measured from the edge of the figure or the edge of the painting. The answer was provided by research in the Moser lab.

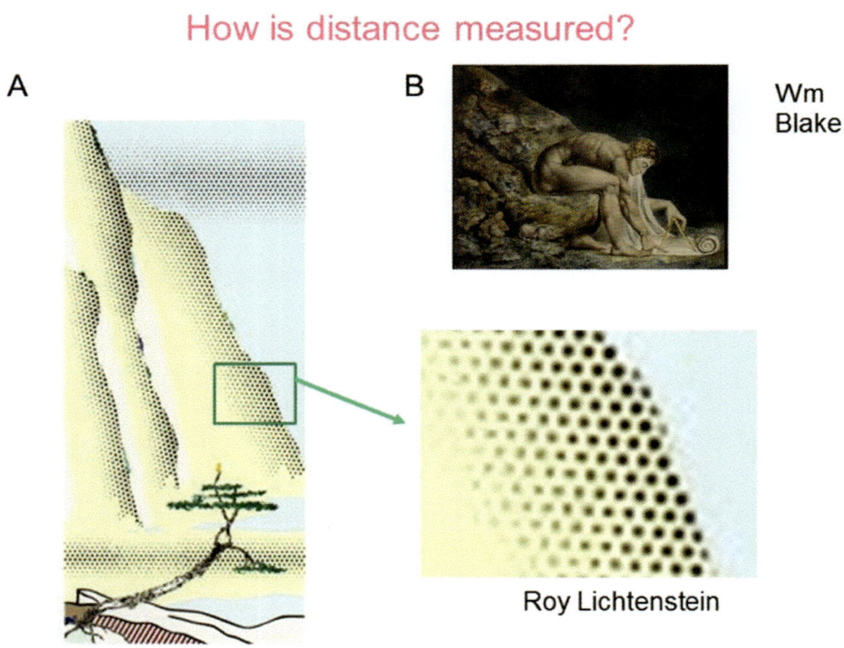

FIGURE 17. Distance within the cognitive map could be measured by a simple one-dimensional calipers as done by William Blake's Newton (B), or by a two-dimensional set of markers laid out on the surface of the environment as in Lichtenstein's painting Yellow Cliffs (A).

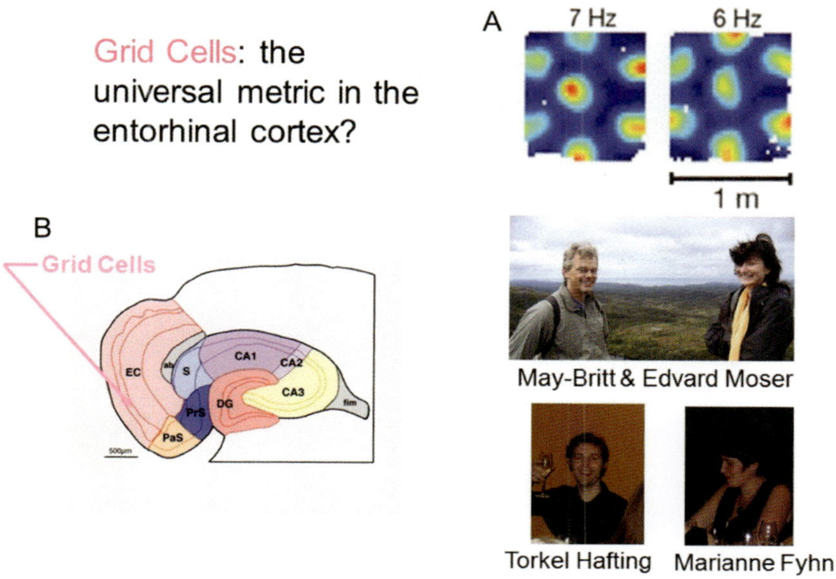

FIGURE 18. The grid cells (A) of the medial entorhinal cortex (B) discovered by the Torkel Hafting, Marianne Fyhn and the Mosers (lower right) are good candidates for the universal metric of the cognitive map. They fire in a repeating hexagonally symmetrical pattern across the surface of the environment. After Hafting et al. (2005).

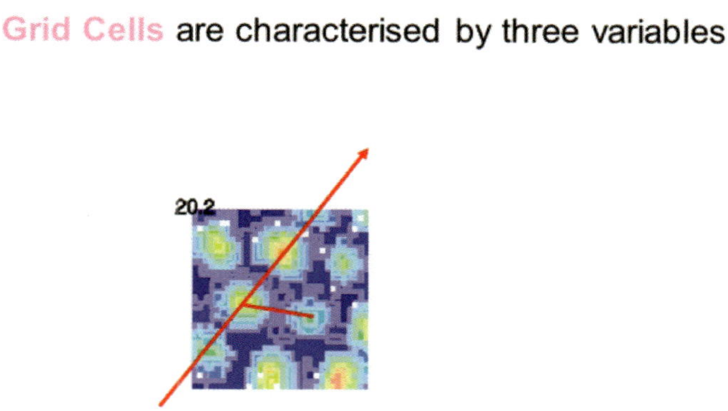

FIGURE 19. The hexagonally symmetrical pattern of grid cell can be described by the distance between two adjacent fields (short horizontal red line), the angle which one of the rows (red arrow) makes with the wall of the box, and the distance of the nearest row from the wall of the box.

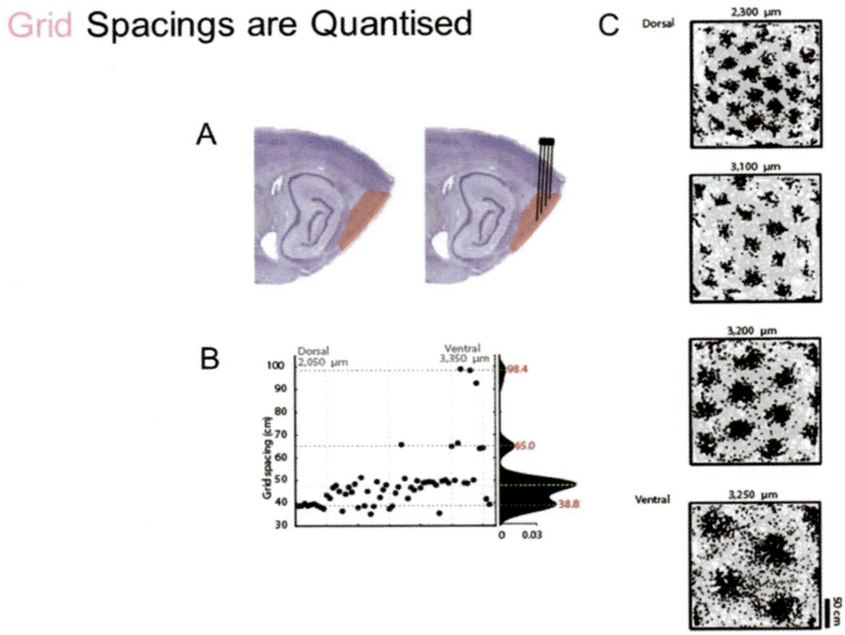

FIGURE 20. The spacings between adjacent peaks of the grid pattern are quantised. Grids more ventral in the entorhinal cortex (A) have a larger metric than ones more dorsal (C) and these changes in metric are quantised, falling into three or four distinct scales (B).

Distance within the mapping system, at least in some environments, could be measured by the entorhinal cortical grid cells (Figure 18). In 2005, the Moser lab reported that there existed in the medial entorhinal cortex (Figure 18B) a set of grid cells which look very much like they represent distances in particular directions: they cover each familiar environment with a set of firing fields which are laid out in a beautiful symmetrical hexagonal pattern and which are reproducible from one trial to next (Figure 18A) (Hafting et al., 2005). It is not hard to see how these patterns could be used to represent distances. As you can see from Figure 19, one can characterise each of these patterns by three variables: the distance between any two adjacent peaks, the smallest offset angle which the orientation of the grid makes relative to the walls and the distance of the grid from the walls of the environment. The cells are grouped into modules with the same orientation and if one looks over a large group of cells in square boxes one finds that they have a preferred orientation relative to the edge of the box with an angle of 8.8° (Krupic et al., 2015). Equally important, the spacing between the peaks of the grid cells varies as a function of location within the entorhinal cortex. As one goes from dorsal to ventral in the entorhinal cortex (Figure 20 A), scale increases in quantum jumps, each animal having three or four different scales (Figure 20 B,C). This is important because if you take two grid cells with different spacings and you simply add them together and do a little bit of mathematical computation you can produce a place cell. (Figure 24). So we have two ways of producing a place cell, one by the addition of information from two or more boundary cells, and the other by the addition of information from two or more grid cells with different scales. Where do the grid patterns come from? One possibility is that they are created by overlaying different striped patterns as suggested by another painting by Lichtenstein (Figure 21 left). Here he has superimposed his pattern of hexagonal dots over the surface of the painting but in addition juxtaposes to them a series of diagonal stripes (upper right) where you can see that each row of dots is actually the extension of a stripe and you can easily imagine that if you had two more stripes of orientations of 60° degrees relative to each other, the intersection of three stripes patterns would effectively produce the grid pattern (lower right, green and red stripes). Surprisingly, one of our colleagues Julija Krupic (Figure 22 upper right) has found cells which look very much like band cells (A) in the parasubiculum (B), an area which has direct connections to the medial entorhinal cortex.

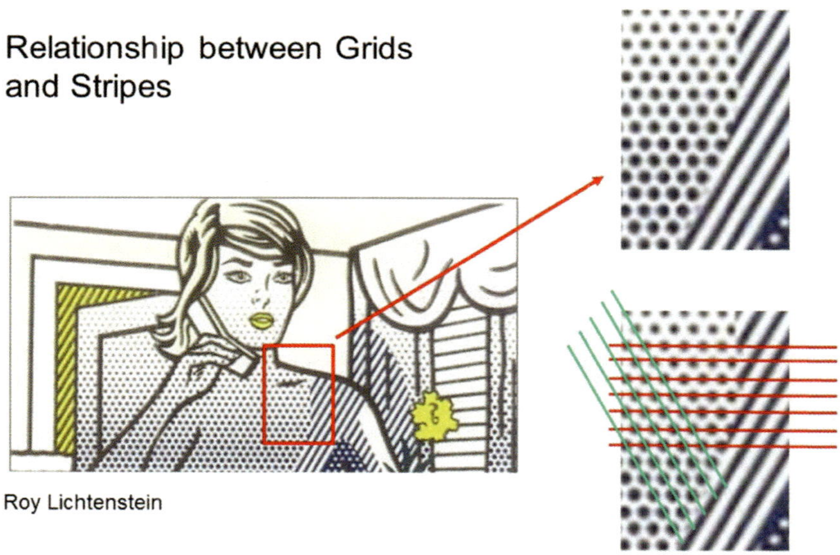

FIGURE 21. A simple relationship exists between grids and regular stripes as shown by the section of the Lichtenstein painting expanded in the upper right hand corner where the stripes are aligned with individual rows of the grid pattern. The addition of extra rows of stripes (red and green) at 60° to the original stripes creates the hexagonal pattern.

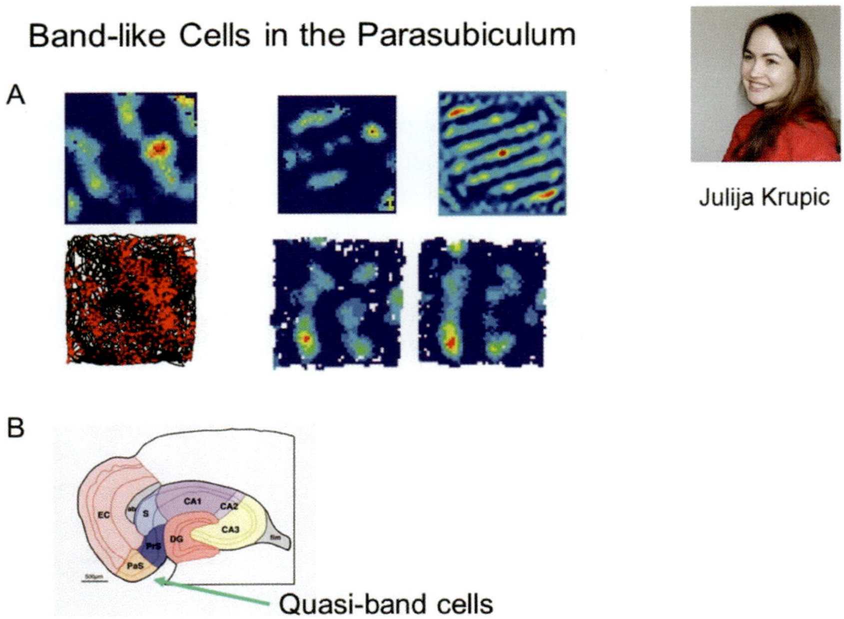

FIGURE 22. Band-like cells (A) were found in the parasubiculum (B) by Julija Krupic (upper right). They and other Spatially Periodic Non-grid cells may be members of a large set of hippocampal formation cells which can be decomposed into Fourier components of which the grid cells are the most stable and symmetrical members. After Krupic et al. (2012).

It is very tempting to assume that the regular pattern laid down by the grid cells across different environments might be the basis for the metric of the cognitive map. However we have to be a little cautious about this conclusion, since most of the studies so far have only recorded in circles and squares i.e., highly symmetrical environments. Furthermore the animals were familiar with most of these environments. In recent studies our group has shown that the grid pattern can be modified when the animal is placed in non-symmetrical environment such as a trapezoid (Krupic et al., 2015) and furthermore that there is an expansion of the pattern even in a symmetrical environment such as a square if the environment is novel (Barry et al., 2007). It is clear that we still have a lot to learn about the grid cells and the types of environmental information they are responding to.

The development of the cognitive map provides evidence for some of the ideas of the philosopher Immanuel Kant (Kant, 1963). Kant believed that space along with time was one of the basic organising principles of the human mind and furthermore that it existed independently and in some sense prior to experience with the objects of the world. He said that "Space is nothing but the form of all appearances of outer sense . . . can be given prior to all actual perceptions, and so exist in the mind *a priori*, and . . . can contain, prior to all experience, principles which determine the relations of these objects" (p. 71). Translated into modern neuroscientific terms, this would predict that some aspects of the cognitive mapping system should be present prior to an animal's having had any experience with the world. With Francesca Cacucci, Tom Wills and Hui Min Tan (Tan et al., 2015; Wills et al., 2010) (Figure 23 right), we decided to test this by recording from three of the major spatial cell types in very young infant rats in the second, third, and fourth week of life. These animals only begin to leave the nest towards the end of the second week around the same time as their eyes open. What we found is summarised in Figure 23 where one can see that the different cell types emerge at different times. Directional cells are present from P12 just before the time the animal leaves the nest and its eyes are opening. They develop their behavioural correlates very rapidly, quickly approximating adult levels. Some of these directional cells can be recorded prior to significant spatial exploration and eye opening, suggesting their properties might be largely experience-independent. Before eye opening, their fields are unstable and cannot be controlled by the usual visual stimuli. Place cells develop later first appearing at

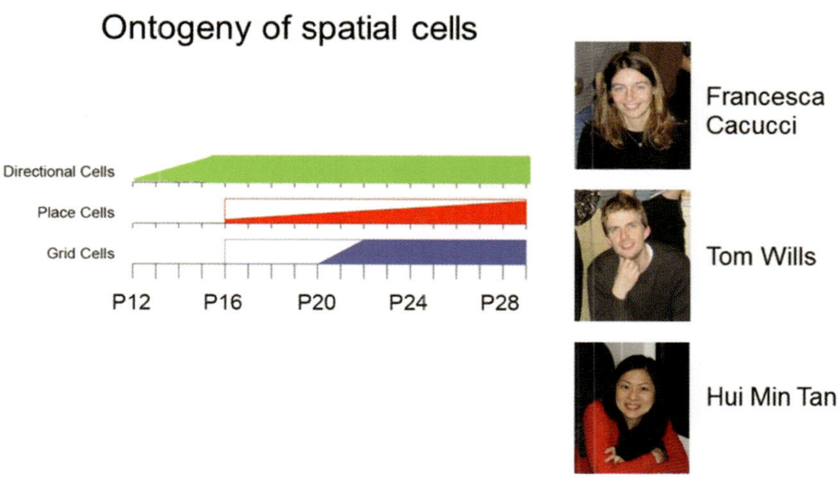

FIGURE 23. Development of spatial cells in the rat. Directional cells appear first as early as postnatal day 12 although they are not stable. They develop rapidly over the next few days to reach adult levels. Place cells first appear around postnatal day 16 and then develop slowly over the next two weeks. Grid cells appear several days later than place cells but develop rapidly. After Wills et al. (2010) and Tan et al. (2015).

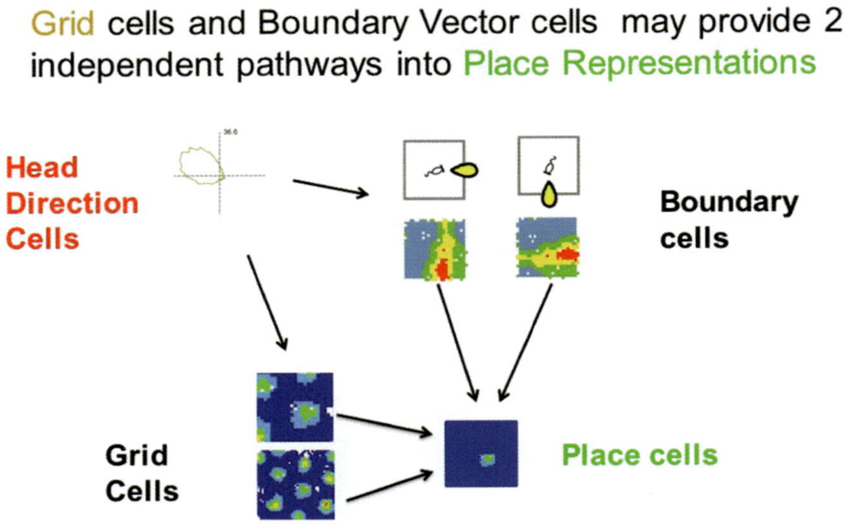

FIGURE 24. Two routes to a place cell. Combinations of boundary cells or grid cells can independently produce a place cell. Both boundary cells and grid cells appear to receive inputs from head direction cells.

P16, and increasing in number and spatiality during the next two weeks. Last to develop are the grid cells, which only appear in significant numbers at P22 but then quickly reach adult levels. Similar findings were published at the same time by the Moser lab (Langston et al., 2010). It appears that one aspect of the cognitive map, the directional system, develops prior to any substantial relevant experience with the environment and it probably provides inputs to the place and grid cells forming the basic substrate for the rest of the cognitive map. The fact that the place cells develop before the grid cells is further support for the idea that there are two or more pathways to create a place cell only of one which is dependent on the grid cell input. Figure 24 shows how place cells can be created either by the intersection of inputs from two boundary cells with stripes oriented at an angle to each other or by the intersection of inputs from two grid cells with different spacings.

Virtual reality technology can be used to test this idea that there are two different ways in which place cells can be generated (Chen et al., 2013). Our setup created by Guifen Chen and John King (Figure 25 right) derives from work originating in Tübingen and perfected in Princeton by David Tank's lab. The animals run on a Styrofoam ball which floats on a cushion of air and the motion of the ball and thus the animal is tracked by a computer mouse (Figure 25 left). Figure 25 (mid right) shows a screenshot of the linear track which is projected onto the

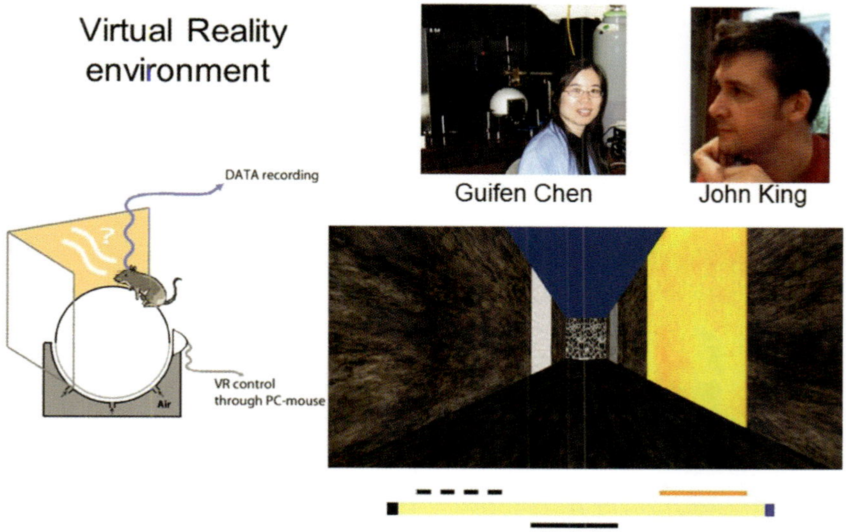

FIGURE 25. A Virtual Reality environment for mice was created by Guifen Chen and John King (upper right) and consists of a Styrofoam ball on top of which the animal runs and where his movements are translated into movements in a virtual environment projected onto VDU screens. A screen shot from the virtual linear track (middle right) shows the visual cues on the ends and sides of the track. The track and visual cues are schematised by the long yellow bar and coloured stripes (below).

two video displays in front of the animal. The linear track and the visual cues are schematically represented as shown in the lower right hand of the figure. The firing fields of 80% of the cells are dependent on the visual cues on the walls of the virtual environment as shown by the loss of the field when these cues are removed (Figure 26A middle). Interestingly it is the side cues which are important and not the cues on the ends of the track (bottom). The importance of the visual cues is confirmed by the maintenance of the place field in 25% of the cells on trials in which the animal is passively moved through the environment at about the same speed as it normally runs (Figure 26B middle). One way in which the path integration system can control the place fields is shown in Figure 27 where the animal was started at the beginning of the track with the visual cues present to allow it to locate itself but then these were turned off as the rat started to move down the track and were turned on again as it reach the goal (Figure 27 bottom). In almost half of the cells the fields were maintained during this procedure showing that once the animal had oriented itself in an environment, information from its own movements was sufficient to update the representation and cause the cell to fire in the correct location. The visual orientation at

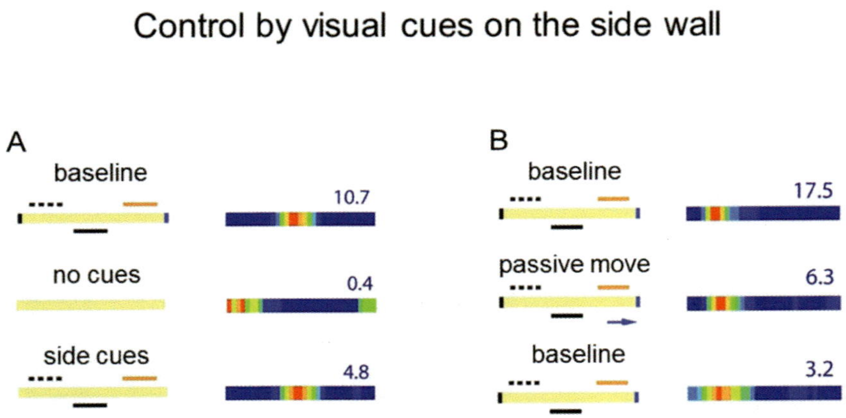

FIGURE 26. Place cells recorded in the virtual environment depend on the visual cues particularly those on the side walls. A, a place cell which stops firing when all the visual cues are removed (middle row) but continued to fire if only the cues on the end walls are removed (bottom row). B, a place cell which continues to fire if the animal is passively moved along the track. After Chen et al. (2013).

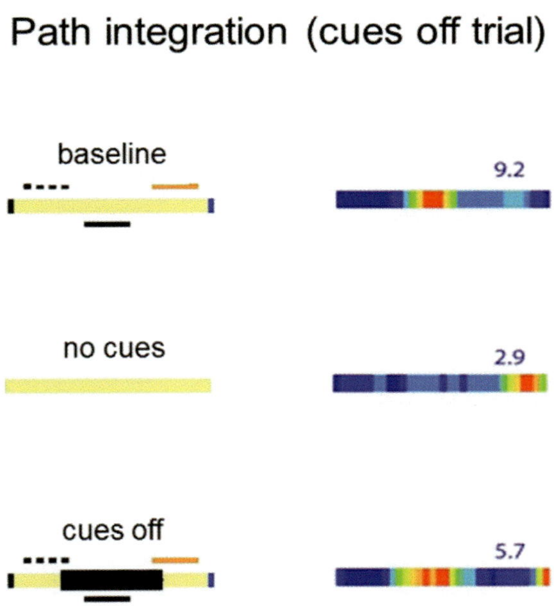

FIGURE 27. Place cells can combine visual and path-integration cues. The cell does not fire if the visual cues are removed throughout the trial (middle row) but does fire appropriately if they are available at the beginning of the run and then turned off when the animal runs through the field (bottom row). After Chen et al. (2013).

the beginning of the trial was necessary, as shown by the fact that the cells did not fire in the correct location if the visual cues were removed throughout the trial (Figure 27 middle).

The human hippocampus is widely believed to store episodic memories and the question arises as to whether it also involved in spatial memory and navigation similar to the rat. It is more difficult to study navigation in humans than in small animals and it was only when virtual reality technology became cheap and widely available in the 1990s that we were in a position to do so. That was when first person video games became available and more importantly came with editing facilities which allowed modifications to be made to the environment. Neil Burgess modified a game called Duke Nukem by removing the guns and monsters leaving us with a 70 × 70 metre environment containing many different rooms (Figure 28) and importantly many different routes by which the participant could move from one location to another (Figure 29 B). Eleanor Maguire (Figure 28 right) and Neil carried out a study in which they allowed normal volunteers to become familiar with this environment and scanned their brains as they found their way around this environment using either a cognitive

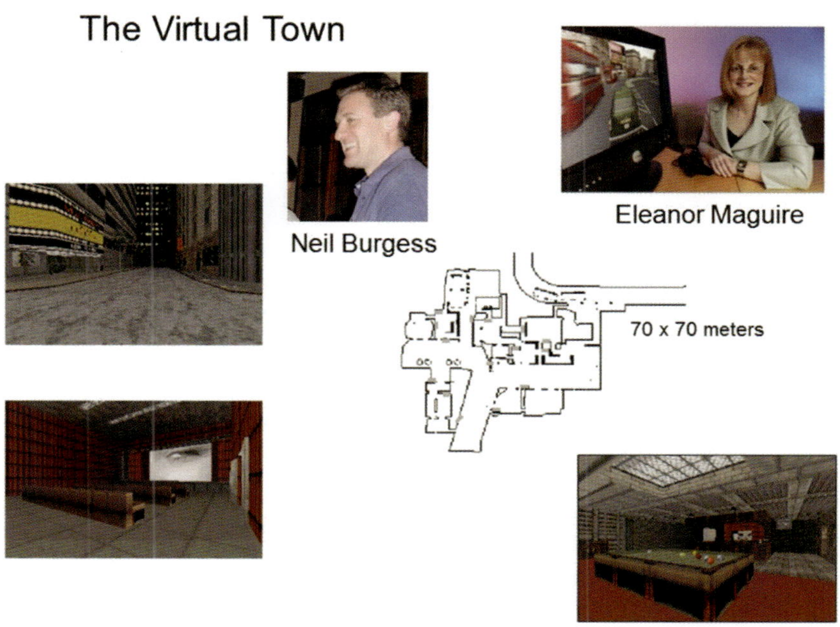

FIGURE 28. Screenshots from the virtual town created by Neil Burgess and used by himself and Eleanor Maguire to test hippocampal function in humans. The centre panel shows the layout of the environment.

map strategy or the route based strategy of following a series of arrows on the floor (Maguire et al., 1998). When we looked at the differences between the activations in these conditions we found the right hippocampus was more active in the cognitive map strategy (Figure 29A). Importantly the amount of activity in the hippocampus increased as a function of the accuracy with which the participant moved from one location to another (Figure 29 C) suggesting that the more active the hippocampus, the better the navigation. Maguire and colleagues (Maguire et al., 2000) then went on to show that London taxicab drivers had a larger posterior hippocampus than controls (Figure 30 A) and that this increase in size was directly related to the amount of time as a cab driver showing that the important factor was the experience of London's complicated street patterns and that London cab drivers are probably not born with bigger hippocampi but develop them.

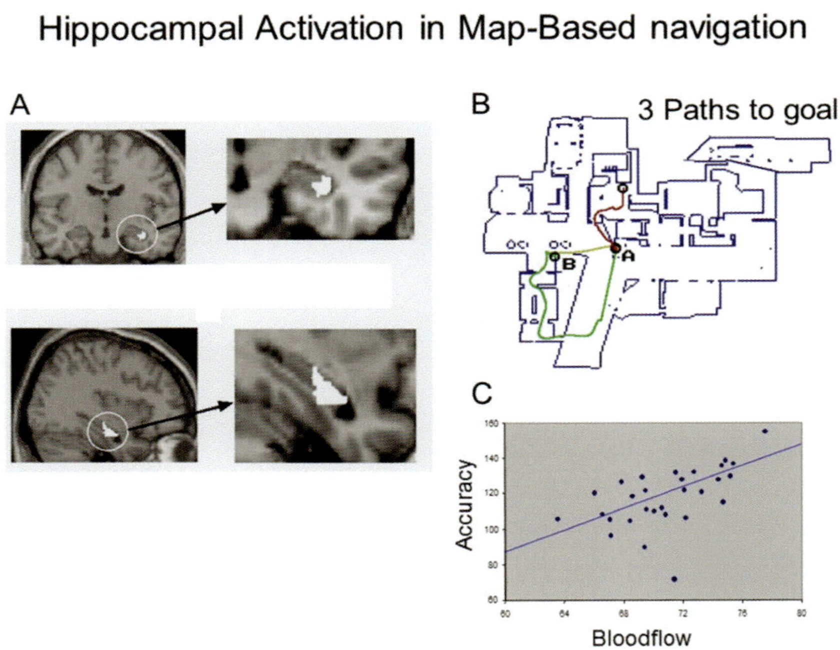

FIGURE 29. Right hippocampus is activated in map-based navigation. PET scans (A) show activation in the right hippocampus when participants used cognitive mapping strategies to find their way around the environment rather than route based ones. More accurate navigation (e.g., yellow line from A to B in panel B) is correlated with more bloodflow in the hippocampus than more circuitous or ineffective routes (green and red lines) (C). After Maguire et al. (1998).

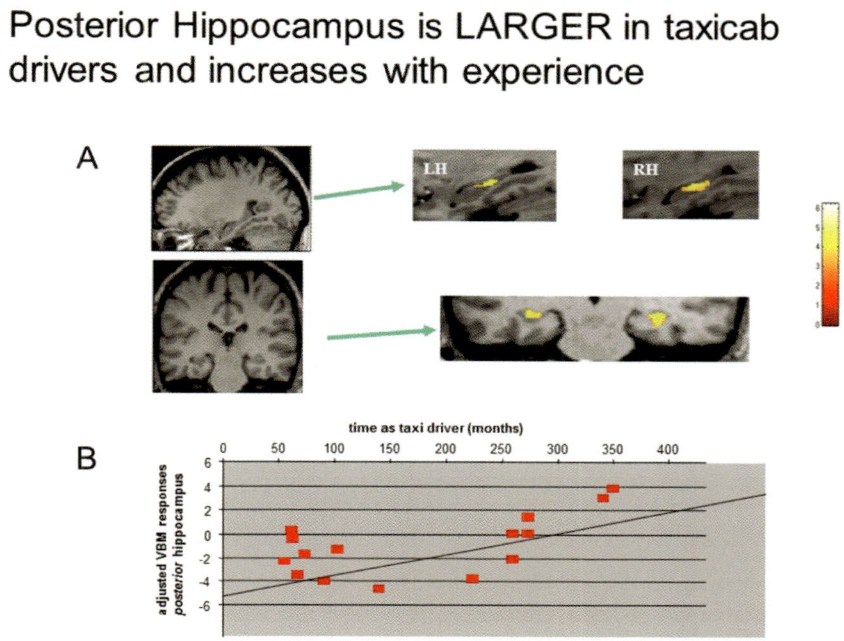

FIGURE 30. The posterior hippocampus is larger in taxicab drivers (A) than in controls and this effect increases with the length of time as a cab driver (B). After Maguire et al., 2000).

In Summary, the Hippocampal Formation provides a cognitive map of a familiar environment which can be used to identify the animal's current location and to navigate from one place to another. The Mapping system consists of a number of different spatial cells including ones which identify the animals place, direction, distance from landmarks such as the walls of an environment in a particular direction (boundary cells) and in some environments a metric for measuring distances between points in the map (grid cells). The grid cells cannot provide a perfect metric in all environments since the grid pattern is distorted in asymmetrical environment such as trapezoids and the scale of the grids is increased in unfamiliar environment. There is evidence for 2 independent strategies for locating places, one based on environmental landmarks probably provided by the boundary cells and the other on a path integration system which uses information about distances travelled in particular directions provided by the grid cells.

A similar spatial system exists in humans which additionally provides the basis for human episodic memory. A prototypical episodic memory system could be achieved by the addition of a sense of linear time to the basic spatial system seen in the rat (Burgess et al., 2002).

REFERENCES

1. Barry C, Hayman R, Burgess N, Jeffery KJ. (2007). Experience-dependent rescaling of entorhinal grids. *Nat Neurosci* **10**:682–684.
2. Burgess N, Maguire EA, O'Keefe J. (2002). The human hippocampus and spatial and episodic memory. *Neuron* **35**:625–641.
3. Chen G, King JA, Burgess N, O'Keefe J. (2013). How vision and movement combine in the hippocampal place code. *Proc Natl Acad Sci U S A* **110**:378–383.
4. Corkin S. (2013). *Permanent present tense.* Basic books.
5. Hafting T, Fyhn M, Molden S, Moser MB, Moser EI. (2005). Microstructure of a spatial map in the entorhinal cortex. *Nature* **436**:801–806.
6. Hartley T, Burgess N, Lever C, Cacucci F, O'Keefe J. (2000). Modeling place fields in terms of the cortical inputs to the hippocampus. *Hippocampus* **10**:369–379.
7. Huxter J, Burgess N, O'Keefe J. (2003). Independent rate and temporal coding in hippocampal pyramidal cells. *Nature* **425**:828–832.
8. Kant, Immanuel. (1963). *Critique of pure reason.* (Translated by N Kemp Smith-original published 1787). London: Macmillan.
9. Krupic J, Bauza M, Burton S, Barry C, O'Keefe J. (2015). Grid cell symmetry is shaped by environmental geometry. *Nature* **518**:232–235.
10. Krupic J, Burgess N, O'Keefe J. (2012). Neural representations of location composed of spatially periodic bands. *Science* **337**:853–857.
11. Langston RF, Ainge JA, Couey JJ, Canto CB, Bjerknes TL, Witter MP, Moser EI, Moser MB. (2010). Development of the spatial representation system in the rat. *Science* **328**:1576–1580.
12. Lever C, Burton S, Jeewajee A, O'Keefe J, Burgess N. (2009). Boundary vector cells in the subiculum of the hippocampal formation. *J Neurosci* **29**:9771–9777.
13. Maguire EA, Burgess N, Donnett JG, Frackowiak RS, Frith CD, O'Keefe J. (1998). Knowing where and getting there: a human navigation network. *Science* **280**:921–924.
14. Maguire EA, Gadian DG, Johnsrude IS, Good CD, Ashburner J, Frackowiak RS, Frith CD. (2000). Navigation-related structural change in the hippocampi of taxi drivers. *Proc Natl Acad Sci U S A.*
15. McNaughton BL, Barnes CA, O'Keefe J. (1983). The contributions of position, direction, and velocity to single unit activity in the hippocampus of freely-moving rats. *Exp Brain Res* **52**:41–49.
16. Morris RGM. (1981). Spatial localisation does not depend on the presence of local cues. *Learning and Motivation* **12**:239–260.
17. O'Keefe J. (1996). The spatial prepositions in English, vector grammar and the cognitive map theory. In: *Language and Space* (Bloom P, Peterson M, Nadel L, Garrett M, eds), pp. 277–316. Cambridge, Mass.: MIT Press.

18. O'Keefe J, Nadel L. (1979). Precis of O'Keefe and Nadel's The hippocampus as a cognitive map. *The Behavioral and Brain Sciences* **2**:487–533.
19. O'Keefe J, Nadel L. (1978). *The hippocampus as a cognitive map*. Oxford University Press.
20. O'Keefe J. (1976). Place units in the hippocampus of the freely moving rat. *Exp Neurol* **51**:78–109.
21. O'Keefe J, Burgess N, Donnett JG, Jeffery KJ, Maguire EA. (1998). Place cells, navigational accuracy, and the human hippocampus. *Philos Trans R Soc Lond B Biol Sci* **353**:1333–1340.
22. O'Keefe J, Dostrovsky J. (1971). The hippocampus as a spatial map. Preliminary evidence from unit activity in the freely-moving rat. *Brain Res* **34**:171–175.
23. O'Keefe J, Recce ML. (1993). Phase relationship between hippocampal place units and the EEG theta rhythm. *Hippocampus* **3**:317–330.
24. O'Keefe J, Speakman A. (1987). Single unit activity in the rat hippocampus during a spatial memory task. *Exp Brain Res* **68**:1–27.
25. Scoville WB, Milner B. (1957). Loss of recent memory after bilateral hippocampal lesions. *J Neurol Neurosurg Psychiatry* **20**:11–21.
26. Solstad T, Boccara CN, Kropff E, Moser MB, Moser EI. (2008). Representation of geometric borders in the entorhinal cortex. *Science* **322**:1865–1868.
27. Tan HM, Bassett JP, O'Keefe J, Cacucci F, Wills TJ. (2015). The development of the Head Direction System before Eye Opening in the Rat. *Curr Biol* **25**:479–483.
28. Tolman EC. (1948). Cognitive maps in rats and men. *Psychol Rev* **55**:189–208.
29. Vanderwolf CH. (1969). Hippocampal electrical activity and voluntary movement in the rat. *Electroencephalogr Clin Neurophysiol* **26**:407–418.
30. Wills TJ, Cacucci F, Burgess N, O'Keefe J. (2010). Development of the hippocampal cognitive map in preweanling rats. *Science* **328**:1573–1576.
31. Yartsev MM, Ulanovsky N. (2013). Representation of three-dimensional space in the hippocampus of flying bats. *Science* **340**:367–372.

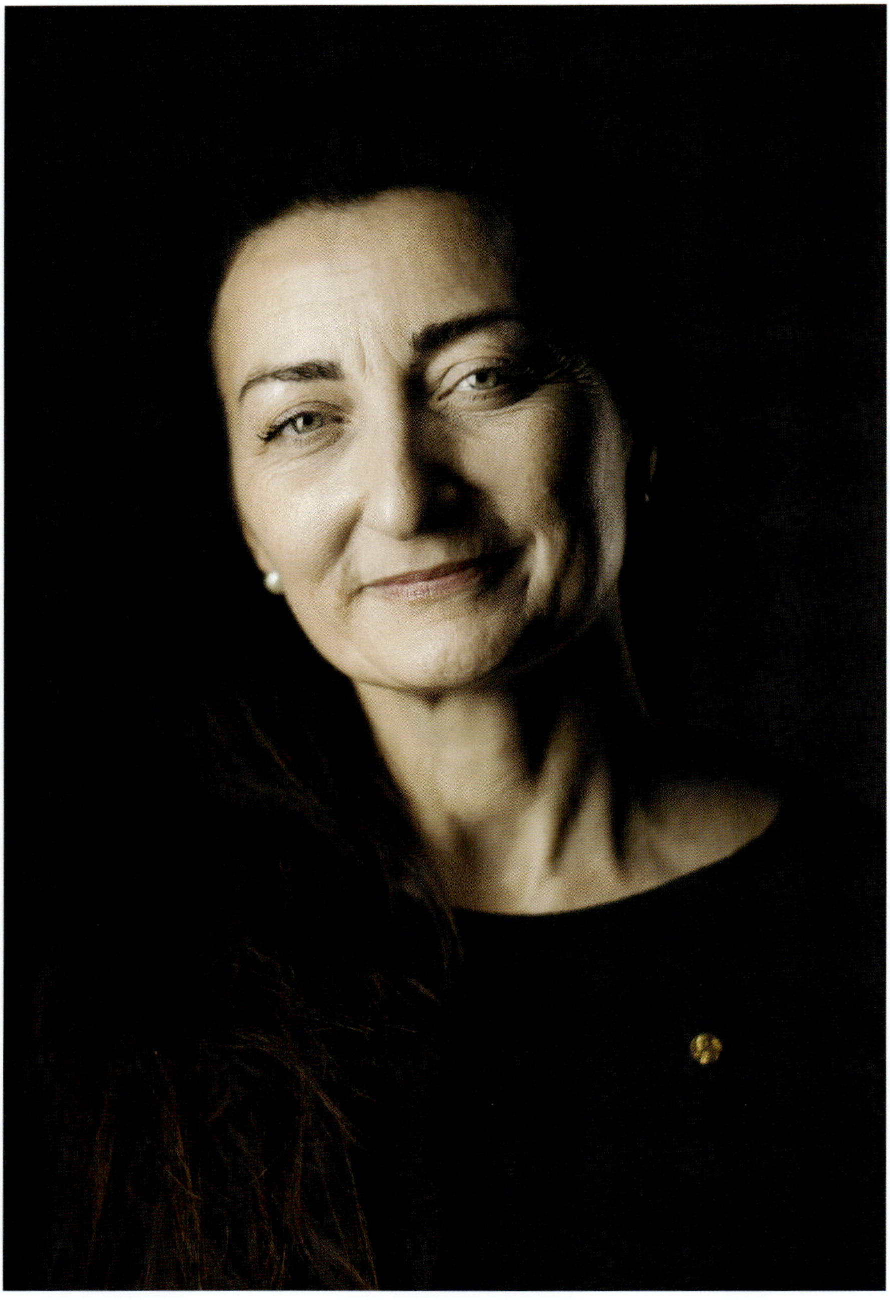

May-Britt Moser. © Nobel Media AB. Photo: A. Mahmoud

May-Britt Moser

I was born and raised in Fosnavåg, a small town on an island on the west coast of Norway, in one of the most beautiful parts of the country (Fig. 1).

My parents owned a small farm, although my father worked as a carpenter. My mother took most of the responsibility for the farm and cared for me and my four older siblings, in addition to having small jobs now and then. Before I was born, we had a lot of animals on the farm, with cows, chickens and a horse, but by the time I was born, we only had sheep. Both my father and mother worked very hard all the time, and I learned at an early age that work makes you happy.

I was a happy, curious child with a lot of dreams and a lucky star above my head. I was also a tomboy who played with the boys a lot. But because we were five children, we didn't have much money and we didn't have a car, so I would stay home during the summers when my friends would go away. I was the youngest child by 10 years, and had a lot of time to myself to study animals on my own, and I loved it. I would spend time out in our fields where I would play by myself. I even studied the behaviour of snails as they ate grass. As I watched, I would always wonder about the reasons behind what the animal was doing.

My mother liked to tell me fairy tales, but she didn't want to frighten me with the scary parts. Instead, she would tell me the parts of the stories that talked about hopes and dreams, like "Askeladden," a boy who had nothing, but he used his head, he was kind and he worked hard—so he succeeded. I loved it when my mother would read me these fairy tales. It also made me believe that even though you have nothing you can become something—it was a bit of the American dream!

My mother had her own dreams, too: she wanted to be a doctor. The area where I grew up is somewhat religious, so I also met missionaries who had travelled to distant countries. My mother's dream and the experience of meeting missionaries made me eager to go abroad so I could work as a doctor and save

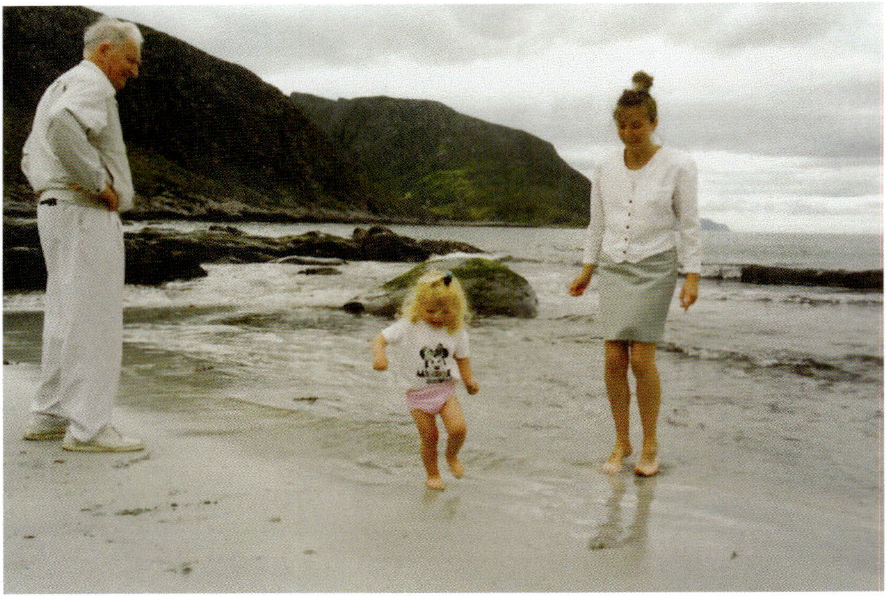

FIGURE 1. My dad, Isabel and me on the beach in Mulevika, on the island where I grew up.

the world. I also loved animals, so I thought perhaps if I didn't study to be a doctor, I could be a veterinarian. My dad had taught me to care for animals, and was a warm, good role model for me.

SCHOOL YEARS

I was not always the best student with the highest grades, but my teachers saw something in me and tried to encourage me. My mother had persuaded the local school officials to let me start school a year earlier than other students because my birthday was in January (the cut-off was the end of December) and because she saw that I was ready. My main primary school teacher would say "Wow, you are the youngest child in the class, and yet you still know this!"

I also had a teacher in high school who would call on me in class and say, "Frøken Andreassen, you know the answer! I believe in you!" And I had a physics teacher who really encouraged his female students by telling us that he wanted us to come back and show him that we had become engineers. There were other teachers, too, like my Norwegian teacher who said she thought my writing was good, but the bottom line is that I felt like I got a lot of special attention, and I was noticed. It made a difference.

At the same time, though, I wasn't that motivated in high school, because I spent too much time with friends, and I didn't have the drive to get the grades I needed to get into medical school. But my grades were still good, because my mother warned me that if I didn't work hard I would have to go to school to study home economics and be a housewife. That thought horrified me.

THE UNIVERSITY OF OSLO

When it came time to go to university, I decided I would go to the University of Oslo, in part because I had two older sisters in the Oslo area. I was also able to live for some time with one sister in Asker, an hour outside Oslo, while I looked for a place to live.

I loved university, it was fantastic—there was so much freedom, and I was very social. But I still wasn't sure what I wanted to do. I loved mathematics and physics in high school, and thought about studying biology or geology and maybe becoming a teacher, but I didn't see myself as a teacher. I also applied to dentistry school, in part because I had a boyfriend at the time who was studying dentistry. The dentistry school accepted me, but I decided not to pursue that either.

It was about that time that I met Edvard with a friend of mine on Karl Johans gate, the main pedestrian mall in downtown Oslo. I recognised him, of course, as the smart kid from my high school. He was visiting before he started at the university, and when I found out that he would be coming back to Oslo to start his studies in January, I told him to look me up so that I could show him around. And he did.

We quickly became friends. We decided that we would study psychology together, so we could learn about the brain. That brought me back to my dreams of my childhood, when I was so eager to understand why we do things. I was in heaven.

During our first year in the main psychology programme we were in the same social psychology class, called Psychology of Small Groups. We published a paper with several classmates and our teacher, Professor Skårdal, as a result of our research from that class. This was our first paper—"The interactional effects of personality and gender in small groups: A missing perspective in research," published in the *International Journal of Small Group Research*. Professor Skårdal liked us so much he tried to encourage us to study social psychology, but we said, "No thanks, we want to study the brain!" We simply burned with eagerness to understand the brain.

TERJE SAGVOLDEN AND PER ANDERSEN

We started in Terje Sagvolden's lab during our second semester. He was studying hyperactivity in rats. At the same time, our own relationship had changed from a friendship to a romance, and we got engaged on top of Mt. Kilimanjaro. It was a dream place for both of us—Edvard loves volcanoes, all volcanoes, and since my childhood encounters with missionaries, I had always wanted to go to Africa.

Working in the Sagvolden lab involved studying pure behaviour for two years. It was quite exciting, and it was interesting to work with rats, to try to understand why these animals were hyperactive. He taught us experimental design, especially the need to have controls in an experiment, and we learned a lot of behavioural theory. But we pushed him very hard, we kept asking him, "Can't you go into the brain?" We had this crazy energy, this drive to know—it wasn't just Edvard, or just me, it was the two of us together.

Eventually it came time for us to do our master's thesis work and we realised that if we were going to have any opportunity to study the brain directly, we needed to work with Per Andersen in the neurosciences group. This was a problem, because we knew he didn't really like psychologists—all the people in the Department of Neurosciences at that time were medical doctors—and that his research group was full.

When we finally got to talk to him, I decided that I was not going to leave the room until he accepted us as graduate students. I felt like I had been glued to the chair. In the end, I think he just realised he couldn't get rid of us. He finally told us, "Fine, if you are going to do your master's research here, you have to read this paper (by Richard Morris on water mazes), see if you understand it, and then build a water maze lab. If that is a success, then you will be allowed to do a master's thesis in my lab." I remember I said, "Oh wonderful, because we want to do a PhD with you, too!"

BUILDING A WATER MAZE LAB

Per wanted us to build a water maze literally from scratch—a tank 2 metres in diameter by 50 cm high. When we left the meeting, I said to Edvard, "This is crazy!" Fortunately my brother-in-law worked at Det Norske Veritas and I called him, and he was able to help us buy a tank. We also had to get a marine pump so we could pump 1,250 litres of water out of the tank—we had a hose so we could pump the water into a toilet across the corridor. The water had to have milk in it because it had to be murky. That meant we had to change the water every day or it would smell, because the water temperature had to be at 25 degrees C so that the rats would feel comfortable in the pool when they searched for the hidden platform.

So we were psychology students during the day, and then worked in our lab at night. Per had a programmer who helped us write a programme so that we could track the rats as they swam in the maze—this was at the point where you couldn't buy anything off the shelf. Early on we realized we had to use hooded rats rather than the albino Wistar rats, because it was easier to track their movement and because they are dark eyed and have better vision than the red-eyed albino rats.

Per showed us how to make tiny lesions in the hippocampus, because he had this idea that he wanted to study LTP in the living brain. Long-term potentiation, LTP, is how the connections between neurons in the brain are strengthened, and had actually been discovered in 1966 by Terje Lømo, in Per's group and supervised by Per. We first had to make lesions in the dorsal and ventral parts of the hippocampus so that a hippocampal slice was left on both sides of the brain. Per's idea was that it would be easier to detect LTP in the living brain if the area where such changes could occur was restricted. This was a brilliant idea, but in order to find out how big this slice had to be to support learning we had to make lesions of different sizes, both in the dorsal and the ventral hippocampus. Theodor Blackstad helped us to figure out where the boundaries of the hippocampus and the subiculum were.

The challenge for us was that we were psychologists, we didn't know much about the brain's anatomy. We first had done one brain dissection on a human cadaver, and that was it. But we learned fast.

LOOKING FOR LTP

Per's idea was to give the animals extensive training in the water maze so after they had learned a lot, we could measure the changes in the tiny hippocampal slice that was left in the brain. He predicted that this slice would have increased synaptic efficiency (LTP) compared to animals who did not learn. He was so excited when he told us about his dream. His excitement was so important for us, and he was a great inspiration.

We thought that we first needed to find out if the animals could learn at all if they had these kinds of lesions, and then we also needed to have controls. We needed to know if we left the middle part of the hippocampus untouched, would the rats be able to learn if we removed the dorsal part, and what would happen if we removed the ventral part.

Once we did this, we found out that when the rats had a lesion in the dorsal part of the hippocampus they didn't learn, but if they had a lesion in the ventral part they were fine—if we made large lesions in the ventral part they could still navigate perfectly well. The hippocampus was known to be involved in this behaviour, but what we found out was that it was only the dorsal part of the hippocampus that was involved in spatial learning and memory, and that the hippocampus was functionally heterogeneous even though it looked like a smooth sausage from the outside.

THE PINK POSTER

Per was president of the European Neuroscience Association (ENA) at that time, and so he allowed us to bring a poster of our research to a meeting of the ENA in Sweden. I have to confess that when I made the poster, I made it pink as a way to tease Per a bit. But maybe the pink also helped it to stand out, because when Richard Morris walked past the poster he commented that he thought our findings on the dorsal-ventral difference were interesting, and he also saw that we had used the water maze.

But he told us that he didn't like our lesion method, because we had used aspiration, which can cut passing axons. He encouraged us to work with Len Jarrard who had just had a sabbatical in Edinburgh and who was an expert in making lesions without removing the fibres, and he thought that was crucial. Richard gave a plenary talk at the meeting and he mentioned our poster, and I thought that was pretty amazing. Edvard and I were so proud!

We published our results in *The Journal of Neuroscience*. This was also our joint master's thesis—we were able to write it together. It was a pretty thick thesis, and a pretty thorough study of the two parts of the hippocampus. We got help from a few external people who came to the lab because Per was an internationally recognised scientist. These visitors included Eric Kandel from Columbia University, who told Per, "You really have to publish this with them," and Larry Squire from the University of California, San Diego, who also encouraged Per to let us publish our results.

FUNDING FOR TWO PhDs

Our experiment also raised the question, if the dorsal part is involved in memory, what does the ventral part do? So we started to read a lot about anatomy, and wondered about the nature of the connections between the entorhinal cortex and the dorsal and the ventral parts of the hippocampus. That was the first time we wrote to Menno Witter at the Free University in Amsterdam, because he had done a lot of work on hippocampal connections.

As we finished our master's thesis, we both wanted to continue with Per on our PhDs, but the challenge was how to get two fellowships to study with him. At the time it was very difficult to get this kind of funding. The Research Council of Norway at the time was concerned about geographic distribution of these grants.

Per had one question that he felt certain would be funded, the relationship between long-term potentiation and memory, which was both a timely and very interesting question. Per told us that we would have to decide which one of us would take the topic and get funded for a PhD. I told Edvard that I thought Per's question was a good topic for him, since he was so interested in the question. Then Per told me that he thought I should also get a PhD, and that he would help me find money.

His plan was for me to collaborate with a colleague of his, Jørg Mørland, in the Toxicology Department, to study what happened to hippocampal synapses if you gave alcohol to an animal. But I didn't like the topic, because I thought the manipulations were too general to learn anything specific about learning and memory and also because I couldn't see myself giving rats the high, high doses of alcohol that you would need to see an effect. So I found a way to convince him that I couldn't do the project—I told him that I was from the Bible Belt of Norway and I simply can't do this. He pushed me but I just refused.

But I was very interested in the fact that we could see synapses with a laser-scanning confocal microscope. This was very new at the time—we had just got the microscope, and it was new enough that people didn't believe that it was possible to see synapses with this equipment. But Per had a dream, and was enthusiastically convinced that it should be possible. Per was still trying to get me to do experiments with alcohol, but I said, no, I'm a psychologist, I want to do exactly the opposite—instead of trying to see if alcohol will reduce the number of synapses, I want to train the animals to see if there is an expansion of the number of synapses with learning. So I started to read, and I was convinced it was possible.

What was interesting was that Per was so sure that this project would be a failure and that it would not be funded that he tried to stop me from sending the grant proposal to the Research Council. I kept going to his office with the application I wrote to see if he had changed his mind, and finally he just gave in—he always had to give in, like my dad typically gave in when I insisted. Then I sent in my application, and both Edvard and I got grants—a surprising and joyful moment in our lives.

PhD RESEARCH

By then we had gotten married, on July 27, 1985 in Oslo. We had the same supervisor, we were studying the same structure in the brain, but we still both got funded from the Research Council of Norway. It was about this time that I realised how insistent I could be—I was always very nice and polite, but if I really wanted something, no one could stop me.

My PhD research involved offering an enriched environment to rats, so I made a big animal enclosure that had different floors. By this time I had Isabel, our oldest daughter, so I made all these toys for the animals when she was there with me, and I changed the environment every day and even moved the floors so that it would be a new environment. I had Isabel on my lap when I observed the animals in the large enclosure.

After 14 days of 4 hours of daily exposures to the enriched environment I took living slices of the hippocampus and filled individual hippocampal cells with Lucifer yellow to stain them. That allowed me to visualise and count the spines in 3-D.

I counted spines blind to the group to which each rat belonged, and found that there was a difference between the rats who lived in the enriched environment and those who didn't. I then trained animals with similar experiences in the water maze, and showed that the animals that had lived in the enriched

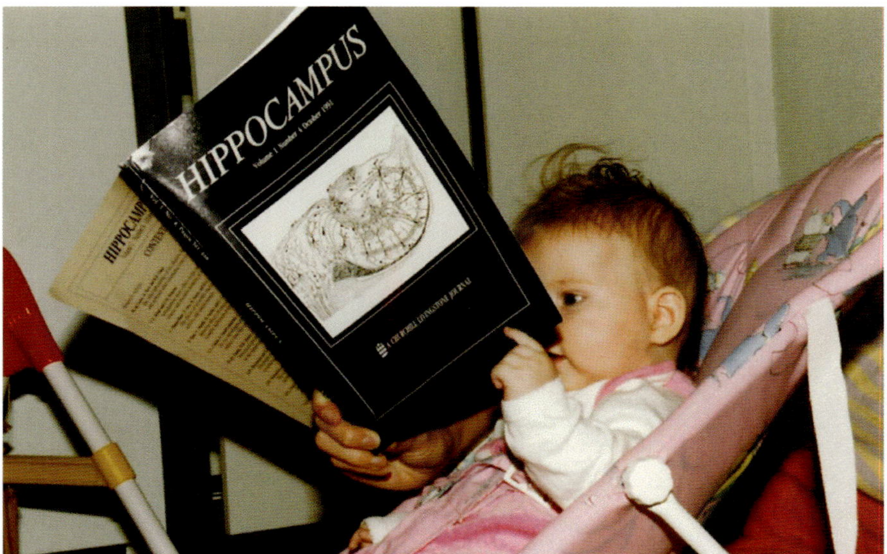

FIGURE 2. Isabel reads the journal *Hippocampus* with great interest. This journal was founded in 1990 by Menno Witter and David Amaral.

environment were faster and better at remembering the hidden platform in the water maze. I published two papers on my work on spines, one in *PNAS* (Proceedings of the National Academy of the Sciences of the United States) and the other in *The Journal of Comparative Neurology*. I also published a third paper on dorsal and ventral differences in the hippocampus in *PNAS*.

CHILDREN AND THE LAB

Many people ask me how I managed to do all this work with two small children—Isabel was born in June 1991, right after we started our PhDs (Fig. 2 and Fig. 3), and Ailin was born in 1995 (Fig. 4), right before we completed our PhDs. The answer is that we were so driven to understand the brain that we simply made things work, we could not see any problems—nothing could stop us. From the earliest days, we took the girls to the laboratory—they were both very good children, very well behaved. Or if I couldn't take them with me, Edvard could take turns watching them. Of course we had nannies and preschool places for the children—both of them attended preschool in Edinburgh, but in the afternoon and in the weekends they often played in the office.

If people objected, I would ask them what was the harm in what I was doing? It wasn't that I had the freedom—I just assumed I could do things, like take my children to scientific meetings and breast-feed them in public, or bring them to the lab. I just didn't see the barriers that others might have seen. We were

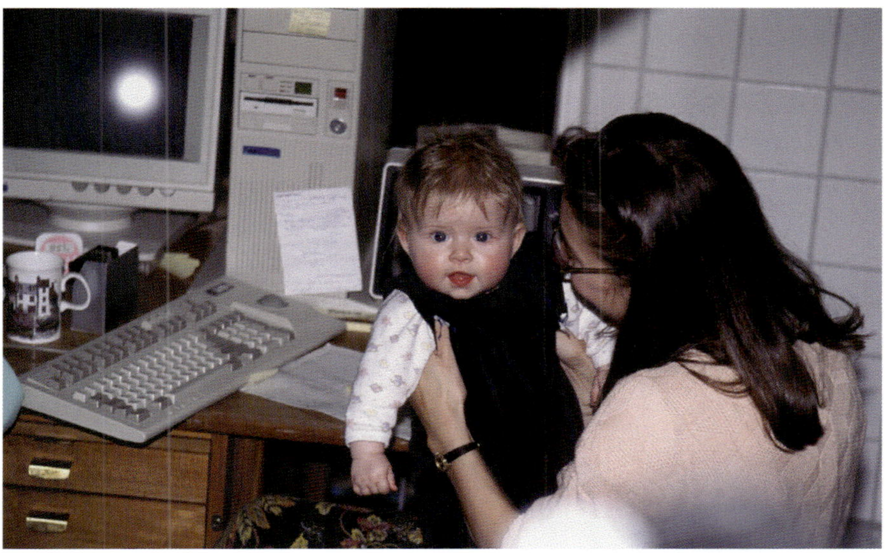

FIGURE 3. Isabel and me in Per Andersen's lab in 1991. I had just started my PhD research.

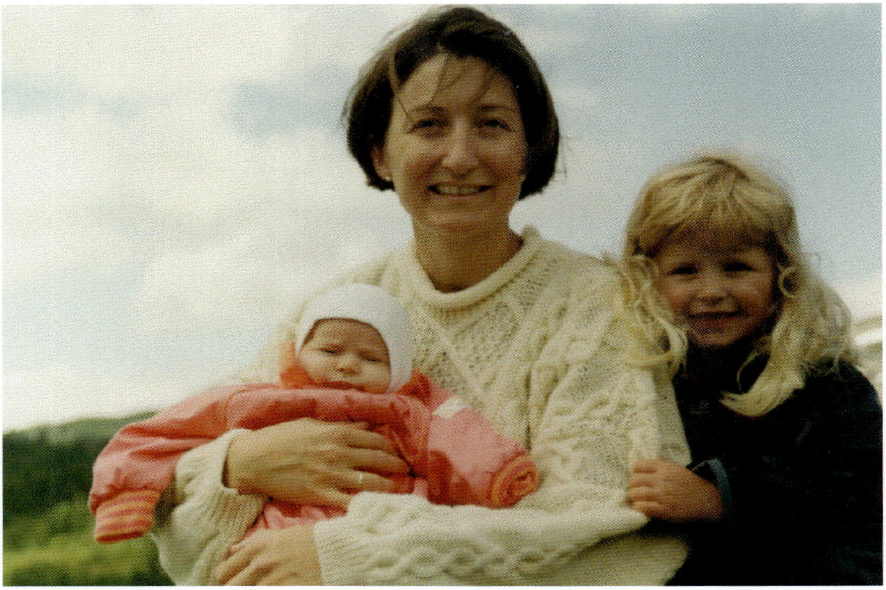

FIGURE 4. Isabel, Ailin and me in 1995, half a year before Edvard and I defended our PhD theses.

somewhat naïve—we couldn't imagine that people would object—so people mostly were very nice and didn't try to stop us.

EDINBURGH AND LONDON

During our PhD work, Richard Morris had invited Edvard and me to the University of Edinburgh to follow up on our master's research findings on the difference between the dorsal and the ventral part of the hippocampus, but using chemical lesions instead of aspiration.

We went there several times during our PhDs, and confirmed our earlier results—that the dorsal and the ventral parts of the hippocampus are different. We also conducted another experiment with him on saturating hippocampal synapses with LTP and testing the animal's ability to learn to find the platform in the water maze. We later completed this work after we came to Trondheim and published the results in *Science*.

We defended our PhDs in Oslo in December 1995, but by that time we were already in Edinburgh with Richard Morris—we even had the girls in a preschool there. In the spring of 1996, Per Andersen and Morris graciously suggested that we go work with John O'Keefe at University College London to learn how to do single cell recordings. We had already met John O'Keefe in Oslo when we defended our PhDs, because he was the opponent for Ole Paulsen, who was one of Per's six students (including us) who defended our theses in the same week.

We had an incredible party after the defences, with all of these top international scientists who served as our opponents, with seminars and sleigh ride! Many of the opponents later became important members of our scientific network, which helped us to win status as a centre of excellence from the Research Council of Norway.

The stay in London, in John O'Keefe's lab, was one of the most learning-rich periods in our lives. John spent an enormous amount of time with us and taught us everything about single cell recordings. He sat with us in the surgery room, showed us how to turn down the tetrodes and do the recordings, how to cluster the data, he talked about the literature—it was all absolutely formative for our future. Edvard had three months with John, and I had just one, in part because of the difficulty of finding care for the children. In Edinburgh we had spots in a preschool for them in Edinburgh only, so in London my brother's wife, Olaug Andreassen, came for a month to help care for them.

TWO POSITIONS AND A LAB

At the same time, one position had opened up at the Norwegian University of Science and Technology in Trondheim, and our former supervisor, Terje Sagvolden, encouraged us to apply for it, just for the experience if nothing else. We knew it was a long shot—when we applied we were still months away from defending our PhDs, and we really weren't thinking that we were ready to settle down just yet.

Suddenly we were called in for an interview, in the autumn of 1995. We told the interview committee that we would not be interested in one position, but Sturla Krekling, the individual at the Department of Psychology who was most involved in the process, really pushed for us and so they offered us two positions. They were in the process of trying to build up the department.

We then said we need a new lab because we wanted to do research—we didn't just want a salary to teach—so we came to them with a list of all the equipment we needed, the prices, the suppliers, because we had been through the process with Per to build the water maze in Oslo. We also knew what was required to build a combined electrophysiology-water maze lab, we had the experience, and we basically got it all. The only condition was that we begin in August of 1996 so that we could teach.

That completely upended our plans, because we had hoped to stay longer with John O'Keefe, or go to the University of Arizona to work with Carol Barnes and Bruce McNaughton's memory and hippocampus group. Both Barnes and McNaughton had been involved with us as PhD examiners, and Arizona was a real neuroscience mecca at the time. We really wanted to go there. But that wasn't possible once we had the offer of positions in Trondheim—the prospect of two jobs and a lab just seemed too good an opportunity to turn down.

(In fairness, we eventually did get a six-week sabbatical in Arizona in 2001, where we learned to do what is called parallel recordings from many dozens of hippocampal cells. It was a technique that was invented by Bruce in the 1990s in Tucson.)

FUNDING FOR COLLABORATION

In parallel with teaching we managed to have our lab operating after a half year of set-up, and after a year or so we had the first results. It took a long time to get data because there was only Edvard and me, and we had to do all the technical aspects of the work along with the actual science—everything from cutting brains to cleaning the rat cages. Our daughters learned to become real "Trøndersk," an expression that describes the residents of mid-Norway in the counties of Nor- and Sør-Trøndelag, where Trondheim is located.

One of the first questions we started with was how are the place cells that O'Keefe discovered generated? What is the basis for the place cells in the hippocampus? To answer this question, we applied for—and received—a collaborative

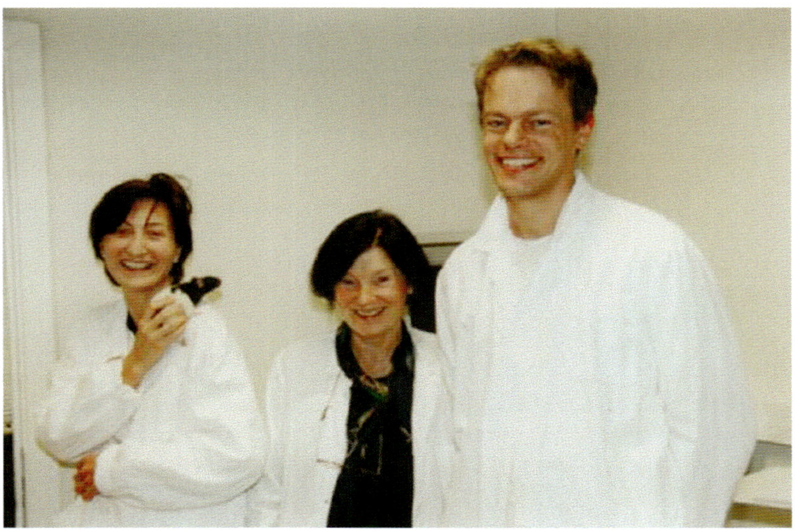

FIGURE 5. Me, Hanna Mustaparta and Edvard at NTNU's Lade campus lab in 2000. This is where we set up our first lab in Trondheim (Photo: Siw Ellen Jakobsen, Forskning.no).

grant from the European Commission in 2000 that gave us three years of funding (Fig. 5).

At the same time, we also applied for funding from the Research Council of Norway's Centre of Excellence programme, a 10-year grant for basic research. This was also approved and as of the December 2002, our group became known as the Centre for the Biology of Memory.

The Centre of Excellence money allowed us to bring internationally recognised researchers to Trondheim for brief but significant periods. We had Menno Witter from the Free University in Amsterdam, Richard Morris from the University of Edinburgh, Bruce McNaughton and Carol Barnes from the University of Arizona, Alessandro Treves from the International School for Advanced Studies in Trieste and Ole Paulsen from Oxford University, all experts in their field, to make a coordinated effort to conduct integrated neural network studies of hippocampal memory. In addition we brought in Randolf Menzel from Freie Universität Berlin who studied neurobiology and spatial memory in the honeybee.

FINDING GRID CELLS

A few weeks after the centre of excellence grant was announced we published a paper that guided us to search for the spatial signal that resulted in place cells in the hippocampus (Brun, Otnæss, Molden, Steffenach, Witter, Moser and Moser, 2002, in *Science*). These exciting data suggested that we should search for the spatial signal in structures upstream of the hippocampus—like the entorhinal cortex. That is what helped us to eventually discover grid cells.

In the Brun et al. (2002) paper we asked where the signal to the place cells came from. The reason this question was so intriguing is that the place signal is buried so deeply in the brain, it really can't be traced back to any sensory input, so how is it made?

We tried to answer this question by making small lesions in the early stages of the hippocampal circuit, in the CA3 area, as a way to interrupt the intrinsic circuit. We then put electrodes in the CA1 area of the hippocampus, which is where most of the place cells had been recorded.

If the place cells were a product of processes that happened at earlier stages of the hippocampus, we should have been able to block those signals by interrupting the hippocampal circuit. But what we found was that we still had spatial signals, even after we made the lesions that should have stopped the signal.

That led us, together with PhD students Marianne Fyhn and Sturla Molden and our colleague Menno Witter, to go to the part of the entorhinal cortex that few other groups had recorded from, the dorso-medial entorhinal cortex. For many reasons people had not worked in the dorsal part of the medial entorhinal cortex before, partly because it was technically difficult, and partly just because of convention.

And this turned out to be the spot, in 2005, where we found grid cells (Fig. 6). Even before we realised that we had discovered a new kind of cell, we realised in 2004 that something was going on in this region with respect to space. The cells there had spatial activity, they had multiple firing peaks and the pattern looked regular—but we really didn't understand what was going on until we extended the size of the environment that we let the rats roam around in a 200-cm-diameter cylinder. And finally, there it was, a clear hexagonal pattern, and that was the discovery of grid cells.

That last sentence makes our discovery sound very simple, but when we first had our results, they were so clear we almost didn't believe them. We thought perhaps that the hexagonal pattern was an artefact of how we made our measurements. But over time we were convinced that this was in fact how the cells were firing.

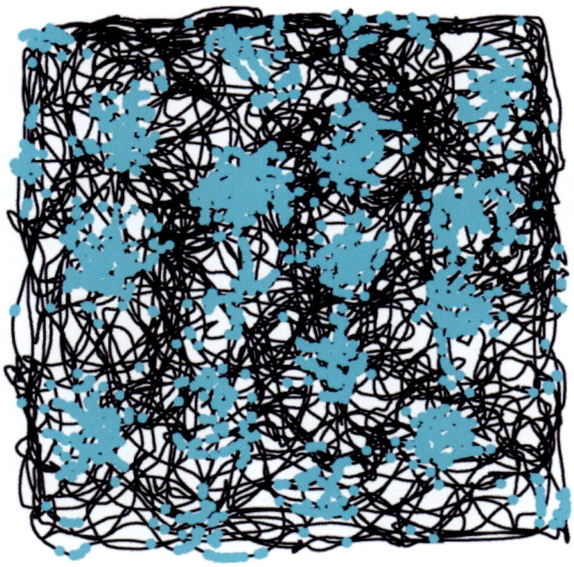

FIGURE 6. A grid cell, recorded by Jonathan Whitlock, a postdoc in our lab some years ago. The rat is named El Burrito. The black trace shows the path of the animal. The blue dots show the firing locations of a single cell in layer II of the medial entorhinal cortex. The activity fields form a hexagonal grid-like pattern that tessellates the whole environment.

We did this research with our students Torkel Hafting, Marianne Fyhn, and Sturla Molden. Marianne came to Trondheim in 2004 to work with us, and Torkel was her boyfriend (and later husband). We offered Torkel a position as a technician in our lab so that they could stay together, and we asked him to work with Marianne on the grid cell project. He later became a postdoc with us. The grid cell results were published in *Nature* in 2005.

THE BRAIN'S OWN INTERNAL CODE

Finding grid cells was exciting because it gave us another piece in the puzzle of how we navigate in space. But the larger significance of the find is that for the first time, we were able to see how the brain takes complex information—in this case, information about where we are and how we move in space—to generate its own internal code to make use of that information. There is no grid pattern out in the world—this is just how the brain makes sense of the environment.

The door was opened on this discovery by John O'Keefe's discovery of place cells, which fire when an animal is at a specific place. In the past, it has been difficult make associations between the firing of neurons deep in the higher parts of the cortex and sensory input, because as the distance between the sensory input and the neuron increases, the firing of the neurons may be triggered by a multitude of converging sensory channels along with intrinsic processes that we don't really understand.

But O'Keefe and his colleagues found that most hippocampal cells had place fields with distinct firing patterns that collectively allowed the brain to create a map of that environment. Here we had neural activity—the firing of the place cell, deep in the hippocampus—that was clearly associated with a property of the environment, the animal's location. The discovery of grid cells took this a step further—and it raised new questions that have continued to shape our research, as we seek to understand how grid cells operate and are generated and how they interact with other cell types and in more distant brain structures. Here, we think, lies a key to unlocking the mystery of how the brain computes.

BORDER CELLS AND BECOMING A KAVLI INSTITUTE

We have made a great deal of progress since our 2005 discovery. In 2006, for example, we and our colleagues, led by Francesca Sargolini, a postdoc, found cells in the medial entorhinal cortex that tell the animal which direction it is facing, called head direction cells. Previously these had been reported in the dorsal presubiculum by Jim Ranck in 1983.

In 2007, we were selected by the Kavli Foundation as the fourth Kavli neuroscience institute, an award that provides funding for basic research in perpetuity. This meant our lab had two names, the Kavli Institute for Systems Neuroscience and the Centre for the Biology of Memory, and a significant increase in funding and support.

In 2008, we and our colleagues, led by then PhD candidate Trygve Solstad, discovered a third type of entorhinal cell type that we called border cells, because they fire at the edges and boundaries of the local environment. We had already seen these kind of cells when Francesca Sargolini discovered the head and conjunctive grid-head direction cells in the medial entorhinal cortex, but we needed a student to search systematically for them and to do the manipulations that were required to call them border cells—like inserting a wall in the box and seeing that the cell would fire again, along the new wall.

GAMMA OSCILLATIONS, MAP RESOLUTIONS AND "A PROTEIN"

Parallel with studying border cells, we asked how CA1 cells in the hippocampus were able to cope with receiving what appeared to be conflicting information from the hippocampus itself—from CA3 and from the upstream structure, the entorhinal cortex, at the same time.

Laura Colgin, our then-postdoc, published a paper in 2009 in *Nature* showing that the brain uses gamma oscillations to route information between grid networks in the entorhinal cortex and the place and memory networks in the hippocampus, which effectively allows the brain to filter out distracting information and focus on one bit of information. We worked for more than five years to finish this amazing story, which shows that passion and persistence go hand-in-hand to produce ground-breaking results.

Also in 2008, with our PhD candidates Kirsten Kjelstrup and Vegard Brun (who were also a couple), we described how the brain makes maps of different resolutions both in the hippocampus and in the entorhinal cortex, thus using place cells and grid cells to create everything from a larger overview map to a finely detailed map. That led the way to the discovery in 2011 led by our colleague Lisa Giocomo that the brain's ability to make these detailed maps at fine resolution was controlled by a single protein. This last paper was published in *Cell* with a companion article in the journal *Neuron*, published by our sister Kavli Institute in New York, headed by our friend and colleague Eric Kandel, whose laboratories had created the mice used in the experiments.

RECORDING FROM MANY GRID CELLS

By 2012, with the ability to record from many grid cells from individual rats, and as many as 186 neurons in one rat called Flekken, we were able to describe how the brain shifts between different map resolutions in a step-wise fashion rather than continuously, and that the brain has at least four difference maps of location, where grid cells are organised into different independent modules in which the scale, orientation and phase relationships are all preserved. These results were published in *Nature* with another fantastic couple and PhD candidates Hanne and Tor Stensola as first authors.

It had not been possible previously to record from so many cells, which is why we suddenly could show that the hippocampal maps were independent. What was also exciting about these data was that we showed in 2007 that when cells in the hippocampus formed statistically significant different ensembles of active cells—different maps for each environment (Fyhn et al., 2007), this was accompanied with a re-anchoring, or shift of the position of the grid cells relative to the boundaries of the boxes in the different rooms.

The models that had already been developed in 2005, just after we discovered grid cells, suggested that place cell activity was the result of the linear summation of grid cell activity (see Solstad, Moser and Einevoll, 2006, for example). Thus, the discovery of different independent grid modules solved the question we faced in 2007, which was to figure out how grid cells could contribute to the activation of several thousands of different ensembles of hippocampal cells if the grid cells were all part of the same map. Independent grid modules suggested that the entorhinal cortex cell activity could trigger the separation of different memories. However, we have not yet been able to prove that this is the way it works.

OPTOGENETICS AND VIRUSES

To address this issue, we first needed to know that grid cells project to the hippocampus. In 2007, we got an email from Sheng-Jia Zhang that eventually led to us being able to answer this question. He asked if we would be interested in having him come to our lab to set up a molecular lab so that we could use a new molecular tool called optogenetics to address questions we were interested in. He came at a moment when we were very eager to understand the entorhinal—hippocampal circuit so we accepted him, his wife Jing Ye and two students he brought with him, Chenglin Miao and Li Lu. They built a molecular lab with the help of a technician in our lab, Alice Burøy.

In 2013 we were able to use defanged viruses to introduce a gene for a fluorescent marker in addition to a gene for the light-sensitive protein channelrhodopsin. The AAV virus was injected into the hippocampus. It was manipulated in a way so that it would go into the axons of cells projecting to the hippocampus. In this way we could examine which neurons in this part of the brain send axons to place cells in the hippocampus. Thus, when we found grid cells, border cells and other cells in the entorhinal cortex responding to the light at a very short latency (less than 10 ms) coming through an optic fibre that we had inserted into the entorhinal cortex along with the electrodes, we started to believe that these cells sent information to hippocampal place cells. Of course we had to do a set of control experiments to be sure. This is why such ground-breaking data usually takes more than four or five years to write up and get published. This story tells us that the way we like to work is not limited by the lack of methods or tools. Either collaborate with other good labs or set up the method in your own lab to follow your dreams!

REMAPPING

We have also worked with cells inside the hippocampus. Since we know from the late 1950s (Scoville and Milner, 1957) that the hippocampus is important for encoding and storing episodic memories, it is exciting to understand how the hippocampus solves problems like not mixing similar information and recognizing an object or an environment with only slight changes. These processes are called pattern separation and pattern completion.

In the mid-1980s, Bob Muller and John Kubie showed that small changes in the environment caused large changes in the hippocampal place maps, in a process they called remapping. In 2005, with Stefan Leutgeb, his wife Jill Leutgeb and others, we found that there are at least two types of these kinds of remapping processes. One we called global remapping and the other rate remapping. Rate remapping is recognised by cells keeping their place preference in the test box, but changing the rate when there is a minor change in the environment, such as changed colours on the wall of the test box.

In contrast, global remapping was typically seen if the changes in environments were big, for example that the test rooms were different even though the test boxes were almost identical. In CA3 of the hippocampus, different cells were active or if they were active in both rooms the spatial preference would be shifted, for example a cell with a place field in the middle of the box in the first room could then have a place field in one of the corners of the box in the other room.

This year we published a study, led by PhD candidate Charlotte Alme, showing that the hippocampus can form ten significantly different new maps when rats were tested in ten new rooms over two days. The ten-room experiment demonstrates that when graduate students are passionate about their work and their animals, impossible data collection is made possible.

TELEPORTATION

The remapping experiments in the lab led us to ask what happens if there is a conflict in the animal's current idea of where it is and the sensory inputs the animals perceives. In order to address this exciting question, Karel Jezek, a postdoc in the lab, ran the animals in a science-fiction inspired experiment. The experiment involved making the animals feel as if they had been teleported from one box to another in a fraction of a second. We were able to create this illusion by training the rats in different boxes that were differentiated only by their lighting schemes. First the rats ran between the boxes, which were connected with a corridor, then the corridor was closed and the rats were tested in only one box where we were able to flip a switch to change the lighting scheme that was associated with one box to the lighting associated with the other box. Thus, while the animal was foraging for chocolate crumbs in one box, we could flip the switch and it would suddenly perceive itself to be located in the other box.

This procedure allowed us to see that each map can be represented in chunks of one theta cycle, or 125 milliseconds, and that the brain's two maps would compete until one took over, and the hippocampus reliably represented the box that was consistent with the landmarks for that given box. This experiment can typically be compared with a situation we all have experienced: We suddenly wake up in the middle of the night in a hotel room. We are confused, and before we realise that we are not at home but in a hotel, our brains have been switching back a forth between the map for the hotel room and our bedroom at home.

SIX RESEARCH GROUPS

Our centre now consists of six research groups, led by Menno Witter (functional anatomy), Yasser Roudi (statistical physics of interference and network organization), Clifford Kentros (transgenic investigation of neural circuits), Jonathan Whitlock (cognitive motor function) and ours (space and memory). Our sixth and newest research group is headed by Emre Yaksi, who studies sensory computations in zebrafish.

The strength of this structure is that we can collaborate across groups. One beautiful example of this was a collaboration between three of the six groups which led us to resolve a question that we had puzzled over for almost eight years. Even with new analyses, new ideas and a lot of discussions of the data both in the lab and at international meetings, we could not figure out what was going on, which is why we did not publish the data.

Menno Witter's group had discovered that stellate cells did not communicate directly with each other, but with a re-route through inhibitory cells. Thus, the grid cells were surrounded by inhibition. At the same time, Yasser Roudi and some of the people from his group had made a computer model of this network and were able to show that this kind of network could produce a functional grid cell network. The excitation could come from the hippocampus and head direction input. The prediction from this model was thus that by removing the excitation from the hippocampus, the grid cells would change from being grid cells to becoming highly head direction modulated.

This is exactly what we found in our lab—but could not explain before the collaboration. We submitted two manuscripts to *Nature Neuroscience* and were lucky enough to get them published back-to-back in 2013. We were so happy and proud to finally be able to publish 8-year-old data that had been so intriguing and yet so difficult to decipher—and to be able to work so closely between the different groups at the centre.

THE NORWEGIAN BRAIN CENTRE

The Norwegian government recognised the importance of neuroscience in Norway by funding the Norwegian Brain Initiative in 2011, which led to us open the Norwegian Brain Centre in 2012 as a collaboration between our lab and research groups working with medical imaging from St Olavs Hospital. The University of Oslo's Centre for Molecular Biology and Neuroscience is a partner in the Norwegian Brain Initiative. We got a new, big, beautiful lab, with the equipment we need to do ground-breaking science.

We are also working hard to make sure that some of our most important lab workers, the rats and mice, have the best environment a science lab can offer. Most of the animals live in big enriched cages, with toys and nests and together with their cage mates. We also try to let animals that wear electrode implants live with their siblings, since rodents are such social creatures. We have a veterinarian who works full-time for our centre, and four well-educated animal caretakers who love animals. In order for them to always remember that the animals

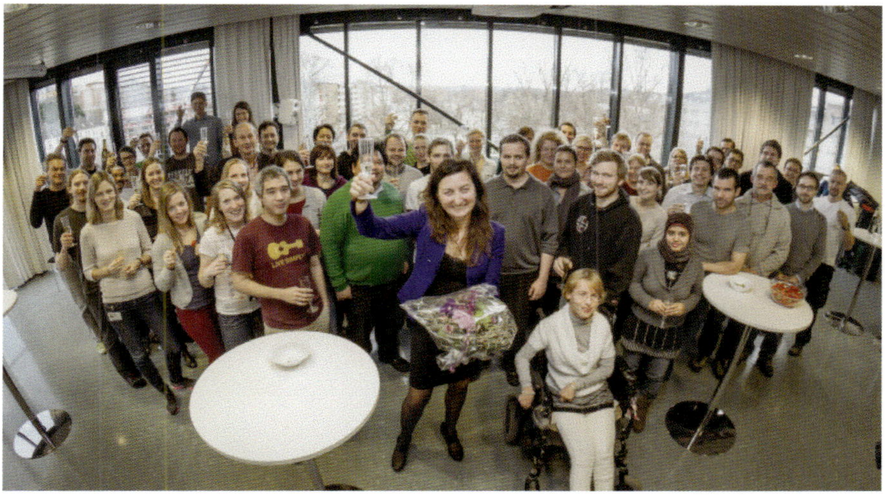

FIGURE 7. Yes, we can! We were awarded a second Centre of Excellence in 2012, the Centre for Neural Computation. This photo is from the celebration, with me, the new Director of our centre in the middle of a wonderful crowd of colleagues (Photo: Tor H. Monsen, *Universitetsavisa*).

are individuals, they have their own pet animals in the animal quarter. Our goal is that our animals be as happy as possible.

A SECOND CENTRE OF EXCELLENCE

Our lab was also awarded funding at the end of 2012 for a second 10-year-long Centre of Excellence by the Research Council of Norway, just as our first decade-long grant ended. Our new centre is called the Centre for Neural Computation, and is directed by me. It was such a relief when we got that grant. We had just ended the first ten year of CoE funding and we were so worried that we could not keep our lab running at the level we had ambitions for if we did not get new funding.

The day the second CoE funding was announced we were euphoric, and we celebrated (Fig. 7)! And celebrations are important as motivation and glue for the team. The support made us even more inspired and enthusiastic than we had been before, and I was handed an exciting new challenge—to serve as director of a centre that had grown from two people to almost one hundred people from different backgrounds and nations (Fig. 8).

The continued support from our colleagues, the Kavli Institute, the Norwegian University of Science and Technology, the Norwegian government, as well

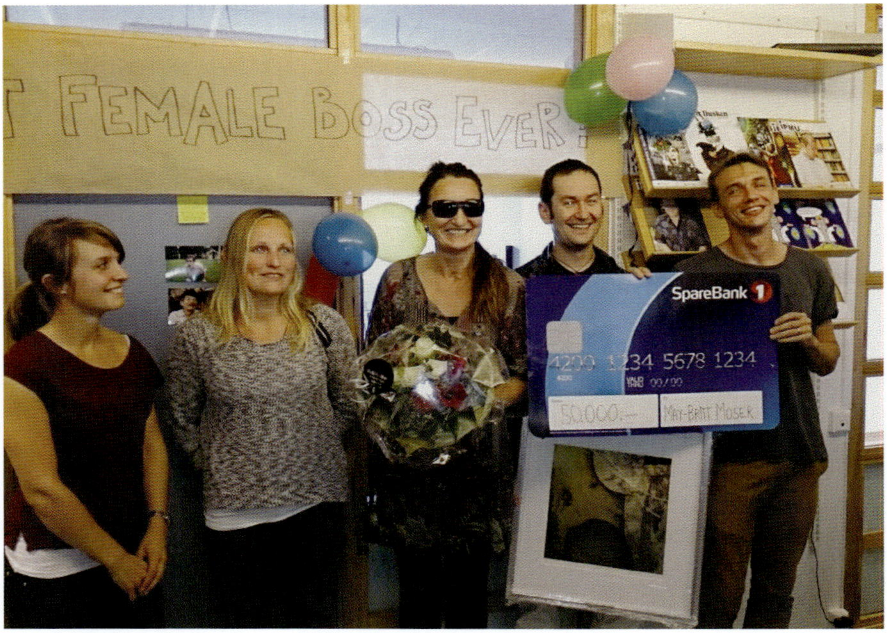

FIGURE 8. Lab members appreciate their new boss! In 2013 I received the Madame Beyer "Best female boss" award. Citation: "in recognition of Moser's superb leadership, scientific achievements, and her high ethical standards, as well as her consistent focus on team work and community spirit." The truth is that it is easy to be the "boss" when you work with the best, from our talented academic colleagues to our amazing technical and administrative staff.

as the city of Trondheim and the county of Sør-Trøndelag has made it possible for us to pursue our dream of unravelling the mysteries of how the brain computes and makes memories and behaviours.

Early on in our careers we realised the importance of bringing in different kinds of expertise in the pursuit of common goals. We also recognise the risks that come from being wedded to only one kind of investigative tool. We're continually looking to expand our neuroscience "toolbox." Our six groups are all eager to work together towards our vision: how does the brain generate cognition and mental function. We have an exciting future in front of us.

TWO CHILDREN AND A LAB

Through hard work and persistence together with fantastic colleagues, I have worked towards my dreams and vision from my childhood: to understand how the neural activity in the brain generates behaviour and cognition. By discovering the grid cell network, we suddenly understood something fundamental about the mystery of the brain—how the brain generates a universal map of the environment. The grid cells that do this are located far away from the senses that tell the animal what is out there. In the same deep structure, the entorhinal cortex, we have also discovered other functional cell types that signal the boundaries of the environment, cells that signal the direction the animal is moving in and cells that combine the head direction and grid signals.

We have shown that with changes of sensory input the universal grid map is shifted and anchored differently to the environment—probably changing the active ensembles of hippocampal place cells. Knowing that the hippocampus contains engrams involved in episodic memories, we have shown that this magic circle of entorhinal and hippocampal cell interactions is part of the mechanism for memory. We are working with findings that are the very essence of being a human being: our conscious memories are what make us who we are, and these memories are anchored in space, in knowing where we are in the environment.

Our two daughters have long joked that our lab is like our third child, and in many ways, they are not wrong. We are proud parents to all three of our

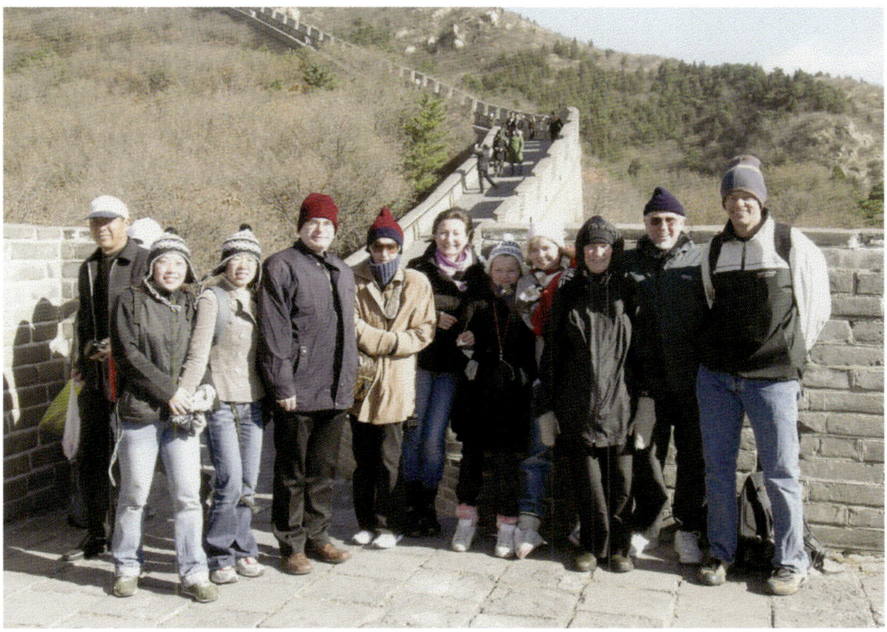

FIGURE 9. As scientists we are expected to travel a lot to give talks. This is from China, in 2006, when we were invited by Joe Z. Tsien to give talks in Shanghai at a symposium he arranged. After the symposium we travelled with two of his students, as well as John O'Keefe and his wife Eileen, Guyry Buzsaki and his wife Veronica, and our children, Isabel and Ailin.

children. Having real "biological" children in addition to our laboratory "child" has brought an amazing happiness to my life. I think that makes it easy for me to do good science.

I have been lucky to live a fairy tale life, with a partner and a long-time collaborator, Edvard Ingjald Moser, who has supported me and helped me fulfil my dreams ever since we met. We have two wonderful daughters, Isabel Maria Moser and Ailin Marlene Moser. They are wise and loving human beings. Being an internationally recognised scientist brings a lot of adventures and a large network of friends and colleagues across the world (Fig. 9). We have travelled to so many different places and learned so much. Our children have come to think it is quite normal to live like this. Ailin was still a pre-teen when she asked us: why haven't we visited Easter Island yet? She could also have asked; why haven't we understood our brains yet?

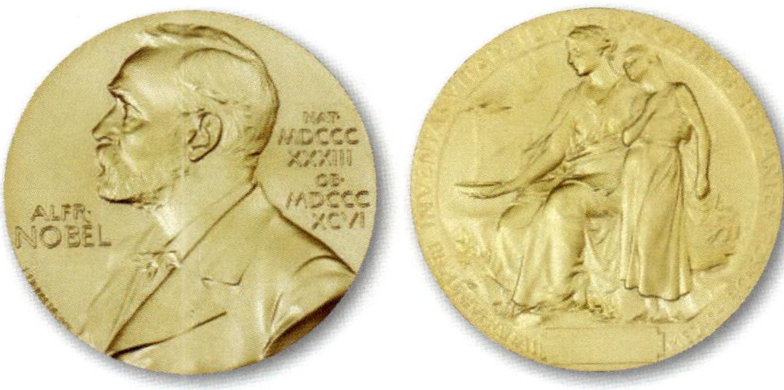

Grid Cells, Place Cells and Memory

Nobel Lecture, 7 December 2014

by May-Britt Moser
Norwegian University of Science and Technology (NTNU), Trondheim, Norway.

On 7 December 2014 I gave the most prestigious lecture I have given in my life—the Nobel Prize Lecture in Medicine or Physiology. After lectures by my former mentor John O'Keefe and my close colleague of more than 30 years, Edvard Moser, the audience was still completely engaged, wonderful and responsive. I was so excited to walk out on the stage, and proud to present new and exciting data from our lab. The title of my talk was: "Grid cells, place cells and memory."

The long-term vision of my lab is to understand how higher cognitive functions are generated by neural activity. At first glance, this seems like an overambitious goal. President Barack Obama expressed our current lack of knowledge about the workings of the brain when he announced the Brain Initiative last year. He said: "As humans, we can identify galaxies light years away; we can study particles smaller than an atom. But we still haven't unlocked the mystery of the three pounds of matter that sits between our ears." Will these mysteries remain secrets forever, or can we unlock them? What did Obama say when he was elected President?

"Yes, we can!"

To illustrate that the impossible is possible, I started my lecture by showing a movie with a cute mouse that struggled to bring a biscuit over an edge and home to its nest. The biscuit was almost bigger than the mouse itself. The mouse tried persistently, without success, but finally took time to sit down and think. This led to success—the mouse got the biscuit up the wall and could bring it to its nest. I think this illustrates the struggle of scientists who are trying to crack

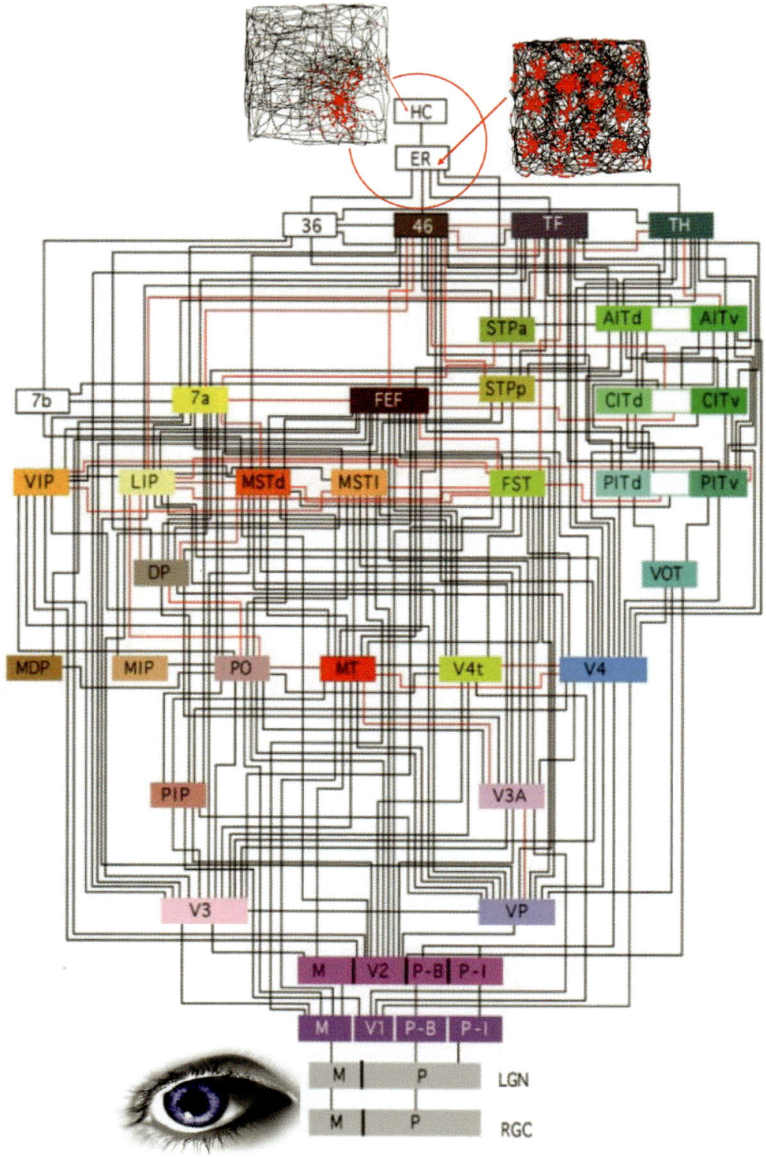

FIGURE 1. Hierarchical map showing complexity and organization of the visual cortices and associated areas. Visual input at the bottom (RGC, retinal ganglion cells; LGN, lateral geniculate nucleus); entorhinal cortex (ER) and hippocampus (HC) at the top. Hippocampal place cells and entorhinal grid cells with trajectory in grey and spike positions in red are indicated. By studying functional cell types at the top of the hierarchy we might understand the computational mechanisms that are responsible for other cognitive functions as well. Reproduced, with permission, from Felleman and van Essen (1991).

the brain's fundamental codes. Occasionally, between long periods of strenuous effort, there is a sense of Eureka when we understand an additional piece of the brain puzzle.

In this lecture, I will show how the discovery of place cells and grid cells has opened our eyes to some of the secrets of the brain, and how work on these cells has put us on the track of the neural computations responsible for perception of space as well as cognitive brain functions in general. Grid cells and place cells comprise a large fraction of the cells in the entorhinal cortex and the hippocampus, respectively—brain regions that are almost as far away from the primary sensory and motor cortices as one can get. The entorhinal cortex and the hippocampus represent the peak of the cortical hierarchy, in the sense that these regions receive highly processed information from nearly all regions of the cortex and that they also project information back to each of these regions (Fig. 1; Felleman and van Essen, 1991; Squire and Zola-Morgan, 1991; Witter and Amaral, 2004). The fact that the characteristic firing pattern of place cells and grid cells cannot be extracted from any particular sensory input suggests that the pattern arises within the hippocampal-entorhinal circuit itself. We have not yet deciphered the neural codes for the grid pattern or the localised firing of the place cells but the presence of experimentally controllable firing correlates, combined with the access to activity patterns of multiple discrete cell types, provides us with a powerful model system. This model system can be used to determine not only how specific activity is generated but also how it gets transformed from one cell type to another. By extracting the principles for formation and transformation of firing patterns in the hippocampal-entorhinal space circuit, we can learn a lot about how the cortex operates in general.

THE RELATIONSHIP BETWEEN GRID CELLS AND PLACE CELLS

The hippocampal-entorhinal space circuit consists of several functionally distinct cell types. The first one to be discovered was the place cell (O'Keefe and Dostrovsky, 1971). As John O'Keefe told you in the first lecture, place cells fire specifically when animals are in certain locations in the environment. Each cell has its own set of preferred firing locations—or place fields. In small enclosures, most cells have only one firing field. Different cells fire at different locations, such that in any ensemble of a few dozen place cells, every single place in the environment is covered by a unique subset of simultaneously active place cells (O'Keefe, 1976; Wilson and McNaughton, 1993). The unique firing patterns associated with every single position led O'Keefe and Nadel (1978) to propose that the hippocampus was the cognitive map of the brain.

The discovery of place cells raised questions about the origin of the place signal. Were the place cells alone, or was there a wider network with different cell types responsible for different functions? As Edvard Moser told you in the second lecture, an obvious place to look for counterparts of the place cells was

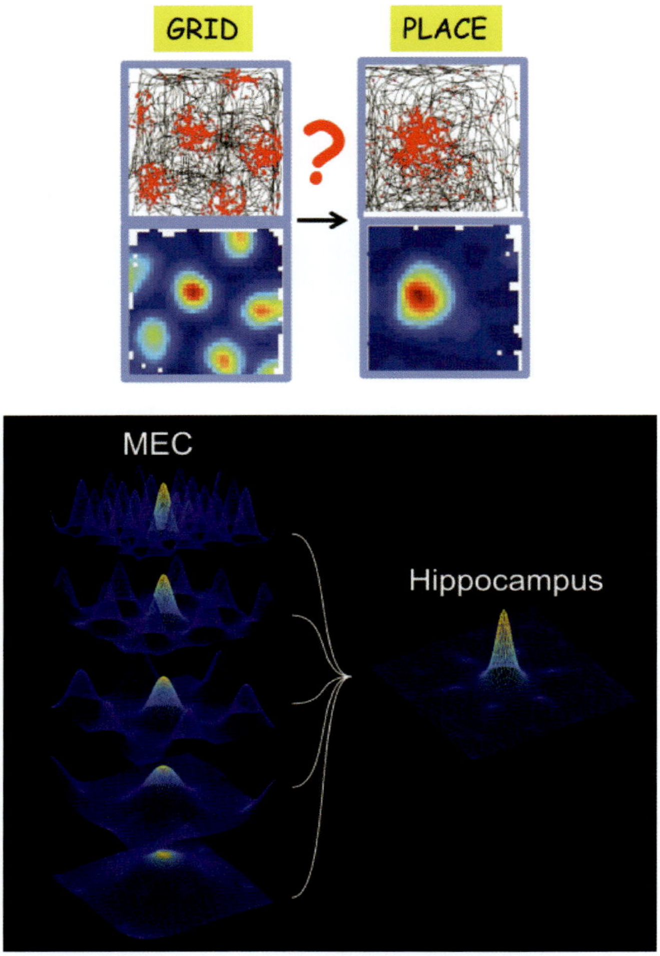

FIGURE 2. Grid cells and place cells are only one synapse apart, but we do not know how grid patterns are transformed to place fields. The bottom part of the figure shows grid fields for five cells and a place field for one cell. Firing rate is represented on the z-axis, position on the x- and y-axes. Place fields may be generated through a Fourier-like process by linear summation of grid fields across a range of grid scales. The coloured central peak will add up to a place field whereas other peaks (in dark blue) will cancel due to different wavelengths. Artwork by Tor Stensola. Modified, with permission, from Solstad, Moser and Einevoll (2006).

the entorhinal cortex, since nearly all cortical input to the hippocampus is mediated via this region (Witter and Amaral, 2004). Our exploration of this area a decade ago led to the discovery of grid cells—cells that fire at discrete locations, like place cells in the hippocampus, but in a unique manner (Fyhn et al., 2004; Hafting et al., 2005). Each grid cell fires at multiple locations and these multiple locations form a periodic hexagonal lattice that covers the entire surface of the local environment.

The presence of grid cells only one synapse upstream of the place cells led us and others to ask whether place cells receive their spatial information from grid cells. Do place cells reflect a transformation of signals from grid cells? Half a century ago, Hubel and Wiesel (1962) suggested that orientation-selective cells in the visual cortex originate by linear summation of inputs from cells with concentric circular receptive fields. In the same way, we and others suggested after the discovery of grid cells that place fields emerge by linear summation of output from grid cells over a range of spatial scales (Fuhs and Touretzky, 2006; McNaughton et al., 2006; Solstad et al., 2006). It was suggested that, via a Fourier-like summation process, inputs from periodic grid fields with different grid scales would be sufficient to generate a single place field (Fig. 2). The periodicity of the grid fields was not inherited by the place cells because the different wavelengths of cells with different grid scales cancelled each other except at the central peak.

Over the subsequent years, we learnt that the story was more complicated. Grid cells were not the only entorhinal cell type with a spatially modulated firing pattern. In 2006, one year after the discovery of grid cells, we found that grid cells co-localised with head direction cells. Head direction cells had been discovered in the 1980s in the presubiculum by Jim Ranck (1985). These cells fire if and only if the rat faces a certain direction in the environment (Taube, 2007). Head direction cells were subsequently found in a number of brain regions (Taube, 2007) and they also turned out to be abundant in the medial entorhinal cortex, primarily in the intermediate and deep layers (Sargolini et al., 2006). Two year later, we found a third cell type in the same circuit—the border cell (Solstad et al., 2008). Border cells fired if and only if the animal was near one or several of the borders of the local environment, for example a wall of a recording enclosure or an edge of a table. Border cells were present in all layers, including layer II, where we found most of the grid cells. Similar cells were reported in the same region by the Knierim group (Savelli et al., 2008) and in the subiculum by the O'Keefe group (Barry et al., 2006; Lever et al., 2009). Grid cells, head direction cells and border cells maintained their firing properties across environments—a grid cell was always a grid cell, a head direction cell was always a head direction cell, and a border cell was always a border cell (Solstad et al., 2008).

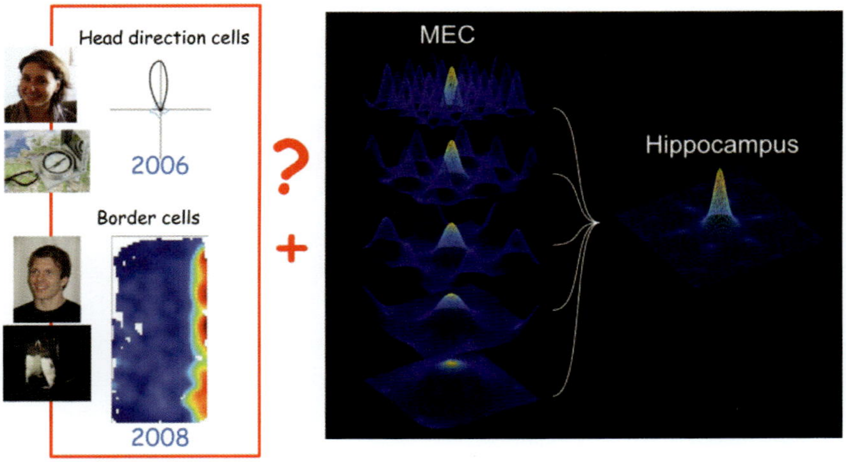

FIGURE 3. Place cells could be computed by the summation of inputs from grid cells over a range of scales (Fig. 2). However, more recent work suggests that both head direction cells and border cells project to the hippocampus (Zhang et al., 2013), suggesting that place fields may be generated by spatial input from a variety of cell types. Top: Francesca Sargolini. Bottom: Trygve Solstad.

The existence of multiple functional cell types in the medial entorhinal cortex led us to ask if place cells receive spatial information not only from grid cells but also from head direction cells and border cells (Fig. 3). The question is particularly relevant because computational models from the late 1990s pointed to cells with boundary-dependent activity as a potential origin of the hippocampal place signal (O'Keefe and Burgess, 1996; Hartley et al., 2000). It was hypothesised, in these models, that place cells receive input from cortical 'boundary-vector cells', cells whose firing rates reflected distance and direction relative to specific boundaries in the local environment. Border cells in the medial entorhinal cortex would represent a subclass of this hypothesised input population.

During the past few years, we have tried to determine which of these cell types project to the hippocampus. We have developed a method for functional tagging of neurons with axonal projections to a target region—in our case the hippocampus (Zhang et al., 2013). Together with Sheng-Jia Zhang and Jing Ye, we developed recombinant adeno-associated virus (AAV) carrying the genes for the light-sensitive cation channel channelrhodopsin-2 (ChR2) as well as a fluorescent marker protein. The virus was infused into the hippocampus, where it transduced not only local neurons but also axons of cells with projections into the hippocampus. Neurons with axonal projections to the hippocampus could subsequently be identified in the superficial layers of the medial entorhinal cortex, as well as other regions with hippocampal projections (Fig. 4). No staining was observed in the deeper layers of the entorhinal cortex, which have limited projections to the hippocampus.

Expression of ChR2 in hippocampus-projecting medial entorhinal cortex neurons made it possible to link the neurons to their functional firing profile. Implanting tetrodes and an optic fibre in the medial entorhinal cortex of animals with hippocampal injections of AAV-ChR2, we first identified ChR2-expressing neurons as entorhinal cells with constant minimal latency responses to a short, locally delivered light pulse (Fig. 4). These cells responded at invariant latencies after the illumination—with a trial-to-trial variation of less than 1 ms. The functional identity of the light-responsive cells was then determined by recording their activity while the animal was running in an open field. As expected, a considerable portion of the responsive neurons—approximately 25%—were grid cells. However, there were also light-responsive border cells (7%) and head direction cells (12%). Because the light-responsive neurons must have axons to the hippocampus (otherwise they would not have been infected), the findings

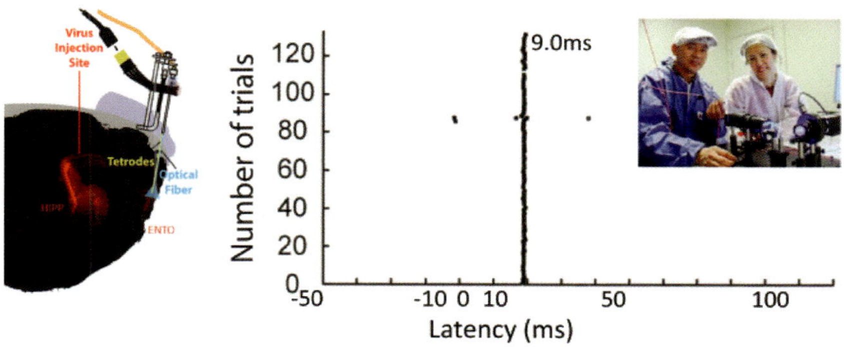

FIGURE 4. The hippocampus receives input from multiple functional cell types in the medial entorhinal cortex. Top right: Sheng-Jia Zhang and Jing Ye. Left: Expression of ChR2 after injection of traffic-improved recombinant adenoassociated virus in the hippocampus. The virus carried the gene for channelrhodopsin (ChR2) as well FLAG (which encodes a peptide sequence that can be identified by fluorescent antibodies). Transduced neurons are labelled in red. Note expression not only in the hippocampus but also in the medial entorhinal cortex, suggesting retrograde transduction of entorhinal cells with axonal projections into the hippocampus. The rats were implanted in the medial entorhinal cortex with a microdrive containing tetrodes for single unit recording as well as an optic fibre for photostimulation of locally infected cells. Right: Raster diagram showing spike times for a single grid cell after laser stimulation on more than 120 trials. The cell fires at a constant latency (9.0 ms), suggesting that it was directly activated by light. Reproduced, with permission, from Zhang et al. (2013).

suggest that the hippocampus receives input from a broad spectrum of entorhinal cell types, including grid cells and border cells, but also a large fraction of cells with no detectable spatial firing pattern.

The retrograde transduction study implies that projections from the medial entorhinal cortex to the hippocampus are functionally mixed. Most likely, place cells can be formed from a variety of spatial inputs, including grid cells and border cells. In this sense, the data provide support for both grid cell and boundary vector cell models of place cell formation. However, the detailed mechanism for place field formation remains elusive. As of today, we do not know if different place cells receive inputs from different cell classes in the medial entorhinal cortex, or if, alternatively, all cells receive the same mix of inputs, with differentiation taking place not at the level of inputs but locally in the hippocampal circuit or at the dendritic level. One possibility is that individual cells receive inputs from a variety of entorhinal cell types with different subsets of inputs predominating at different times. A number of more recent models have proposed that place fields can be generated from any pattern of spatially modulated input, regardless of whether it is periodic or modulated by distance from boundaries. The condition is that selected inputs can be amplified by local circuit activity or Hebbian plasticity (Rolls et al., 2006; de Almeida et al., 2009; Savelli et al., 2010; Monaco and Abbott, 2011). It will remain for the future to determine to what extent place cells are formed by hard-wired connections between entorhinal cells and hippocampal cells, but the functional tagging study suggests that place fields can be formed in more than one way and that intrahippocampal processes contribute to the transformation mechanism.

ENTORHINAL SPEED CELLS

I have told you that the entorhinal cortex contains spatially modulated cell types such as grid cells and border cells. These cell types provide accurate information about the animal's current location, but how is this information updated in accordance with the animal's movements in the environment? A number of observations point to grid cells as part of a path integration-based representation of space, where displacement is obtained by constantly integrating running velocity over short intervals (Hafting et al., 2005; McNaughton et al., 2006). In this scheme, new grid cells are recruited, in a periodic manner, as the animal moves from one place to another, with the selection of cells dependent on information about the animal's current speed and direction. But is such information available to the grid cells? Directional information is expressed in head direction cells, but while speed has been observed to correlate weakly with the firing rates

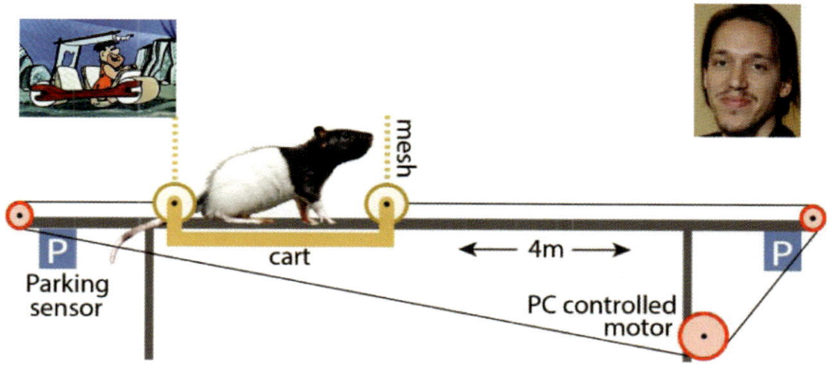

FIGURE 5. Experimental set-up for identification of speed cells. Spike activity was monitored as a rat ran along a linear track with its body confined inside a computer-driven frame without a bottom (a 'Flintstone car') that was moved along the track at a pre-set speed. Top right: Emilio Kropff.

of some grid cells (Sargolini et al., 2006; Wills et al., 2012), the existence and nature of a local speed signal in the entorhinal microcircuit has remained unclear. In the following section, I will present new data suggesting that a population of cells in the medial entorhinal cortex is dedicated to the representation of speed.

To estimate the relationship between firing rates and speed, we recorded neuronal activity under strict control of the animal's running speed (Fig. 5). Together with postdoc Emilio Kropff, we monitored activity in the medial entorhinal cortex while rats ran across a linear track with their body confined inside a frame without a bottom—a Flintstone car. The frame was moved along the track at a computer-determined speed. The recordings showed that among the cells recorded in the medial entorhinal cortex, approximately 15% had firing rates that correlated strongly with the running speed of the animal, irrespective of where the animal was on the track. In these cells, a change in running speed was always accompanied by a change in firing rate. The faster the speed, the higher the firing rate (Fig. 6). The relationship was linear. The observations in the Flintstone car suggested that we had come across a new functional cell type—speed cells.

But if speed cells represent speed, and nothing else, they should also do so in the open field environments where we identified both grid cells and border cells. This led us to record, in 17 rats, from more than 2000 cells in the medial entorhinal cortex while the rats foraged randomly in standard square enclosures. The rats covered a wide range of instantaneous running speeds, from 0 cm/s to more than 50 cm/s. For each cell, we plotted firing rate as a function of running speed.

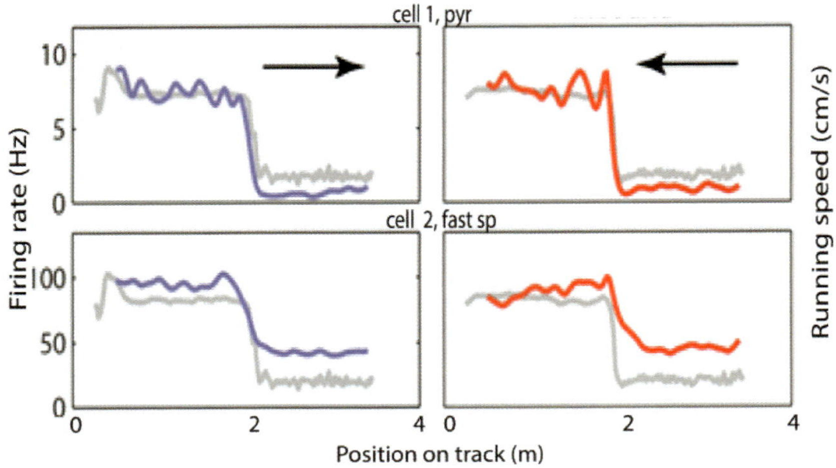

FIGURE 6. Firing rate and running speed as a function of position for two representative speed cells. Pyramidal cells (pyr); fast spiking cell (fast sp). The speed of the Flintstone car is changed abruptly at the middle of the track. Top: Curves show the mean firing rate of the cell (blue and red, left axis) and the mean running speed of the rat (grey, right axis). Bottom: Pearson correlation between instantaneous running speed and mean firing rate for different car speeds.

As in the Flintstone car, many cells had firing rates that increased linearly with speed (Fig. 7). Approximately 15% of the cells had speed-rate relationships exceeding the correlations obtained in a shuffled distribution of spike-time pairs. Virtually none of the cells exhibited any spatial preferences; mean firing rates were similar across the entire recording environment.

Having established that a considerable number of entorhinal cells respond to instantaneous running speed, we asked whether these cells form a population of their own, or if they overlap with other cell types. Grid cells, head direction cells and border cells were classified by standard statistical criteria, and speed cells were identified as cells with speed-rate correlations exceeding the 99th percentile of the shuffled distribution. Speed cells were found in all cell layers (Fig. 8). Throughout the circuit, the speed cells formed a discrete cell category (Fig. 9). The overlap between speed cells and any of the other cell types was significantly lower than expected by chance from random category assignments. For example, only 8 out of 518 grid cells had significant responses to speed. The overlap with head direction cells and border cells was similarly low. These analyses suggest that speed cells are functionally distinct from other entorhinal cell classes. The spatial and directional information expressed by these cells is an order of magnitude lower than that of all other entorhinal cell types.

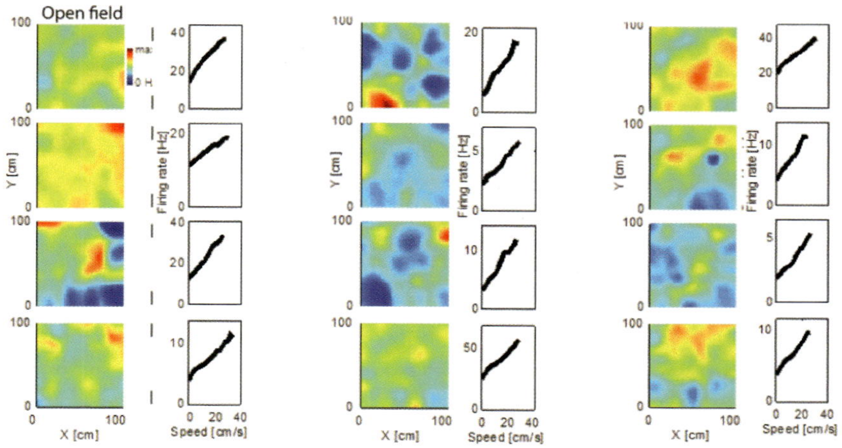

FIGURE 7. Firing rate as a function of position and running speed in 12 representative medial entorhinal speed cells recorded during chocolate cereal-motivated free foraging in a square open field. Left for each cell: colour-coded spatial rate map showing maximal activity in red and minimal activity in blue. Right for each cell: Mean firing rate as a function of running speed. All speed cells demonstrated a linear relationship between running speed and firing rate.

Taken together, our findings show that the medial entorhinal cortex has a large dedicated population of speed cells, characterised by a linear response to firing rate. The linear nature of the speed-rate relationship makes the temporal integration of the signal proportional to the displacement of the animal in the environment. The information encoded by these speed cells provides exactly what grid cells need for position to be updated dynamically during movement. We do not know yet how the speed signal is generated, but observations of speed-representing cells in the mesencephalic locomotor region (Lee et al.,

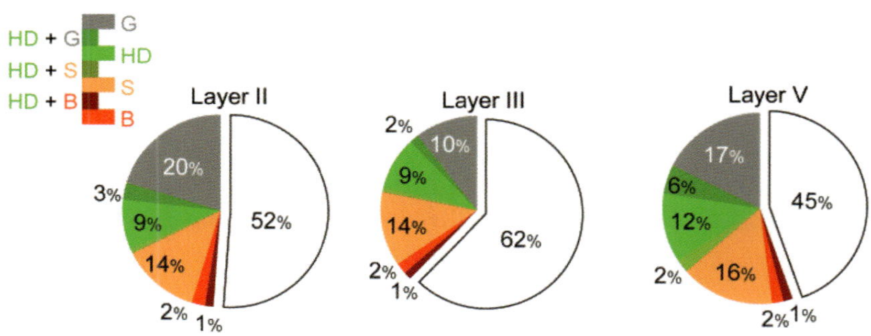

FIGURE 8. Pie charts showing distribution of speed cells across layers of the medial entorhinal cortex. Speed cells were located in all cell layers.

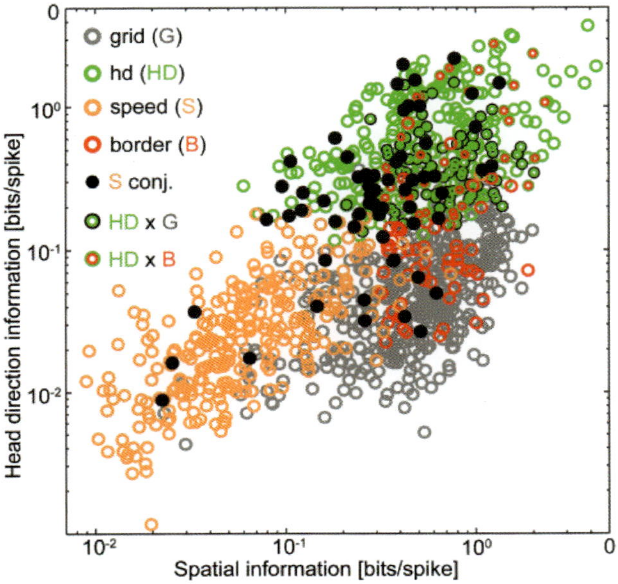

FIGURE 9. Speed cells form a population of their own. The scatter plot shows head direction and spatial information for more than 1,200 neurons classified as grid, head direction, speed, or border cells. The scale is logarithmic. Each dot corresponds to one cell. Cell identity is colour-coded as indicated; colour code as in Fig. 8. Black dots represent speed cells that met at least one additional criterion. Note the low number of speed cells that satisfy criteria for other cell types.

2014) point to efference copies in this region as a potential source of speed information in the entorhinal cortex as well as other cortices.

THE HIPPOCAMPUS—MEMORY OR SPACE?

Until now the focus of my talk has been on hippocampal and entorhinal circuits for spatial representation. However, are these circuits only important for space? In fact, modern studies of the hippocampus began with a different approach to the function of the hippocampus. More than half a century ago, Scoville and Milner (1957) reported, in patient H.M., that surgical removal of the two hippocampi was accompanied by a severe disruption of memory for daily life events. They described the loss of memory as follows:

> After operation this young man (HM) could no longer recognize the hospital staff nor find his way to the bathroom, and he seemed to recall nothing of the day-to-day events of his hospital life.

For the next 55 years, each time he met a friend, each time he ate a meal, each time he walked in the woods, it was as if for the first time.

But how can the same brain structures be responsible for two so apparently different functions as spatial mapping and memory? The link between space and memory has been known since ancient times. The Greek invented the Method of Loci as a mnemonic device to recall large quantities of information (Yates, 1966). In this technique the subject memorises the layout of a building (a 'memory palace'), or a path through a familiar environment (Fig. 10). The subject then encodes items by placing them at unique locations in the palace, or along the path, as he or she walks through the environment. Retrieval of items

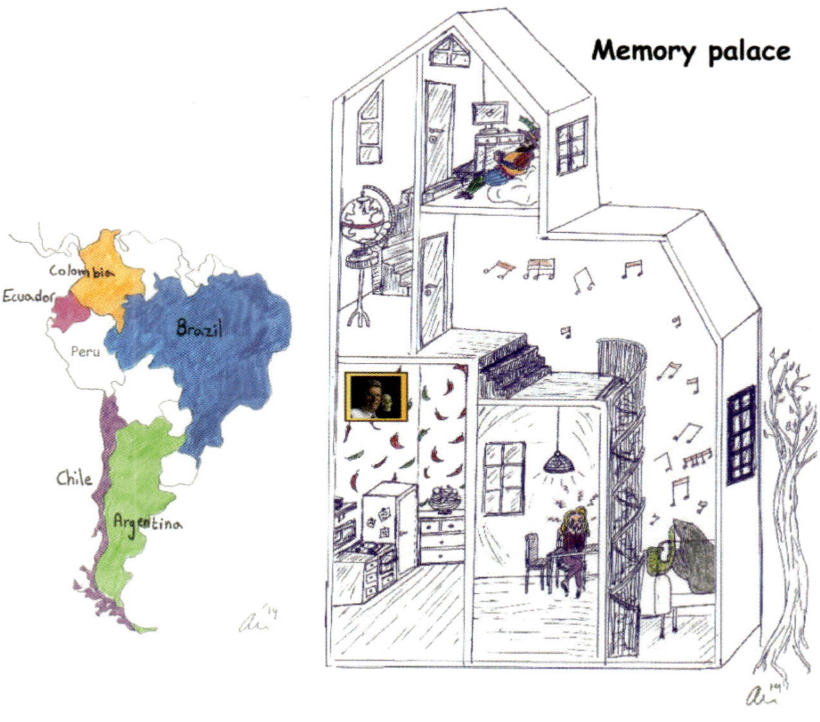

FIGURE 10. Space is used as a framework for storing memories. A cartoon of a 'Memory Palace' can be used to illustrate the Method of Loci. Different countries in South America (left) are associated with symbols placed at unique locations in the memory palace (right). For example, Chile is placed in the room at the bottom left that has chilli wallpaper. Peru is placed in a room with a photo of my former supervisor Per Andersen. The method exploits the natural tendency for memories of objects and events to be associated with space and is widely used as a method for remembering long lists of items. Illustration: Ailin Moser.

is subsequently achieved by walking through the palace once again, which will activate the items in order. The method is efficient in that it increases substantially the number of items that can be recalled, at the same time as interference between the items is reduced. The successful use of this method for over two thousand years points clearly to a link between space and memory.

So if space and memory linked, and the link occurs in the hippocampus, what are the mechanisms? O'Keefe and colleagues observed early on that place cells do not exclusively represent the animal's current location. Place cells may also reflect the memory of a location, expressed as a position-correlated firing pattern in the absence of the sensory inputs that originally elicited the firing (O'Keefe and Speakman, 1987). Reactivation of past place field patterns has subsequently been reported in a variety of circumstances (Pavlides and Winson, 1989; Wilson and McNaughton, 1994; Jarosiewicz and Skaggs, 2004; Leutgeb et al., 2005a). The expression of past locations in the activity of place cells is consistent with a huge clinical and experimental literature pointing to the hippocampus as a key element of the brain's network for declarative memory (Squire, 1992; Squire and Wixted, 2011). Presumably, each memory stored in the hippocampus contains information about place, expressed in firing locations of place cells, as well as the events that take place in each of those places, expressed in the form of rate variations (O'Keefe and Nadel, 1978; Leutgeb et al., 2005b).

If we accept that place cells merge spatial and nonspatial information, from present and past, let us then put the hippocampal memory circuit in a wider anatomical context. So far I have spoken much about the medial entorhinal cortex as a major cortical determinant of neural activity in the hippocampus. However, the hippocampus receives an equally large projection from the lateral entorhinal cortex (Fig. 11). The lateral entorhinal cortex is likely to provide the hippocampus with information about discrete objects as well as olfactory information, considering that cells in this area have been reported to fire specifically in response to discrete objects (Deshmukh and Knierim, 2011; Fig. 12) as well as specific odours (Petrulis et al., 2005; Igarashi et al., 2014).

Motivated by the presence of object-responsive cells, we decided, with graduate student Albert Tsao, to examine whether cells in the lateral entorhinal cortex respond not only when an object is present but also when an object has been in a certain location in the past (Tsao et al., 2013) (Fig. 13). A LEGO toy was placed at an arbitrary location in a standard square open field. Activity was recorded from the lateral entorhinal cortex while the animal investigated the environment. Activity was also recorded during subsequent trials, when the object was no longer there. A small number of cells responded to the presence of the

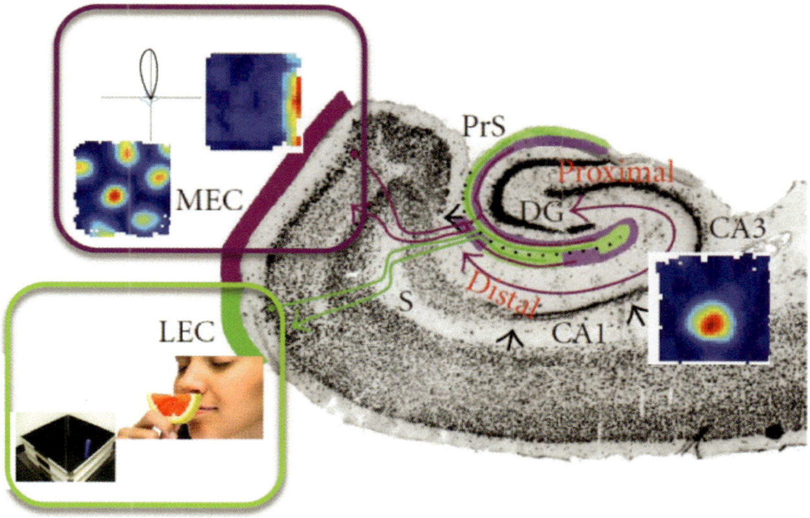

FIGURE 11. Association between position and memory cues. A horizontal section of the entorhinal cortex and hippocampus with cartoons suggesting different functions encoded in the medial and the lateral entorhinal cortex and place cells in the CA region. The firing field of a place cell is indicated over the hippocampus (as in Fig. 1 and 2). Medial entorhinal cortex (MEC), lateral entorhinal cortex (LEC), presubiculum (PrS), dentate gyrus (DG) and subiculum (S). Brain section with projections: Courtesy of Menno Witter.

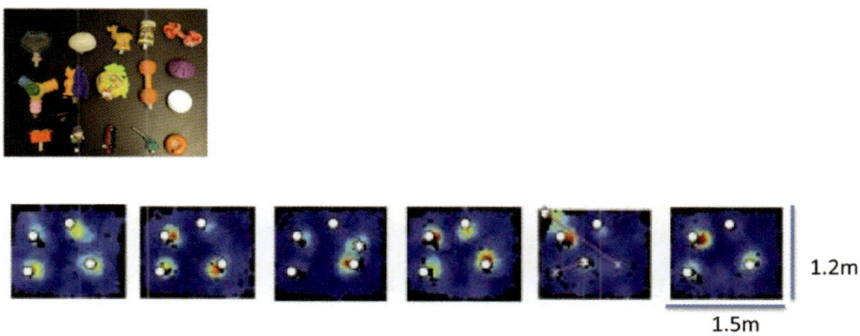

FIGURE 12. Cells in the lateral entorhinal cortex (LEC) respond to objects. Top: Samples of toys used as objects in the box where the rat chased after pieces of food. Bottom: colour-coded rate maps showing the response of a lateral entorhinal cell to objects placed at different positions in the box. The cell responds specifically to the presence of toy objects (objects: white circles, arrows: subsequent object location). Reproduced, with permission, from Deshmukh and Knierim (2011).

object but other cells, intermingled among the object-sensitive cells, responded only after the object had been removed. The response was sometimes transient, lasting for only a few exposures after the presentation of the object, but after repeated exposures, the response could be generally be followed for a long time, in some cases two weeks, as long as the cells could be monitored (Fig. 14). When the object was moved to new locations on successive trials, traces of activity were left at each of those locations (Fig. 13). These findings suggest that cells in the lateral entorhinal cortex are not only involved in encoding of discrete elements of the current spatial environment but also express the memory of objects or events associated with past locations.

Whether trace cells project to the hippocampus remains to be determined but assuming that a large fraction of the lateral entorhinal cells project to the hippocampus, place cells are likely to receive information about discrete objects and events in addition to the spatial information they receive from grid cells and border cells in the medial entorhinal cortex. In the hippocampus, these types of information are likely brought together to form a coherent spatial-nonspatial memory. The Method of Loci may work so well because it exploits the preparedness of the hippocampus for associating space with individual items and experiences.

MECHANISMS FOR ASSOCIATING EVENTS WITH PLACE—ODOURS AS A GATEWAY

I would now like to present some recent data that illustrate potential mechanisms for interaction between the lateral entorhinal cortex and the hippocampus. I present them because they may help us understand how cortical areas communicate in general.

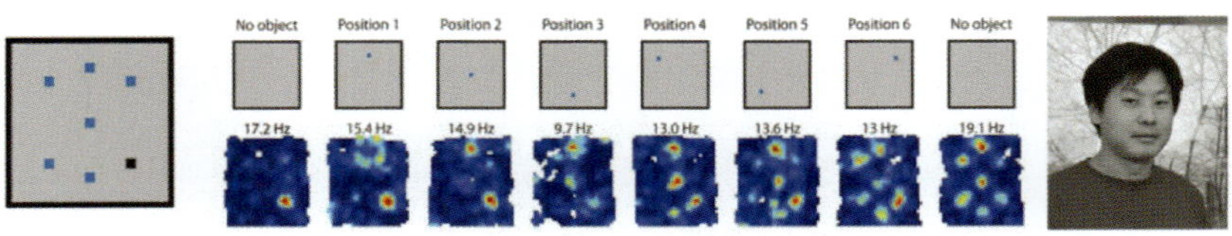

FIGURE 13. Colour-coded firing rate maps showing neural activity in response to past locations of a LEGO toy object. Left: successive positions of LEGO object in the recording enclosure. Black, training position. Blue, new positions on test day (one per trial). Right: object locations on successive trials (top). All rate maps (bottom) are for the same cell. Activity cumulates at places where the object has been located. Right: Albert Tsao. Reproduced, with permission, from Tsao et al. (2013).

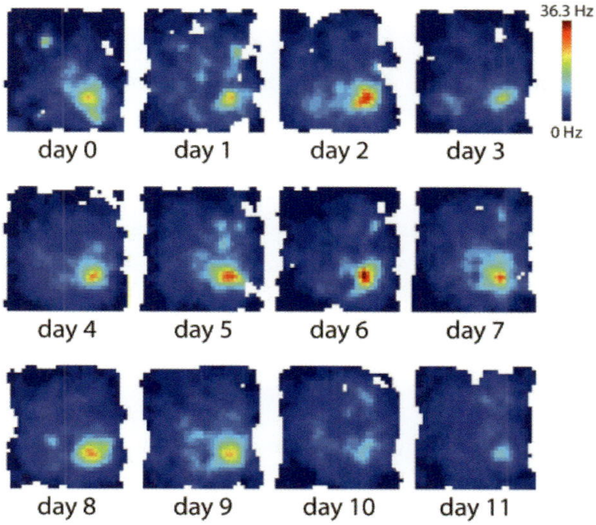

FIGURE 14. Colour-coded rate maps showing long lasting trace of activity in a lateral entorhinal trace cell following exposure to an object at a single location in the recording box. The object was placed for consecutive days at the bottom right of the box. The object was then moved before the recordings in the figure started. Object traces could be seen for almost two weeks after the object was removed. Reproduced, with permission, from Tsao et al. (2013).

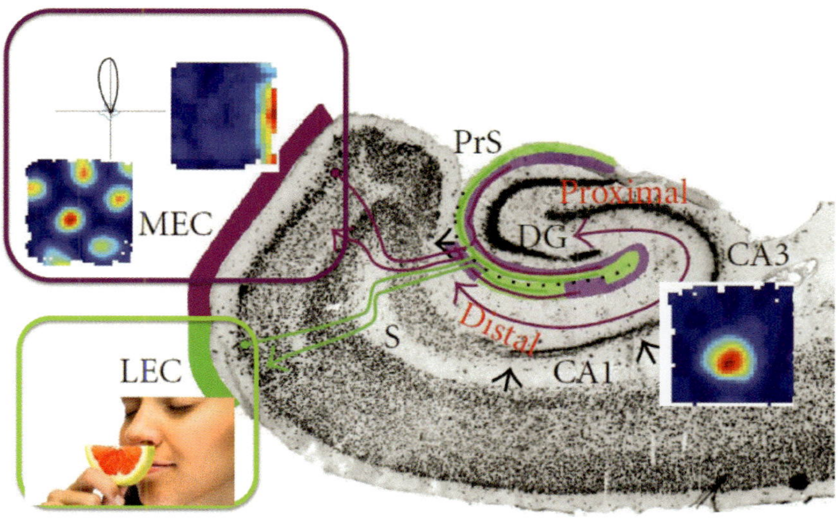

FIGURE 15. The hippocampus receives olfactory information via the lateral entorhinal cortex. Abbreviations as in Fig. 11.

To examine how cells in the lateral entorhinal cortex interact with cells in the hippocampus, let us take advantage of the strong connections that this part of the entorhinal-hippocampal circuit has with the olfactory bulb and the piriform cortex (Burwell, 2000; Witter and Amaral, 2004). When we experience a situation and there are strong odours associated with this situation, the odours are likely encoded in the hippocampus along with the place and other aspects of the experience (Fig. 15). When we re-encounter the odour, it may function as a retrieval cue, and the entire situation may be re-experienced in memory. The power of odours as retrieval cues is beautifully illustrated by Marcel Proust in his novel "In search of lost time," where he declares that ". . . the smell and taste of things remain poised a long time, like souls, ready to remind us, waiting and hoping for their moment . . ." (Fig. 16).

To study the mechanisms of odour-induced memory retrieval in the lab, we teamed up with postdoc Kei Igarashi and trained rats in an odour-place association task (Fig. 17; Igarashi et al., 2014). When odour A (for example, chocolate) was presented in the odour port, the rat had to run to a food cup in location A¢ to obtain the reward. When odour B (for example, banana) was presented,

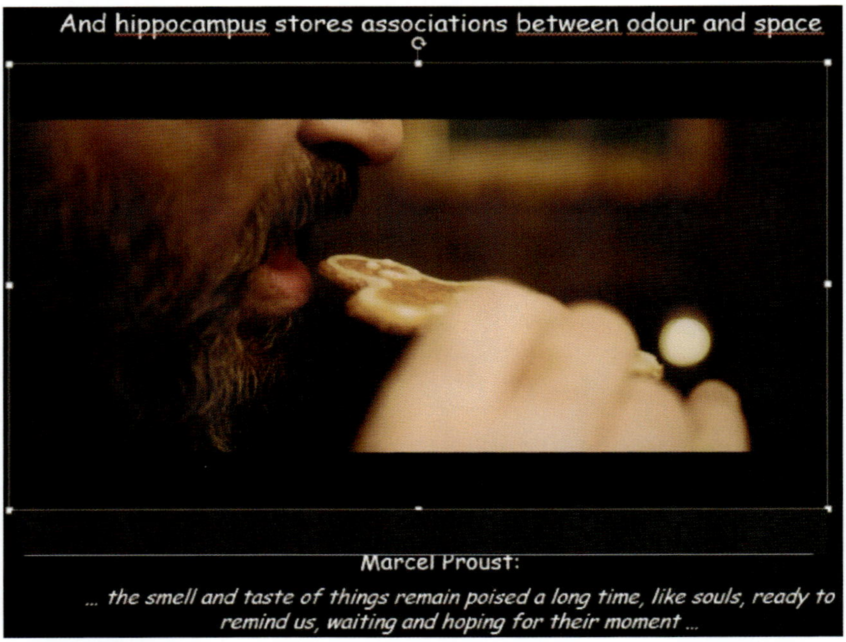

FIGURE 16. Movie illustrating associations between odour and space, as described in Marcel Proust's *In Search of Lost Time*. The movie was produced by Helmet Movie and can be viewed at www.nobelprize.org.

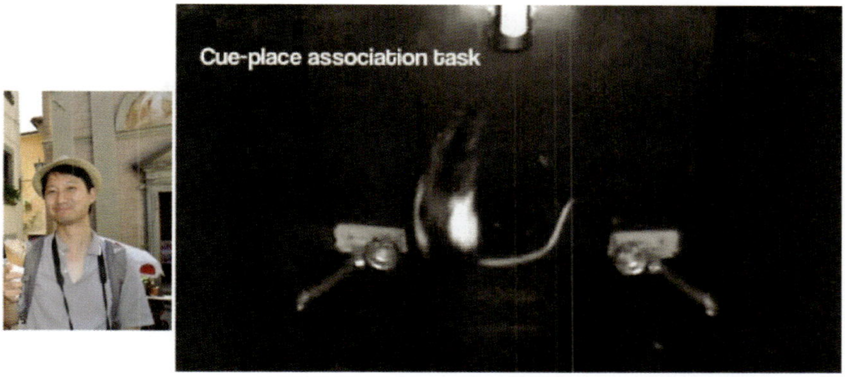

FIGURE 17. Odour-place association task. Left: Kei Igarashi. Right: Movie illustrating performance in a rat trained to discriminate odours with unique associations to food locations. If Emma the rat sniffed chocolate in the odour port, she had to go to position A to get a reward. If she sniffed banana, she would have to go to position B for her reward. The rats reached asymptotic performance (more than 85% correct) after a few weeks of training. Reproduced, with permission, from Igarashi et al. (2014). The movie can be viewed at www.nobelprize.org.

it received a reward only after running to location B¢. After some training, the rats ran to the correct location on nearly all trials. Performance stabilised at 85% correct performance. While the rats acquired the odour-place task, we recorded spike activity and field potentials from the lateral entorhinal cortex and hippocampus, often simultaneously.

Task acquisition was associated with a gradual increase in the number of cells with odour-selective firing in the odour port (Fig. 18). For each cell, we calculated odour selectivity as the difference between firing rates during odour A and odour B as a fraction of the sum of these rates. Odour selectivity in the hippocampus and the lateral entorhinal cortex increased strongly during the cue period when the rat was sniffing in the odour port. During the first training stages, few cells fired differentially to odours A and B but at the end, when the rats had reached asymptotic performance, odour-selective firing was observed in approximately half of the cells, both in lateral entorhinal cortex and in the distal part of CA1, which has strong connections with the lateral entorhinal cortex. The selectivity of the odour representations was entirely abolished on error trials, when the rat subsequently ran to the wrong food location.

The change in firing preferences was accompanied by a selective increase in the power of 20–40 Hz beta-gamma oscillations in the lateral entorhinal cortex and the distal CA1 (Fig. 19). The power increase was associated with an increase in the coherence of 20–40 Hz oscillations between field potentials in the

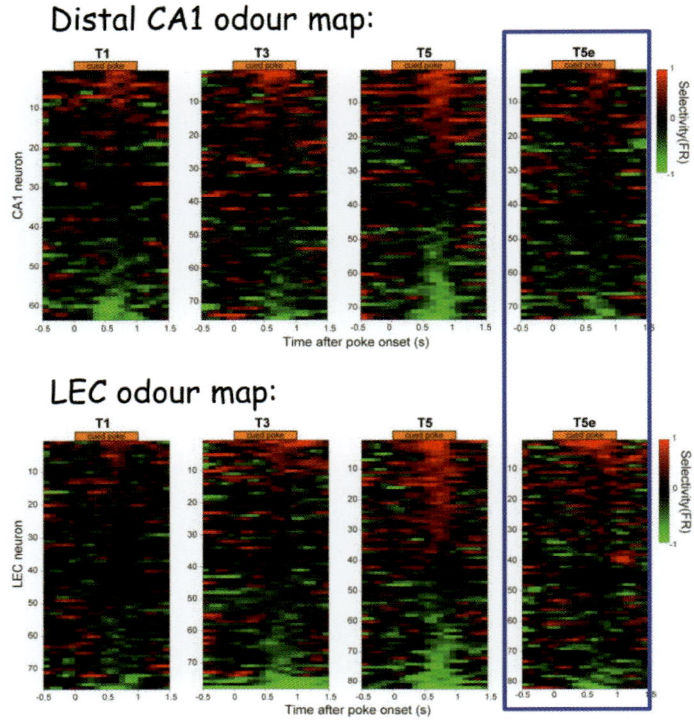

Selective firing to one odour =

(Firing rate to odour A – Firing rate to odour B)
(Firing rate A + Firing rate B)

Red –more firing to odour cue A (max 1)

Green- more firing to odour cue B (max -1)

FIGURE 18. Response of all cells with activity at the odour port. Cells were recorded in the distal CA1 and the lateral entorhinal cortex at times T1–T5 of odour-place training (T5 is above 85% correct criterion), and on error trials at T5 (T5e). Each row shows data for one cell around the time of odour sampling. Selectivity for odour cues is expressed for each cell as the difference in firing rate in the presence of left- and right-associated odours, divided by the sum of these rates. Selectivity is colour-coded from –1 to +1. Cells were sorted along the y-axis according to selectivity. Reproduced, with permission, from Igarashi et al. (2014).

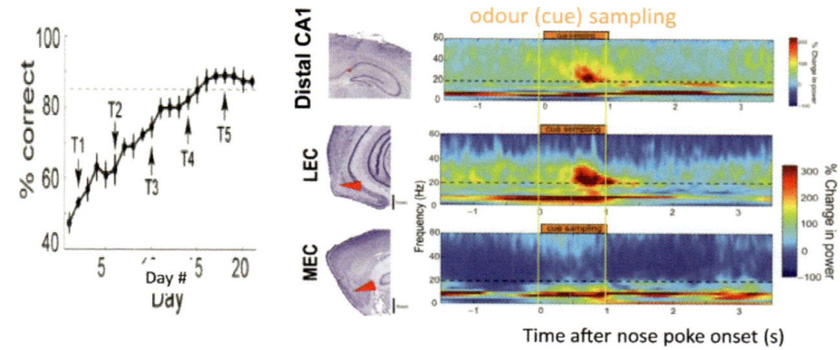

FIGURE 19. Well-trained animals exhibited strong 20–40 Hz oscillations in the distal CA1 and the lateral entorhinal cortex. Left: Percentage of correct choices as a function of training day. Arrows indicate different stages of training (T1–T5). Middle: recording locations in the distal CA1, the lateral entorhinal cortex, and the medial entorhinal cortex. Right: Time-resolved power spectra averaged across tetrodes in the distal CA1, the lateral entorhinal cortex, and the medial entorhinal cortex. Change in power is colour-coded. T5e indicates power spectra for error trials; T5d shows spectra for correct trials down sampled to the number of error trials. Note strong 20–40 Hz activity during presentation of the odour cue. Reproduced, with permission, from Igarashi et al. (2014).

two areas (Fig. 20). Again, the increase occurred gradually, in parallel with task performance and development of odour selectivity. At the beginning of training, there was no detectable coherence at all, but as the rats approached asymptotic performance, strong coherence developed (Fig. 20). On error trials, the coherence was abolished. The increase in power and coherence on correct trials was confined to the cue sampling interval in the odour port, when retrieval of odour-paired target locations was likely to take place. In CA1, the increase in coherence preceded the formation of odour-selective representations, suggesting that the CA1 activity was imposed by the emergence of coherent activity between cells in distal CA1 and lateral entorhinal cortex.

Taken together, these findings demonstrate a form of hippocampal learning where improvement in associative performance coincides with increased coupling of 20–40 Hz oscillations in connected cell populations. The increase in functional coupling was associated with the development of unique odour representations in each area. Error trials were invariably accompanied by reduced coupling and reduced odour selectivity, suggesting that the changes are necessary for successful odour-cued place retrieval. The results point to 20–40 Hz oscillations as a mechanism for the formation of functional circuits between the

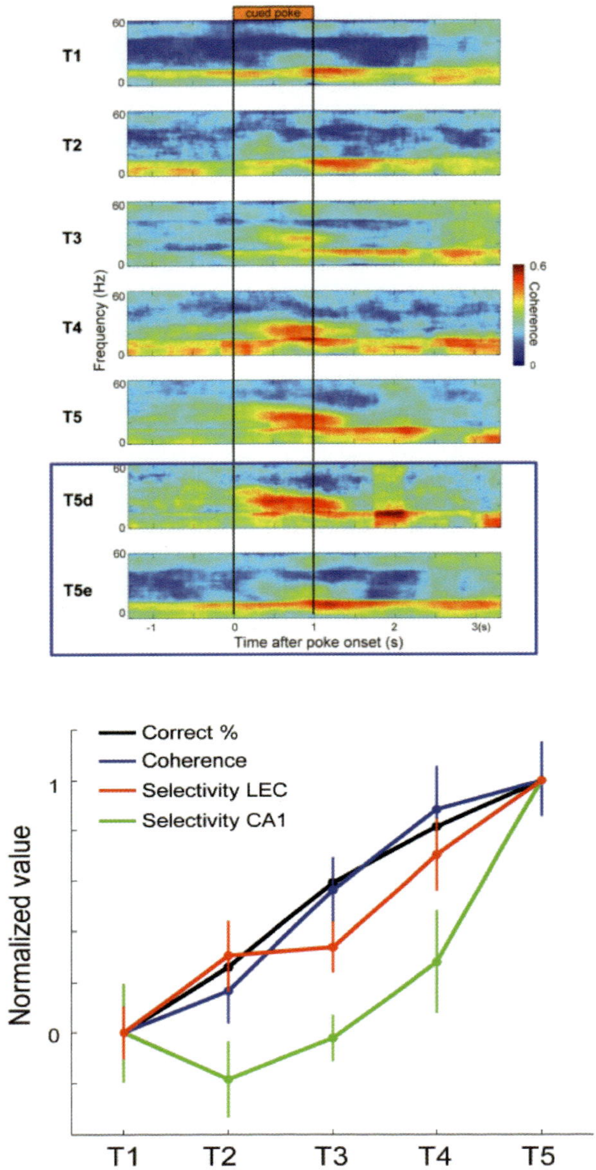

FIGURE 20. Coherence between field potentials in the lateral entorhinal cortex and the distal CA1 at successive stages of training (T1–T5). Top: Time-resolved coherence spectra for EEG recorded simultaneously in the lateral entorhinal cortex and the distal CA1. T5e indicates coherence spectra for error trials; T5d shows spectra for correct trials downsampled to the number of error trials. Note the development of 20–40 Hz coherence as animals learn the task, as well as the loss of coherence on error trials. Reproduced, with permission, from Igarashi et al. (2014).

lateral entorhinal cortex and the hippocampus during encoding of associative memory. Coherent firing in the lateral entorhinal cortex and CA1, mediated by coherent neural oscillations, may provide sufficient presynaptic and postsynaptic coincidence for changes in entorhinal-CA1 synapses to take place (Singer, 1993; Bi and Poo, 1998).

REMAPPING KEEPS MEMORIES APART

One of the greatest challenges for a memory system is to keep memories apart. Avoiding memory interference is particularly a challenge for the hippocampal system, given its involvement in episodic memory. Every day we experience thousands of episodes—episodes that must be stored as overlapping patterns of activity if the hippocampus is to have capacity for them all. If the storage involves overlapping activity, how can we then avoid mixing up memories that involve similar subsets of neurons, and what does this mean for the storage capacity of the hippocampus?

The overlap of hippocampal representations has until now been tested by recording place cells in pairs of environments—in two differently shaped recording enclosures, or in boxes located in two different rooms. It was shown by Bob Muller and John Kubie in the 1980s that place cells form distinct maps for different recording environments (Muller and Kubie, 1987). The replacement of activity patterns between environments was referred to as 'remapping'. In 2004, with postdoc Stefan Leutgeb, we showed that, in the CA3 area of the hippocampus, representations for environments in two different rooms are no more similar than expected by chance, with the chance level determined by scrambling the distribution of neurons that were active in the two rooms (Leutgeb et al., 2004). These recordings suggested that pairs of hippocampal representations are fully orthogonalised, raising the possibility that the hippocampus has mechanisms for decorrelating new representations from existing ones. The generality of this assumption has not been tested, however.

With graduate student Charlotte Alme we thus set out to determine whether there is a limit to the number of orthogonal representations that can be stored in the CA3 network. Place cells were recorded in CA3 while animals explored a series of 11 environments, 10 of which were novel to the animal. All environments consisted of black square recording boxes placed in rooms with similar background cues. With this setup, we were able to compare 55 pairs of recording environments. The results were striking. All pairs were completely uncorrelated (Fig. 21), except when an environment was presented twice (Fig. 22). Thirty per cent of cells fired in only one environment, 13% fired in two rooms, and only

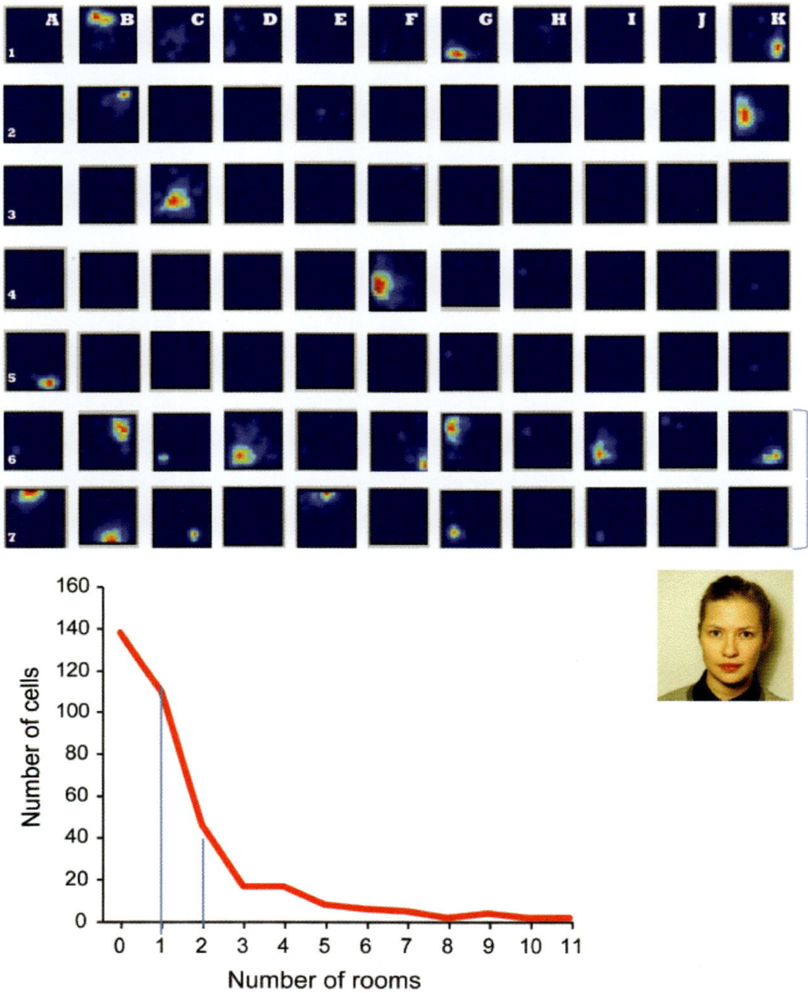

FIGURE 21. Independence of place representations in CA3 of the hippocampus. The rat was tested in 11 different rooms (A–K). Data are shown for seven representative simultaneously recorded CA3 cells. Colour-coded firing rate maps show high rates in red and low rates (no activity) in blue. Note different patterns of activity across pairs of rooms. Most cells are active only in one or few rooms, and the combination of active cells differs from room to room. The bottom graph shows the number of cells with activity in different numbers of rooms. The majority of cells are active in either no rooms or only one room. Bottom right: Charlotte Alme. Reproduced, with permission, from Alme et al. (2014).

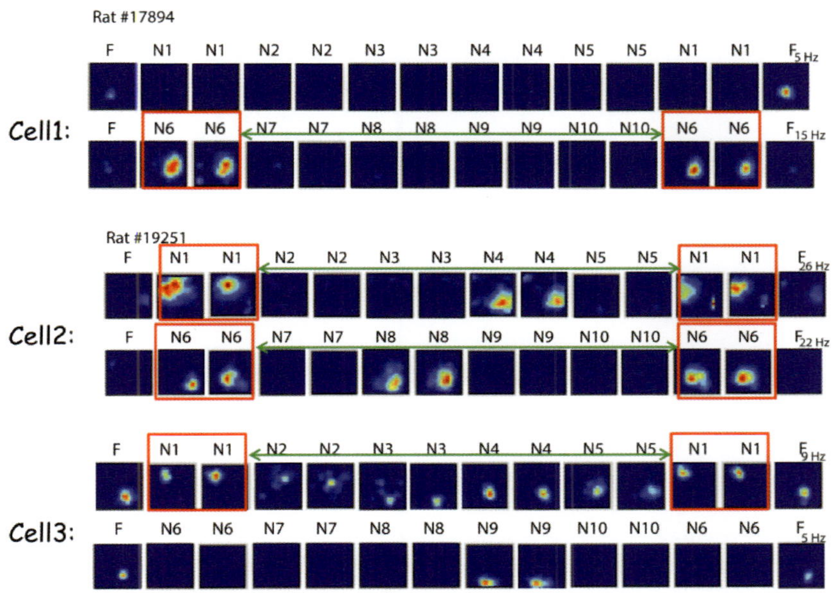

FIGURE 22. Stability of place cells in the 11-room protocol. Room number is indicated at the top of each row (N, novel; F, familiar). Colour maps show firing rate across the recording box. Repeated recordings in N1 and N6 show stability of new representations. Reproduced, with permission, from Alme et al. (2014).

6% fired in 6 rooms or more. Population vector analyses further showed that the pattern of spatial firing across the cell sample was completely uncorrelated between each of the rooms (Fig. 23). In sum, these findings suggest that hippocampal place cells have the capacity to form large numbers of independent representations. Spatial patterns never carried over between environments. This independence among representations is exactly what is needed for a memory system to minimise interference.

FROM SPATIAL MAPPING TO NAVIGATION

In the final part of my talk I would like to ask how the brain uses hippocampal and entorhinal maps for navigation. For animals to get from one place to another, there must be mechanisms for reading out the information expressed in place cells and grid cells. These mechanisms are not well understood. We do not

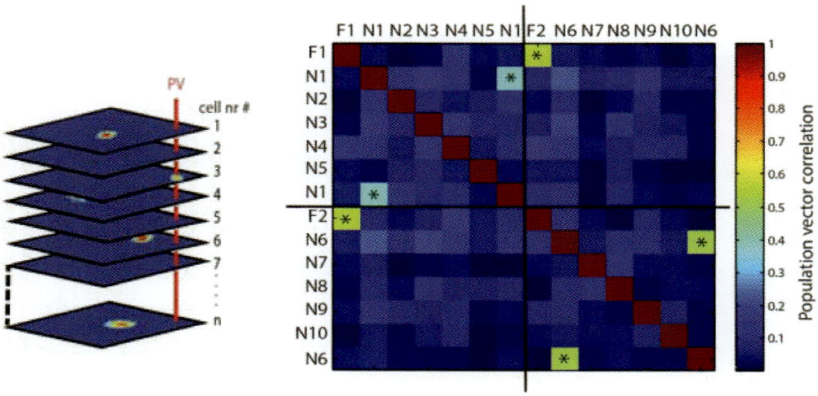

FIGURE 23. Population vector correlations across all pairs of test rooms in the 11-room experiment. Left: Definition of population vectors. Rate maps for all CA3 cells were stacked and 400 population vectors (PVs) were defined, one for each of the 20×20 pixels of the recording box. Right: Colour-coded matrix showing average dot product values for pairs of population vectors across all 55 room pairs. Room symbols as in Fig. 22. Note low dot products between all different pairs of rooms but high dot products between repeated trials in the same room (asterisks). Reproduced, with permission, from Alme et al. (2014).

know, at present, how place cells or grid cells are used for animals to get from their current location to a goal location elsewhere in the environment.

Some important clues were obtained when scientists in the Eichenbaum lab reported, more than a decade ago, that place cells in hippocampal area CA1 express information about where the animal is coming from or where it is going (Wood et al., 2000). Rats were trained in a T-maze-based alternation task, in which they were trained to take alternating left or right turns at the junction (Fig. 24). Place cells on the stem of the maze fired at different rates on left- and right-turn trajectories. Later work showed that the dependence on trajectory had both retrospective and prospective components (Ferbinteanu and Shapiro, 2003), reflecting both the preceding and the succeeding choice of trajectory, with prospective components dominating near the end of the stem, before the decision point (Catanese et al., 2014). The source of this trajectory-dependent information has not been identified, however. In the final set of experiments, we asked whether the expression of trajectory choices depended on a wider circuit including not only the CA1 but also the medial prefrontal cortex and the nucleus reuniens of the thalamus, which projects selectively to the CA1 subfield of the hippocampus (Witter and Amaral, 2004; Cassel et al., 2013).

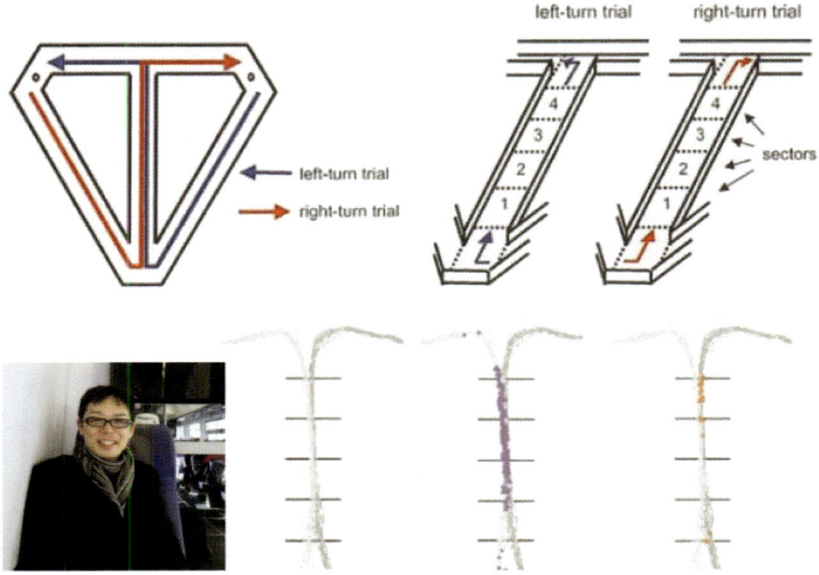

FIGURE 24. Trajectory-dependent firing in CA1 of the hippocampus. Left: Hiroshi Ito. Top right: Modified T-mazes used for the continuous alternation task. The stem of the maze was divided into successive sectors. Bottom right: Trajectory of animal (grey) and spike positions of a single CA1 place cell. Left: trajectory only; middle: left-turn trials; right: right-turn trials. Reproduced, with permission, from Wood et al. (2000).

First, to test the impact of inputs from the nucleus reuniens, we compared trajectory-dependent firing in CA3 and CA1 of the hippocampus (Fig. 25; Ito et al., 2015). CA3 does not receive inputs from the nucleus reuniens, so if the latter is the source of trajectory-dependent firing, it should not be expressed strongly in the CA3 region. This prediction was verified in the data. While 55% of the cells in CA1 showed trajectory-dependent firing, with significantly higher firing rates on left turns than right turns, or vice versa, only 18% of the CA3 cells showed such activity.

We then tested the contribution of reuniens activity more directly by monitoring activity in this nucleus, at the same time as spikes were recorded in CA1 (Fig. 26). Nucleus reuniens neurons were active across the entire maze but nonetheless exhibited differential firing on left- and right-turn trajectories. Forty-two per cent of the reuniens cells showed significant trajectory-dependent firing.

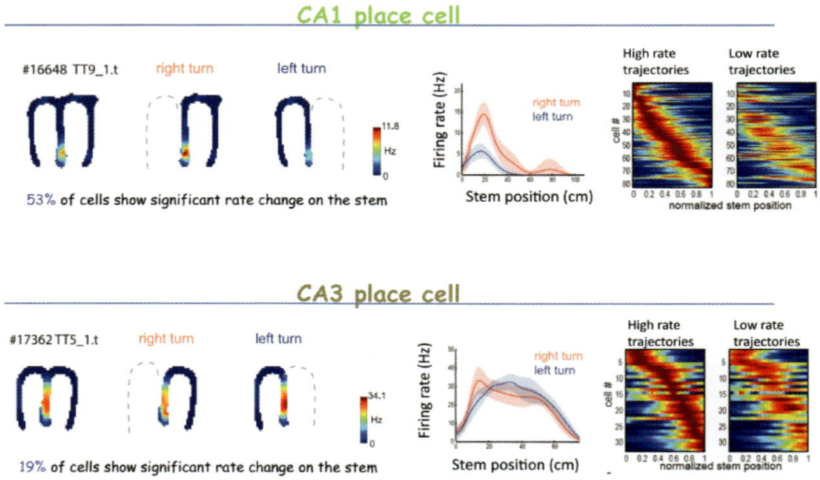

FIGURE 25. Trajectory-dependent firing in CA1 (top) but not CA3 (bottom). Left panels: Rate maps for representative place cells during running in the continuous alternation task (left to right: all laps, right-turn laps, left-turn laps). Right panel: means (solid lines) and 95% confidence intervals (shaded) for spike rates of a single cell across the stem of the maze. Left-turn runs in blue, right-turn runs in red. Right: Left- and right-turn trajectories were classified as high-rate or low-rate depending on which direction had the highest mean peak rate on the stem. Spike rates were normalised to the peak firing rate of each cell and sorted according to field position on the high-rate trajectory. Each line shows one cell. Normalised spike rate is colour-coded. Reproduced, with permission, from Ito et al. (2014).

Because the nucleus reuniens receives strong projections from the medial prefrontal cortex (Cassel et al., 2013), we next hypothesised that trajectory-dependent firing in the reuniens is imposed by activity on this nucleus by inputs from the medial prefrontal cortex. To test this, we recorded activity in the anterior cingulate cortex and the prelimbic cortex (Fig. 27). Trajectory-dependent firing was found in both of these medial prefrontal areas, despite the lack of discrete firing fields in the rate maps. Approximately one-third of the cells showed significant differences in firing rate between left and right-turn trajectories.

Finally, we asked if activity in the nucleus reuniens is necessary for trajectory-dependent firing in the CA1, or if alternatively trajectory-dependent firing patterns are expressed independently across a variety of brain regions. The question was addressed in two ways. First we used ibotenic acid to induce selective lesions in the nucleus reuniens. Activity was then recorded in CA1 (Fig. 28). The

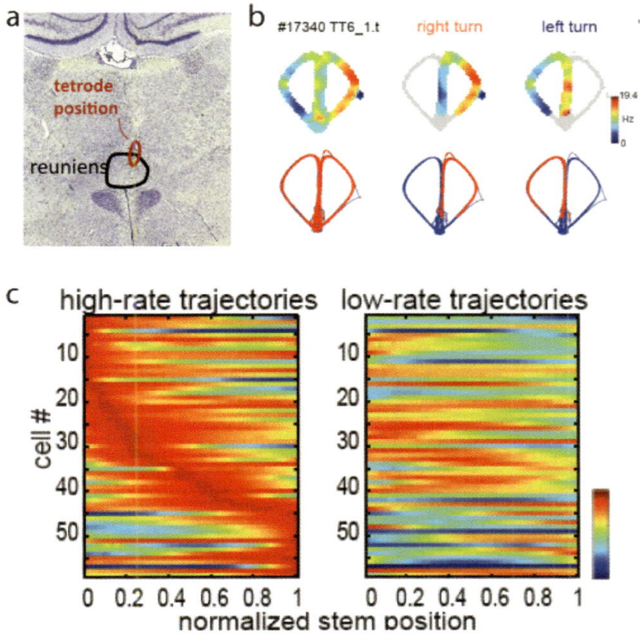

FIGURE 26. Trajectory-dependent firing in the nucleus reuniens. a: Nissl-stained coronal section showing tetrode track (red circle) in the nucleus reuniens (outline). b: Rate maps of a representative nucleus reuniens cell in the continuous alternation task. Top, colour-coded rate maps, with scale bar; bottom, spike locations (red) on trajectory (blue). c: Normalised spike rate on the stem for all cells recorded in nucleus reuniens, plotted as in Fig. 25. Reproduced, with permission, from Ito et al. (2014).

lesions reduced the number of cells with trajectory-dependent firing. Only 16% of the cells passed the criterion for trajectory dependence, a level almost identical to the percentage recorded in the CA3 region of control animals. In a second series of experiments, we inactivated parts of the nucleus reuniens using optogenetic methods. The enhanced halorhodopsin eNpHR3.1 was expressed selectively in the nucleus. Light was then applied over the injection site, and spikes were recorded in CA1. Again the percentage of trajectory-dependent cells decreased. These data demonstrate that nucleus reuniens activity is required for goal-directed firing in the CA1 area of the hippocampus.

Collectively, our findings identify the medial prefrontal cortex, the nucleus reuniens and CA1 as part of an interconnected circuit for representation of goal-directed activity during spatial navigation. The data point to this circuit as

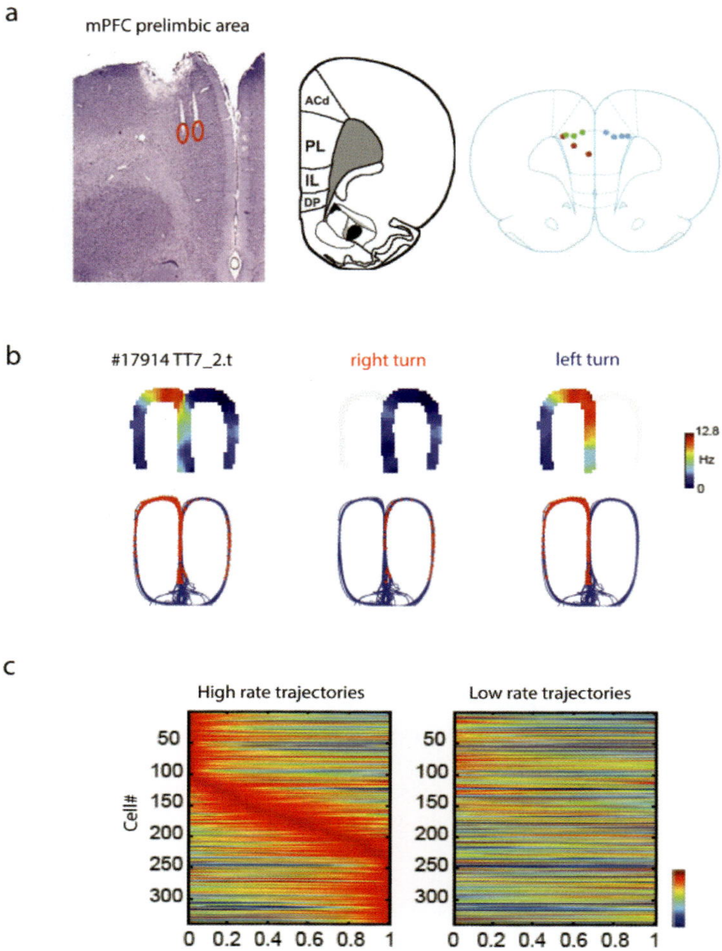

FIGURE 27. Trajectory-dependent firing in the medial prefrontal cortex. a: Nissl-stained coronal section showing tetrode positions (red circles) in the dorsal prelimbic area. b: Rate maps for a representative cell recorded at the location in a. c: Normalised rate on the stem for all cells in the medial prefrontal cortex, as in Fig. 25 and 26. Reproduced, with permission, from Ito et al. (2014).

part of the animal's representation of the intended direction of movement, and suggest that activity in this circuit is imposed by activity in the medial prefrontal cortex via connections through the nucleus reuniens. The data also provide evidence for a role of the thalamus in long-range communication between cortical regions.

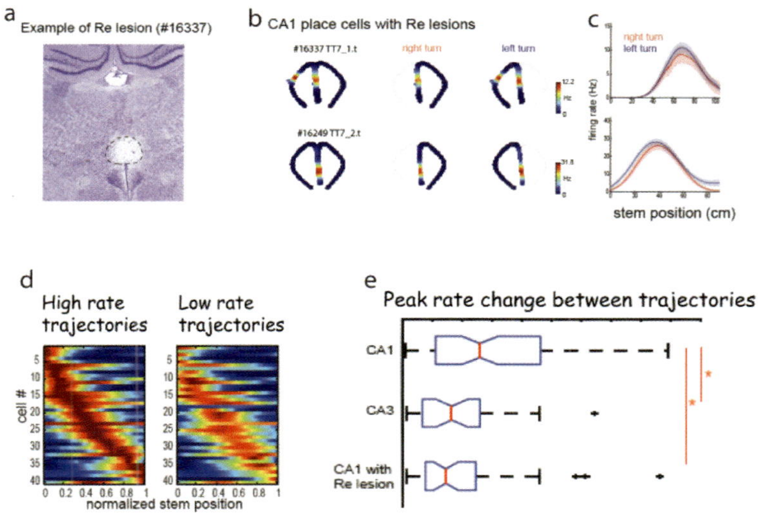

FIGURE 28. Impaired trajectory coding after lesions in the nucleus reuniens. a: Nissl-stained coronal brain section showing a bilateral nucleus reuniens lesion. Outline shows the nucleus reuniens. b: Colour-coded rate maps for a representative CA1 place cell in a nucleus reuniens-lesioned animal. c: Mean rate, 95% confidence intervals and rasters for the cell in b. d: Normalised firing rate on the stem for all CA1 place cells from animals with nucleus reuniens lesions, plotted as in Fig. 25–27. e: Box plot showing change in peak rate between left- and right-turn trajectories for CA1 place cells with trajectory-dependent firing. Note that in nucleus reuniens-lesioned animals, the number of CA1 cells with trajectory-dependent firing is no larger than in CA3 of control animals. Reproduced, with permission, from Ito et al. (2014).

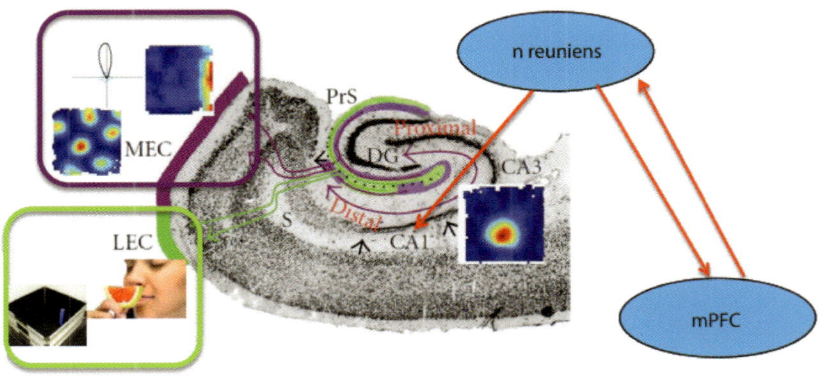

FIGURE 29. Illustration of the medial prefrontal—nucleus reuniens—CA1 circuit for trajectory-dependent activity. Goal-directed information through this circuit is mixed in the hippocampus with information from the medial and lateral entorhinal cortices.

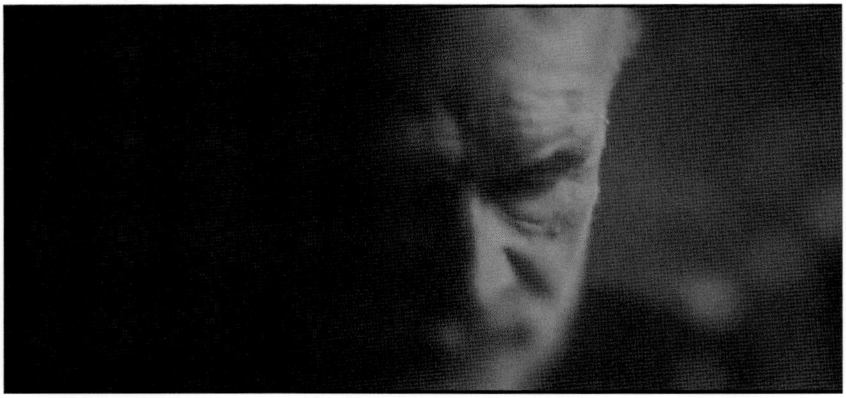

FIGURE 30. Movie illustrating with music the search for insight in the brain sciences. The search occurs in a foggy landscape but for the one who searches persistently there are openings. Music composed and performed by musicians at the Norwegian University of Science and Technology (Helmet; names at the end of the movie). The movie can be viewed at www.nobelprize.org.

THANK YOU!

Edvard, John and I would like to thank the Nobel committee and the assembly for awarding us the 2014 Nobel Prize. I want to celebrate the event by sharing a movie with music made especially for this event. The music is made by jazz musicians at my institution, the Norwegian University of Science and Technology. It is inspired by our search for knowledge—a search that sometimes feels like wandering in a fog landscape where we see things close to us but fail to obtain a global view. Research is a bit like that but sometimes we make breakthroughs and see far. During the past few decades there have been many breakthroughs in systems and circuit neuroscience. The prize to the three of us is recognition of this exciting development.

REFERENCES

1. Alme CB *et al.* (2014). Place cells in the hippocampus: Eleven maps for eleven rooms. *Proc. Natl. Acad. Sci. USA*, **111**, 18428–18435.
2. Barry C *et al.* (2006). The boundary vector model of place cell firing and spatial memory. *Rev. Neurosci.* **17**, 71–97.
3. Bi GQ and Poo MM (1998). Synaptic modifications in cultured hippocampal neurons: dependence on spike timing, synaptic strength, and postsynaptic cell type. *J. Neurosci.* **18**, 10464–72.

4. Burwell RD (2000). The parahippocampal region: corticocortical connectivity. *Ann. N. Y. Acad. Sci.* **911**, 25–42.
5. de Almeida L, Idiart M and Lisman JE (2009). The input-output transformation of the hippocampal granule cells: from grid cells to place cells. *J. Neurosci.* **29**, 7504–7512.
6. Cassel JC *et al.* (2013). The reuniens and rhomboid nuclei: neuroanatomy, electrophysiological characteristics and behavioral implications. *Prog. Neurobiol.* **111**, 34–52.
7. Catanese J, Viggiano A, Cerasti E, Zugaro MB and Wiener SI (2014). Retrospectively and prospectively modulated hippocampal place responses are differentially distributed along a common path in a continuous T-maze. *J. Neurosci.* **34**, 13163–13169.
8. Deshmukh SS and Knierim JJ (2011). Representation of non-spatial and spatial information in the lateral entorhinal cortex. *Front. Behav. Neurosci.* **5**, 69.
9. Felleman DJ and van Essen DC (1991). Distributed hierarchical processing in the primate cerebral cortex. *Cereb. Cortex* **1**, 1–47.
10. Ferbinteanu J and Shapiro ML (2003). Prospective and retrospective memory coding in the hippocampus. *Neuron* **40**, 1227–1239.
11. Fuhs MC and Touretzky DS (2006). A spin glass model of path integration in rat medial entorhinal cortex. *J. Neurosci.* **26**, 4266–4276.
12. Fyhn M, Molden S, Witter MP, Moser EI and Moser M-B (2004). Spatial representation in the entorhinal cortex. *Science* **305**, 1258–1264.
13. Hafting T, Fyhn M, Molden S, Moser M-B and Moser EI (2005). Microstructure of a spatial map in the entorhinal cortex. *Nature* **436**, 801–806.
14. Hartley T, Burgess N, Lever C, Cacucci F and O'Keefe J (2000). Modeling place fields in terms of the cortical inputs to the hippocampus. *Hippocampus* **10**, 369–379.
15. Hubel DH and Wiesel T (1962). Receptive fields, binocular interaction, and functional architecture of cat striate cortex. *J. Physiol. (Lond.)* **160**,106–154.
16. Igarashi KM, Lu L, Colgin LL, Moser M-B and Moser EI (2014). Coordination of entorhinal-hippocampal ensemble activity during associative learning. *Nature* **510**, 143–147.
17. Ito HT, Zhang S-J, Witter MP, Moser EI, Moser M-B (2015). A prefrontal-thalamo-hippocampal circuit for goal-directed spatial coding. *Nature*, in press.
18. Jarosiewicz B and Skaggs WE (2004). Hippocampal place cells are not controlled by visual input during the small irregular activity state in the rat. *J. Neurosci.* **24**, 5070–7.
19. Lee AM *et al.* (2014). Identification of a brainstem circuit regulating visual cortical state in parallel with locomotion. *Neuron* **83**, 455–466.
20. Leutgeb S, Leutgeb JK, Treves A, Moser MB and Moser EI (2004). Distinct ensemble codes in hippocampal areas CA3 and CA1. *Science* **305**, 1295–1298.
21. Leutgeb JK *et al.* (2005a). Progressive transformation of hippocampal neuronal representations in "morphed" environments. *Neuron* **48**, 345–358.
22. Leutgeb S, Leutgeb JK, Moser M-B, Moser EI (2005b). Place cells, spatial maps and the population code for memory. *Curr. Opin. Neurobiol.* **15**, 738–746.
23. Lever C, Burton S, Jeewajee A, O'Keefe J and Burgess N (2009). Boundary vector cells in the subiculum of the hippocampal formation. *J. Neurosci.* **29**, 9771–9777.

24. McNaughton BL, Battaglia FP, Jensen O, Moser EI and Moser M-B (2006). Path integration and the neural basis of the 'cognitive map'. *Nature Rev. Neurosci.* **7**, 663–678.
25. Monaco JD and Abbott LF (2011). Modular reealignment of entorhinal grid cell activity as a basis for hippocampal remapping. *J. Neurosci.* **31**, 9414–9425.
26. Muller RU and Kubie JL (1987). The effects of changes in the environment on the spatial firing of hippocampal complex-spike cells. *J. Neurosci.*, 1951–1968.
27. O'Keefe J (1976). Place units in the hippocampus of the freely moving rat. *Exp. Neurol.* **51**, 78–109.
28. O'Keefe J and Burgess N (1996). Geometric determinants of the place fields of hippocampal neurons. *Nature* **381**, 425–428.
29. O'Keefe J and Dostrovsky J (1971). The hippocampus as a spatial map. Preliminary evidence from unit activity in the freely-moving rat. *Brain Res.* **34**, 171–175 (1971).
30. O'Keefe J and Nadel L (1978). *The Hippocampus as a Cognitive Map* (Oxford: Clarendon Press).
31. O'Keefe J and Speakman A (1987). Single unit activity in the rat hippocampus during a spatial memory task. *Exp.Brain Res.* **68**, 1–27.
32. Pavlides C and Winson J (1989). Influences of hippocampal place cell firing in the awake state on the activity of these cells during subsequent sleep episodes. *J. Neurosci.* **9**, 2907–2918.
33. Petrulis A, Alvarez P and Eichenbaum H (2005). Neural correlates of social odor recognition and the representation of individual distinctive social odors within entorhinal cortex and ventral subiculum. *Neurosci.* **130**, 259–274.
34. Ranck J Jr. (1985). Head direction cells in the deep cell layer of dorsal presubiculum in freely moving rats. In *Electrical Activity of the Archicortex*, ed. G. Buzsáki, CH Vanderwolf, pp. 217–20 (Budapest: Akademiai Kiado).
35. Rolls ET, Stringer SM and Ellio T (2006). Entorhinal cortex grid cells can map to hippocampal place cells by competitive learning. *Network* **17**, 447–465.
36. Sargolini F, Fyhn M, Hafting T, McNaughton BL, Witter MP, Moser M-B and Moser EI (2006). Conjunctive representation of position, direction, and velocity in entorhinal cortex. *Science* **312**, 758–762.
37. Savelli F and Knierim JJ (2010). Hebbian analysis of the transformation of medial entorhinal grid-cell inputs to hippocampal place fields. *J. Neurophysiol.* **103**, 3167–3183.
38. Savelli F, Yoganarasimha D and Knierim JJ (2008). Influence of boundary removal on the spatial representations of the medial entorhinal cortex. *Hippocampus* **18**, 1270–1282.
39. Scoville WB and Milner B (1957). Loss of recent memory after bilateral hippocampal lesions. *J. Neurol. Neurosurg. Psychiatry* **20**, 11–21.
40. Singer W (1993). Synchronization of cortical activity and its putative role in information processing and learning. *Annu. Rev. Physiol.* **55**, 349–74.
41. Solstad T, Boccara CN, Kropff E, Moser M-B and Moser EI (2008). Representation of geometric borders in the entorhinal cortex. *Science* **322**, 1865–1868.
42. Solstad T, Moser EI, Einevoll GT (2006). From grid cells to place cells: A mathematical model. *Hippocampus* **16**, 1026–1031.

43. Squire LR (1992). Memory and the hippocampus: A synthesis from findings with rats, monkeys, and humans. *Psychol. Review* **99**, 195–231.
44. Squire LR and Wixted JT (2011). The cognitive neuroscience of human memory since H.M. *Annu. Rev. Neurosci.* **34**, 259–288.
45. Squire LR and Zola-Morgan S (1991). The medial temporal lobe system. *Science* **253**, 1380–1386.
46. Taube JS (2007). The head direction signal: origins and sensory-motor integration. *Annu. Rev. Neurosci.* **30**, 181–207.
47. Tsao A, Moser M-B and Moser EI (2013). Traces of experience in the lateral entorhinal cortex. *Curr. Biol.* **23**, 399–405.
48. Wills TJ, Barry C and Cacucci F (2012). The abrupt development of adult-like grid cell firing in the medial entorhinal cortex. *Front Neural Circuits* **6**, 21.
49. Wilson MA and McNaughton BL (1993). Dynamics of the hippocampal ensemble code for space. *Science* **261**, 1055–1058.
50. Wilson MA and McNaughton BL (1994). Reactivation of hippocampal ensemble memories during sleep. *Science* **265**, 676–679.
51. Witter MP and Amaral DG (2004). Hippocampal Formation. In: *The Rat Nervous System*, edited by Paxinos G, p. 635–704.
52. Wood ER, Dudchenko PA, Robitsek RJ and Eichenbaum H (2000). Hippocampal neurons encode information about different types of memory episodes occurring in the same location. *Neuron* **27**, 623–633.
53. Yates, FA (1966). *The Art of Memory*. Chicago: University of Chicago Press.
54. Zhang SJ *et al.* (2013). Optogenetic dissection of entorhinal-hippocampal functional connectivity. *Science* **340**, 1232627.

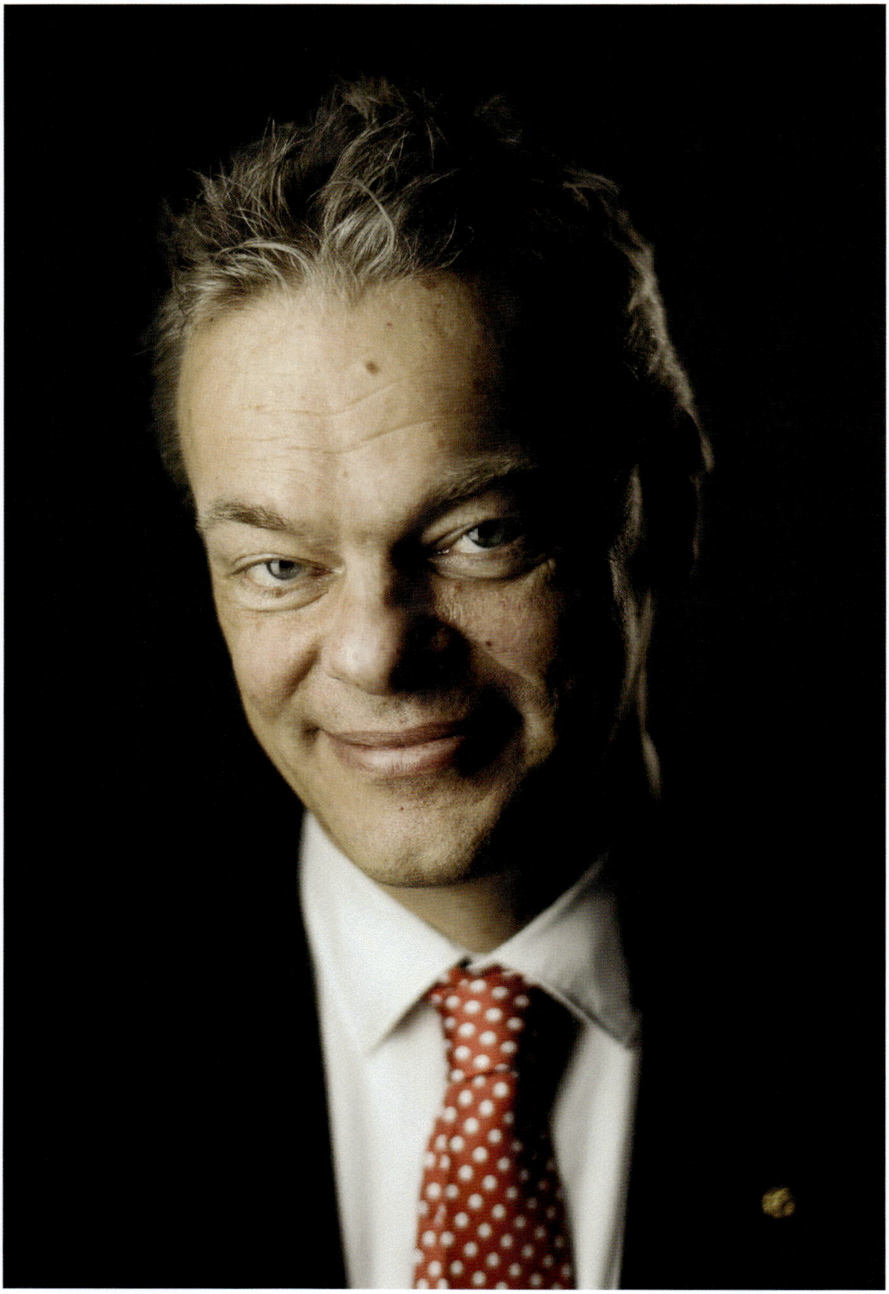

Edvard I. Moser. © Nobel Media AB. Photo: A. Mahmoud

Edvard I. Moser

I was born in 1962 on the west coast of Norway, about 200 kilometres north of Bergen. I spent the first 9 months of my life on Haramsøy (Fig. 1), an island with fewer than 500 inhabitants and, at that time, only a single daily ferry connection to the mainland. In 1963 my parents and I moved to a more urban environment, relatively speaking, and settled on another island, in Hareid, a village with about 4,000 inhabitants spread across four different settlements (Fig. 2). My two younger sisters were born there, and I lived there until I finished high school at age 18 in Ulsteinvik, on the same island.

MY GERMAN ROOTS

My parents were German immigrants, a rare species in Norway during the first decades after World War II. They met during the war in Kronberg im Taunus, a small village north-west of Frankfurt am Main. My father was the oldest son of the pastor in Kronberg; my mother was the daughter of a famous butcher in Essen, in the Ruhr area near the Dutch border. Together with her siblings, my mother was sent out of Essen when the bombing of the Ruhr area began in 1943. Her father could afford to send his children to a private family in Kronberg through a teacher they knew in the village. The children were brought back to Essen in 1944 because my grandfather feared that Germany would be divided, with Kronberg and Essen going to different territories. After the war, my parents met again in Kronberg and later in Bonn.

Both of my parents wanted an education but did not get an opportunity to pursue one. In my father's family, the oldest son was expected to be a pastor, which had been the tradition for the last six or seven generations. My father, however, liked to play cello and wanted to study music. After the war there was no money for him to pursue a formal education, so instead he learned a trade in

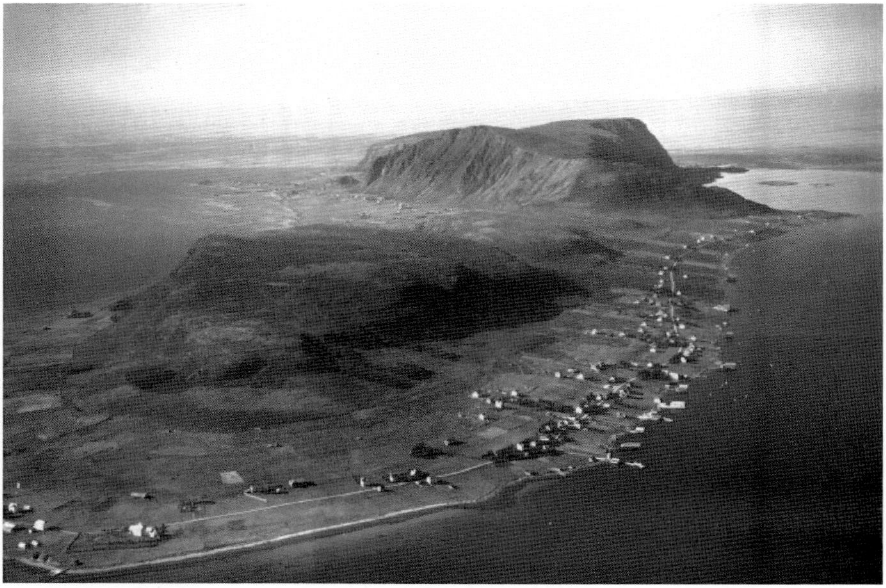

FIGURE 1. Haramsøy, where I lived the first year of my life. Taken in 1953, the year when my father moved to the island. Wideroe air photo, with permission from the Haram Public Library.

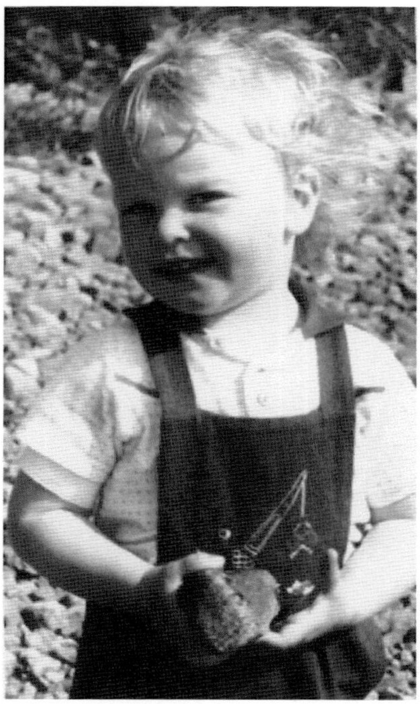

FIGURE 2. Me on the island of Hareid in 1963. I lived in Hareid from age 1 to age 19. Photo taken by my father Eduard Paul Moser.

Bonn, with Klais Orgelbau, where he made church organs. After a few years, he came across an advertisement by a small organ factory on an island off the west coast of Norway that was looking for skilled labour. My father applied for the job, got it and moved to Haramsøy in 1953.

My mother wanted to become an interior designer but this type of career was all but closed to her because it required work experience and companies were not willing to accept women for training. Instead she went to a business college and subsequently got a job in Essen as a secretary with AEG, a large German producer of electrical equipment. While she was working at AEG, she came in contact with my father again. He had by then moved to Norway, and my mother visited him on a nice summer day in 1957. In 1958 she gave up her AEG job and moved to Haramsøy.

Norway was a big change for my mother. She came from quite a wealthy family in a big city in Germany. In Haramsøy, she was expected to be a housewife like all other women at the time. The shops had only three types of vegetables—cabbage, turnips and carrots, and there was still outdoor plumbing, which my mother had never experienced before. The weather was harsh and the laundry often flew off the outdoor line where she hung it to dry.

SCHOOL DAYS

I was born into two different worlds—a poor community on an isolated but beautiful island that offered little more than was needed for work and survival, and a rich cultural tradition that had its roots in the European continent. A third dimension was added when we moved to Hareid, which in spite of its small size, had an exceptionally active community life centred around the church and the Christian meeting house. But I was still in the middle of the Norwegian Bible Belt—no alcohol, no playing cards, no dancing. My parents' love for good wines remained a well-kept secret.

I went to primary school in Hareid. As was the practice at that time, all students were taught at the same level, and I had to learn everything at the same pace as everyone else. I was the only child who wanted to learn French, so I was put in a bookkeeping class instead. Occasionally I got a few extra assignments to feed my academic interests, but it was my mother who saved me, by giving me tons of books. I started with Donald Duck comics, which my mother gave me when she wanted me to be quiet during the early morning hours. At the age of 4 or 5, I was so motivated to understand the content of the speech bubbles that I cracked the reading code largely on my own. Later, after I started school at the age of 7, which was when children commonly began school at the time, I got real books—with a strong emphasis on science. I read a lot—about geology, meteorology, palaeontology, astronomy, all of the sciences—and I asked for more. I was totally absorbed by these books.

The books introduced me to science and it became my passion. With a friend I started an astronomy club where we learned everything we could about planetary systems, and we memorised the distances between all of the planets and the Sun (I had an affection for numbers). I bought a globe with the first money I ever earned from mowing the lawn. I learned about all of the countries on that globe, all the capitals, the mountains and rivers, and dreamed about visiting all these places.

My father took me around in Norway in his travels to tune church organs, and we visited remote islands and mountain areas, which fuelled my interest in exploration. I collected stones, I had a herbarium, and I got a chemistry set, which enabled me to create some noxious gases in the bathroom. I played school with my younger sisters—I was the teacher and taught them about everything I had read. My parents encouraged my interests further by feeding me more books. As I got older, I even sent my mother to the university bookstore in Tübingen to get astrophysics books that I could not buy in Norway.

It became clear to me that someday I might become some sort of scientist, but I didn't really know what kind, nor did I have any idea about what it really meant to be a scientist. Scientists in the books I read spent their time digging up dinosaurs. During summer holidays in Germany, I visited the Senkenberg Museum in Frankfurt, every time—it was my favourite holiday destination. I saw dinosaurs, fossils, mummies, rock collections, and insects. I wanted to understand evolution and natural history and in my imagination, scientists were people who provided things for the natural history museum.

High school offered me more challenges. The school was in Ulsteinvik, on the same island as Hareid, but on the other side of the mountains. The teachers there were really warm and motivated and suddenly school was much more fun. I was no longer the only one who liked to learn and I could study without disguising it. I liked mathematics and natural sciences but was also fascinated by history and literature, perhaps due to my teachers in these subjects, in particular my form teacher Gunder Runde. With him as a guide, I wrote my thesis about Ibsen. My fascination with Ibsen is still alive to this day. I graduated from high school in 1981 with a top grade in all subjects except physical education (I was never very good at football).

And—I met May-Britt at Ulsteinvik. We were in the same mathematics, physics and chemistry classes, but since she came from another island, and high school cliques were defined by islands, and I was quite shy, we did not interact all that much. When I was not at school and not studying (which I did most of the time), I walked in the mountains on the island. I visited every single peak.

LEAVING THE ISLAND

I grew up during the Cold War. Military service was compulsory for men who were not absolute pacifists. Most men from my region of Norway were sent to stations in the far north of the country, near the Russian border, and I was no exception. After working for three months at a local shipyard when I had finished high school, I was ready for military service in October 1981. I was trained as a communications officer and worked in an underground bunker in Kautokeino, a Sami village near the border of Northern Finland, in the far north of Norway. I got to know a few people in the village and enjoyed their openness and different life style. I also liked the endless open country, and took long walks when I was not on duty. My task in the bunker was to receive and send secret messages about military activity in the airspace near the Russian border. Not much happened though, so I had time to study differential equations and think about my future.

My year-and-a-half of military service meant that I had to start at the University of Oslo in the middle of the academic calendar, in January 1983. By this

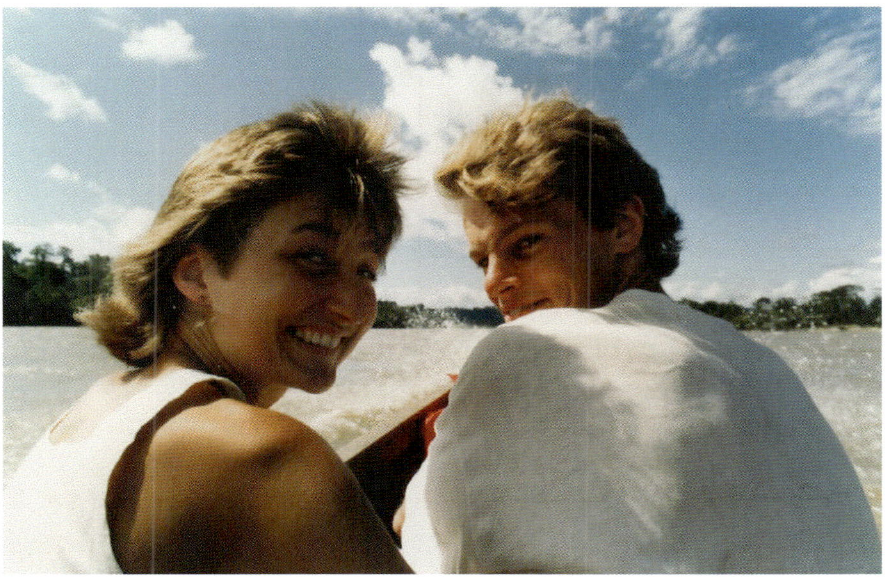

FIGURE 3. May-Britt and me on a tributary of the Amazon in Ecuador in 1986.

point I was still unsure of what I would study but certain that it would be in the sciences. I considered elementary particle physics and nuclear physics but signed up for a course in chemistry. I was fascinated by biochemistry and genetics but had to start with the basics. The first course was in inorganic chemistry. I thought there was too much rote learning and I felt like I wanted to use my energy on other things.

It was about this time that I bumped into May-Britt again by chance. Just before I had moved to Oslo, we met on Karl Johans Gate, Oslo's main pedestrian zone, and she offered to show me the university. She had been there for a year-and-a-half already and was an obvious guide. It turned out she had also puzzled over studying different science topics—she had taken courses in mathematics, physics and astronomy and was considering a future in geology, since the oil adventure had just started on the Norwegian continental shelf. She even considered becoming a dentist but none of the subjects were as interesting as she thought they would be. So we had something in common (Fig. 3).

TURNING TO PSYCHOLOGY

At the time I had just finished reading Freud's *The Interpretation of Dreams*, and I found it fascinating. May-Britt was also attracted to psychology. In August 1983, we signed up for a one-year bachelor's programme in psychology. The coursework covered the entire field of psychology, which was much broader than we had imagined. We became aware of behaviourism, which had a scientific rigour that we thought outshined other subfields of psychology. We saw that behaviour could be broken down into elementary laws and that behaviour could be predicted based on the correct timing of discrete stimuli in relation to the animal's behaviour. At the same time we realised that behaviourist psychology was simple—too simple—and we missed explanations that involved the underlying neural mechanisms.

During our studies, we attended a lecture by Svein Magnussen, in which he described the pioneering work of David Hubel and Torsten Wiesel, who by the early 1960s had already shown how the visual image was broken down into elementary neural responses in the visual cortex. We went to see our teacher in behaviourism, Carl Erik Grennes, and asked how we could learn more about the interface between psychology and physiology. He gave us a copy of a special issue of *Scientific American*, published in September 1979, which was all about the brain. The magazine included Eric Kandel's demonstration of synaptic mechanisms of memory in *Aplysia californica*, and the characterisation of the mechanisms for feature analysis in the visual cortex done by David Hubel and

Torstein Wiesel. There was even a piece by Francis Crick, who at the end of his career argued for neural circuit studies and speculated about what was needed for the discipline of neural circuits neuroscience to be born. It was enough to tell us that there was science there to be done.

But in order to get any further, we had to wait a year after our bachelor's courses before we could start our professional studies in psychology. At that time, psychology was such a popular subject that there was a one-year waiting list, even for those who passed the admission threshold. That year I worked in a psychiatric hospital. I had a full-time job, working with psychotic patients at an acute ward, before they received medication. In my spare time, I studied mathematics, statistics and programming. I took these courses only because I thought mathematics was fun but it turned out to be very useful for my later work, although I did not realise it at that time. While I was at the psychiatric hospital, May-Britt worked in a geriatric institution while she also took classes. During this waiting period, our interests merged and we started thinking about a common future. We went to Kilimanjaro to get engaged in 1984 and decided to marry in 1985, just before we took up psychology again.

The first semester of the professional studies programme in psychology focused on social psychology. May-Britt and I got involved in a research project on small group dynamics and even contributed to a paper—our first publication. But our interest in the brain persisted and we continued to bug Carl Erik Grenness. Carl Erik advised us to approach Terje Sagvolden, the only psychologist at the university with research projects in neuroscience at that time. Terje was working with neurochemical mechanisms of attention deficit disorder in rats. His idea was that if he found out why a certain strain of rats was hyperactive, that might give us some clues about what causes hyperactivity in children. We learned how to design experiments, we learned behavioural analysis, and we learned more statistics in Terje's lab. The work resulted in three papers on behaviour in hyperactive rats. The results were perhaps not all that revolutionary but we were proud to see our own work published.

But we were impatient. The focus was still too much on behaviour while the underlying neural operations remained in the dark. Terje saw our willingness to go further and sent us to Uppsala for a collaborative project on neurochemical modulation in hyperactive rats. We stayed for a month but in the end concluded that there was no reason to go all the way around the barn to find the door. In Oslo, there was a famous professor at Terje Sagvolden's department who was working on the neural mechanisms of memory—Per Andersen. We had seen Per on TV but had never dared to approach him. One day though, after he and his group gave a seminar on the mechanisms of long-term potentiation (LTP) of synaptic transmission and the possible relationship between LTP and memory, we decided that this just might be our future. LTP might be the bridge between physiology and psychology that we had searched for so long.

WORKING WITH PER ANDERSEN

One day in 1998, we went to Per's office and asked if he could take us on as master's students in preparation for a PhD. Per was quite sceptical. He really didn't want new people, because he already had enough students. Moreover, he might not have had the highest opinion of psychologists, although he also wanted to make the connection to behaviour. But we were persistent and shared our ambitions with him. In the end he gave us a paper by Richard Morris, who was at the University of Edinburgh and had invented the water maze, and issued us a challenge: he told us that if we successfully built a water maze laboratory, he would take us on.

A water maze is a big tank, roughly 2 metres across, filled with milky water. There is a platform in the tank that is hidden by the water, which rats can learn to find. As part of our "test," Per wanted us to actually construct the tank in the basement, but we convinced him that it would be acceptable to buy a tank from a plastic factory on the West Coast that made fish tanks. A few months later the water maze was in place in a small room in the basement. The pool was filled with 1200 litres of water and 3 litres of milk. Every day we emptied the pool, filled again with water, and went to the shop to buy new milk.

We used the water tank to address one of Per's greatest dreams. He wanted to make an *in vivo* hippocampal lamella that was as small as possible but at the same time large enough to support learning. The idea was that synaptic changes would be denser in such a preparation—dense enough to be detected by physiological recordings or microscopic analyses. To make this lamella, we removed the remaining hippocampal tissue by aspiration under the microscope. Per wanted the *in vivo* lamella to be in the dorsal hippocampus but to be sure that the enhanced plasticity of the lamella did not reflect the location of the lamella, we asked Per to include a control group where the lamella was in the ventral part of the hippocampus. We also agreed that we might need to try lesions of different sizes, since we did not know how large the lamella had to be to be functional.

The control group turned out to be the key to our first success in the lab. We found it took only quite small lesions to impair navigation, and we were not able to make the *in vivo* lamella that Per wanted so much, but there was an interesting dependence on the location of the lesion. The rats with dorsal lesions (ventral remnants) were not able to find the platform but those with ventral lesions (dorsal remnants) could actually navigate very well.

As it became clear that there was a difference between the dorsal and ventral hippocampus in their involvement in water-maze learning, we searched the literature to try to understand it. We came across the work of Menno Witter, who with David Amaral had shown that the dorsal and ventral hippocampus have quite different cortical inputs, and we were able to put the findings into a meaningful context. We wrote up the master's thesis as a joint thesis of 127 pages and published the results in the *Journal of Neuroscience*. It was the first behavioural study from Per's lab and he was probably a bit anxious about publishing it, but after some strong encouragement from several visitors, including Eric Kandel and Larry Squire, we submitted it. It was published in 1993, 3 years after we completed our thesis.

As we finished our master's thesis in 1990, we both wanted to continue with Per on our PhDs, but the challenge was how to get two fellowships to study with him. At the time it was very difficult to get this kind of funding. There were not many fellowships to hand out and it was not like today, when the labs have the money themselves and get to decide. The Research Council of Norway at the time was concerned about geographic distribution of their fellowships.

My proposed dissertation research was about the relationship between LTP and memory, which was what really got us interested when we first started working with Per, and which had motivated our dorso-ventral hippocampal lesion study. LTP had been discovered 20 years earlier, in Per's group, and it seemed like the right place to pursue the question.

There were several indications that LTP might be involved in memory, but what Per wanted, and what I also found very interesting, was to see if this phenomenon could be directly observed *in vivo*. At that time, Carol Barnes had shown that LTP decay correlated with forgetting, Bruce McNaughton had shown that saturation of LTP blocked subsequent memory formation, and Richard Morris had found that learning could not take place if LTP was blocked by an NMDA receptor antagonist. But no one had observed changes in hippocampal excitatory postsynaptic potentials (EPSP) as a direct consequence of learning. So that was the PhD funding I applied for.

At the same time, May-Britt applied for a project where she wanted to see if learning and memory involved changes in the number of synaptic connections, in the same way as seen after induction of LTP. Against all odds, we both did get fellowships.

In 1991, we were ready to learn how to make electrodes and implant them in the brain. We got help with this skill from Bolek Srebro at the University of

Bergen. He showed us how to make electrodes, how to implant them into the hippocampus, and how to read out the field potentials in an awake, freely moving animal. Once I had learned the technique, I implanted chronic electrodes in the performant path and dentate gyrus and let the rats wander around in a box. As they learned about their environment, the EPSPs got stronger, usually for 20–30 minutes. That was by itself no surprise and had been reported previously, but what was strange was what happened when I put the same animals in the water maze. The animals learned to find the platform but the EPSPs got consistently smaller, which really did not make sense. The hypothesis was that they should be larger as a result of naturally occurring LTP.

We finally figured out that the reason for the decrease in EPSPs was that they are very sensitive to the temperature of the brain, so the higher the temperature, the larger the potentials. The water maze was room temperature, much below the body temperature of the rat. I varied the temperature of the water maze and found that the lower the temperature, the more the EPSP was reduced. Per advised me to insert a thermistor in the rat's brain to monitor the temperature directly and in collaboration with master's student Iacob Mathisen, I was soon able to show that the strength of the synaptic connection was determined directly by the temperature of the brain. I showed that exploration and other learning behaviours increased brain temperature sometimes by more than 2 degrees and that EPSP changes previously reported to accompany learning were due to temperature, not LTP. We published these findings in *Science* in 1993. I defended my thesis in 1995, with Bruce McNaughton and Tim Bliss as public examiners, or opponents as they are called in Norway. The thesis defence was part of Per's 'Grand Slam', where 6 of his students publicly defended their work within a week, with an impressive collection of 12 world-leading scientists as thesis opponents (Fig. 4).

I was able to show in my thesis that if temperature was subtracted, there remained small components of EPSP enhancement that reflected behaviour and possibly learning. However, the findings that temperature could so dramatically affect EPSP shook the field. Like several other scientists, when I submitted my PhD thesis in 1995, I was inspired to move on to individual cell recordings, which were much less temperature dependent. This is what finally led me to John O'Keefe's lab at the University College of London.

EDINBURGH INTERMEZZO

Long before we submitted our theses, May-Britt and I had decided to do our postdocs with Richard Morris at the University of Edinburgh. We met Richard

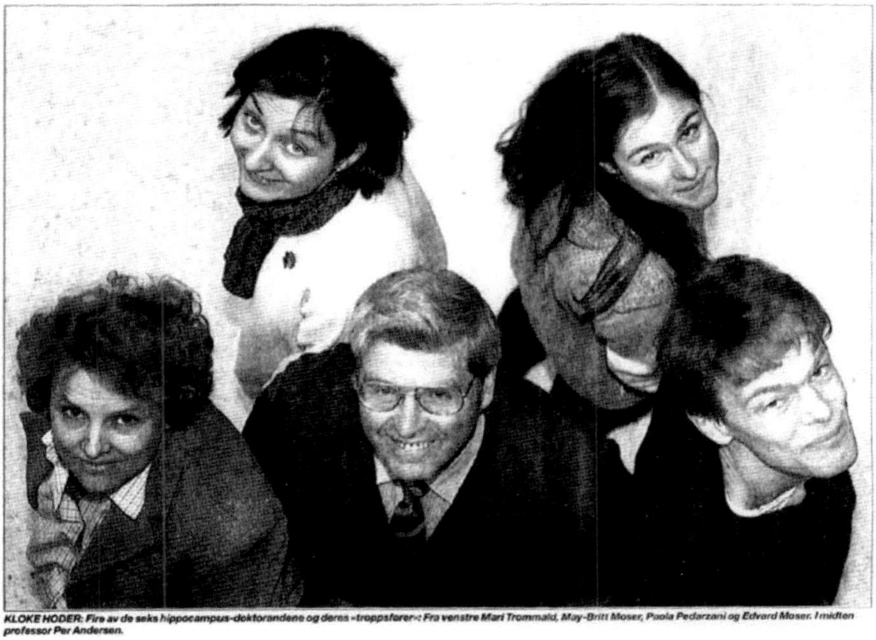
KLOKE HODER: Fire av de seks hippocampus-doktorandene og deres «troppsfører»: Fra venstre Mari Trommald, May-Britt Moser, Paola Pedarzani og Edvard Moser. I midten professor Per Andersen.

FIGURE 4. Per Andersen and four of the students who participated in his Grand Slam, where six students defended their dissertations during the same week in 1995. Left to right: Mari Trommald, May-Britt, Per, Paola Pedarzani, and me. Photo credit: Universitas.

for the first time at the European Neuroscience Meeting in Stockholm in 1990. This was the first time we presented our dorsal-ventral lesion study at a conference and we were extremely proud when Richard referred to our poster in his plenary lecture. Later he invited us to repeat the study with more selective ibotenic acid lesions in his lab, in order to rule out the possibility that behaviour was impaired by dorsal lesions simply because those aspiration lesions severed bypassing fibres. At the same time, ibotenic acid lesions gave us another opportunity to make the *in vivo* lamella that Per wanted. Perhaps, with more selective lesions, it would be possible to get animals to learn with only a small remaining piece of the hippocampal circuit.

The collaboration between Oslo and Edinburgh started in 1991, when we went to Richard for a month to make the first ibotenic acid lesions. We brought our first daughter Isabel, who was less than a year old, and Richard's wife Hilary looked after her. We visited several times, and Per visited Edinburgh, and in 1995 we published the results, showing the same dorso-ventral difference in spatial learning, but now with intact learning even with quite small remnants in the dorsal part of the hippocampus. The remnant was still a lot thicker than Per had hoped for but it showed that hippocampal learning could be maintained with minimal hippocampal circuitry.

Finally, in 1995, after we had submitted our PhD theses in Oslo, we went for a longer visit to Edinburgh. By this time, we had two small girls: Isabel, now 4 years old, and Ailin, who was only 4 months old. Our focus was now on LTP. The aim was to saturate LTP using a protocol developed by Bruce McNaughton and colleagues some years before. Many studies had failed to replicate the learning impairments Bruce and colleagues had demonstrated, but we suspected that the induction of LTP was incomplete and so devised an electrode array that covered a much larger part of the perforant path input to the hippocampus. We struggled a lot to obtain saturation, and I am not sure we ever got it, but at least our induction protocol produced a learning impairment much like that seen in Bruce's early studies. It took a while to complete this particular project, however. We worked on it in Edinburgh in 1995, then in Oslo during Richard's winter sabbatical in 1995–96, then in Edinburgh in 1996, and finally in Trondheim in 1996–97, where we got it to work. We did not spend many months in Edinburgh but we learned a lot, met scientists from all over the world, and had great discussions that helped us define and refine our goals. Moreover, I developed a life-long friendship with Richard.

A QUICK VISIT TO LONDON

My postdoc in Edinburgh was paid for by a Human Frontiers grant that Richard Morris had obtained for a group of labs interested in synaptic plasticity. The LTP saturation experiment was part of this project, but based on my experiences from Oslo, I wanted to go ahead with single unit recording and look for changes in neural activity related to memory. I had hoped eventually to set up unit recording in Edinburgh but it was expensive and at that time, the lab had no experience with single units. Richard understandably hesitated but suggested that I instead go work with John O'Keefe at University College London to learn how to do single cell recordings. This suggestion was especially gracious since by this time we were already committed to moving to Trondheim later in 1996. It would also allow us to set up our own single-unit recording lab there.

I have often described the period with John as the most learning-rich time in my life, and it was. John spent an enormous amount of time with me so that I could learn everything about how to make single cell recordings. He showed me how to do the surgery, how to make the electrodes, how to do the recordings, and how to analyse the data. I had a little desk inside his office, which gave me almost unlimited opportunities to ask all the questions I wondered about.

In his office, and while I was recording, we discussed what was known and not known about place cells and he alerted me to all the pitfalls in the field—it was all absolutely formative for my future.

I moved to London in March, while May-Britt stayed in Edinburgh to run LTP saturation experiments, but two months later May-Britt came too, as well as our two young daughters, along with May-Britt's brother and sister-in-law as babysitters. Our visit was a training visit and nothing more but the animals we implanted ran on tracks that could be shortened and extended to dissociate the contributions of landmarks and path integration, a question that we have continued to pursue in our research to this very day. In July, finally, we flew back to Norway, ready to set up our own lab.

THE UNEXPECTED MOVE TO TRONDHEIM

Many things happened in parallel in 1995–96. During the course of completing our PhDs and preparing for our postdocs, May-Britt and I were called in for an interview at the university that would become the Norwegian University of Science and Technology (NTNU), in Trondheim, right before Christmas in 1995. Earlier that year, Terje Sagvolden had advised us to apply for a faculty position at NTNU's Psychology Department and we did so, mostly just to test the waters. We were confident that we would not even be shortlisted, given that we had only a few papers and had not yet defended our PhDs. Yet they were indeed interested and we went to check out the location, even though our plan was to spend at least a few years abroad, in London with John O'Keefe and perhaps later at the Centre for Neural Systems, Memory and Aging in Tucson with our PhD thesis opponents from 1995, Bruce McNaughton and Carol Barnes. At that time, this centre was the mecca for neural population codes for memory.

We told the search committee that we would not be interested in only one position, but Sturla Krekling, the head of the committee, really pushed for us and so they soon offered us two positions. We then said we needed a new lab, and we came to them with a list of all the equipment that such a lab required—right down to the prices and suppliers. We had, after all, been partly through the same process before, both in Oslo and in Edinburgh. They basically gave us everything we asked for and we were offered lab space in an empty bomb shelter in the basement under the department. The only condition was that we begin in August of 1996 so that we could teach.

The request for us to start almost immediately completely upended our plans. But the prospect of two jobs and a lab just seemed too good an opportunity to turn down.

TRONDHEIM—FROM BOMB SHELTER TO LAB

May-Britt and I started work in Trondheim on August 1, 1996. We bought a small house near the lab, so that we could run back and forth between the lab and our home to feed the rats and start deprivation at appropriate times, sometimes late in the evening. There were no animal experiments at the department at that time, so we had to build an entire vivarium at the same time as we ordered and set up equipment for place cell recording. We ordered our first recording system from a company associated with the O'Keefe lab—Gignomai, now Axona Ltd—and Jim Donnett and Kate Jeffery came for a few days to help us set up the equipment.

After about a year, we had our first place cell. This was an exciting moment. We brought Sturla Krekling to the lab and he was as proud as we were. With his background from visual-cortex neurophysiology in cats, Sturla was perhaps the only one at the department who really appreciated the spike sounds from the loudspeaker. But the Dean of the Faculty, Jan Morten Dyrstad, a social economist, also showed interest. He was impressed and has since then been one of the strongest supporters of our work. Today he is the chairperson of the Kavli Institute fundraising committee.

It took a long time to collect data because there was only May-Britt and me, and we had to handle routine technical work in addition to the experiments—everything from making cables to cleaning rat cages. In addition, we did most of the teaching in biological psychology, which was quite a lot. The students were excited, and we enjoyed lecturing, but most students were still interested in a clinical career—none of them wanted to spend the rest of their life in a rat laboratory. Thus recruitment was minimal.

In 1999, three years after we started, we managed to attract one student, though. Stig Hollup was different from the other psychology students and liked the technical challenges in our lab. At the same time, we got one part-time technician—Kyrre Haugen, who is still with us. He was able to join our lab because at the end of the year, in 1999, Hans Hellebostad at the Research Council called us and said that they had NOK 100,000 of extra money (about 11,000 euros) that they thought we might be interested in. We were euphoric. Suddenly we had a part-time technician who could section brains and do the histology for us.

But our luck did not end there. At about the same time, the department needed a technician to administer test batteries in the human neuropsychology section. Luckily for us the HR section misunderstood what a test battery was and recruited an electronics engineer for the job. His name was Raymond

Skjerpeng. He knew nothing about neuropsychological test batteries but was an expert on the type of batteries we used in our lab. Since the neuropsychologists could not use him, we convinced the department to let him join our lab. He was extremely creative and spent day and night in the bomb shelter, helping us build up a state-of-the-art neurophysiology lab.

At the turn of the millennium, May-Britt and I recorded routinely from place cells but the cell yield was quite modest. We knew that to understand memory, we needed simultaneous recordings from large numbers of cells. The place to go to learn large-scale parallel recording at that time was the Barnes-McNaughton lab in Tucson, Arizona, where we had wanted to go as postdocs. In 2001, we were able to take a six-week sabbatical in Tucson where we learned to do parallel recordings from many dozens of cells in the hippocampus. It was a technique that had been developed by Bruce in the 1990s.

The visit in Tucson was another intense learning period. During the day, we wired electrode arrays and used them to record from hippocampus cells while the rats ran on circular tracks. In the evening, we went home with Bruce and Carol, lived in their guest house in the saguaro-studded desert next to the Catalina Mountains, and enjoyed long discussions over a glass of wine in the Jacuzzi in their garden. In the early morning, before it got too hot, we went for a walk in the desert, with their dogs (or half wolves, really) every day. Our two girls went to a Baptist school—the only school that could offer them a place for just 6 weeks. The school was radically different from anything they were used to—the children had to walk in the streets to proclaim the gospel—a different way of expressing religion than what I was used to from the Norwegian west-coast islands—but our two girls learned tolerance and the visit was as formative for them as for us.

During our first years in Trondheim, we were primarily interested in hippocampal mechanisms of memory. We set up a water maze and started recording place cells while rats navigated in a water maze. This was a technically challenging task, as we had to keep water away from the animal's headstage, but the electrical silence of the bomb shelter helped, and in 2001 we could report our first findings in *The Journal of Neuroscience*. We showed that place fields were not evenly distributed in the water maze but were more abundant in the area where the animals found the platform. Many experiments failed though, because water leaked through the insulation around the headstage, so we gradually turned our focus to simpler behavioural paradigms, while at the same time we switched to multi-tetrode parallel recording, based on our experiences from the visit in Tucson.

FROM FOUR HANDS TO TWO DOZEN

One of the questions that intrigued May-Britt and me most was quite fundamental: What was the origin of the place signal in the hippocampus? With CA1 and CA3 cell recordings up and running in our lab, we saw early on that place cells could be used not only to understand place coding as such but also to more generally understand computation in the hippocampus.

There is no place signal in the sensory inputs to the brain, so how does it come about? Is it generated by the hippocampus itself? Since John O'Keefe discovered place cells in 1971, almost all studies had been performed in the CA1 subfield, the last stage of the hippocampal intrinsic circuit. We wondered if the earlier subfields—the dentate gyrus and CA3—played any role in the formation of place correlates, and if any part of the signal came from the outside, from the entorhinal cortex, which provides most of the cortical input to the hippocampus.

To address this and related questions we applied for funding from the European Commission's Framework V programme. This programme funded only collaborative grants. I had never before applied for a consortium, just for May-Britt and myself. To put together an application that succinctly addressed the criteria of the call, we got enormous help from Bruce Reed, a highly intelligent and knowledgeable advisor quite different from any other grant consultant I have worked with. Unlike most of his colleagues, he gave us feedback on the content of our proposal and helped us shape it into an application that pointed directly to the experiments that so tremendously changed our understanding of spatial representation a few years later. In one of the proposal's work packages, we aimed specifically to determine the nature of the entorhinal inputs to the place cells, in order to find out how they were generated.

The proposal was submitted in 1999, the reviews were positive, and in 2000 I was suddenly the coordinator of a consortium of 7 groups. Among the members in the group were Richard Morris, our postdoc advisor, and Menno Witter at the Free University of Amsterdam, an expert on entorhinal-hippocampal anatomy whom we had already approached in 1990 as we wrote up our master's thesis on dorso-ventral gradients in hippocampal function. He wrote a long and helpful reply to our letter in 1990, which encouraged us to maintain contact.

The EU grant came at a time when many funding agencies started to get interested in our work. Just a year later, we applied for 'strategic' money from the Research Council of Norway. They had a programme to strengthen research in pre-selected areas, and neuroscience was certainly not among those areas. A group of deans at NTNU was responsible for selecting proposals in the right areas. They chose our proposal, despite the fact that it was completely outside of the Research Council's pre-selected areas. This group included several people who later became rectors of NTNU, including Eivind Hiis Hauge, Torbjørn Digernes and Gunnar Bovim. They all had confidence in our work from the very beginning. I am very grateful for their ability to see the potential in our proposal at a time when we had little published evidence of scientific excellence.

At about the same time, May-Britt and I moved our lab to the Faculty of Medicine. The Psychology Department had given us exceptional start-up conditions, and we are forever grateful to Sturla Krekling, who saw our potential, but psychology is a diverse field, our work was expensive, and we were too different to remain there. To compensate for the lack of biology-minded individuals at the Psychology Department, we had first met regularly with Arne Valberg, a visual neuro-psychophysicist, and Hanna Mustaparta, a biologist who studied neural coding in insect olfactory systems. Based on these encounters, in 2001, after extensive lobbying by Jon Lamvik, a former Dean of Medicine, we were offered lab space at the Medical-Technical Centre, where most of the Faculty of Medicine's basic experimental research was conducted. The building was immensely crowded at that time, and we are grateful to Jon Lamvik as well as the Dean in 2001, Gunnar Bovim, for making that space available.

As we moved in, our lab was transformed in many ways. Not only did we get an opportunity to build a lab more suited to our increasing interest in the basic computational mechanisms of the hippocampus, but we suddenly had lots of money—from the EU and from the Strategic Research Programme. In 2002, our success continued. The Research Council inaugurated a new funding scheme where 13 Centres, selected among all fields of science and technology, were given extensive funding for 10 years. This was a new funding scheme meant to boost performance among highly selected research groups. We applied for one of these grants. It was a long application process, involving two stages of selection, and our research plans for the next decade were considerably refined as we wrote the application.

A Christmas and New Year's visit in 2001 by Carol Barnes and Bruce McNaughton helped improve our application. We talked and wrote, went skiing, and celebrated the holidays together. Bruce even dressed up as Santa for the two girls. In the end our proposal was selected, again before we had much of a track record. But I believe the research plans convinced the committee, as well as the proposal to hire 7 internationally recognized scientists as visiting members of the Centre: Carol and Bruce, Richard Morris, Alessandro Treves, Menno Witter, Randolf Menzel and Ole Paulsen.

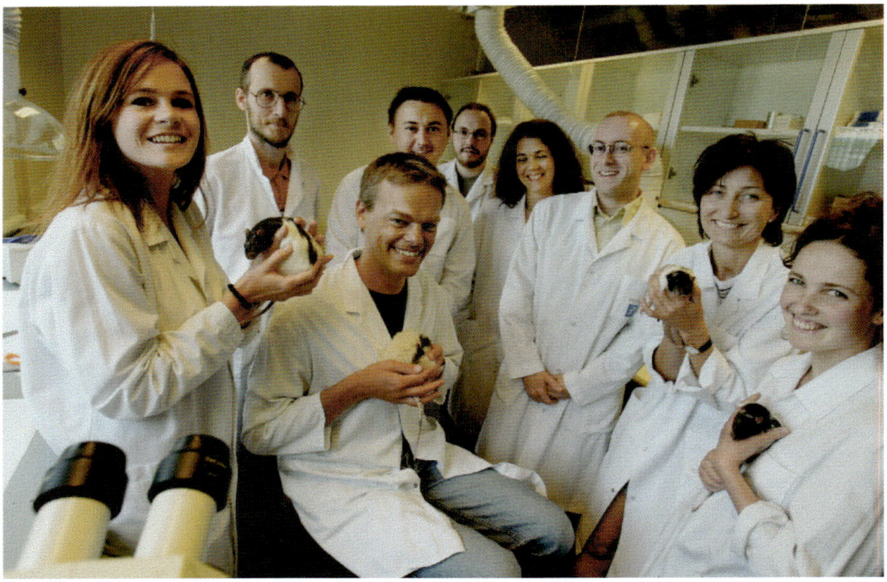

FIGURE 5. Our research group in 2002, just after the award of the Centre of Excellence grant. I am in the middle, May-Britt is second from the right. Credit NTNU Info/ Rune Petter Ness.

The idea was that these researchers would visit the lab once or twice per year to participate directly in experiments. So starting in December 2002, the Centre for the Biology of Memory became a reality and all of a sudden we had enough money to address all of our favourite questions. We could buy equipment, we could recruit just the right number of students, and we had some of the world's best advisors coming periodically to our lab to help us plan and conduct cutting-edge experiments. From late 2002, we were a group with about 10 motivated and talented students and technicians as well as a wonderful international network (Fig. 5).

THE PATH TO THE ENTORHINAL CORTEX

The discovery of grid cells began with the study of intrahippocampal origins of the place cell signal. In the 1990s, it was commonly believed that localised firing emerged within the hippocampus, based on weakly spatial inputs from the entorhinal cortex. This belief was based on several studies showing that cells in the entorhinal cortex had large and diffuse firing fields, very different from those in the CA1 of the hippocampus. Spatial selectivity was thus thought to originate somehow and somewhere in the intrahippocampal circuit. To find out how and where, May-Britt and I joined forces with Menno Witter, one of the members of the EU consortium that I coordinated. Along with Vegard Brun, a talented medical student, we selectively lesioned the CA3 of the dorsal hippocampus, or we used small knife cuts to interrupt connections from CA3 to CA1. With Menno Witter, we used fluorescent tracers to show that after both interventions, intrahippocampal inputs to the CA1 were absent, leaving only the direct connections from the entorhinal cortex.

We expected the lesions to severely disrupt place signals in CA1 but in fact they did not. Despite effective cuts, the cells exhibited localised firing, suggesting that place signals emerged either within the CA1 circuit itself, or were based on spatial signals from the only remaining cortical source—the entorhinal cortex. These findings, published in *Science* in 2002, suggested it was high time to record within the entorhinal cortex itself—a dormant goal in the EU grant that we wrote in 1999.

Until around 2001, the entorhinal cortex had seemed scary but now we were motivated to get started as soon as possible. We needed students. Vegard Brun was an obvious choice but he had medical exams and was only available part-time so we looked around. A year earlier we had recruited Marianne Fyhn. She applied for a position as a technician but we saw her potential and offered her a fellowship instead. For a while she recorded place cells in the water maze but the task was challenging and we considered alternatives. She was the perfect candidate for entorhinal cortex recordings.

In 2002 we got started. Menno Witter was by now a visiting member of the Centre for the Biology of Memory. Based on his early work on dorso-ventral gradients in entorhinal-hippocampal connectivity, which I had read in the finest detail, and based on the many discussions we had in person as we started our collaboration, it became clear that there was an alternative interpretation to the difference between entorhinal and hippocampal spatial selectivity reported in previous *in vivo* recording studies. It turned out that these earlier recordings had all been conducted in the intermediate-to-ventral part of the entorhinal cortex, which is primarily connected to the ventral hippocampus, where place fields are large and difficult to identify when rats run in standard-sized laboratory environments.

We reasoned that it would make much more sense to record in the dorsal part of the entorhinal cortex, from which the dorsal place cells get most of their input. It would also make sense to target the medial part of the entorhinal cortex, considering that much of the visual-somatosensory input reaches this region. Thus, Menno sat down with Marianne and May-Britt and showed them how to access the dorsomedial entorhinal cortex, a chunk of cortex never targeted before in any *in vivo* study, due to its location at the very back of the rat cerebrum, close to the transverse sinus. It was also not easy to localize in standard atlases of the rat brain, which at time mostly showed coronal and horizontal sections, without a sagittal orientation, which is the only suitable one for localizing electrode traces so far back in the brain.

It did not take long before interesting results surfaced. The recordings showed that entorhinal cells had discrete firing fields much like those of hippocampal place cells but each cell had multiple fields scattered all around in the box. The animal's location could not be inferred from a single cell alone, but collectively the cells provided a pretty good estimate. It was also clear that the multiple firing fields were not arranged randomly. The distance between neighbouring fields was strikingly constant and clearly different from what could be expected by chance. We published these findings in *Science* in 2004, knowing now that the dorsomedial entorhinal cortex provided much of the spatial input to CA1 but without being able to understand the neural code of these inputs.

But we were on the right track. At the end of 2004, we presented our findings at the Society for Neuroscience meeting in San Diego. We knew our results contained much of what O'Keefe and colleagues had searched for in their work on the cognitive map and we changed the title of one of our posters to 'The Entorhinal Cortex as a Cognitive Map', in order to highlight the connection to John O'Keefe and Lynn Nadel's work on hippocampal maps more than 25 years earlier. The poster attracted a lot of attention and excitement from the place cell community and from modellers interested in the neural basis of path integration-mediated spatial representation. We got many insightful suggestions during the poster presentation.

One of the most helpful poster session participants was Bill Skaggs, then at the University of California at Davis. After his many useful suggestions on the poster floor, May-Britt and I invited him for a breakfast meeting in order to discuss how such a pattern could arise, in the context of his understanding of continuous attractor mechanisms for place cells, and we discussed ways to follow up on the findings. Bill clearly suggested how hexagonal firing could arise from an attractor mechanism not too different from the ones he had proposed with Bruce McNaughton for place cells and head direction cells. During the course of a few days, it all became clear to us. We needed to expand the size of the environment, to be sure that the pattern was really hexagonal, the way it appeared to be. We also needed to test animals in darkness, to show that the pattern was path integration-dependent, and we needed to show that the pattern was anchored to visual inputs by testing whether rotation of salient cues also rotated the grid pattern.

GRID CELLS

Returning from the Society meeting we had a package of experiments to do, and we again asked Marianne for help, along with her boyfriend Torkel Hafting, who had by then moved to Trondheim. The two of them ran the majority of the experiments, with May-Britt stepping in periodically, working with Marianne in the lab on a daily basis and taking over experiments during weekends or holidays when they were away. My role was to analyse data, write it up, and not least, read, to try to understand. Sturla Molden, the fifth person on the project, wrote code and helped with statistical analysis, including the use of spatial autocorrelation procedures to identify spatial periodicity.

We suspected that there might be something like a hexagonal firing pattern as this was already evident from the recordings in the 2004 paper. However it seemed too good to be true and we needed data from larger environments to be sure that this periodicity was not just coincidental. The turning point was the recording from the circular environment that was two metres in diameter and that we had adopted for this purpose. The arrangement of the firing fields looked strikingly hexagonal—and this became particularly clear when Sturla Molden had finished the autocorrelation program. Within a few weeks, on several occasions, we had multiple Eureka experiences, where it became clearer and clearer that the hexagonal pattern was neither a coincidence nor a technical artefact. The firing fields tiled the entire space available to the rat, in a pattern reminiscent of the holes of a beehive. We had several names for our baby, but because of the grid-like nature of the firing pattern, I suggested we called them grid cells. It was a simple and descriptive term.

The fact that firing fields were so regular despite changes in the animal's speed and direction suggested that their location was determined by path integration and that grid cells were part of the mechanism for path integration-based spatial mapping—a mechanism envisaged by O'Keefe as early as 1976, but with no evidence for it until now. I was convinced that we had found an important element of the cognitive map—something completely different from anything known elsewhere in the brain. Our journey to this point was aided by important input from the visiting members of the centre. In particular, Bruce McNaughton's insights in computational neuroscience were really transformative for me. His earlier work on attractor mechanisms inspired me and is still the basis for much of my thinking about how space is represented. With this as a background we felt that we could not only describe a new cell type but we could also put it in a historical and theoretical context. We submitted the paper to *Nature*, the reviews were positive, and in the summer of 2005 the paper was out.

Finding grid cells was exciting because it gave us another piece in the puzzle of how we navigate in space. But the larger significance of the find is that we were able to see how the brain generates one of its own internal codes, with mechanisms that reflect the inner workings of a cortical system, quite independently of any particular sensory inputs. In the past, it had been difficult to make associations between the firing of neurons deep in the higher parts of the cortex and properties of the external world, because as the distance between the sensory input and the neuron increases, the firing of the neurons is triggered by a multitude of converging sensory channels along with intrinsic processes that we don't really understand.

But with the grid cells, and the place cells that O'Keefe had discovered, we had neural activity that was clearly associated with a feature of the environment, the animal's location. Here, we think, lies a key to unlocking the mystery of how the brain computes. There is no grid pattern in the external world so the pattern must originate from activity in the entorhinal cortex itself, or in adjacent structures. Having access to data from these cells felt like a great reward, as it might put us on the track of the more general computational operations of the cortex.

FROM LAB TO INSTITUTE

When we found the grid cells, we were still a medium-sized research group, and we had only our own group to care for. But soon after, things started to change. Just before the grid cell results were published, the philanthropist Fred Kavli visited NTNU, along with David Auston, the President of the Kavli Foundation at that time. They were in Norway to prepare for the inauguration of the Kavli Prize, which would be awarded for the first time in 2008. At the same time, they used the opportunity to visit research groups in the fields they were interested in. They came to our lab and were totally struck by the grid cell discovery. At the same time, Eric Kandel, who himself was head of a Kavli Institute at Columbia, argued strongly for a Kavli Institute at NTNU. He was tremendously excited about our work.

Soon after they left, May-Britt and I were invited to submit an application, and in 2007, we became the 15th Kavli Institute in the world and the fourth in neuroscience (Fig. 6). In the end, Fred was enormously proud that a Kavli Institute had been established at his alma mater, although it was important for him, to the very end, that the institute had not been established for that reason but only because it satisfied the foundation's strict criteria for quality. The inauguration of the institute not only gave us funding and support but also opened doors to some of the best neuroscience groups in the world. Many individuals made

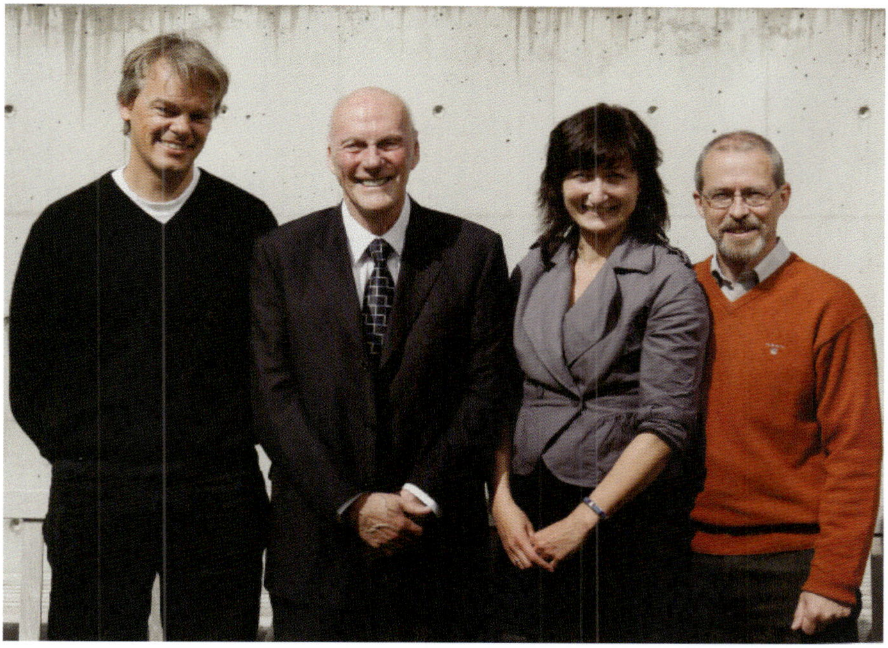

FIGURE 6. In 2007, we became the Kavli Institute for Systems Neuroscience. The picture was taken during Fred Kavli's visit in 2008. Left to right: me, Fred, May-Britt and Menno Witter. Photo credit Grom Kallestad / SCANPIX.

important contributions to the formation of the institute. In Norway, these individuals include two NTNU rectors—first Eivind Hiis Hauge, and then Torbjørn Digernes, who was the rector during the negotiations—as well as the secretary general of the Ministry of Education and Research, Trond Fevolden, and Arvid Hallén, Director of the Research Council of Norway.

The establishment of the Kavli Institute represented the beginning of a transition from a single-group centre to an institute. Menno Witter was the first new faculty to join us. Menno had collaborated with us almost from the beginning, when we got our first EU grant in 1999. He became a member of the Centre for the Biology of Memory and participated in some of the most important studies in the Centre's history—studies that led up to the grid cell discovery and several studies that investigated their properties. In 2007, with the Kavli Institute in place, and with the help of the Dean of the Faculty of Medicine, Stig Slørdahl, we were able to offer Menno conditions that convinced him to move his entire research group to NTNU.

A few years later, in 2010, we recruited Yasser Roudi, a theoretical and computational neuroscientist, and a student of Alessandro Treves, who is a visiting member of our institute. In 2013, Cliff Kentros moved from the University of Oregon to set up a group for studies of memory using transgenic mouse technology, and in 2014 we recruited Emre Yaksi to set up a lab for zebrafish studies of the nervous system. Jonathan Whitlock joined the faculty when he received a Starting Grant from the European Research Council.

THE CONNECTION TO MEMORY

The discovery of grid cells opened the door on understanding the brain's system for spatial mapping. However, the brain regions containing place cells and grid cells are also crucial for everyday memory and it was the relation to memory that motivated our first studies in the hippocampus. What could be the link between space and memory? Are the same neurons involved and if so, how can they perform both functions? To understand this relationship, May-Britt and I maintained our interest in memory and conducted a number of studies, in parallel with the entorhinal work, which made it easier to understand how the two phenomena are related.

By 2002, when we moved out of the Psychology Department, we had realized that place cell recording in the water maze was too ambitious. The problem was not primarily the contact with water but rather the complexity of the task. Recording while rats learned to find the hidden platform might reveal activity specifically related to storage of spatial information but the task could be solved in many ways, and it was difficult to rule out the contribution of trivial sensory or motor contributions to changes in firing rates. Thus we were increasingly attracted to simple reductionistic paradigms such as the old open field that we started out with during our work on hyperactive rats with Terje Sagvolden. After a few years in the new lab at the Faculty of Medicine, we made sure that all the rooms in the lab had open fields.

So how could we address spatial memory in an environment with no goal to search for? In the late 1980s, Bob Muller and John Kubie at SUNY Downstate had shown that place cells 'remap' between environments. They trained animals in different versions of the same enclosure, in the same place, and found that each enclosure was associated with a different subset of active cells. Along with later work from a number of laboratories, including that of Bruce McNaughton and Carol Barnes in Tucson, they showed that hippocampal ensembles switched between quite different firing patterns as animals moved from one environment to another, and sometimes even when only task factors were changed within the same environment.

It became clear to them, and to us, that remapping might serve as a window on the mechanisms underlying memory storage in the hippocampus. Each environment had its distinct representation, mediated by different combinations of active cells. It seemed like the hippocampus had one map for each environment, operating much like a catalogue for all environments that the animal had encountered. Studying how these representations are formed and how they are segregated from one another felt like an interesting set of questions to pursue.

For our studies of remapping, May-Britt and I recruited Stefan Leutgeb, one of the postdocs who participated in our first EU grant. Stefan shared our interest in neural substrates of memory, as well as computational differences between the hippocampal subfields. We started out by comparing CA3 and CA1 and found, in collaboration with Alessandro Treves, a visiting member of the Centre, that place representations in CA3 cells were much more decorrelated than those typically recorded in CA1. Later work, with Jill Leutgeb, who joined the lab a year later, as well as with Bruce McNaughton and Carol Barnes, showed that CA3 networks had attractor properties, although transitions between representations were not always as sharp as envisaged if the hippocampus contained only discrete attractors.

Our work showed that there are two types of remapping—sharp transitions similar to those seen by Muller and Kubie, which we referred to as global remapping—and more gradual transitions, in which firing rates changed smoothly as external inputs were altered, whereas firing locations remained the same. The latter was dubbed rate remapping. The studies of remapping were possible because we could record large numbers of cells at the same time, using the multitetrode technology that we had learned from Bruce and Carol during our 2001 visit in Tucson.

The use of remapping as a way to understand hippocampal memory begged an obvious question: how was hippocampal memory, expressed through remapping, influenced by inputs from grid cells in the entorhinal cortex? Grid cells are the most abundant cell type in layer II of the entorhinal cortex, and it was very likely, as shown in more recent work from our lab, that they provide a significant share of the projections from the medial entorhinal cortex to the hippocampus.

This led us to compare representations across environments in grid cells, at the same time as cells were recorded in the hippocampus. Again with Marianne Fyhn in the lab, we recorded grid cells and place cells in different enclosures in the same place or in different enclosures in different rooms. With the help of Alessandro Treves, we cross-correlated ensemble maps from each environment to see if relative firing locations and orientations were maintained. The striking finding was that the map structure was maintained in grid cells whereas no similarity was preserved in the hippocampus, suggesting that as information is passed from grid cells to place cells, it is completely transformed—from a single universal map in the entorhinal cortex to a multitude of almost-orthogonal maps in the hippocampus, with apparently one map for each environment.

In this sense, the grid cell map was similar to maps of head direction cells in other areas, which also maintained their intrinsic structure across environments. The data suggested there were two types of spatial maps—a rigid map in the entorhinal cortex that maintained a single metric independent of the nature of the environment, and a much richer map in the hippocampus with representations individualised to each environment, much as one would like for a memory storage system. The relationship between the two maps intrigued us, and with Laura Colgin, we showed that spatial maps in the entorhinal cortex and CA1 are temporarily synchronised via oscillations in the fast gamma range. Between these short moments of entorhinal-CA1 synchronisation, CA1 cells synchronise with CA3 cells possibly involved in the internal storage of spatial representations. Finally, using new molecular and optogenetic tools, we also showed, with Sheng-Jia Zhang and Jing Ye, that grid cells project directly to the hippocampus, as hypothesised by our work on remapping. Thus, by approximately 2012, we felt that we had an improved understanding of how grid and place cells interact, although there remain major questions yet to be answered.

GRID CELLS: FROM SINGLE CELLS TO NETWORKS

The discovery of grid cells also led us to ask what the intrinsic network of the entorhinal cortex is like. How is the grid pattern formed? How do grid cells interact; what can they achieve together that they cannot do alone? What other cell types are there and how do they all interact?

Since the discovery of grid cells, my fascination with their crystal-like firing pattern and its potential mechanisms has not flagged. In 2005, we were able to record only a few grid cells at the time and it was difficult to infer how they operated at the ensemble level. This has changed. In 2009, Hanne and Tor Stensola, another couple, joined our lab. Hanne had a talent for recording large numbers of grid cells in the same animal and Tor a talent for devising clever analyses to infer their systems properties. They were able to record almost 200 grid cells per animal, enough to demonstrate that grid cells are organised into a small number of functional modules, each with its own unique grid spacing. This result was published in *Nature* in 2012. We found that modules can operate independently in the presence of changes to the geometry of the environment.

Two years later, during the Nobel celebrations in Stockholm, *Nature* accepted a second major finding from their work. We were able to show that grid cells align with borders of the local environment through a shearing-like mechanism that causes both deformation and rotation of the grid pattern. The asymmetry of grid cells is completely predictable by the shearing mechanism that we described.

But what was behind the mechanism of the grid pattern? Early on, Bruce McNaughton alerted us to the significance of attractor network mechanisms in spatial representation. Our interest in these kinds of representations grew as Yasser Roudi joined the faculty to start a theoretical physics group. Shortly after Yasser moved to Trondheim in 2010, Menno Witter's group had shown that stellate cells—most of which are likely to be grid cells—lacked excitatory recurrent connections. The lack of such connections was a puzzle for attractor theories of grid cells but Yasser and his colleagues showed that hexagonal symmetries could also be obtained by purely inhibitory interconnections.

The attractor model explained some key features of the data. The observed independence of the grid modules, for example, was exactly as predicted. For grid patterns to appear as an equilibrium state in a network of interconnected neurons, and for such patterns to be updated in accordance with the animal's movement, interconnected cells may need to share both grid spacing and grid orientation. This means that the network must be organised in a modular fashion, with each module corresponding to a semi-independent attractor network. The data have convinced me that grid cells do, to some extent, reflect attractor mechanisms but the detailed implementation of the mechanism is clearly not well understood. Digging deeper into the mechanism of the grid pattern will certainly be among our major goals in the years to come.

Grid cells do not operate in isolation, however. Soon after the discovery of grid cells in 2005, Francesca Sargolini came to the lab. She showed that there are head direction cells in the medial entorhinal cortex, especially in the deeper and intermediate layers, and that they intermingle with grid cells in these layers. Head direction cells are cells that fire selectively when animals face a certain direction, with activity similar to a compass, except that the firing direction is determined by local cues, not magnetic inputs. Head direction cells were discovered by Jim Ranck at SUNY Downstate in 1985, in the dorsal presubiculum, adjacent to the medial entorhinal cortex, but Francesca's head direction cells were the first in the entorhinal cortex. Many head direction cells were grid cells at the same time. We called them conjunctive cells. The combined spatial and directional signal of these cells obviously pointed to a close link between the metrics for direction and location.

The search for additional cell types also led us to discover border cells in the entorhinal cortex. With Trygve Solstad and others in our lab, we found that approximately one-tenth of our cells fired selectively along walls or edges of the recording environment. They did so in every single environment, and their firing also lined up along small wall inserts within an open field. Border cells were functionally different from their more abundant counterparts, the grid cells. Entorhinal border cells were also observed by Jim Knierim's group, then at the University of Texas in Houston, and cells with similar properties, referred to as boundary vector cells, had been reported by John O'Keefe and colleagues in the subiculum. The entorhinal border cells were intermingled with head direction cells and grid cells, and they were also present in layer II.

Finally, quite recently, we have shown that grid cells, border cells, and head direction cells co-localise with speed cells, cells that fire linearly in relation to the animal's instantaneous speed. This is work we have conducted with Emilio Kropff, who worked as a postdoc in our lab. Combined, these many cell types form a network of diverse cells with distinct functions, all embedded in the same network. Understanding how this network of cell types operates to form a holistic representation of space will keep us busy for many years to come.

THE NEXT DECADE

After the 10-year lifetime of the Centre for the Biology of Memory ended in 2012, we were awarded another decade of funding. The Centre for Neural Computation, with May-Britt as the Director, will be alive until 2023 and we expect the number of faculty at this centre to increase. The rapid expansion of our activity is the result of generous support from Stig Slørdahl, the Dean of the Faculty of Medicine, who has used every opportunity to help us to further improve and extend the centre. At the same time, the Research Council and NTNU have given us funding for an almost ten-fold expansion of the lab space of the institute, and the Ministry, in collaboration with the Research Council, gave us more or less permanent support for technical and administrative staff—support that is generally not easy to obtain through regular grants. Because of this support, the team has been transformed from a single entity with a strong focus on a single cluster of questions to an entire institute consisting of multiple research groups covering a broad range of systems questions, well beyond the domain of space and memory.

With the new centre funding, we are also establishing new collaborations. One of these is with Tobias Bonhoeffer from the Max Planck Institute for Neurobiology outside Munich. He joined us as a visiting professor in 2014 and works with us on using two-photon imaging to establish the detailed functional organisation of the grid cell network. A student of ours, Albert Tsao, has been working in his lab for almost two years and I have visited Tobias' lab frequently. At the same time we are setting up imaging technology in our own lab. The collaboration re-establishes a friendship that started almost 50 years ago, when the two of us used to play in a sandbox in a residential area in Tübingen in Germany. I used to spend parts of the summer with my parents visiting my aunt and uncle, Ulrike and Hermann Lange, who lived just a few houses away from the Bonhoeffer house. We rediscovered our friendship when Tobias's mother told him about the Norwegian boy who came to visit every summer. Today Tobias is the external collaborator who is most strongly transforming our lab, via his help to introduce imaging technology for population studies of grid cell activity. He is not the only one, however. Pico Caroni is also a very valuable member, as is John O'Keefe, who is, and always has been, a thoughtful and forward-looking discussion partner.

THE CALL FROM STOCKHOLM

On October 6, 2014, I was on the plane to Munich for an extended research visit to Tobias Bonhoeffer's group at the Max Planck Institute for Neurobiology near Munich. While I was in the air, working on a manuscript, my life changed dramatically, without me knowing. My first surprise was the encounter with a representative from the Munich Airport who met me with flowers and an airport car at the gate when we landed. She told me I had won a prize but mixed up things and said it was a prize from the Max Planck Society.

It was only when I checked my iPhone that I started to understand (Fig. 7). There was a text message from Göran Hansson, the secretary of the Nobel Committee, as well as hundreds of other emails and text messages. Then Tobias called and congratulated me. A few minutes later I was met by Tobias and his lab, with champagne in the arrivals hall, and an hour later there was a press conference and even more champagne. After an hour or so was I able to connect with May-Britt, who got the call from Göran Hansson two hours before I became aware of the news from Stockholm. On the day after, on October 7, I was back in Trondheim, to celebrate the event with the family, the lab and the rest of the university (Fig. 8).

The subsequent weeks were crazy. It took a while to get organised and find a way to handle the steady flow of requests to lecture, open conferences, and give interviews and comments. In the end I learned to prioritise and life got back to normal, with the brain at the centre. Then, in December, the celebrations

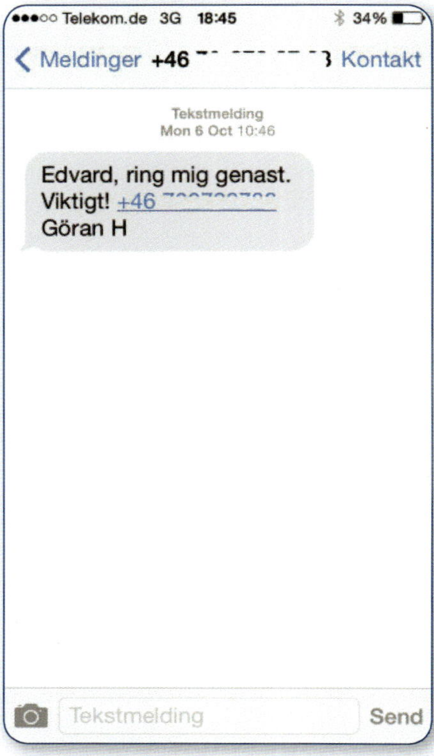

FIGURE 7. The text message from Göran Hansson, the secretary of the Nobel Committee, which I received when I landed at Munich airport on October 6, 2014. English translation: "Edvard, call me as soon as possible. Important!"

started again. The Swedes treated us like kings. Each laureate had his or her own attaché who took care of all appointments and guided us from event to event. The ceremony was moving. Receiving the medal from King Carl Gustaf on the stage, with applause from a packed audience, is imprinted in my memory, as is the Nobel lecture in the new Aula Medica, in front of 1,200 attentive listeners.

It was delightful to share the experience with John, our generous mentor from the 1990s and such a thoughtful scientist. I liked the other laureates. By the end of the Nobel week, we felt we knew all of them a little bit. And I must add that the Swedes really know how to celebrate science. Torsten Wiesel and Eric Kandel had come to celebrate with us, as had numerous colleagues and collaborators. When we left on December 13, I believe everyone in the country knew what a grid cell was. Our research had reached the public and I got the impression that they all celebrated with us. It was a prize not only for systems neuroscience but also for research in Norway and Scandinavia, and everyone was part of it.

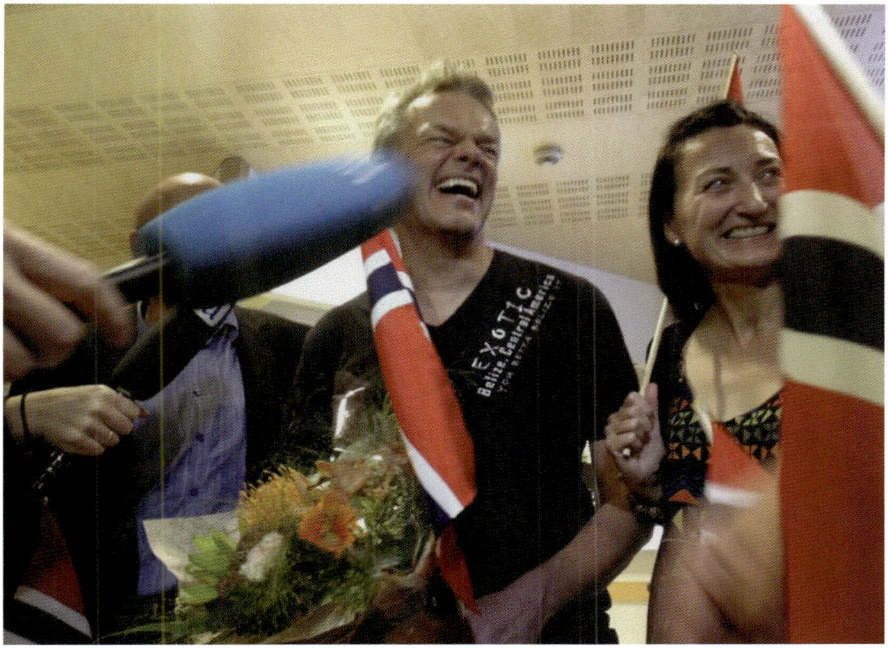

FIGURE 8. Welcome at the Trondheim airport upon my return on October 7.

PERSPECTIVE

My journey from Haramsøya—that small island off the coast where I was born—to Stockholm has been quite an adventure. Who would have predicted this when I entered the world from our modest house on that little windy island of farmers and fishermen? I am still not entirely certain what made it possible. The academic interests of my parents certainly contributed, but in the absence of an external intellectual environment, and with no extra stimulation in primary school or secondary school, the fact that I became a successful scientist was perhaps somewhat against the odds.

Even after I knew that I wanted to spend my life doing research, success was far from guaranteed. Finding the right research group is an essential part of any science career, and I can say that my choices were fortuitous. I learned behavioural analysis with Terje Sagvolden but switched to neuroscience with Per Andersen at the right time, when we—and the field—were ready to bring psychology and physiology together.

Since our PhD days, May-Britt and I have been helped by individuals and institutions, all of whom saw the potential in our work and supported us. Perhaps my personality also helped a little bit. I have a strong will and can be extremely

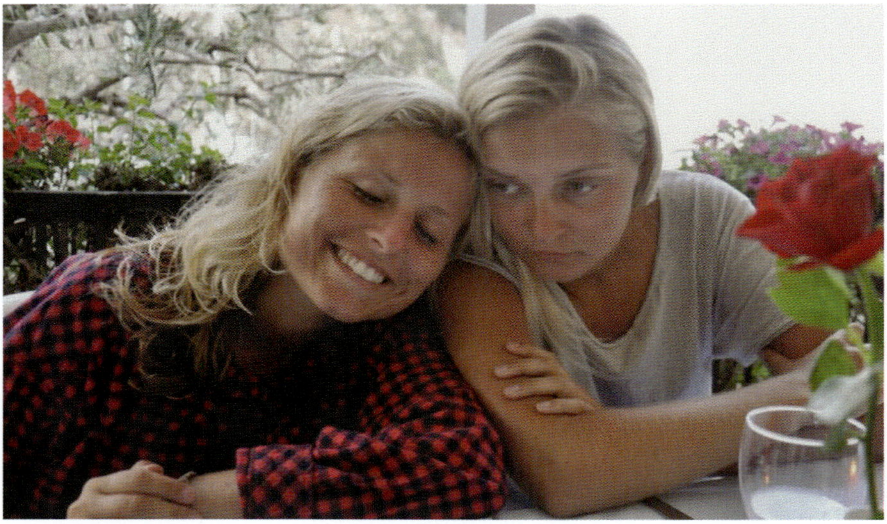

FIGURE 9. My daughters Isabel and Ailin from a tour in France in 2012.

focused on a particular goal, even if it is decades away. My slight enthusiasm for mathematics has been useful, as well as my passion for putting together disparate pieces of information. With the help of May-Britt I felt I could sometimes see the whole picture and the path forward. However, it remains for the historians to put it all together.

Let me finally add that my scientific journey did not happen in a vacuum. I have had a wonderful partner and we in turn have two remarkable daughters—Isabel and Ailin. They were born in 1991 and 1995, respectively, and came with us as we travelled the world—to Edinburgh where we worked with Richard Morris, to John O'Keefe in London, and to Bruce McNaughton and Carol Barnes in Tucson. Together we have explored the planet, not only laboratories and conference auditoriums, but also beaches, rainforests, volcanoes, reefs and remote islands. Today our two girls are mature, thoughtful and warm young women who continue to bring happiness to my life (Fig. 9). That is a gift that is even greater than the Nobel Prize.

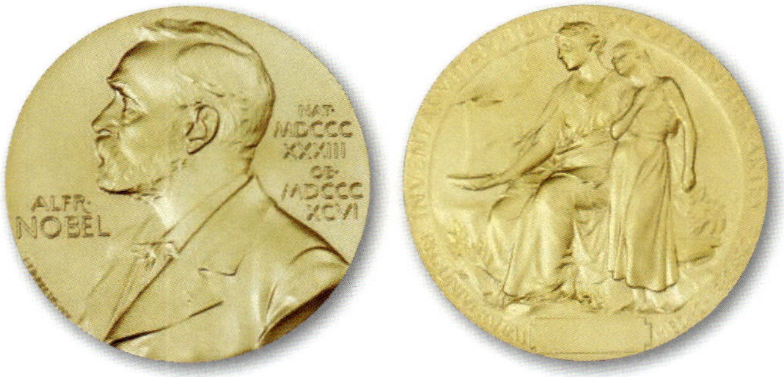

Grid Cells and the Entorhinal Map of Space

Nobel Lecture, 7 December 2014

by Edvard I. Moser

Centre for Neural Computation and Kavli Institute for Systems Neuroscience;
Norwegian University of Science and Technology, Norway.

1. FROM PSYCHOLOGY TO NEUROPHYSIOLOGY—AND BACK

In 1983, May-Britt and I signed up for psychology studies at the University of Oslo. We wanted to understand the neural basis of behaviour. We were intrigued by the great learning theories from the 1930s, 1940s and 1950s and studied the work of J.B. Watson, C.L. Hull, B.F. Skinner and E.C. Tolman (Fig. 1). We found it fascinating that psychology had reached a level where application of the basic laws of the field made it possible to control long sequences of behaviour in animals.

Yet, while the scientific rigour of behaviourism attracted us, we were at the same time disappointed by the fact that physiology was deliberately left out from most behaviourist theories, due to lack of both methods and concepts. Karl Lashley's search for the neural basis of memory at the peak of the behaviourist era was a brave exception and defined the beginning of the merge between psychology and physiology (Lashley, 1929, 1950). However, it was only with Donald O. Hebb, from the end of the 1940s, that behaviour was linked conceptually to neurophysiology (Hebb, 1949). Hebb's ideas on cell assemblies and plasticity inspired an entire new generation of physiologists and psychologists with an interest in learning and memory. The new interest in learning culminated decades later by the discovery of key synaptic mechanisms of memory, as recognised by the 2000 Nobel prize to Eric Kandel (Kandel, 2000).

The potentials of this development—from the laws of learning to its detailed synaptic implementation—really caught May-Britt and me. The wish to bring

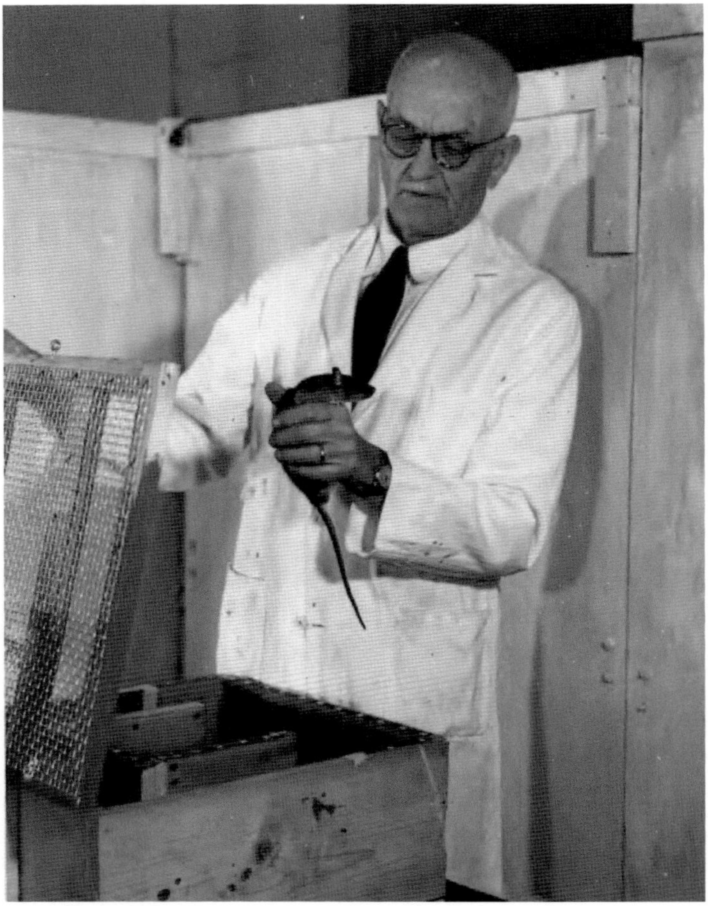

FIGURE 1. All three 2014 Nobel Prize winners in Physiology or Medicine stand on the shoulders of E.C. Tolman. Based on experiments on rats running in various types of mazes, Tolman suggested from the 1930s to the 1950s that animals form internal maps of the external environment. He referred to such maps as cognitive maps and considered them as mental knowledge structures in which information was stored according to its position in the environment (Tolman, 1948). In this sense, Tolman was not only one of the first cognitive psychologists but he also directly set the stage for studies of how space is represented in the brain. Tolman himself avoided any reference to neural structures and neural activity in his theories, which was understandable at a time when neither concepts nor methods had been developed for investigations at the brain-behaviour interface. However, at the end of his life he expressed strong hopes for a neuroscience of behaviour. In 1958, after the death of Lashley, he wrote the following in a letter to Donald O. Hebb when Hebb asked him about his view of physiological explanations of behaviour in the early days of behaviourism: "I certainly was an anti-physiologist at that time and am glad to be considered as one then. Today, however, I believe that this ('physiologising') is where the great new break-throughs are coming." Photo: courtesy of the Department of Psychology, UC Berkeley. Letter: Steve Glickman, UC Berkeley.

physiology to psychology was a wish that we shared with many of our forerunners (Fig. 1), and it was the beginning of a long journey for the two of us, a journey that was aided tremendously, at different stages, by many mentors and collaborators, particularly our Ph.D. supervisor Per Andersen.

Somewhat independently of Hebb's approach to physiology, the psychology-physiology boundary was broken from the other side—by two pioneers of physiology—David Hubel and Torsten Wiesel (Fig. 2)—who in the late 1950s bravely started to record activity from single neurons in the cortex, the origin of most of our intellectual activity. Inserting electrodes into the primary visual cortex of awake animals, they discovered how activity of individual neurons could be related to specific elements of the visual image (Hubel and Wiesel, 1959, 1962, 1977). This work set the stage for decades of investigation of the neural basis for vision and helped the emergence of a new field of cortical computation. Their insights at the low levels of the visual cortex provided a window into how the cortex might work. As a result of Hubel and Wiesel's work, parts of the coding mechanism for vision are now understood, almost 60 years after they started their investigations.

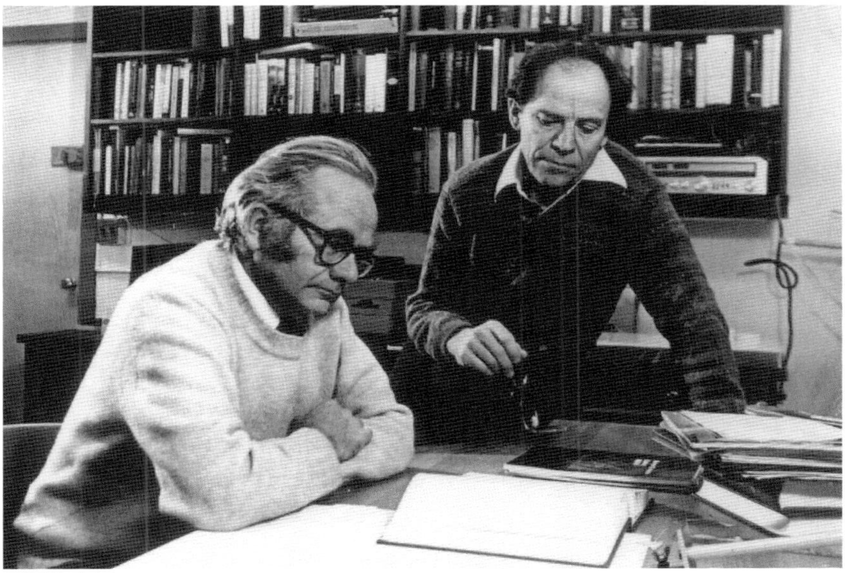

FIGURE 2. David H. Hubel and Torsten N. Wiesel broke the physiology-psychology boundary from the physiology side. By identifying the elementary neural components of the visual image at low levels of the visual cortex, they showed that psychological concepts, such as sensation and perception, could be understood through elementary interactions between cells with specific functions. Courtesy of Torsten N. Wiesel.

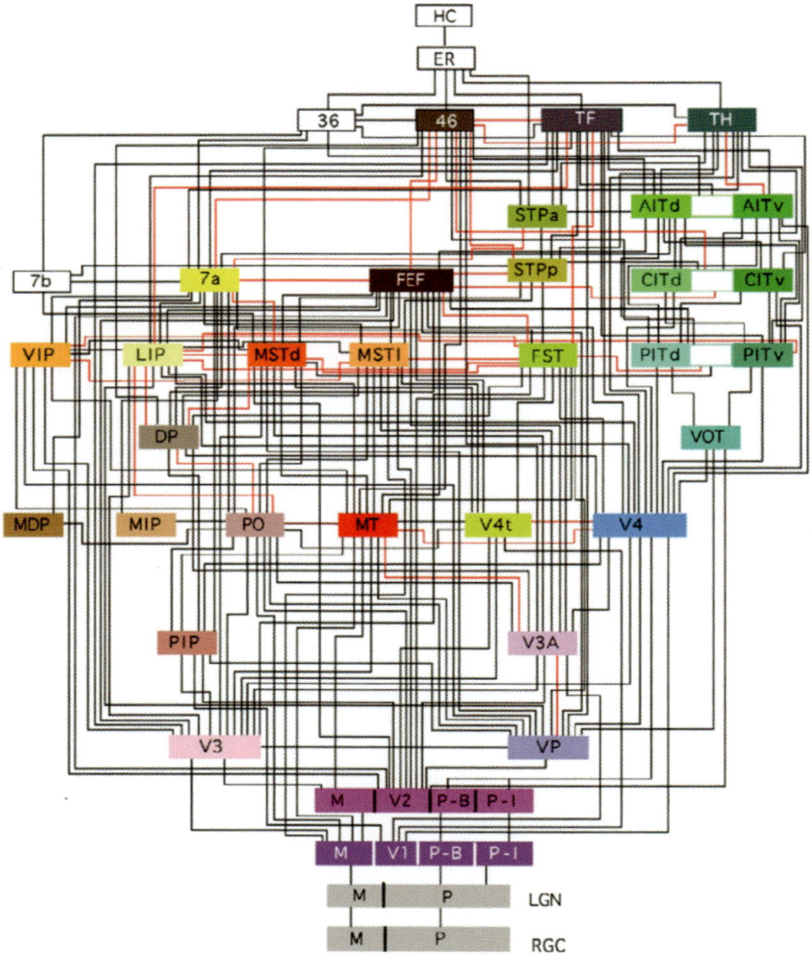

FIGURE 3. Hierarchical map of visual regions of the cortex showing visual input at the bottom (RGC, retinal ganglion cells; LGN, lateral geniculate nucleus) and entorhinal cortex (ER) and hippocampus (HC) at the top. Hubel and Wiesel's work led to revolutionary insights at the low levels of the hierarchy. As we move upwards in the hierarchy, correlations between neural activity and events or patterns in the outside world disappear rapidly. The cells of the hippocampal-entorhinal space system, at the peak of the hierarchy, represent a rare exception. Reproduced, with permission, from Felleman and van Essen (1991).

However, most of our knowledge of the cortex is confined to the entry level, at the early stages of sensory systems. As we move upwards in the cortical hierarchy (Fig. 3), clear correlates to the external world become rare and scientists often get lost or they avoid these areas. There are a few exceptions though. At higher levels of the visual system, there are cells that respond to sophisticated combinations of elementary features, as well as ethologically important objects such as hands and faces (Gross et al., 1969, 1972; Bruce et al., 1981; Perrett et al., 1982; Tanaka et al., 1991; Tsao et al., 2005). The most striking example, perhaps, appears at the very peak of the sensory hierarchy, in the hippocampus, as deep into the cortex as you can get. In 1971, John O'Keefe and John Dostrovsky discovered that hippocampal cells tend to fire specifically when animals are at certain locations of the environment (O'Keefe and Dostrovsky, 1971; O'Keefe, 1976; Fig. 4). In small environments, each cell usually has a single firing location. Collectively a bunch of co-localised cells cover all areas of the environment, giving rise to the idea that place cells are part of an internal Tolmanian map of space (O'Keefe and Nadel, 1978). The strong relationship between neural activity and a property of the outside world—the animal's location—suggested that it was indeed possible to link physiology and psychology even in brain systems far away from sensory inputs and motor outputs.

The potential for understanding a higher brain function brought May-Britt and me to John O'Keefe's lab in 1996. During a period of three months, John generously taught us everything about place cells and how they were studied and we then went back to Norway, to Trondheim, to set up our own new lab. One of our hopes was to find out how the place signal was generated.

In this overview, I will first review the events that led up to the discovery of grid cells and the organisation of a grid cell-based map of space in the medial

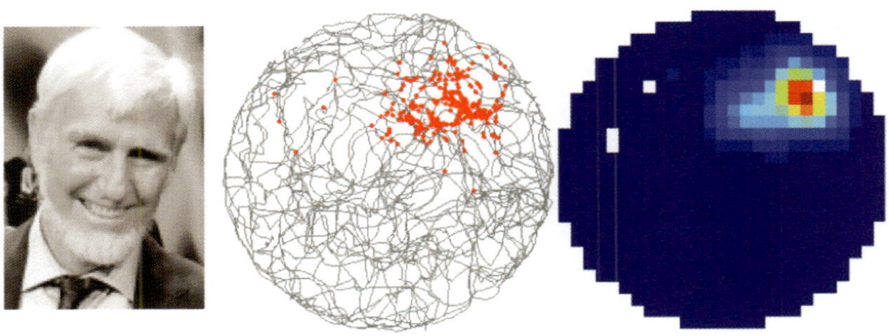

FIGURE 4. John O'Keefe (left) discovered place cells in the hippocampus (O'Keefe and Dostrovsky, 1971). Place cells (middle and right) are cells that fire specifically when an animal is at a certain location in its local environment. In the middle diagram, the animal's path in a circular recording enclosure is shown in grey; firing locations of individual spikes are shown for a single place cell in red. To the right, the firing rate of the same cell is color-coded (blue, low rate; red, high rate). In larger environments, place cells usually have more than one firing field (Fenton et al., 2008).

entorhinal cortex. Then, in the second part, I will present recent work on the interactions between grid cells and the geometry of the external environment, the topography of the grid-cell map, and the mechanisms underlying the hexagonal symmetry of the grid cells.

2. MOVING INTO UNKNOWN TERRITORY—THE ENTORHINAL CORTEX

The hippocampal circuit consists of several stages—including dentate gyrus, CA3 and CA1—which are connected more or less in a unidirectional sequence parallel to the transverse axis of the hippocampus (Andersen et al., 1971; Fig. 5). Each stage in this circuit receives additional direct input from the entorhinal cortex. In the 1990s, neural recordings from the entorhinal cortex suggested that cells in this area have broad and dispersed firing fields, quite different from the sharp and confined fields of the CA1 area of the hippocampus (Barnes et al., 1990; Quirk et al., 1992; Frank et al., 2000). A common idea until the end of the 1990s was therefore that the place signal was computed, or at least sharpened, between the entorhinal cortex and CA1, within the intrinsic circuit of the hippocampus, at the level of dentate gyrus and CA3.

To determine if place fields were formed in the intrahippocampal circuit, we worked together with neuroanatomist Menno Witter, then at the Free University of Amsterdam. Our first project was to isolate the CA1 from the earlier stages of the hippocampus, using chemical inactivation (Brun et al., 2002; Fig. 5). Following isolation of CA1 from the earlier stages, we could demonstrate that only direct inputs from the entorhinal cortex were left. We then recorded place cells in CA1 of this preparation. In spite of the rather complete removal of intrinsic excitatory input, cells with place fields could still be identified in CA1, although the firing fields were often somewhat more blurred than in control animals (Fig. 6). The findings suggested that spatial information was computed either by the CA1 circuit alone, which we thought was unlikely due to its predominant feed-forward architecture, or that the signal came in to the CA1 via direct inputs from the entorhinal cortex that bypassed the CA3. It made sense to record activity in the entorhinal cortex to settle this issue.

In collaboration with Menno Witter and our two students Marianne Fyhn and Sturla Molden, we then implanted electrodes in the dorsocaudal part of medial entorhinal cortex, far dorsal to the region where entorhinal activity had been recorded in earlier studies. We chose this region of the entorhinal cortex because it projects to the dorsal hippocampus, which is where most of the place-cell activity had been recorded at that time (Witter et al., 1989; Dolorfo and Amaral, 1998). Cells in this area of the entorhinal cortex had clearly defined

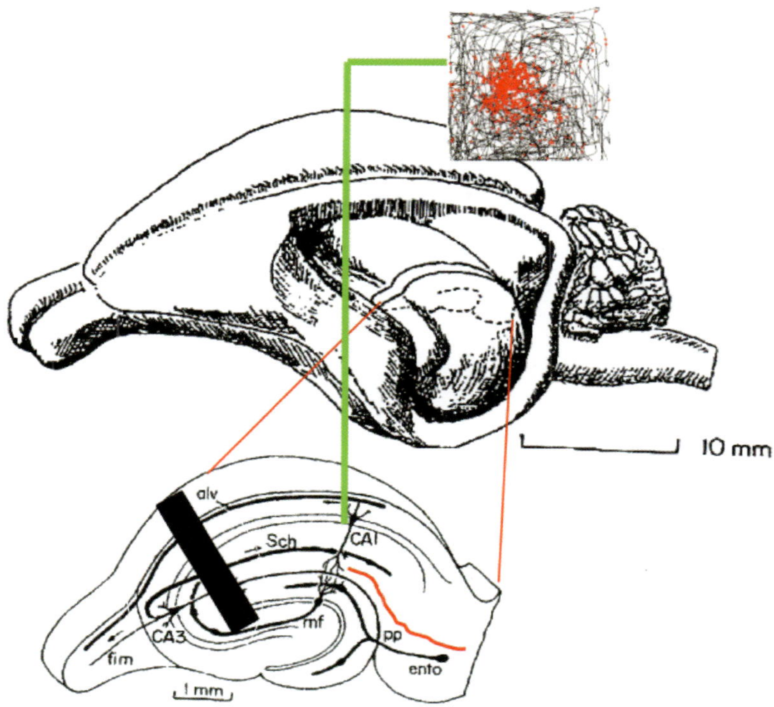

FIGURE 5. Location of recording electrode and lesion in the experiment that led us to move out of the hippocampus, to the entorhinal cortex (Brun et al., 2002). The upper image shows the hippocampus as a cashew nut-shaped structure underneath the cortical surface in a rodent brain. The lower image shows a transverse transection through the hippocampus. The major subfields of the hippocampal region, including entorhinal cortex (ento), CA3 and CA1, are indicated. Connections through the hippocampus are largely unidirectional, from entorhinal cortex through dentate gyrus and CA3 to CA1 (the intrinsic circuit) or directly from entorhinal cortex to each individual subfield, as indicated in red for the connection to CA1. The position of a tetrode in the CA1 area is indicated, as is the place field for a cell in this area (spike locations shown as red dots on black trajectory, as in Fig. 4). The black bar indicates the location of lesions that interrupted the intrinsic circuit and disconnected CA1 from the CA3 in the Brun study. The hippocampus diagram is modified from Andersen et al. (1971).

firing fields (Fyhn et al., 2004). Many cells had firing patterns that were as sharp as those of place cells in the CA1 of the hippocampus but they were different (Fig. 7). First of all each cell had many firing fields. Second the fields were not at random positions in the environment but neighbouring fields rather seemed to be separated by a constant distance. There was a peculiar regularity about this pattern but we did not understand the underlying algorithm.

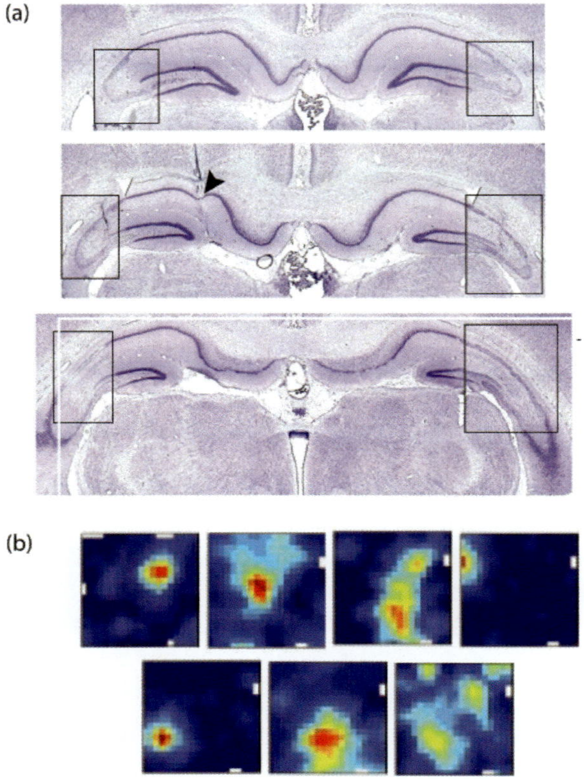

FIGURE 6. Place cells in CA1 after interruption of the intrinsic hippocampal circuit. (a) Nissl-stained coronal brain sections showing location of lesion and tetrodes in a single animal. CA3 of the dorsal hippocampus was almost entirely removed (outline of lesion indicated by rectangular boxes). Arrowhead indicates location of tips of the tetrodes in the CA1 pyramidal cell layer. (b) Colour-coded firing rate maps showing place fields of 7 representative CA1 pyramidal cells in a square enclosure (red, peak rate; dark blue, no firing; colour code as in Fig. 4). Same animal as in (a). Reproduced, with permission, from Brun et al. (2002).

3. GRID CELLS AND THEIR FUNCTIONAL ORGANISATION

In 2005, with our students Torkel Hafting, Marianne Fyhn and Sturla Molden, we were able to describe the structure of the firing pattern. Using larger environments than in the past, we could clearly see that the firing pattern was periodic (Hafting et al., 2005). The multiple firing fields of the cell formed a hexagonal grid that tiled the entire surface space available to the animal, much like the holes in a bee hive or a Chinese checkerboard (Fig. 8). Many entorhinal cells

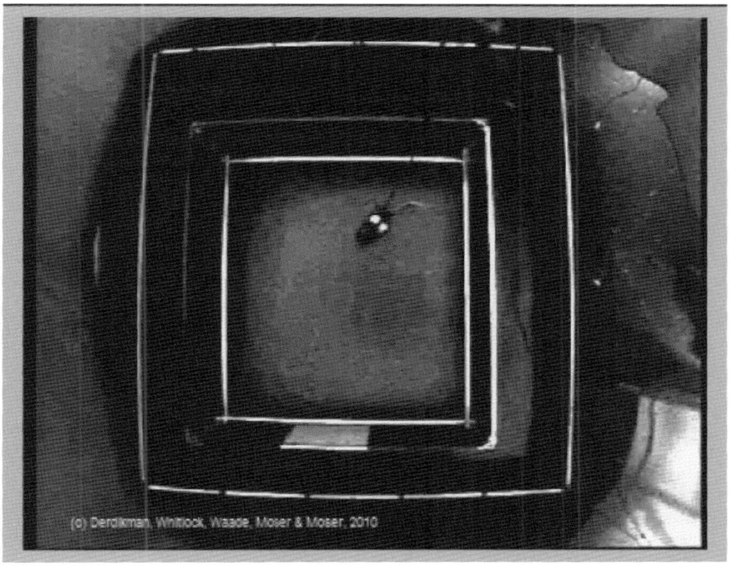

FIGURE 7. Movie showing firing location of a single cell in the medial entorhinal cortex while the rat is chasing chocolate sprinkles in a square recording enclosure. Individual spikes are displayed as white dots at the location of firing. Note the appearance of multiple firing fields and the apparently fixed distance between neighbouring fields. See nobelprize.org for the movie.

fired like this, and we named them grid cells. We were excited about the grid-like firing pattern, both because nothing like it exists in the sensory inputs to the animal, suggesting that the pattern is generated intrinsically in the entorhinal cortex or neighbouring structures, and because such a regular pattern provides a metric to the brain's spatial map—a metric that had been missing in the place map of the hippocampus (O'Keefe, 1976).

Grid cells were abundant in all cell layers of the medial entorhinal cortex (Sargolini et al., 2006). The most regular cells were in layer II, where approximately half of the cell population passed the criteria for grid cells. But grid cells came in different varieties (Fig. 9). There were at least three parameters of variation (Hafting et al., 2005). First, the cells differed in phase, or the *x-y* locations of the grid vertices. All possible grid phases were represented. Second, grid cells differed in scale, or spatial frequency, or the size of the fields and the spacing between them. In the grid cells with the smallest scale, the distance between the firing fields was only 30 cm. Other cells had field distances of more than a meter. Finally, grid cells sometimes had different orientations, i.e., the axes of the grid

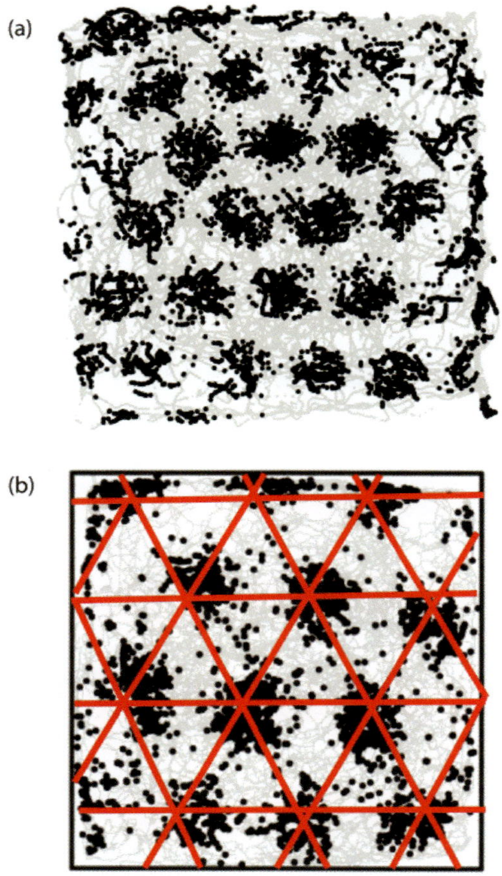

FIGURE 8. Firing pattern of grid cells. (a) Spatially periodic firing pattern of an entorhinal grid cell during 30 min of foraging in a 220 cm wide square enclosure. The trajectory of the rat is shown in grey, individual spike locations in black. (b) Firing pattern of a grid cell in a 1 m wide enclosure. Symbols as in (a) but with red lines superimposed to indicate the hexagonal structure of the grid. Modified from Stensola et al. (2012) and Hafting et al. (2005), respectively.

were tilted at different degrees from a reference axis such as a wall of the recording environment.

Following the discovery of the new cell type, we set out to determine how the grid map was organised according to parameters such as phase and scale (Hafting et al., 2005). Let me begin with the phase of the grid cells, i.e. the locations of the grid vertices. Do neighbouring cells have the same phase, or are their phase relationships random? Cells that were recorded on the same tetrode generally had different grid phases (Fig. 10). The firing locations of cells from

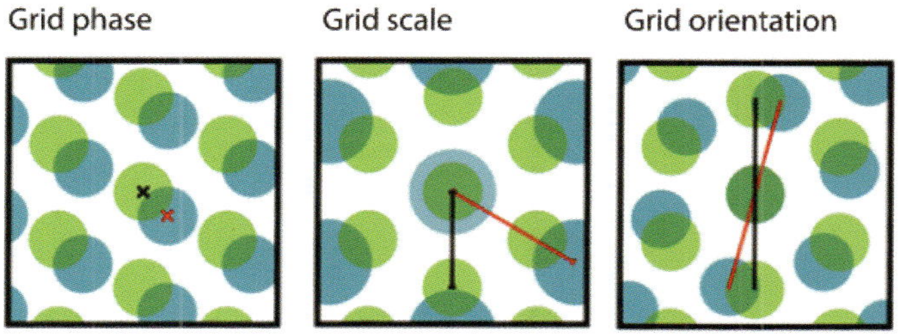

FIGURE 9. There are at least three parameters of variation among grid cells: grid phase, grid scale and grid orientation. Differences in phase, scale and orientation are illustrated for a pair of grid cells—one in green and one in blue. Grid phase refers to the *x-y* locations of the firing fields, grid scale is reflected in size of the firing fields and the distance between them (grid spacing), and grid orientation is determined by the angle of the grid axes relative to an external reference line (e.g. a wall of the recording box).

the same tetrode were apparently no more similar than those of cells that had been recorded on widely dispersed tetrodes. The findings suggested that, within the spatial resolution of the tetrode technique, grid phase is represented non-topographically. All grid phases appeared to be present within a small patch of the entorhinal network. The scattered representation is reminiscent of the

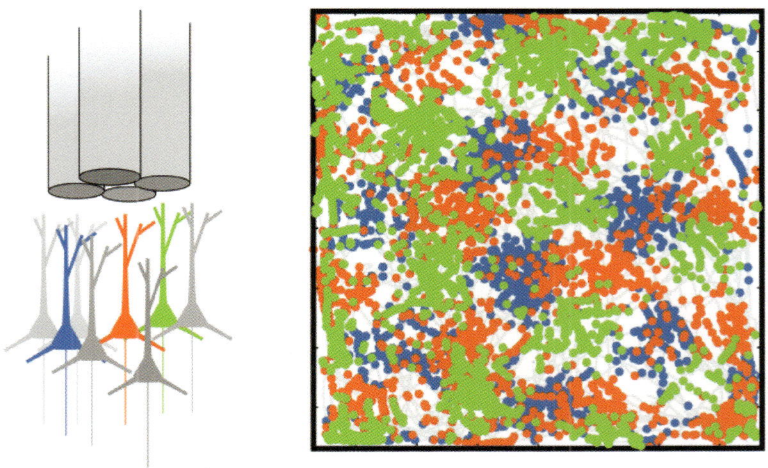

FIGURE 10. Grid phase appears to be organised non-topographically, at least within the resolution of the tetrode technique. Left, tetrode with cells that give rise to signals on the tetrode. Three grid cells are indicated with different colours. Right, firing fields of three grid cells recorded at the same tetrode location. There is apparently no correspondence between the grid phases of the three cells. The exact location of the three cells within the recording field of the tetrode cannot be determined from the tetrode signals. Modified from Hafting et al. (2005).

salt-and-pepper organisation of orientation-selective cells in rodents (Ohki et al., 2005; van Hooser et al., 2005), and of a number of other neural cortical representations such as odour maps in the piriform cortex (Stettler and Axel, 2009) or the place-cell map of the hippocampus (O'Keefe, 1976; Wilson and McNaughton, 1993).

In contrast to grid phase, the scale of the grid was mapped topographically at the macroscopic level. On average, grid spacing increased from dorsal to ventral medial entorhinal cortex. As the electrodes were moved downwards, we saw a progressive increase in the mean scale of the grid, reflected in the size of the fields as well as their separation (Fig. 11). The earliest data were not able to tell us whether this increase was smooth and gradual, or whether the grid increased in discrete steps. Because of limited cell sampling, we had to average the data across animals (Fyhn et al., 2004; Hafting et al., 2005), and it remained possible that averaging wiped out step-like increases that were present in individual animals.

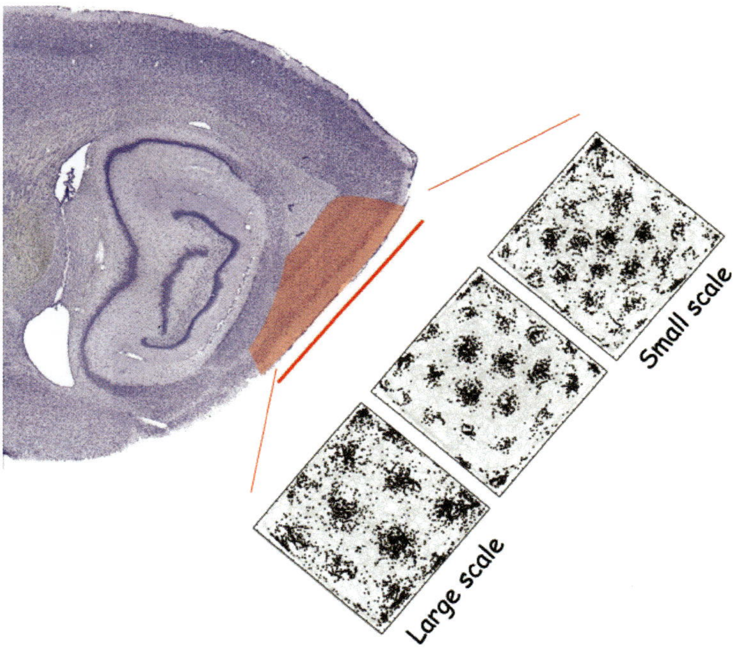

FIGURE 11. Topographical organisation of grid scale. The figure shows a sagittal brain section with medial entorhinal cortex indicated in red. Firing maps are shown for three grid cells recorded at successive dorso-ventral levels in medial entorhinal cortex. Note change from small scale to large scale along the dorso-ventral axis. Modified from Stensola et al. (2012).

In 2012, with Hanne and Tor Stensola and several other students, we were eventually able to determine the nature of the scale change (Stensola et al., 2012). We were now able to record up to almost 200 grid cells from the same animal, enough to determine if grid scale increases continuously or in a step-like manner. The recordings showed indeed that grid spacing increases in discrete steps (Fig. 12a). On average, grid spacing increased from dorsal to ventral, as we had observed before, but there were only four or five levels of spacing. We referred to each level as a module. As the electrodes were moved from dorsal to ventral, new modules were recruited in an additive manner, such that the most dorsal levels of medial entorhinal cortex had only the smallest module (M1), whereas more ventral levels had both M1 and M2, and even more ventral levels M1, M2 and M3. The number of cells in each module decreased substantially from M1 to M4 and M5. Thus, grid scale is organised topographically but the map consists of anatomically overlapping modules. The organisation is quite different from the strict anatomical separation of functionally similar cells in some primary sensory cortices.

What is the relationship between the grid scales of successive modules? To determine this we measured the ratio between values for grid spacing of each successive pair of modules (Fig. 12b). Despite considerable variation in the scale ratios, the mean ratio was almost constant, between 1.40 and 1.43. For each pair of modules, the scale of the larger module could be obtained by multiplying the scale of the smaller module by a constant factor, just like in a geometric progression. This way of organising grid scale might, according to theoretical analyses, be the optimal way to represent space at maximal resolution with a minimum number of cells (Mathis et al., 2012; Wei et al., 2013).

4. A UNIVERSAL MAP

As I approach the end of the historical part of my lecture, I want to draw your attention to the functional rigidity of the grid modules. In 2007, with our close collaborator Alessandro Treves from SISSA in Trieste and our students Marianne Fyhn and Torkel Hafting, we found that simultaneously recorded grid cells maintained scale, phase and orientation relationships across environments and experiences (Fyhn et al., 2007; Fig. 13a). We assessed the similarity of grid maps in square and circular environments, in the same room or in different rooms, by cross-correlating the rate maps of all recorded grid cells (Fig. 13b). Cross-correlation maps of cells from different environments had vertices that were spaced in a hexagonal grid pattern reminiscent of the grid pattern in individual cells (Fig. 13c). The maintenance of grid structure in the cross-correlation maps,

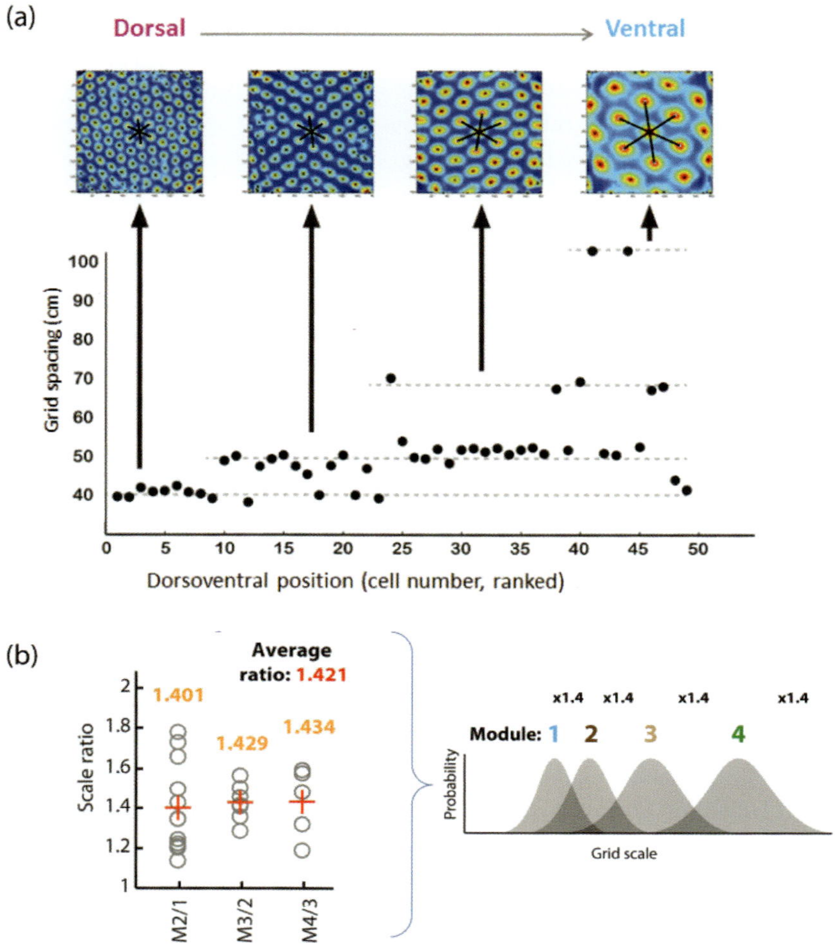

FIGURE 12. The grid map is modular. (a) Grid scale increases in discrete steps. Top, autocorrelograms for four cells belonging to different modules. Bottom, grid spacing for all grid cells of a single animal as a function of recording position along the dorso-ventral axis of medial entorhinal cortex. Each dot corresponds to one cell. Cells are rank-ordered from dorsal to ventral. Stippled lines indicate mean values for four discrete modules (modules M1-M4). Cells were assigned to modules through a k-means clustering algorithm. Arrows indicate module identity for the four example cells at the top. (b) Left, scale ratio of successive module pairs. Circles correspond to individual module pairs (32 modules, 11 rats). Mean scale ratios for module pairs are indicated in orange, grand mean in red. Right, schematic illustration of increase in grid scale across 4 modules. For each module, the mean scale value can be obtained by multiplying the scale of the preceding module by a fixed factor (1.4), as if module scales formed a geometric progression. Modified from Stensola et al. (2012) and Moser et al. (2014).

despite shifts in the absolute positions of the vertices, implies that cells keep spatial relationships across environments. If two cells have overlapping grid vertices in one environment, they will have overlapping vertices in another environment too; if their phases are opposite in one environment, they will be opposite in the other too. In 2012, after the discovery of modules, we observed that this rigidity always applied to cells within the same module, whereas cells from different modules might have unpredictable spatial relationships (Stensola et al., 2012). These findings suggested that a grid module operates like a universal map that does not care about the detailed content of the environment, much unlike maps of place cells, which change to completely different configurations whenever the animal moves to a different environment (Muller and Kubie, 1987). Simultaneous recordings from the hippocampus verified this difference. Cross-correlograms for hippocampal cells showed no reliable peaks (Fig. 13d), suggesting that the structure of simultaneously active place cells was highly different in the two environments (Fyhn et al., 2007).

Taken together, these observations point to a key difference between grid cells and place cells. Grid modules are universal and rigid—as would be expected by a metric for space—whereas place cells take on a variety of patterns, as would be expected if they also participate in memory for events associated with the locations stored in the place-cell maps (Moser et al., 2008, 2014).

Finally, how universal are grid cells across species? I can reassure you that grid cells are not unique to rats (Fig. 14). Grid cells also exist in mice (Fyhn et al., 2008). In 2011, Nachum Ulanovsky's group found them in Egyptian fruit bats (Yartsev et al., 2011), on a different branch of the phylogenetic tree (Fig. 14), then Elisabeth Buffalo's group found them in macaque monkeys (Killian et al., 2012), and then Iszhad Fried and Mike Kahana's group found them in humans (Jacobs et al., 2013). Thus, grid cells, like the other spatial cell types, exist across many mammalian orders and probably originated early in mammalian evolution, or before.

5. GRID CELLS AND THE GEOMETRY OF THE ENVIRONMENT

During the remainder of this lecture, I wish to share with you what trajectories our lab is following at the moment. I will briefly touch on three sets of new questions and data, much of which is still unpublished.

First I would like to ask how the grid pattern interacts with the environment. Grid cells are generated by intrinsic computations but to be useful for spatial mapping and navigation, they need to maintain a consistent relationship to the

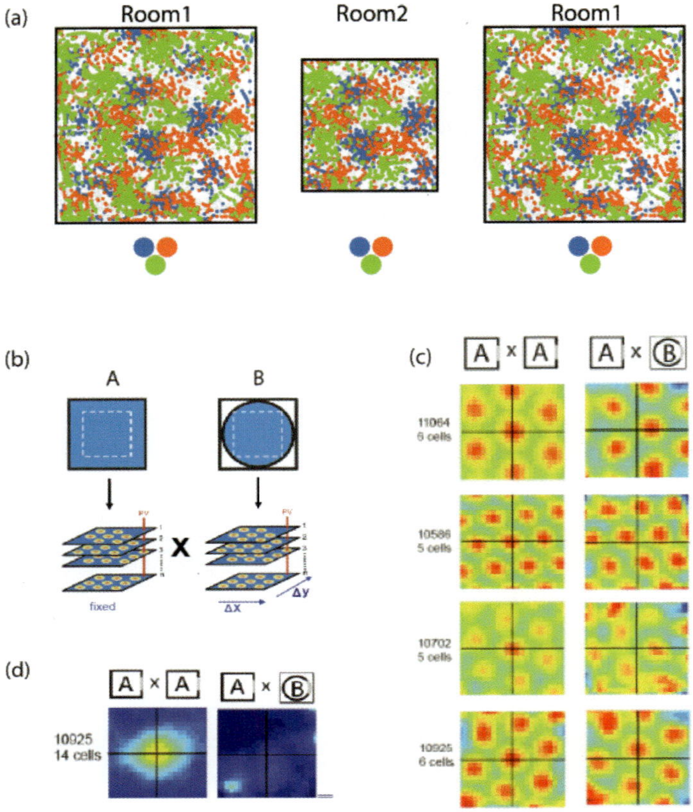

FIGURE 13. Universality of the grid map. (a) Schematic illustrating preservation of scale, phase and orientation relationships among grid cells when animals are tested in different environments. Firing patterns of three grid cells, each with a different colour, are copied across environments to illustrate that pattern relationships are maintained across rooms. (b) Illustration of cross-correlation method. For each environment A and B, rate maps for different cells were stacked into a three-dimensional matrix with space defined by x and y and cell identity by z. For each stack a population vector was defined for every single bin of x-y space. Pairs of population vectors were then correlated across environments by shifting one of the stacks in small increments along the entire x and y axes. (c) Cross-correlation matrices for ensembles of simultaneously recorded grid cells in the medial entorhinal cortex. Left, repeated trials in the same environment (A × A); right, trials in different environments (A × B). The peak of the cross-correlogram remains at the origin on repeated trials in the same environment but shifts to a different location in comparisons of different environments, at the same time as the grid structure of the correlation map is retained. This indicates that phase, scale and orientation relationships are maintained across the two environments whereas absolute phase or orientation are different (vertices are shifted). (d) Cross-correlation matrices for cells that were recorded in CA3 of the hippocampus. Note lack of structure in the hippocampal cross-correlation matrix for different environments, suggesting that decorrelated maps are retrieved in the two environments. Modified from Fyhn et al. (2007).

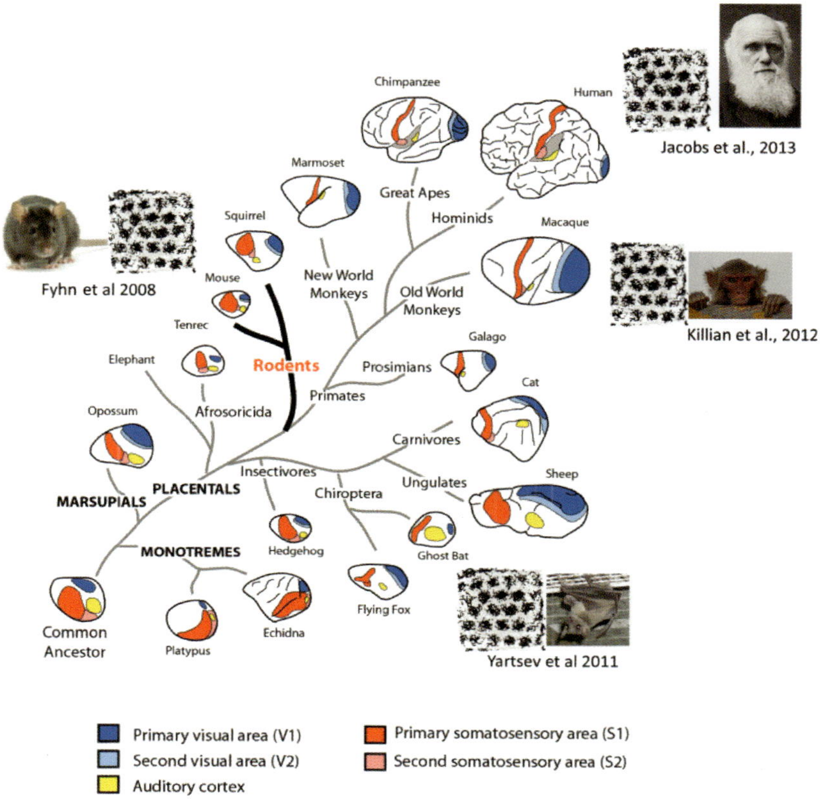

FIGURE 14. Grid-like cells have been reported in rodents, bats, monkeys and humans, suggesting they originated early in mammalian evolution. Adapted, with permission, from Krubitzer et al. (2011).

surroundings. They need to fire in the same locations each time the animal visits a particular place. They do so (Hafting et al., 2005) but how is this anchoring to the environment accomplished?

One clue to the mechanisms underlying the anchoring process is that the orientation of the grid pattern relative to the environment seems to be non-random (Stensola et al., 2012; Krupic et al., 2014). With our students Tor and Hanne Stensola we set out to explore this further (Stensola et al., 2015). Early on we were struck by the fact that the grid axes of different cells are more similar than expected by chance (Fig. 15a). In most cells the grid axes were slightly tilted with respect to the wall axes and the tilt seemed similar even between animals. In a sample of 587 grid cells from 6 different rats, tested in a 1.5 m wide square

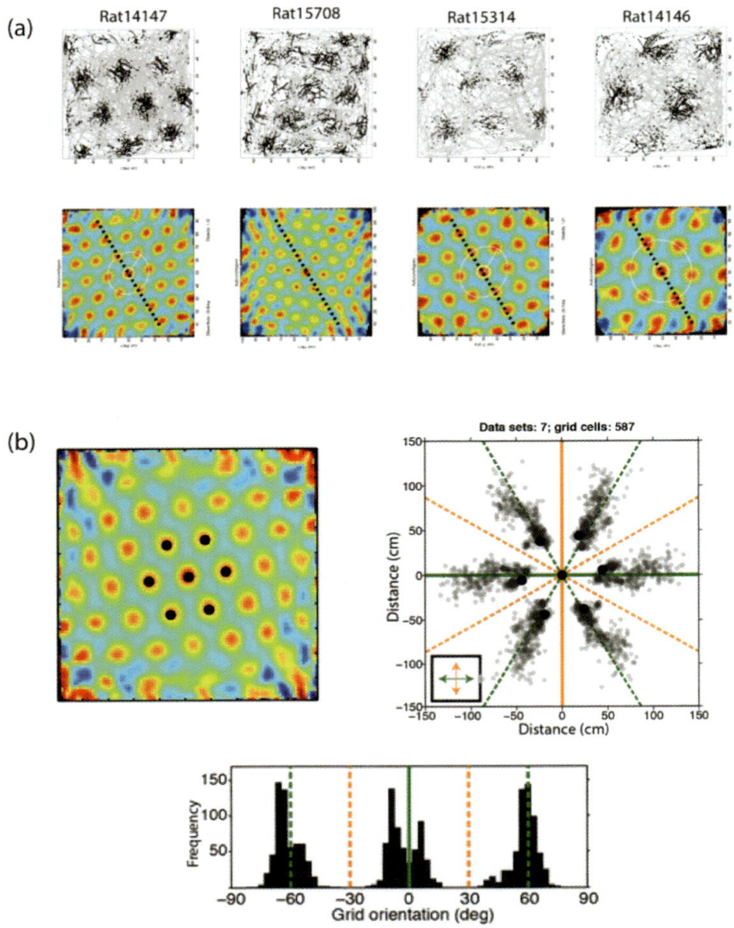

FIGURE 15. Alignment of grid patterns to external geometry. (a) Spike plots (top row) and spatial autocorrelograms (bottom row) for four representative grid cells recorded in different animals in the same 1.5 m wide square enclosure. Spike plots show trajectory in grey, with individual spike locations superimposed as black dots. Autocorrelogram is colour-coded, with correlation increasing from blue to red. Stippled line indicates orientation of one grid axis. Note similar orientation across cells and animals. (b) Top left: Spatial autocorrelogram of a single cell. Central peak and surrounding 6 peaks are indicated by black dots. Top right: Polar scatterplot showing distribution of grid orientation and grid spacing for 587 grid cells in the 1.5 m wide square enclosure. For each cell, the location of the 1+6 innermost fields in the spatial autocorrelogram (black dots in the left diagram) is shown (1+6 dots per cell; darkness indicates overlap). Distance from the centre is proportional to grid scale. Cardinal axes of the box are shown in orange and green. Stippled lines indicate 60-degree multiples of the cardinal axes. Bottom: Frequency distributions showing clustering of data in the polar scatterplot around each of the 3 axes defined by 60-degree multiples of the east-west orientation. Modified, with permission, from Stensola et al. (2015).

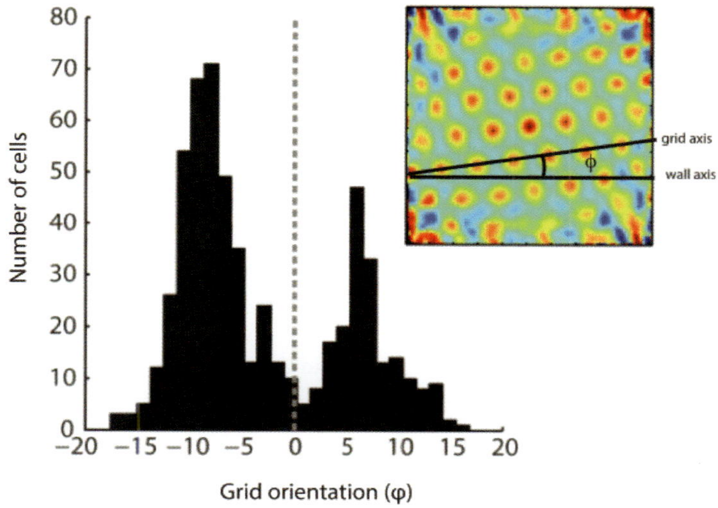

FIGURE 16. Frequency distribution showing orientation of the grid axis with the smallest offset from any of the box walls. This orientation is defined by the angle from the wall axis, as illustrated in the inset. Modified, with permission, from Stensola et al. (2015).

environment, only a limited range of grid orientations was represented. To illustrate the distribution, we made spatial autocorrelograms for each cell, identified for each autocorrelogram the centre and the surrounding 6 vertices, and then transferred, for each cell, these 7 points to a common circular scatterplot (Fig. 15b). The distribution was highly clustered, suggesting not only that grid cells had a small number of scale values, as would be expected from their scale modularity, but also that grid cells within a module had a similar orientation. Orientation was also shared across modules in many cases.

At first glance, it seemed as if grid cells line up with the symmetry axes of the environment, i.e. the north-south or east-west walls of the recording environment (Fig. 15b). Closer inspection suggested this was not the case, however (Fig. 16). On average, the grid axis nearest any of the wall axes had an offset of 5–10 degrees in either direction from the wall axis. In the 1.5 m box, grid orientations clustered around + or −7.5 degrees relative to the east-west wall. Almost no cells at all had offsets of 0 and 15 degrees. This invariant rotation of the grid pattern of course led us to ask if there is anything advantageous about 7.5 degree offsets and if 0 and 15 degrees were somehow disadvantageous.

The answers may be yes. 7.5 degrees is the offset that minimises symmetry between the grid pattern and the axes of the environment; it is *the* orientation

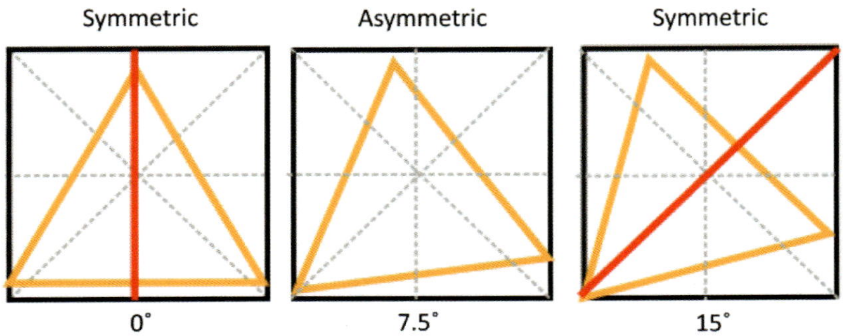

FIGURE 17. Overlap between symmetry axes of box and grid at 0° and 15° but not 7.5°. Stippled lines show symmetry axes of the box (2 cardinal axes and 2 diagonal axes). Orange lines indicate symmetry axes of the grid pattern at different degrees of offset. Red lines show symmetry axes common to box and grid. Note that symmetry axes of box and grid are maximally different when the grid is rotated 7.5° from one of the walls. 7.5° rotation may thus cause maximal disambiguation of grid patterns along orthogonal walls of the environment. Reproduced, with permission, from Stensola et al. (2015).

that causes maximal dissimilarity between patterns along the two wall axes (Fig. 17). In contrast, at 0 and 15 degrees, the box and the grid have common axes, and the grid pattern would look similar along some of the wall pairs. It might be then, that the offset is developed and maintained by the fact that it causes maximal disambiguation of activity patterns across similar regions of the environment.

What could generate such a consistent rotation of the grid pattern? One clue is that the rotation differs between the three grid axes. For the axis that is nearest one of the wall axes, the offset is on average 7.5 degrees, as I have shown. For the two other axes, however, the offset is smaller, with the axis furthest away from the wall axes showing only a 2–3-degree rotation (Fig. 18ab). The differential rotation means that the grid must have lost its hexagonal symmetry and that the inner fields form an ellipse instead of a circle. A comparison of the ellipticity of the grid pattern and the rotational offset of the grid showed that the two effects were closely correlated, suggesting that they are caused by a single underlying mechanism (Fig. 18cd). So—what could this mechanism be?

We hypothesised that rotation and deformation of the grid could be due to shearing—a type of deformation where points on a plane are shifted along the shear axis in proportion to the distance from this axis (Mase, 1970). Shearing can be explained by starting out with an initially symmetric grid pattern, where the vertices of 6 neighbouring grid fields define a circle (Fig. 19, left). In the next

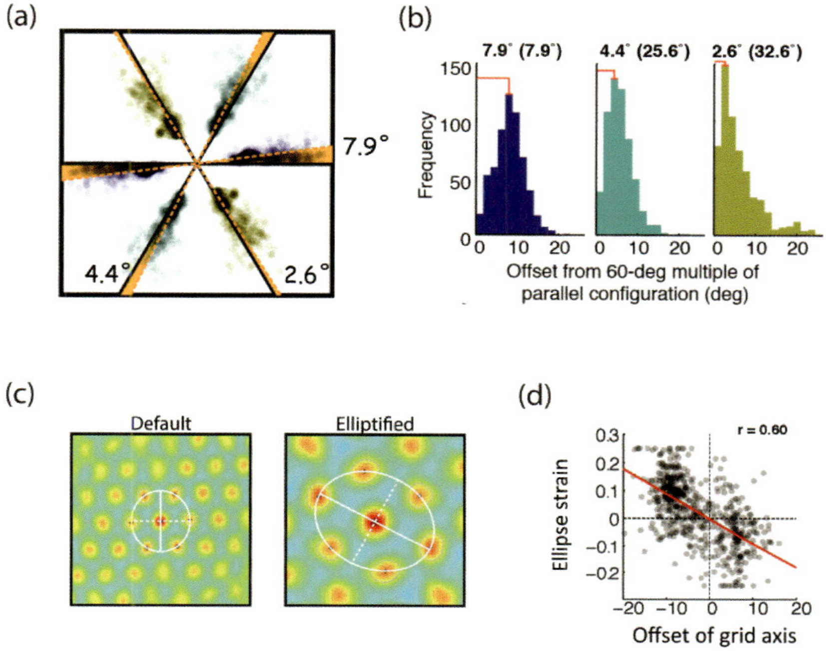

FIGURE 18. Rotational offset is accompanied by deformation. (a) Polar scatter plot (same data as in Fig. 16) showing axis-specific offset from the nearest wall axis or 60-degree multiples of it. Grids are reflected around the horizontal alignment axis for visualisation of differences between grid axes. Orange dashed lines show peak angular offset from 60° multiples (black lines) of parallel wall alignment (0°) for each axis. (b) Distribution of angular offset from nearest wall axis or 60-degree multiples of it. Peak angular offsets from nearest 60°-multiples are indicated at the top of each distribution (offset from respective nearest wall axis in brackets). (c) Spatial autocorrelogram showing symmetric and distorted grid pattern. Symmetry of the grid pattern is indicated by a white circle connecting the inner vertices of the autocorrelogram to the left. For the autocorrelogram to the right, which shows a deformed grid pattern, the vertex locations are defined instead by an ellipse. (d) Scatter plot showing strong correlation between angular offset of the grid and the strain of the ellipse fit shown in (c). Taken together, the covariation of grid rotation and grid deformation raises the possibility that they are reflections of a single mechanism. Modified, with permission, from Stensola et al. (2015).

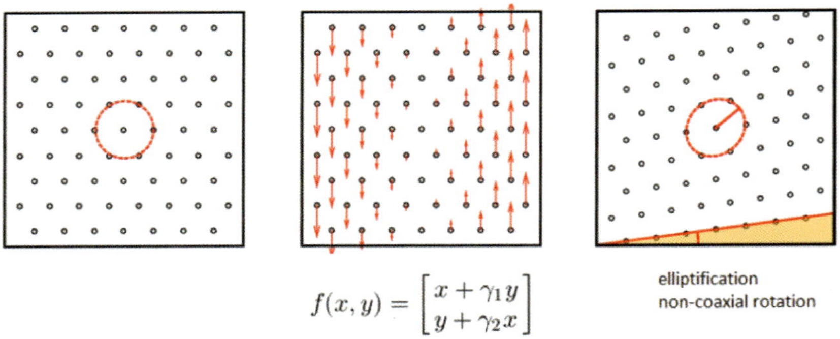

FIGURE 19. Rotation and deformation of the grid pattern may be caused by shearing, a type of deformation where points on a plane are shifted along a given axis in proportion to the distance from the axis. Shearing is illustrated here in three diagrams. The diagram to the left shows a grid pattern before any deformation. The inner vertices are identified by a red circle. The middle diagram shows the operation of shear forces. Red arrows indicate direction and strength of forces (length of arrow is proportional to strength). Shear forces are parallel to the east and west walls and operate in opposite directions on the two sides of the box. Transformation of the grid pattern due to simple shearing is given by the equation below. The result of the shear transform is shown to the right. Note strong rotation of the grid axis orthogonal to the shear forces (7.5° rotation, as illustrated by the red axis line) as well as deformation of the grid pattern (as indicated by transformation of the inner circle to an ellipse). Illustration by Tor Stensola.

step (Fig. 19, middle) we introduce shear forces, parallel to each of the east and west walls, and in opposite directions, with decreasing amplitude as we depart from the walls. Applying these forces converts the circle to an ellipse, at the same time as the axes of the grid pattern are rotated, with the strongest rotation occurring on the grid axis that is most offset from the shear axis (Fig. 19, right). The transformation of the pattern can be described as:

$$T(x,y) = \begin{bmatrix} 1 & \gamma_1 \\ \gamma_2 & 1 \end{bmatrix} \begin{bmatrix} x \\ y \end{bmatrix}$$

where γ_1 is the shear parameter along the y-axis, γ_2 the shear parameter along the x-axis, and x and y row vectors of initial coordinates of points in the plane. For simple shearing, only one of the shear parameters has a non-zero value. The strong relationship between elliptification and rotation in the simulations is reminiscent of the data. In fact, if simulated grids are elliptified exactly to the extent observed in the data, the accompanying rotation is 7.5 degrees, just as in the data, strongly pointing to shearing as a mechanism for both the elliptic deformation and the rotational offset.

Thus, given that the effects could be reproduced by shearing on simulated grids, we turned to the real data and applied shear forces until we had minimised the ellipticity of the inner circle of the autocorrelogram, in the reverse direction of the forces that likely operated when the pattern was distorted in the first place (Fig. 20). As predicted, shearing completely removed the grid offset when the forces were applied with a direction that was orthogonal to the alignment axis,

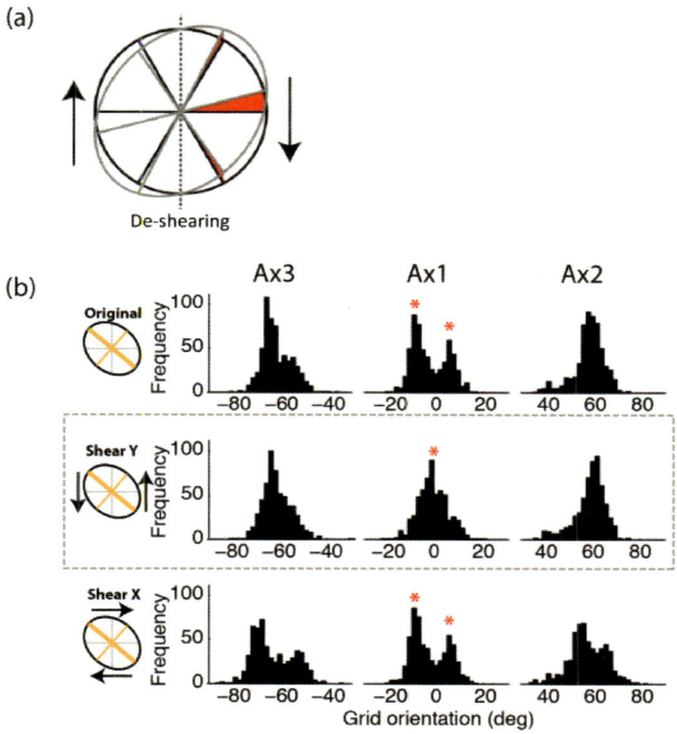

FIGURE 20. Effects of shearing are axis-specific. (a) Deformation and rotation of grid axes following shearing in the north-south direction. Shearing was applied in the reverse direction of the forces thought to operate as the grid was aligned in the first place. Shearing completely removed not only the deformation but also the offset of the grid axes. (b) Frequency distribution showing orientation for each grid axis before and after minimisation of ellipticity by simple shearing along the cardinal axes of the environment. Asterisks indicate peaks of the distribution for the axis nearest one of the cardinal axes. Note disappearance of orientation peaks at 7.5° following north-south shearing. Shearing in the orthogonal direction had minimal effects on the angular offset of the same grid axis. Modified, with permission, from Stensola et al. (2015).

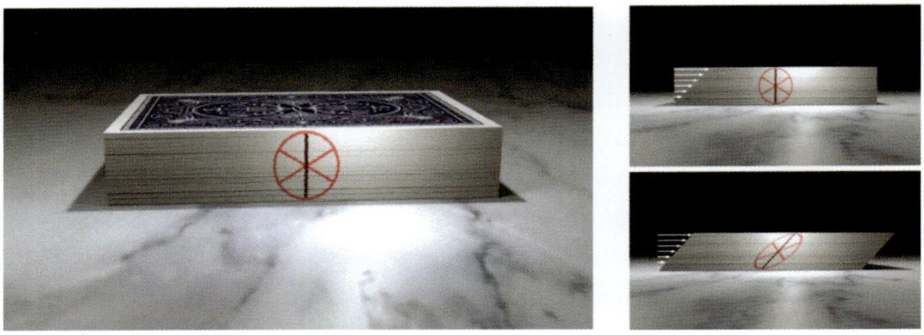

FIGURE 21. Effects of shearing on rotation and deformation of a pattern can be illustrated with a stack of cards. Note grid axes on the side of the stack. Shear forces are imposed horizontally, with decreasing amplitude as distance from the top of the stack increases (top right; white arrows indicate strength of shear forces). The result of the shear transformation is shown at the bottom right. Note strong rotation of the grid axis orthogonal to the direction of the shear forces (black axis). The two other axes, with smaller offsets from the shear direction, show less rotation (red). Illustration by Tor Stensola.

i.e., with a north-south shear direction. Shearing in the east-west direction, parallel to the alignment axis, had no effect. The effect of shearing on rotation of the grid pattern can be illustrated in a stack of cards with grid axes displayed on the side of the stack (Fig. 21). When shear forces are applied along the top surface of the stack, with decreasing amplitude towards the centre, the grid is elliptified and the orthogonal axis is rotated more than the two other axes, which deviate less from the shear axis.

Taken together, these analyses clearly point to shearing as the mechanism for grid deformation and grid rotation. The findings imply that local boundaries exert distance-dependent effects on the grid pattern. Whether these forces are mediated through the existence of border cells, which intermingle with the grid cells (Savelli et al., 2008; Solstad et al., 2008), remains to be determined—but it is certainly a possibility (Hartley et al., 2000).

6. FINE-SCALE TOPOGRAPHY OF THE GRID-CELL NETWORK

In the next state-of-the-art part of my lecture, I wish to return to the anatomical organisation of the grid network. I showed you that within the resolution constraints of the tetrode technique, there seems to be no topography of grid phase, i.e. grid cells with different grid phases seem to be scrambled, at least at a macroscopic scale. However, tetrodes are thought to pick up spike signals within a range of as much as 50–100 um (Gray et al., 1995), corresponding to several cell widths. Thus we need other methods if we are to determine the topography of the grid-cell network at single-cell resolution.

One approach that *has* sufficient spatial resolution is two-photon fluorescent calcium imaging, which for some years has been applied to superficial cortical structures in anaesthetised animals (Stosiek et al., 2003; Kerr et al., 2005; Ohki et al., 2005, 2006) and awake head-fixed animals (Dombeck et al., 2007). With graduate student Albert Tsao we joined forces with Tobias Bonhoeffer at the Max Planck Institute for Neurobiology in Martinsried to image grid cells in head-fixed mice during navigation in a virtual environment where mice move forward in the environment in correspondence with their running movements on a stationary ball (Dombeck et al., 2007).

The first problem to solve was to get access to the medial entorhinal cortex. The medial entorhinal cortex lies at the worst possible place, at the back of the cortex, adjacent to the cerebellum, under the transverse sinus—apparently not readily accessible to surface imaging. The solution to the problem was to insert a prism between the cerebral cortex and the cerebellum, pushing back the cerebellum and leaving cortex, cerebellum, and sinus fully intact (Fig. 22; see also Heys et al., 2014, and Low et al., 2014). This allowed us to image the back surface of the cortex, i.e. the medial entorhinal cortex, from the top of the brain. Mice with prisms could then be injected in the medial entorhinal cortex with AAV virus encoding the fluorescent calcium indicator GCaMP6f, and three weeks later, when the indicator had expressed, the mice could be head-fixed and allowed to run in the virtual environment.

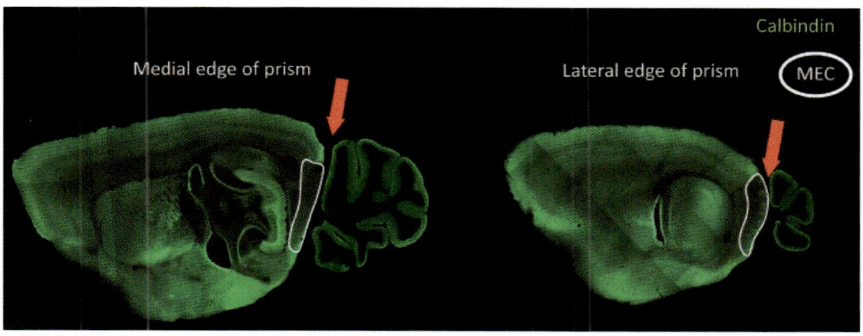

FIGURE 22. Calbindin-stained sagittal brain section showing that medial entorhinal cortex can be imaged from the local cortical surface by inserting a prism between the cerebral cortex and the cerebellum (red arrow). Stained by Flavio Donato.

With the prism approach the activity of individual cells in layer II of the medial entorhinal cortex could be viewed as the mouse ran through the virtual environment (Fig. 23a). Hundreds of cells could be imaged at the same time at cellular or subcellular resolution. A large fraction of the cells had spatial firing patterns in that they always lit up at constant positions on the track (Fig. 23b). Most cells had multiple firing fields. In some cases, the fields appeared at regular distances, suggesting that the cells were grid cells; however, in the majority of the space-modulated cells, the inter-field distances were variable (Fig. 23b, right). Could these non-periodic cells be grid cells? One problem is that the running track is one-dimensional whereas grid patterns are two-dimensional. Given what we now know about grid rotation, we cannot take for granted that grid cells line up with the direction of the track. If instead the activity on the track corresponds to a slice through a two-dimensional grid, in more than one direction, it might be difficult to tell if a cell is a grid cell or not, because in most slices the field distances would no longer be equal (Fig. 23b). Using an approach inspired by David Tank and colleagues (Domnisoru et al., 2013), we tried to solve this problem by determining the Euclidean distance between the firing pattern of a cell on the track and patterns in slices through all possible locations, orientations and deformations in a simulated two-dimensional grid pattern. Cells with low Euclidean distances between observed and simulated patterns were classified as grid cells.

Having a way to separate out grid cells, we then asked how they are organised in anatomical space. First we asked if grid cells were clustered. A circular window was moved across the entire available surface of the medial entorhinal cortex. For each step, we counted the number of grid cells inside the window. The number of grid cells counted per window was clearly higher than the number of grid cells in a shuffled image, where the identity of the cells in the image was scrambled randomly (Fig. 24), suggesting that the medial entorhinal cortex is organised as entangled small clusters of functionally similar cells. Whether grid cells within a cluster belong to the same grid module remains to be determined.

Finally, now that entorhinal two-photon imaging is operative, let me return to the question I started out with, which was whether neighbouring cells have a more similar grid phase than expected. So far the data suggest that the correlation between firing locations of neighbouring cells, spaced by 50–100 um or less, is indeed higher than between randomly selected cell pairs. A recent report from another lab has shown the same (Heys et al., 2014). Thus, there is, in fact, some fine-scale topography in the grid map, but at a scale so small that tetrodes

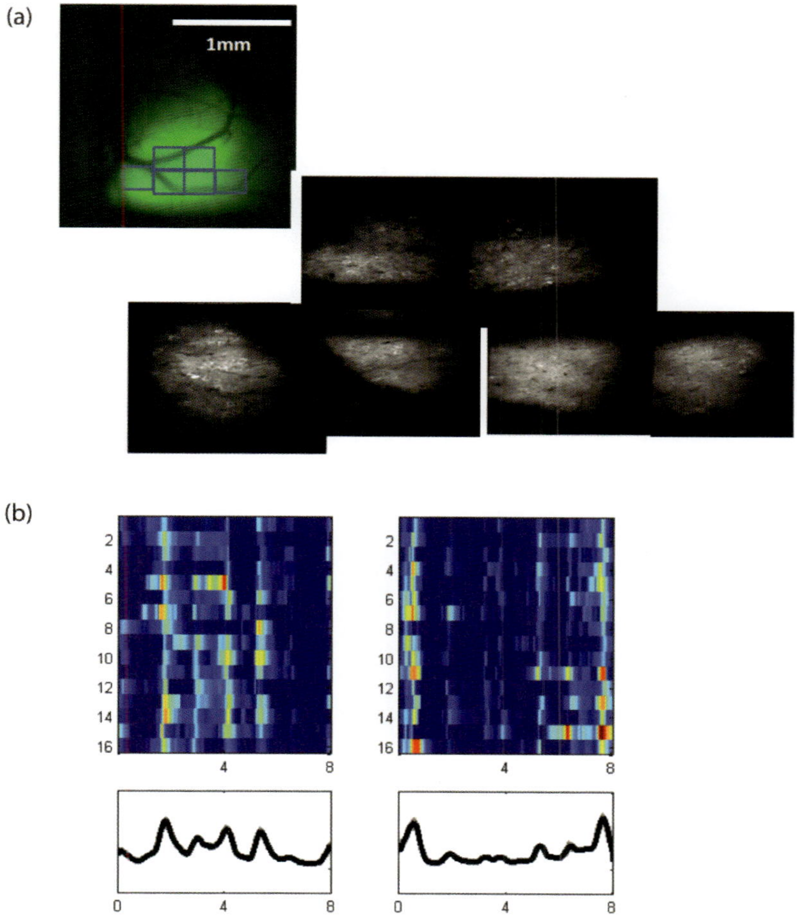

FIGURE 23. Two-photon imaging of medial entorhinal cortex cells during navigation in a virtual environment. (a) Top left: Surface view of medial entorhinal area seen through the prism. Note intact blood vessels. Bottom: magnified images showing instantaneous activity in each of the 6 rectangular windows of the top left image. White implies strong fluorescence. (b) Grid cells can be identified in the virtual linear environment as cells with periodic fields. Each colour-coded diagram shows activity as a function of distance along the track (0 to 8 m). Activity is colour-coded, with red indicating maximum activity and blue minimum. Each row shows one lap (all same cell). Left and right diagrams display opposite running directions for the same cell. Mean activity is shown in line diagrams below the colour plots. Note periodicity in the left diagram but not so much in the right diagram. Whether the sequence of activity fields corresponds to a slice through a two-dimensional grid was determined by comparing the activity on the virtual track with slices across all directions and locations of a simulated grid pattern. Euclidean distances between the observed pattern and the optimal slice through the simulated pattern were determined and cells were classified as grid cells if this distance was below a certain threshold. Illustrations made by Albert Tsao (Bonhoeffer-Moser collaboration).

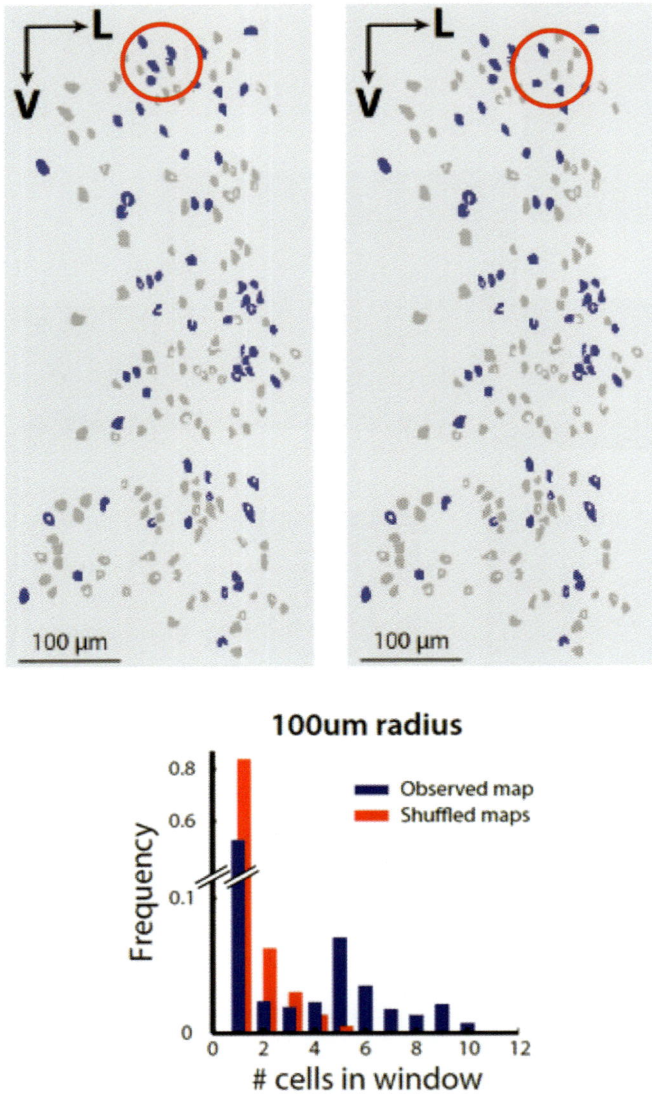

FIGURE 24. Grid cells are distributed but form functional clusters. Rectangles show an imaging window; blue cells are grid cells. Clustering of grid cells was determined by moving a circle in steps across the entire imaging window and counting, for each step, the number of grid cells in the window. Two example steps are shown (red circles). The number of grid cells was compared to the number obtained after random shuffling of cell identities (grid vs. non-grid) within the imaging window. The histogram shows the result of the counts. Note more frequent occurrence of large cell numbers in the real data than after shuffling, suggesting that grid cells are anatomically clustered. Illustrations made by Albert Tsao (Bonhoeffer-Moser collaboration).

do not detect it. The nature of this fine-scale topography, and its relation to cell identity, is still to be determined.

7. HOW IS THE GRID PATTERN GENERATED?

In the final part of my lecture, I would like to address one of the most important questions raised by the discovery of grid cells, which is how these hexagonal patterns are generated. There is a variety of computational models for the formation of grid patterns but most researchers now believe that attractor mechanisms are somehow involved. In a continuous attractor network, localized firing can be generated by mutual excitation between cells with similar firing locations (Fig. 25a; Tsodyks et al., 1995; McNaughton et al., 1996; Samsonovitch et al., 1997). Mutually connected cells may or may not be co-localised. When cells in the network are organised according to firing location, not anatomical location, excitatory connections between cells with similar firing fields maintain a localised bump of activity in the network, which is prevented from spreading in an uncontrolled manner by a surrounding ring of inhibition in a Mexican hat-like

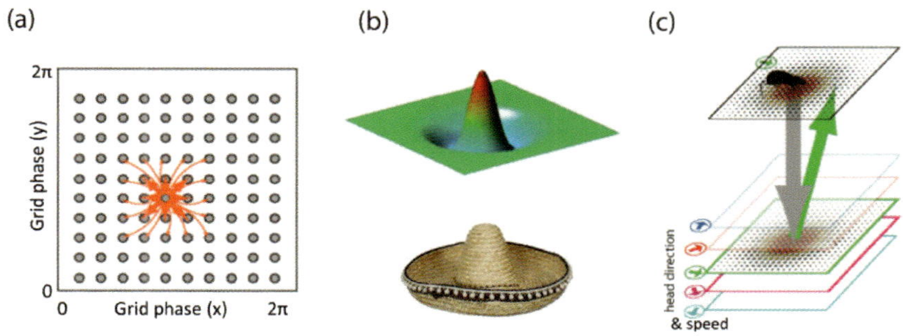

FIGURE 25. Mechanisms of spatially localised firing. Place-cell formation has been explained by continuous attractor dynamics (Tsodyks et al., 1995; McNaughton et al., 1996; Samsonovitch and McNaughton, 1997). In a continuous attractor network localized firing is generated by mutual excitation between cells with similar firing locations. In the network in (a), cells (circles) are arranged according to firing location in the square recording environment. Red arrows indicate excitatory connections. In addition, for each cell, there is an inhibitory surround that is wider than the radius of excitation. The inhibitory surround prevents uncontrolled spread of excitation and maintains a localised bump of activity. (b) The excitatory-inhibitory connectivity is often referred to as Mexican-hat connectivity. (c) Translation of the bump of activity across the network in accordance with movement in the external environment. Information about instantaneous displacement may reach grid cells via cells that monitor the animal's speed and direction in the environment. Modified, with permission, from McNaughton et al. (2006).

pattern (Fig. 25b). This bump of activity is then moved around in the neural network in accordance with the animal's movement in external space though inputs from cells that carry information about instantaneous speed (Fig. 25c). However, there is one problem with this model, which was originally developed for place cells. It explains localised activity but not the formation of hexagonal patterns.

During the years after the discovery of grid cells, several models were developed to explain how hexagonal firing could emerge in a continuous attractor network (Fuhs and Touretzky, 2006; McNaughton et al., 2006; Burak and Fiete, 2009). A common idea was that blobs of activity could emerge many places in the network, through mutual excitation and inhibitory surrounds, and that competitive interactions, i.e. inhibition, would keep these blobs away from each other. Mutual inhibition would then force the pattern into an equilibrium state where the blobs are as far away from each other as possible, which would be a hexagonal pattern (Fig. 26 and 27).

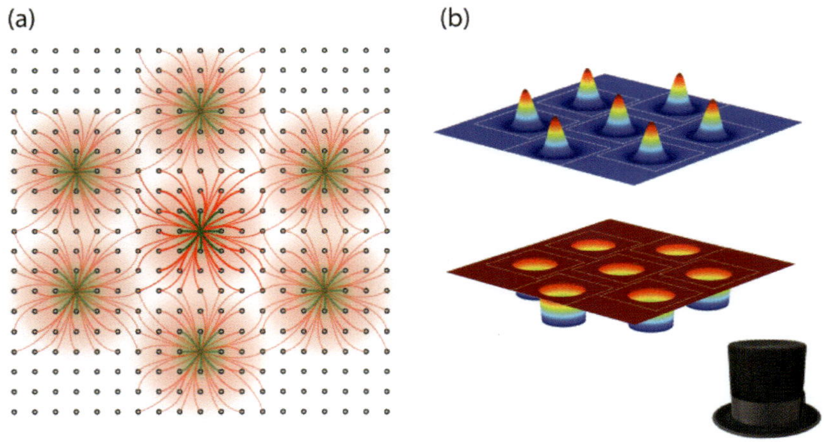

FIGURE 26. Continuous attractor models may explain origin of hexagonal structure in the grid pattern. (a) Competition between multiple self-exciting activity bumps on a neuronal lattice, each with an inhibitory surround. The competition may cause the network to self-organise into a hexagonal pattern, in which distances between bumps are maximised. Excitatory connections are green, inhibitory connections red. (b) Self-organization into hexagonal patterns has been demonstrated not only for Mexican hat connectivity but also for networks consisting of cells that have all-or-none inhibitory connections with each other, without additional recurrent excitation (inverted Lincoln hat connectivity). Excitation is colour-coded (red is strong excitation; blue is strong inhibition).

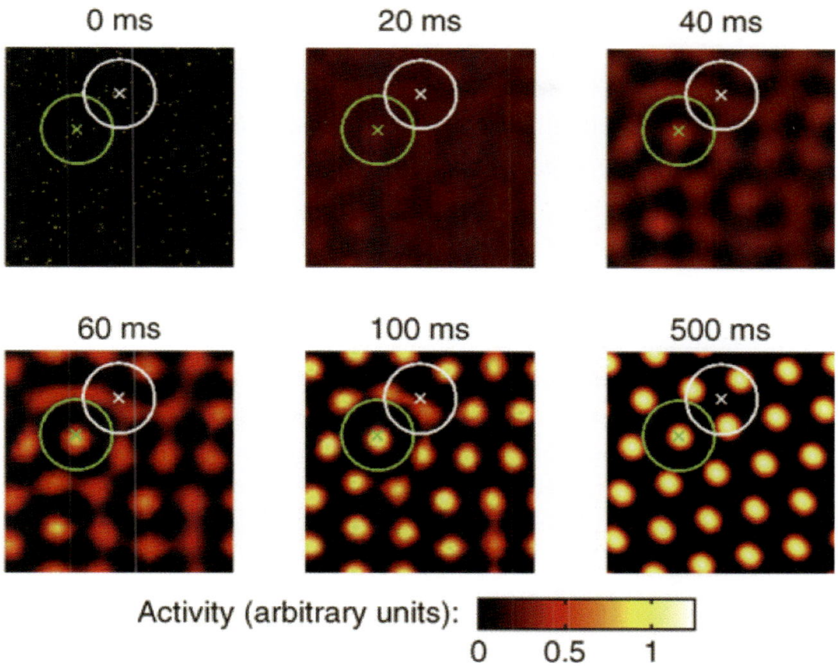

FIGURE 27. Hexagonal pattern formation on a two-dimensional lattice of stellate cells that have all-or-none inhibitory connectivity within a given radius. Neurons are arranged on the lattice according to their spatial phases. Connection radii for two example neurons are indicated by white and green circles. Activity is colour-coded, as indicated by the scale bar. Note low activity where circles overlap. Regions of low activity are regularly spaced. Note that hexagonal patterns are formed.

A problem with these models, in their original form, is that, at least among stellate cells in layer II of the medial entorhinal cortex, there is no recurrent excitation (Dhillon and Jones, 2000; Couey et al., 2013). However, in collaboration with Yasser Roudi and his colleagues, we have shown that hexagonally spaced patterns can be obtained exclusively by inhibitory surrounds, converting the Mexican hat of excitation and surrounding inhibition to an inverted Lincoln hat with only inhibition (Fig. 26b; Couey et al., 2013; Bonnevie et al., 2013). Once hexagonal firing is generated in a network with inverted Lincoln-hat all-or-none inhibitory connectivity, the network activity can be updated in accordance with the animal's position based on inputs that tell the network about the instantaneous speed of the animal (Fig. 25c) and, as a result, the grid pattern of the network will be reflected in the firing of individual neurons (Bonnevie et al., 2013).

Thus possible mechanisms of grid cell formation have been outlined. Data in support of these models are still scarce but new methods and technologies allow key predictions of the models to be tested. Testing the models, and developing them further, will certainly be among the main endeavours of scientists interested in grid cells during the years to come.

8. GENERAL PRINCIPLES OF NETWORK FUNCTION

Although a lot remains to be explored, I think we can say that the thousands of neuroscientists who have worked on cognitive maps have learnt much about the neural basis of space and maybe also cognition more generally. The entorhinal-hippocampal space system is one of the first cognitive functions to be understood in some mechanistic detail at the cell and cell-assembly level. In some sense the network of grid cells, border cells, head direction cells and place cells provides the components of the neural computations envisaged at the behaviour level by Tolman (1948) and at the cell assembly level by Hebb (1949). Moreover, what is particularly fascinating about grid cells is that they may inform us about general principles of neural pattern formation. Grid cells may for example offer a window to understanding continuous attractor mechanisms in the cortex, mechanisms that may be applied in different forms across the entire brain.

Studies of the space system may pave the way for quantitative analyses of neural ensemble coding, analyses that may draw on properties analysed in other physical systems that have been studied in more depth. Grid cells provide an example of this potential as hexagonal patterns are abundant in nature, appearing in widely different systems, as illustrated by chemical concentrations in reaction-diffusion systems (Turing, 1953; Edelstein-Keshet, 1988) and current vortices in superconductors (Abrikosov, 1957; Essman and Träuble, 1967). In many systems, the patterns are thought to arise as an equilibrium state following competitive interactions between the elements. In a superconductor, for example, current vortices may arrange themselves in a hexagonal pattern because of repulsive interactions between the vortices in the presence of an external magnetic field into the superconductor (Fig. 28; Essman and Träuble, 1967). It is our view that the principles underlying pattern formation in other physical and biological systems can shed light on pattern formation processes in the brain. The exploration of such common principles has barely started but I believe that, in the years to come, we will see many examples of neural computation where systems self-organise according to principles known to apply far beyond a particular brain system.

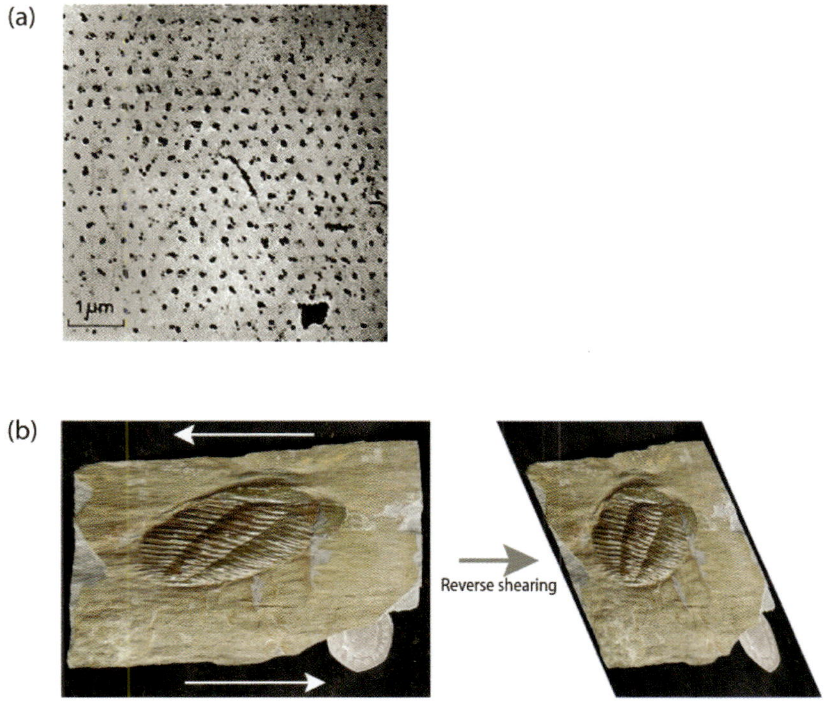

FIGURE 28. Neuroscience is beginning to understand some aspects of brain function in terms of underlying general principles of physics, as illustrated in (a) by the formation of Abrikosov current vortices through repulsive interactions in a superconductor exposed to an external magnetic field (Abrikosov, 1957; Essman and Träuble, 1967), and in (b) by inference of the original shape of a body, e.g. a trilobite, through reverse application of the shearing forces that once operated upon it. (a) is reproduced from Essman and Träuble (1967); (b) with permission from Pete Lawrance (www.bigfossil.com).

REFERENCES

1. Abrikosov AA (1957). Magnetic properties of superconductors of the second group. *Sov. Phys.-JETP (Engl. Transl.)*, 5:6.
2. Andersen P (1971). Lamellar organization of hippocampal pathways. *Exp. Brain Res.* **13**, 222–238.
3. Barnes CA, McNaughton BL, Mizumori SJ, Leonard BW and Lin LH (1990). Comparison of spatial and temporal characteristics of neuronal activity in sequential stages of hippocampal processing. *Prog. Brain Res.* **83**, 287–300.
4. Bonnevie T *et al* (2013). Grid cells require excitatory drive from the hippocampus. *Nature Neurosci.* **16**, 309–317.

5. Bruce C, Desimone R and Gross CG (1981). Visual properties of neurons in a polysensory area in superior temporal sulculs in the macaque. *J. Neurophysiol.* **46**, 369–384.
6. Brun, VH, Otnass MK, Molden S, Steffenach HA, Witter MP, Moser M-B and Moser EI (2002). Place cells and place recognition maintained by direct entorhinal-hippocampal circuitry. *Science* **296**, 2243–2246.
7. Burak Y and Fiete IR (2009). Accurate path integration in continuous attractor network models of grid cells. *PLoS Comput. Biol.* **5**, e1000291.
8. Couey JJ *et al* (2013). Recurrent inhibitory circuitry as a mechanism for grid formation. *Nature Neurosci.* **16**, 318–324.
9. Dhillon A and Jones RS (2000). Laminar differences in recurrent excitatory transmission in the rat entorhinal cortex in vitro. *Neuroscience* **99**, 413–422.
10. Dolorfo CL and Amaral DG (1998). Entorhinal cortex of the rat: topographic organization of the cells of origin of the perforant path projection to the dentate gyrus. *J. Comp. Neurol.* **398**, 25–48.
11. Dombeck DA, Khabbaz AN, Collman F, Adelman TL and Tank DW (2007). Imaging large-scale neural activity with cellular resolution in awake, mobile mice. *Neuron* **56**, 43–57.
12. Domnisoru C, Kinkhabwala AA and Tank DW (2013). Membrane potential dynamics of grid cells. *Nature* **495**, 199–204.
13. Edelstein-Keshet L (1988). *Mathematical models in biology.* Vol. 46. New York: Birkhäuser-McGraw-Hill.
14. Essman U and Träuble H (1967). The direct observation of individual flux lines in type II superconductors. *Physics Letters* **24A**, 526–527.
15. Felleman DJ and van Essen DC (1991). Distributed hierarchical processing in the primate cerebral cortex. *Cereb. Cortex* **1**, 1–47.
16. Fenton AA *et al.* (2008). Unmasking the CA1 ensemble place code by exposures to small and large environments: more place cells and multiple, irregularly arranged, and expanded place fields in the larger space. *J. Neurosci.* **28**, 11250–11262.
17. Frank LM, Brown EN and Wilson M (2000). Trajectory encoding in the hippocampus and entorhinal cortex. *Neuron* **27**, 169–178.
18. Fuhs MC and Touretzky DS (2006). A spin glass model of path integration in rat medial entorhinal cortex. *J. Neurosci.* **26**, 4266–4276.
19. Fyhn M, Molden S, Witter MP, Moser EI and Moser M-B (2004). Spatial representation in the entorhinal cortex. *Science* **305**, 1258–1264.
20. Fyhn M, Hafting T, Treves A, Moser M-B and Moser EI (2007). Hippocampal remapping and grid realignment in entorhinal cortex. *Nature* **446**, 190–194.
21. Fyhn M, Hafting T, Witter MP, Moser EI and Moser M-B (2008). Grid cells in mice. *Hippocampus* **18**, 1230–1238.
22. Gray CM, Maldonado PE, Wilson M and McNaughton B (1995). Tetrodes markedly improve the reliability and yield of multiple single-unit isolation from multi-unit recordings in cat striate cortex. *J. Neurosci. Methods* **63**, 43–54.
23. Gross CG, Bender DB and Rocha-Miranda CE (1969). Visual receptive fields of neurons in inferotemporal cortex of the monkey. *Science* **166**, 1303–1306.

24. Gross CG, Rocha-Miranda CE and Bender DB (1972). Visual properties of neurons in inferotemporal cortex of the Macaque. *J. Neurophysiol.* **35**, 96–111.
25. Hafting T, Fyhn M, Molden S, Moser M-B and Moser EI (2005). Microstructure of a spatial map in the entorhinal cortex. *Nature* **436**, 801–806.
26. Hartley T, Burgess N, Lever C, Cacucci F and O'Keefe J (2000). Modeling place fields in terms of the cortical inputs to the hippocampus. *Hippocampus* **10**, 369–379.
27. Hebb DO (1949). *The Organization of Behavior*. New York: Wiley.
28. Heys JG, Rangarajan KV and Dombeck DA (2014). The functional micro-organization of grid cells revealed by cellular-resolution imaging. *Neuron* **84**, 1079–1090.
29. Hubel DH and Wiesel T (1959). Receptive fields of single neurones in the cat's striate cortex. *J. Physiol. (Lond.)* **148**, 574–591.
30. Hubel DH and Wiesel T (1962). Receptive fields, binocular interaction, and functional architecture of cat striate cortex. *J. Physiol. (Lond.)* **160**,106–154.
31. Hubel DH and Wiesel T (1977). Functional architecture of macaque monkey visual cortex. *Proc. R. Soc. B* **198**, 1–59.
32. Jacobs J *et al.* (2013). Direct recordings of grid-like neuronal activity in human spatial navigation. *Nature Neurosci.* **16**, 1188–1190.
33. Kandel ER (2000). Nobel Lecture: The Molecular Biology of Memory Storage: A Dialog between Genes and Synapses. *Nobelprize.org*. Nobel Media AB.
34. Kerr JND, Greenberg D and Helmchen F (2005). Imaging input and output of neocortical networks in vivo. *Proc. Natl. Acad. Sci. U. S. A.* **102**, 14063–14068.
35. Killian NJ, Jutras MJ and Buffalo EA (2012). A map of visual space in the primate entorhinal cortex. *Nature* **491**, 761–764.
36. Krubitzer L, Campi KL and Cooke DF (2011). All rodents are not the same: A modern synthesis of cortical organization. *Brain Behav. Evol.* **78**, 51–93.
37. Krupic J, Bauza M, Burton S, Lever C and O'Keefe J. How environment geometry affects grid cell symmetry and what we can learn from it. *Philos. Trans. R. Soc. Lond. B Biol. Sci.* **369**, 20130188 (2014).
38. Lashley KS (1929). *Brain Mechanisms and Intelligence: Quantitative Study of Injuries to the Brain*. Chicago: University of Chicago Press.
39. Lashley KS (1950). In search of the engram. *Society of Experimental Biology Symposium* **4**, 454–482.
40. Low RJ, Gu Y and Tank DW (2014). Cellular resolution optical access to brain regions in fissures: Imaging medial prefrontal cortex and grid cells in entorhinal cortex. *Proc. Natl. Acad. Sci. U.S.A.* **111**, 18739–18744.
41. Mase, G. *Continuum Mechanics*, p. 44–53 (McGraw-Hill Professional, 1970).
42. Mathis A, Herz AV & Stemmler M (2012). Optimal population codes for space: grid cells outperform place cells. *Neural Comput.* **24**, 2280–2317.
43. McNaughton BL *et al* (1996). Deciphering the hippocampal polyglot: The hippocampus as a path integration system. *J. Exp. Biol.* **199**, 173–185.
44. McNaughton BL, Battaglia FP, Jensen O, Moser EI and Moser M-B (2006). Path integration and the neural basis of the 'cognitive map'. *Nature Rev. Neurosci.* **7**, 663–678.
45. Moser EI, Kropff E and Moser M-B (2008). Place cells, grid cells, and the brain's spatial representation system. *Annu. Rev. Neurosci.* **31**, 69–89.

46. Moser EI et al. (2014). Grid cells and cortical representation. *Nature Rev. Neurosci.* **15**, 466–481.
47. Muller RU and Kubie JL (1987). The effects of changes in the environment on the spatial firing of hippocampal complex-spike cells. *J. Neurosci.* **7**, 1951–1968.
48. Ohki K, Chung S, Ch'ng YH, Kara P and Reid RC (2005). Functional imaging with cellular resolution reveals precise micro-architecture in visual cortex. *Nature* **433**, 597–603.
49. Ohki K, Chung S, Kara P, Hübener M, Bonhoeffer T and Reid C (2006). Highly ordered arrangement of single neurons in orientation pinwheels. *Nature* **442**, 925–928.
50. O'Keefe J (1976). Place units in the hippocampus of the freely moving rat. *Exp. Neurol.* **51**, 78–109.
51. O'Keefe J and Dostrovsky J (1971). The hippocampus as a spatial map. Preliminary evidence from unit activity in the freely-moving rat. *Brain Res.* **34**, 171–175 (1971).
52. O'Keefe J and Nadel L (1978). *The Hippocampus as a Cognitive Map* (Oxford: Clarendon Press).
53. Perrett DI, Rolls ET and Caan W (1982). Visual neurones responsive to faces in the monkey temporal cortex. *Exp. Brain Res.* 47, 329–342.
54. Quirk GJ, Muller RU, Kubie JL and Ranck JB Jr (1992). The positional firing properties of medial entorhinal neurons: description and comparison with hippocampal place cells. *J. Neurosci.* **12**, 1945–1963.
55. Samsonovich A and McNaughton BL (1997). Path integration and cognitive mapping in a continuous attractor neural network model. *J. Neurosci.* **17**, 5900–5920.
56. Sargolini F, Fyhn M, Hafting T, McNaughton BL, Witter MP, Moser M-B and Moser EI (2006). Conjunctive representation of position, direction, and velocity in entorhinal cortex. *Science* **312**, 758–762.
57. Savelli F, Yoganarasimha D and Knierim JJ (2008). Influence of boundary removal on the spatial representations of the medial entorhinal cortex. *Hippocampus* **18**, 1270–1282.
58. Solstad T, Boccara CN, Kropff E, Moser M-B and Moser EI (2008). Representation of geometric borders in the entorhinal cortex. *Science* **322**, 1865–1868.
59. Stensola H, Stensola T, Solstad T, Frøland K, Moser M-B and Moser EI (2012). The entorhinal grid map is discretized. *Nature* **492**, 72–78.
60. Stensola T, Stensola H, Moser M-B and Moser EI (2015). Shearing-induced asymmetry in entorhinal grid cells. *Nature* **518**, 207–212.
61. Stettler DD and Axel R (2009). Representations of odor in the piriform cortex. *Neuron* **63**, 854–864.
62. Stosiek C, Garaschuk O, Holthoff K and Konnerth A (2003). In vivo two-photon calcium imaging of neuronal networks. *Proc. Natl. Acad. Sci. U.S.A.* **100**, 7319–7324.
63. Tanaka K, Saito H, Fukada Y and Moriya M (1991). Coding visual images of objects in the inferotemporal cortex of the macaque monkey. *J. Neurophysiol.* **66**, 170–189.
64. Tolman EC (1948). Cognitive maps in rats and men. *Psychol. Rev.* **55**, 189–208.
65. Tsao DY, Freiwald WA, Tootell RB and Livingstone MS (2005). A cortical region consisting entirely of face-selective cells. *Science* **311**, 670–674.

66. Tsodyks M and Sejnowski T (1995). Associative memory and hippocampal place cells. *Int. J. Neural Syst.* **6** (Suppl.), 81–86 (1995).
67. Turing A (1953). The chemical basis of morphogenesis, *Phil. Trans. Royal Soc. (part B)* **237**, 37–72.
68. Van Hooser SD, Heimel JA, Chung S, Nelson SB and Toth LJ (2005). Orientation selectivity without orientation maps in visual cortex of a highly visual mammal. *J. Neurosci.* **25**, 19–28.
69. Wei X-X, Prentice J and Balasubramanian V (2013). The sense of place: Grid cells in the brain and the transcendental number e. arXiv:1304.0031 [q-bio.NC].
70. Wilson MA and McNaughton BL (1993). Dynamics of the hippocampal ensemble code for space. *Science* **261**, 1055–1058.
71. Witter MP, Groenewegen HJ, Lopes da Silva FH and Lohman AHM (1989). Functional organization of the extrinsic and intrinsic circuitry of the parahippocampal region. *Prog. Neurobiol.* **33**, 161–254.
72. Yartsev MM, Witter MP and Ulanovsky N (2011). Grid cells without theta oscillations in the entorhinal cortex of bats. *Nature* **479**, 103–107.

Physiology or Medicine 2015

William C. Campbell and Satoshi Ōmura

"for their discoveries concerning a novel therapy against infections caused by roundworm parasites"

Tu Youyou

"for her discoveries concerning a novel therapy against Malaria"

The Nobel Prize in Physiology or Medicine

Speech by Professor Hans Forssberg of the Nobel Assembly at Karolinska Institutet.

Your Majesties, Your Royal Highnesses, Esteemed Laureates, Ladies and Gentlemen,

All around us – in nature, on our skin and in our bodies – a constant power struggle is under way between myriads of microscopically small creatures that are fighting for their survival. Many are important constituents in nature's ecosystems, while others attack us humans and cause disease and death. This year's Nobel Prize in Physiology or Medicine is awarded to scientists who have enlisted the help of nature and made use of weapons from this power struggle in order to develop drugs against parasites that have plagued humankind since ancient times.

Parasitic roundworms cause lymphatic filariasis and river blindness. These are life-long diseases that have afflicted hundreds of millions of people in the poorest parts of the world. Satoshi Ōmura of Japan and William Campbell of the United States have made discoveries that have led to a drastic decline in these diseases and that will hopefully eradicate them within ten years.

It began with Satoshi Ōmura's search for natural substances that could be used in producing new drugs. He became an expert in culturing Streptomyces, a type of soil bacteria known to produce antibiotic substances. He travelled around and collected thousands of soil samples from all over Japan which he used for culturing bacteria. In one of Ōmura's bacteria cultures, which was sent to William Campbell's laboratory, a whole new strain of Streptomyces was discovered – one that would change the world.

In Campbell's laboratory, extracts from these cultures were given to mice that had been infected with roundworms. One of the extracts was remarkably effective, killing all the worms. Campbell purified the active component, which was given the name Avermectin. With the help of chemists, it was modified to become even more effective. The new substance was called Ivermectin, and it turned out to have an extremely powerful effect on parasites in farm and domestic animals. Campbell now wanted to test whether this drug was equally effective in humans, and he helped start clinical studies on patients with river blindness. A single dose was enough to kill the larval form of the worm that infects the eyes. This was the beginning of an anti-parasite drug that has saved hundreds of millions of people from severe disabilities.

Malaria is caused by parasites that are spread by mosquitos. The disease infects the red blood cells and leads to fever, shivering and in severe cases encephalitis. Every year half a million people die of malaria: most of them children. During the 1960s and 70s, Tu Youyou took part in a major Chinese project to develop anti-malarial drugs. When Tu studied ancient literature, she found that the plant Artemisia annua, or sweet wormwood, recurred in various recipes against fever. She tested an extract from the plant on infected mice. Some of the malaria parasites died, but the effect varied. So Tu returned to the literature, and in a 1700-year-old book she found a method for obtaining the extract without heating up the plant. The resulting extract was extremely potent and killed all the parasites. The active component was identified and given the name Artemisinin. It turned out that Artemisinin attacks the malaria parasite in a unique way. The discovery of Artemisinin has led to development of a new drug that has saved the lives of millions of people, halving the mortality rate of malaria during the past 15 years.

Professors William Campbell, Satoshi Ōmura and Tu Youyou: Your discoveries represent a paradigm shift in medicine, which has not only provided revolutionary therapies for patients suffering from devastating parasitic diseases, but also promoted well-being and prosperity for individuals and society. The global impact of your discoveries and the resulting benefit to mankind are immeasurable.

On behalf of the Nobel Assembly at Karolinska Institutet, I wish to convey to you our warmest congratulations. May I now ask you to step forward to receive the Nobel Prize from the hands of His Majesty the King.

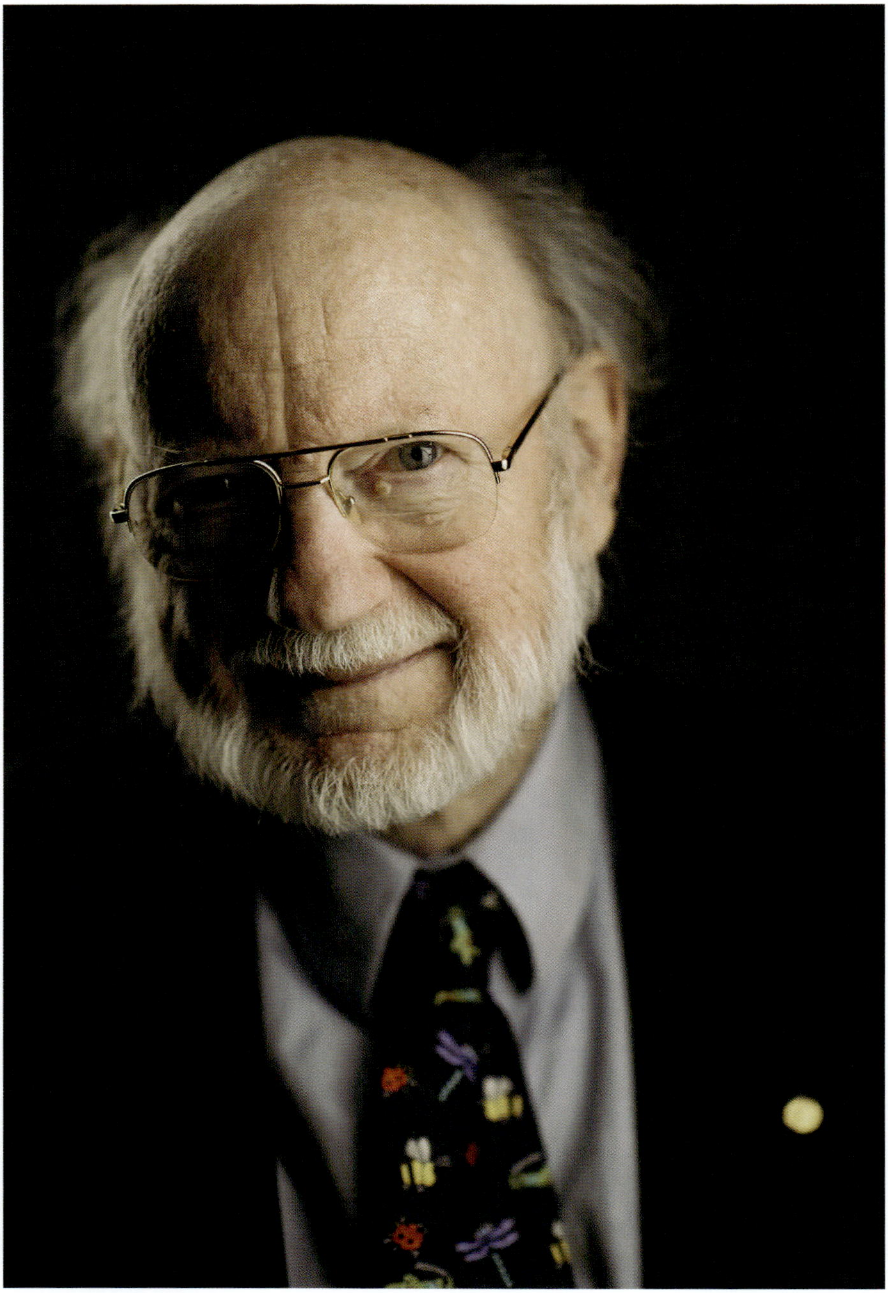

William C. Campbell. © Nobel Media AB. Photo: A. Mahmoud

William C. Campbell

Before any of the present fuss I was, of course, born; and that turned out to be slightly complicated—not in an obstetrical sense, but in a political one.

Several years before the event, an international border was created between my parents' rural town and the nearby city where maternity facilities were available at a price. Thus it came about that I was born in Northern Ireland, U.K. (in Londonderry city) but was raised in Eire, the Irish Republic (in Ramelton town, County Donegal). The year was 1930, and that was a long time ago (the Great Depression was in full swing, but I did not learn about that until much later).

My parents were strong believers in the value of education. My father, having had little formal education himself, went so far as to employ a professional teacher, Miss Elisabeth Letitia Martin, as a live-in tutor for me, my two brothers and my sister. (There were cultural factors at play as well as educational values.) For a considerable period I was the only pupil in school (my sister being too young for school and my brothers having departed for boarding school). Miss Martin instilled in me a desire to learn, and to remember the things that were considered good. Science was not mentioned. In those years before and during World War II, it did not, I think, occur to either of us that a multicultural, multidisciplinary transformation was taking place in the tumultuous world outside our attic classroom. I do not think that anyone now cares that I still remember a few lines of Wordsworth and Tennyson; but learning to love learning, through Miss Martin's influence, was a gift for which I shall be forever grateful.

Having been taught by Miss Martin from the age of 6, I moved at the age of 13 to a boarding school: Campbell College, Belfast, Northern Ireland. The school had a reputation for excellence; it was said to be "the Eton of Ulster" and indeed it was run on the lines of a classic British boarding school. It had been evacuated from Belfast to the seaside resort of Portrush because of the war, and for the same reason the teaching faculty was composed largely of teachers brought out

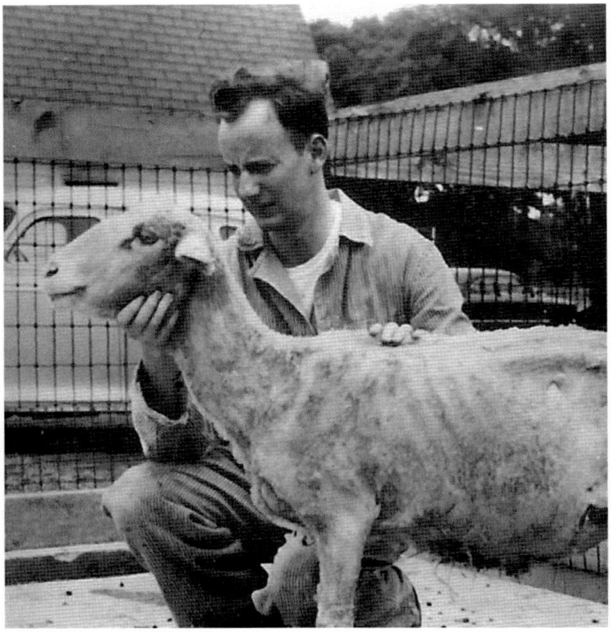

FIGURE 1. University of Wisconsin *circa* 1954, holding a sheep infected with *Fascioloides magna.*

of retirement. On arrival, I did not even know the difference between physics and chemistry (today I begin to suspect that there might not be one). I was thrown into those subjects very much as I was thrown into rugby football—without even a rudimentary instruction as to which way to run. Physics was hard; chemistry seemed like magic. Biology, however, I found fascinating. I was not robust enough or pugnacious enough to be good at contact sports, and playing tennis was not an option until the final years. Perhaps it was that factor, combined with the rather solitary prior period under Miss Martin's tutelage, that I became more interested in learning than in sports. In those school-days, and especially in the college years that were to follow, there was a great deal of peer pressure to be knowledgeable and "cultured." Certainly, my scholarly interests did not arise from any effusion of intellectual brilliance.

Life at Campbell College was an awesome adventure for a country boy who had led a rather sheltered life. It was not always fun (nor should it have been) but it was never boring. It meant making new friends in a regimented and hierarchical system. Traveling to school at the beginning of each term meant traveling to a country at war. It meant carrying a gas-mask in a little box slung around my shoulder. As a member of the Air Training Corps, I trained in the methods of, and at camps of, the Royal Air Force. I used to see fighter planes rising from

RAF airfields, and I longed to be old enough to fly them. I pictured myself an ace fighter pilot, strolling nonchalantly in my beribboned uniform and impressing the girls. In reality I was sequestered in an all-boys school and didn't know what I would say to a girl if I met one. The war ended while I was still a school-boy, and with it ended my dream of soaring into the sky in my trusty Spitfire. Campbell College moved back to Belfast.

It was at Campbell College that I first learned of the existence of a parasitic worm. It was *Fasciola hepatica*, the common liver-fluke of sheep and cattle. In the course of a school outing to an agricultural show, I was fascinated to learn that a drug could be used to treat liver-fluke disease. When it was time to move on to university, my biology teacher, Mr. Wells, advised me to go into biology while the head master advised me to go into medicine. I took Mr. Well's advice, but devoted my subsequent career to biology in the context of human and veterinary medicine.

Upon entering Trinity College, Dublin University in the autumn of 1948, I was again confronted with sciences that were not much to my liking. Swedish chemist Thomas Lindahl recalls that when he was a child a teacher gave him

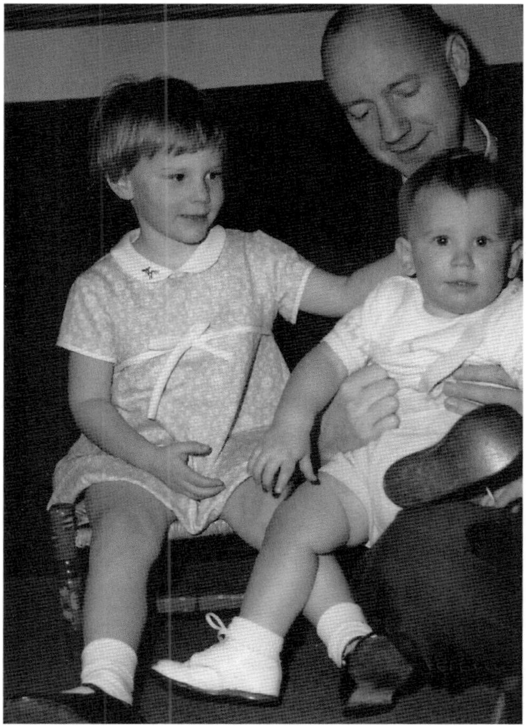

FIGURE 2. With daughter Jenifer and son Peter. New Jersey, 1967.

a failing grade in chemistry, but he went on to get a Nobel Prize in Chemistry (as recorded in Nobel speeches). When I was a university freshman, the standard grade for passing was 40%—and my final mark in chemistry was 39.7%. Fortunately the mark was rounded up to the nearest whole number. But for me chemistry remained mysterious. Physics, too, was a challenge. Perhaps my physics professor (Ernest Walton) was distracted by the news that he had just won the Noble Prize in Physics; but I cannot blame my teachers for the fact that I found the "hard sciences" hard. Biology was about to become vastly more chemical and physical: across the Irish Sea, Watson and Crick were building models with a novel twist. Luckily for me, my strong interest in zoology carried me through to graduate from Trinity with first-class honors.

Even in the earlier Trinity years, the pleasures of botany and zoology more than made up for the struggles in other sciences. Soon I came under the influence of Dr. J. D. Smyth, about whom I have written elsewhere [1]. Desmond Smyth was making a name for himself in the field of invertebrate physiology and especially in the area of experimental parasitology. He became (informally, of course) my mentor; and he changed my life. Among the things that Professor Smith did for me as I approached graduation was to respond positively to inquiries from Professor Arlie Todd of the University of Wisconsin, USA. The result

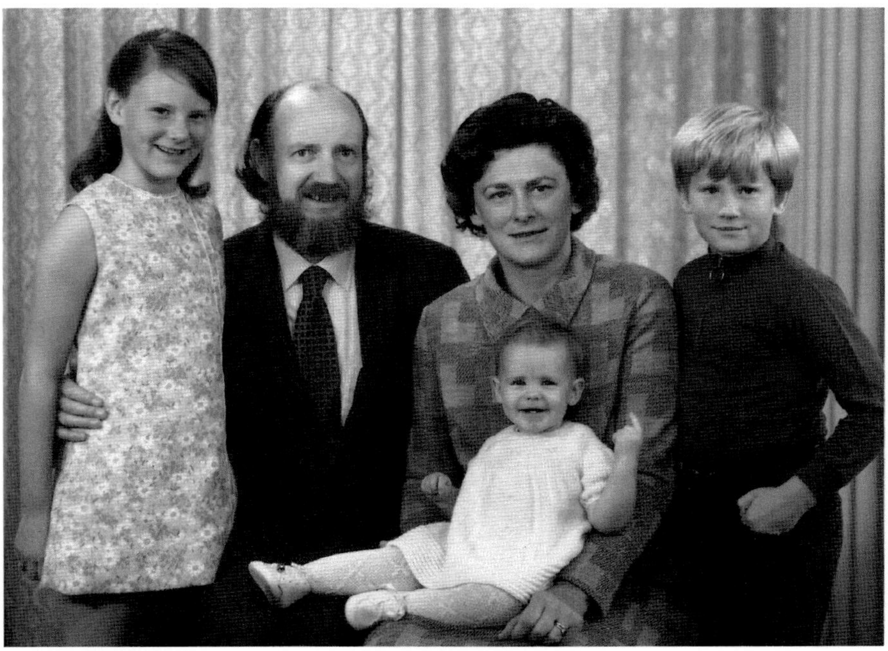

FIGURE 3. Family in Australia, 1973. Jenifer, Bill, Mary, Betsy, Peter. Photo by Eyre.

of that communication was my application for graduate school at the University of Wisconsin along with two other Trinity students. Both of the others dropped out, and before I set out on that journey alone, one of them sent me a note saying, "For God's sake, don't panic when you get off the boat." I thought that was a very easy thing for him to say.

As it turned out, getting on and off the boat (which turned out to be the liner *Britannic*) was made easier by two wonderful organizations. Prof. Smyth encouraged me to apply for a Fulbright Travel Grant, which led to various complications relating to the foundation of the Fulbright grants and my rather confusing British and Irish citizenship. All was settled favorably and I set off on my big adventure to the New World and graduate school, with all my travel expenses covered by the Fulbright grant. I was therefore one of the innumerable beneficiaries of the generous impulse and astute insight of United States Senator William Fulbright and his conjuring of international good will from the horrors and economics of war. Getting off the boat in the dockyards of New York City (in January 1953) would indeed have been a fearsome affair had it not been for the other organization, the Committee on Friendly Relations Among Foreign Students (founded in 1915, with funds given by Andrew Carnegie and Cleveland Dodge). Its angelic Mrs. Minucci met me on the dock and soon had me installed in a nearby hostel where I was assigned to one of the many beds in a large dormitory room, and was advised to keep my belongings close about me. I am still haunted by the realization that I always intended to write that kind woman a thank-you note, but never did.

I was dismayed to find that the U.S. system required graduate students to take many academic courses, but the requirement proved advantageous. My doctoral program was a "joint major" program in Veterinary Sciences (supervised by Arlie Todd) and Zoology (supervised by Chester Herrick). Professor Todd's laboratory in the Department of Veterinary Sciences was my campus 'home'. Since I knew something about the trematode *Fasciola hepatica*, I was delighted to learn that my research project would be on a giant relative, *Fascioloides magna*.

Todd's method (unspoken by him, unsuspected by me) was to set a new student to some routine task such as tending the snail tanks where the vector snails were raised, and waiting for the student's curiosity to take its course. Gradually and unwittingly I discovered the joy of being able to do something in the lab to test some item of casual curiosity—the fun of actually doing an experiment that no one had done, to answer a question no one had asked. Those graduate school explorations led to half a dozen scientific papers.

For most of my years in Madison, Wisconsin, I lived rent-free in the old Governors' Mansion on the edge of Lake Mendota! This extraordinary bit of good

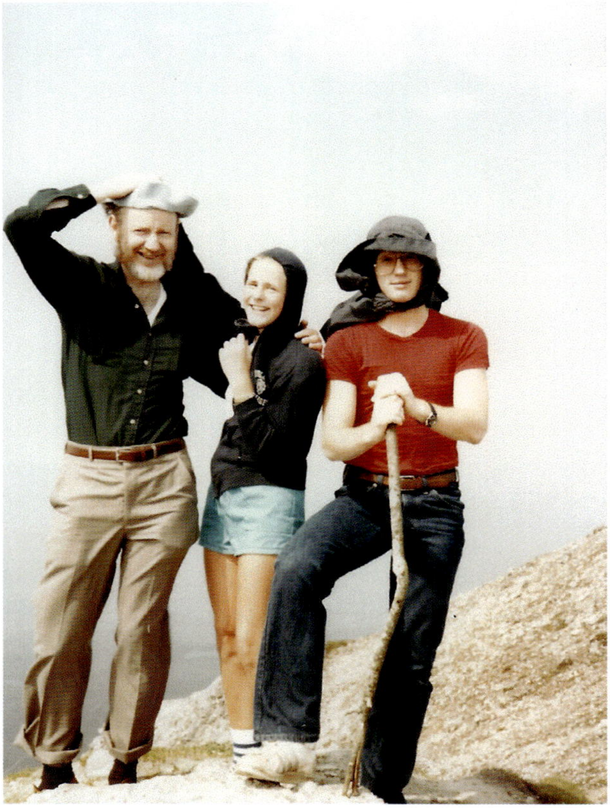

FIGURE 4. Climbing Mt. Errigal (County Donegal) with family. 1983. The photo shows the author with Betsy and Peter.

fortune resulted from being awarded a Kemper K. Knapp Fellowship—a grant that enables a group of graduate students from various disciplines to live together in a an environment conducive to intellectual 'cross-fertilization.' The "Knapp House" experience was a major highlight of my University of Wisconsin years.

In 1957, as the graduate school experience came to an end, Professor Todd responded positively (echo of the end of my Trinity days) to an enquiry from Dr. Ashton C. Cuckler, Director of Parasitology at the Merck Institute for Therapeutic Research. Todd encouraged me to at least go for an interview at the Merck organization in Rahway, New Jersey. With considerable misgiving I decided to give the pharmaceutical industry a try—and stayed for 33 years. It was a marvelous experience—challenging, exciting and (at least in the early years!) remarkably free of workplace politics. I am deeply indebted to Cuckler for his leadership in those early years [2]. Sharply focused research was exactly what I needed to keep me from wandering indefinitely into tangents and sub-tangents of a project;

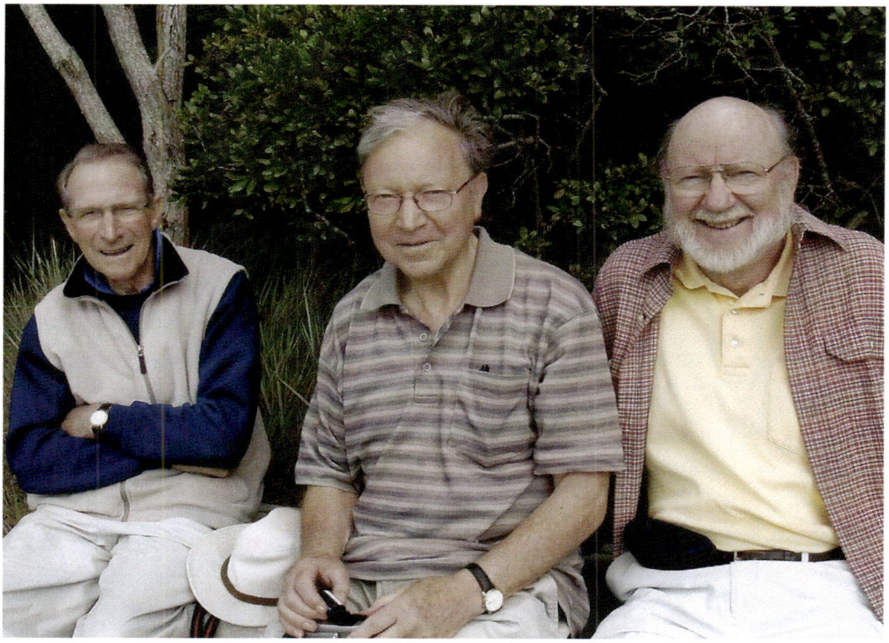

FIGURE 5. With brothers Lexie (left) and Bert (center) Ramelton, Ireland, 2006.

yet at the same time I was always free to make refreshing forays into the most enticing tangential byways.

Given my struggles with chemistry as a student, it is ironic that I went on to have a career in experimental chemotherapy. That happened quite naturally because at the Merck Institute I was surrounded by brilliant chemists and close interdisciplinary collaboration was a way of life. During my years at Merck, collaboration between Parasitology and many other scientific disciplines enabled the company to introduce several anthelmintic (anti-worm) drugs: thiabendazole (Thibenzole^R, TBZ^R); cambendazole (Camvet^R); rafoxanide (Ranide^R); clorsulon (Curatrem^R); ivermectin (Mectizan^R, Ivomec^R); eprinomectin (Eprinex^R). For several years I had administrative responsibility for the Merck poultry coccidiosis program, and the amebiasis and trypanosomiasis programs, but my contribution to protist biology was essentially nil.

It was a chemist who imbued me with confidence in the empirical approach to drug discovery. The parasitologists and chemists at Merck had weekly lunch meetings, co-chaired by Cuckler and Dr. Lewis H. Sarett. Sarett was one of the great medicinal chemists of that era (he was renowned especially for his partial synthesis of cortisol). He quickly deflated my naïve assumption that the best way to find a new antiparasitic drug was to devise a rational therapy based on the latest discoveries in the field of parasite biochemistry. Sarett convinced me that, at least in the near term, the probability of finding a drug by empirical screening (for which there was much historical precedent) was higher than the probability of finding one through research on the biochemical processes of parasites (for which there was no precedent). That assessment has, of course, no bearing on the importance of research on parasite biochemistry. Cuckler placed great faith in the use of animal (*in vivo*) models, and dietary medication, for the routine screening of test substances. In the era of biochemical biology there was a high price to pay for adherence to such traditional assay methodology; but I do not regret my espousal of it.

Chemotherapy has by no means been my only parasitological interest, and I will mention just a few of the others. I devoted a lot of time to the study of Trichinella and trichinellosis, including much "burning of midnight oil" to produce a

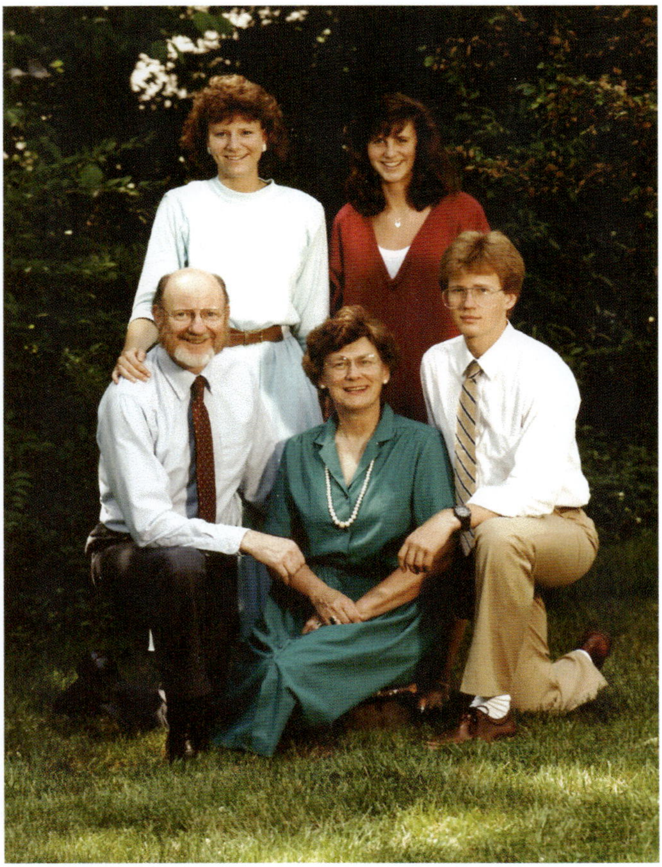

FIGURE 6. Family in the US. 1987. Photo by DRM Photo.

book on that subject. I was privileged to become deeply involved in the activities of the International Commission on Trichinellosis. My passion to be the first person to deep-freeze worms without killing them led to the discovery of a laboratory manipulation that allowed the cryopreservation of strongyle nematodes for at least 10 years [3, 4]. It turned out to be useful because it made possible the maintenance of species and strains of nematodes without the enormous cost of serial passage in sheep, cattle or other large animals. My close association with chemotherapy prompted me to use drugs as tools for the study of stage-specific immunity to helminth parasites. The first of these was a demonstration of the protection conferred by pre-pulmonary migration of *Ascaris suum* in rats [5].

My decades of work at the Merck labs in Rahway NJ were punctuated by two leaves of absence and one temporary re-assignment. I requested, and was granted, leave to travel to the University of Cambridge to become a visiting researcher in the laboratory of Lawson Soulsby (now Lord Soulsby, Baron of Swaffham Prior), who is recognized as an outstanding pioneer in the field of immunity to helminth parasites. My wife and I sailed on the *Queen Elizabeth* in 1963, and our life in England was marked by immunological studies on trichinellosis, many new friendships, and the birth of our daughter Jenifer. Our son Peter was born in the US at the beginning of 1966; and later that year I was granted a brief second leave—this time to accept an Inter-American Fellowship in Tropical Medicine

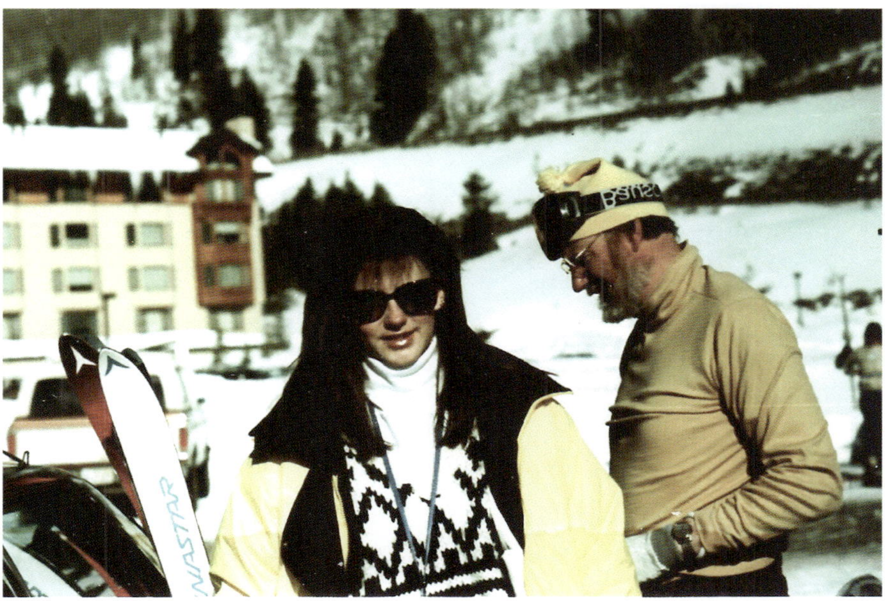

FIGURE 7. Skiing in Colorado with family (the photo shows Betsy and the author).

under the auspices of the Louisiana State University. Previously this fellowship had not been open to scientists employed in industry. Professor Harold Brown, a legendary parasitologist at Columbia University, appealed for a lifting of that restriction and I had the great benefit of visiting laboratories and hospitals in Central and South America. A third departure from the United States (1972–73) was not a leave of absence, but rather a temporary transfer from Company headquarters in New Jersey, USA to Australia to assume directorship of the Merck, Sharp and Dohme Veterinary Research and Development Laboratory in Campbelltown, N.S.W. That, too, was a memorable and instructive period, with novel administrative responsibilities, research on the use of cambendazole for the control of tapeworm in sheep (with colleague Richard Butler); further research on the cryopreservation of strongyle nematodes [6, 7], lasting new friendships—and the birth of our daughter Betsy.

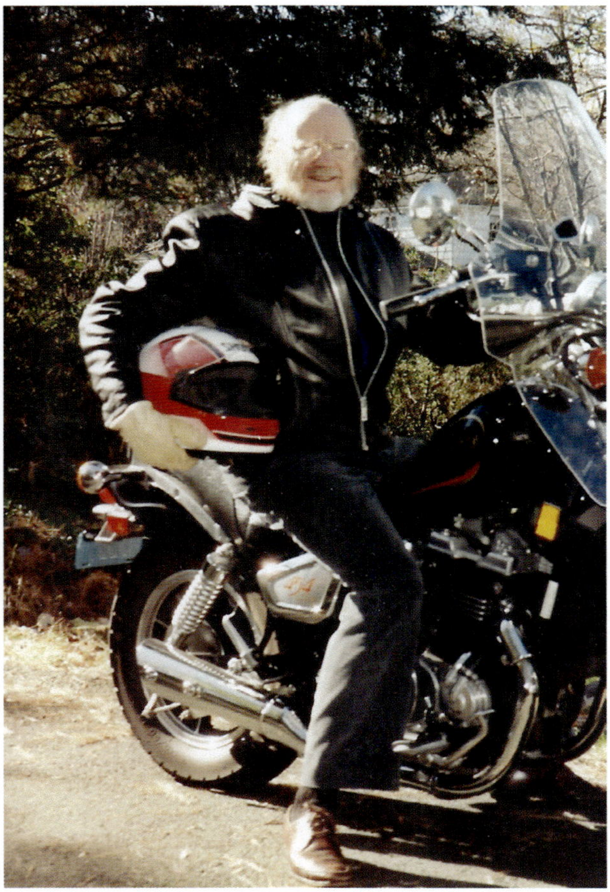

FIGURE 8. Approaching retirement.

Beginning in 1975, and continuing for a period of 15 years, I was mostly preoccupied with matters relating to ivermectin [8]. Advancing years and perturbations in career pathway brought thoughts of retirement. There was no doubt about what to do. I knew that Drew University in Madison, NJ had an unusual program that enables retired industrial scientists to turn their years of experience to the benefit of undergraduate students, while at the same time enabling the scientists to continue to be active in their fields of interest. In doing this, the scientists give up much in absent salary, and they gain much in an incomparable "job satisfaction." The Charles A. Dana Research Institute for Scientists Emeriti had been founded at Drew University to provide this sort of opportunity. In 1990, Merck and Company announced an offer of increased retirement benefits to employee scientists who opted to take early retirement in order to teach mathematics or science. I therefore moved quickly, at the age of 59, to Drew University. Few experiences are as gratifying as that of mentoring undergraduate students as they discover the joy of doing an experiment that is not a classroom exercise but an experiment that constitutes real research. Several of my undergraduate students have published their research findings in reputable peer-reviewed journals by the time they graduated. I had always enjoyed teaching and had held adjunct professorships at University of Pennsylvania, New York Medical College

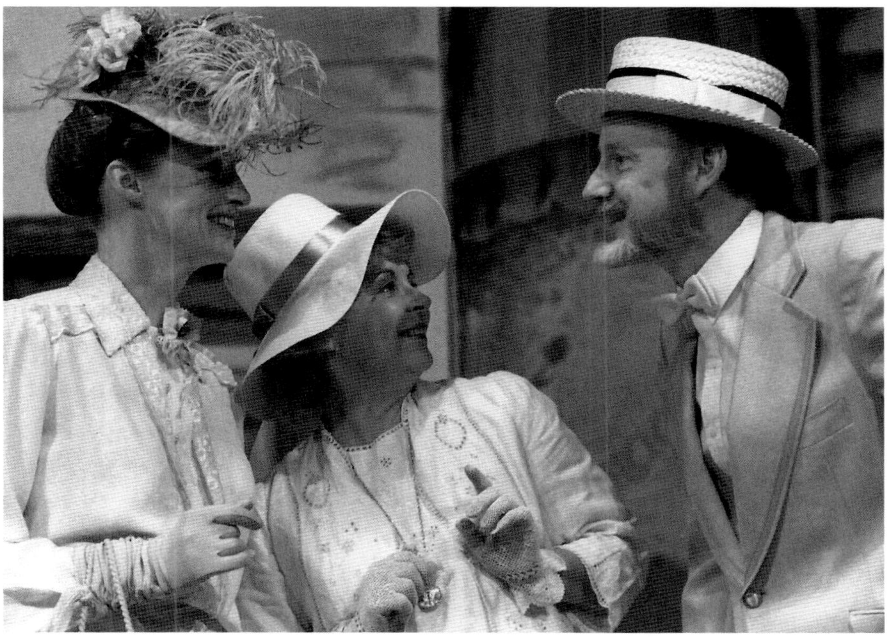

FIGURE 9. On stage, Summit Playhouse, with Lesley Fischer, Norma McGuff. Photo by Playhouse.

and Drew University for many years. I was delighted to find new opportunities to teach at Drew University: teaching a course on Parasitology (in the Biology Department) and a course on the History of Biomedical Science (in the graduate school). I cannot imagine a more rewarding professional *finale* than retiring a bit early to profess one's calling in such an environment.

Leaving the land of my birth (Northern Ireland) and of my upbringing (Ėire) had never been my intent; but circumstances changed and the New World got hold of me. The people of the United States welcomed me, and in 1964 I became a citizen.

In accord with instructions, I have devoted these pages to education and career. Recreational, avocational and social activities have been left out. But that sort of limitation is not the hardest part of writing such a biographical sketch. The hardest part of all is coping with the realization that one is evading the most important part. Without family (at least in the ancestral sense), there would be no biography to write. With family, there is no way a really true biography can be written. I have no words to say how much I love my wife and children; and how much, magically, I feel loved by them. My wife Mary, and my children Jenifer, Peter and Betsy must be counted in whatever honors come my way. And then there is the love that emanated (unspoken, in the manner of the time and place) from my parents Robert and Sarah Campbell, and was shared by my sister Marion and my brothers Bert and Lexie. Without my being aware of it, my younger self must have been molded by the nurturing care of my parents, their commitment to honest and industrious living, their stalwart religious faith and their admiration of learning. Beyond the family circle and our extended families, many other people have granted me the blessing of friendship. I may not be able to express my gratitude here, but of this I am certain: I have a great deal to be thankful for.

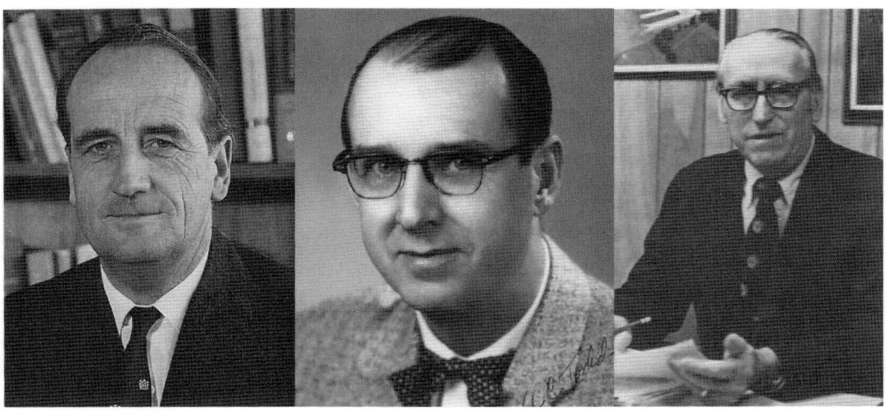

FIGURE 10. Three mentors: Dr. J.D. Smyth, Dr. A.C. Todd, Dr. A.C. Cuckler.

LITERATURE

1. Campbell, W.C. 1999. In Memoriam: James Desmond Smyth, Honorary Member ASP. *J. Parasitol.* **85**:992–993.
2. Campbell, W.C. 2001. In Memoriam: Ashton C. Cuckler. *J. Parasitol.* **87**:466–467.
3. Campbell, W.C., Blair, L.S. and Egerton, J.R. 1973. Unimpaired infectivity of the nematode Haemonchus contortus after freezing for 44 weeks in the presence of liquid nitrogen. *J. Parasitol.* **59**: 425–427.
4. Rew, R.S. and Campbell, W.C. 1983. Infectivity of Haemonchus contortus in sheep after freezing for ten years over liquid nitrogen. *J. Parasitol.* **69**:251–252.
5. Campbell, W.C. and Timinski, S.F. 1965. Immunization of rats against Ascaris suum by means of non-pulmonary larval infections. *J. Parasitol.* **51**:712–716.
6. Campbell, W.C. and Thomson, B.M. 1973. Survival of nematode larvae after freezing over liquid nitrogen. *Australian Vet. J.* **49**:110–111.
7. Kelly, J.D. and Campbell, W.C. 1974. Survival of Nippostrongylus brasiliensis larvae after freezing over liquid nitrogen. *Internat. J. Parasitol.* **4**:173–176.
8. Campbell, W.C., Fisher, M.H., Stapley, E.O., Albers-Schonberg, G. and Jacob, T.A. 1983. Ivermectin: A potent new antiparasitic agent. *Science* **221**:823–828.

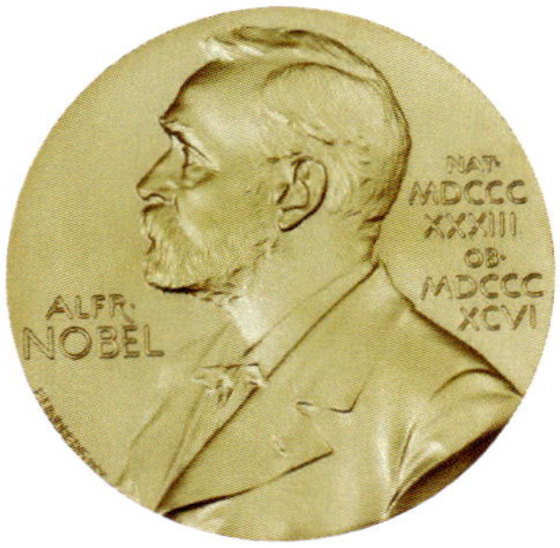

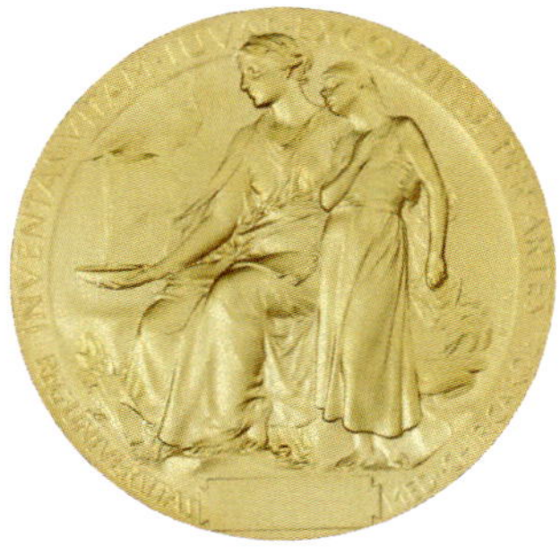

Ivermectin: A Reflection on Simplicity

Nobel Lecture, December 7, 2015

by William C. Campbell
Research Institute for Scientists Emeriti, Drew University, Madison, New Jersey, USA.

THE BEGINNING

I am using the word "simplicity" here in the context of science, but I do not mean to suggest that science is simple; nor will I suggest that the development of the drug ivermectin was an exercise in simplicity. I want rather to call attention to the element of simplicity within science—and I want to do that by pointing out the prominence of simplicity in the genesis of the drug ivermectin. It has long been acknowledged that simplicity has an intrinsic appeal to scientists (as to others), and indeed simplicity is widely celebrated in science as a matter of beauty. But I want to speak of it, not as a matter of beauty, but as a matter of practical utility.

Consider an actual real-life event. On a particular day, the ninth of May 1975, there was a mouse in a mouse-box in a laboratory. It had been purposely infected with worms—but not enough to cause illness. On that day its diet was altered—some liquid was stirred into its regular food. And the mouse ate that food for almost a week. Then its normal diet was restored. And about a week after that—its worms had gone! From that moment a train of events was set in motion. It would lead, some years later, to an advance in medical and veterinary science; and *that*, in turn, would lead to practical changes in the management of parasitic disease. To a very large extent the drug ivermectin was brought about by simple science. It was not conventional science; it was not obvious science; but it was simple science.

There is a question that warrants a slight digression here. In the past few weeks I have often been asked how I felt when I heard that I had won the Nobel

Prize. I can say without hesitation that my mind was instantly flooded by two emotions. One was a sense of joy and gratitude. The other was a feeling of sadness—sadness that so many of the people who made this discovery a success could not be named individually. But I represent the research team at Merck & Co., Inc., and in that role I feel honored and grateful beyond imagining.

The mouse I mentioned a moment ago was a single mouse. I do not mean that the mouse was unmarried. I mean that the special diet that proved to be so very special was tested, not in a conventional experimental group of mice, but rather in just one mouse. The diet was special because it had been supplemented with a liquid in which a bacterium had been allowed to flourish. Other solitary mice got other diets supplemented with other liquids in which other bacteria had flourished. But the bacterium that cured the mouse of its worm infection was the only one that did so. This method of testing "fermentation broths" for anti-worm (anthelmintic) efficacy had been developed by Dr. John Egerton and his technical staff in the Merck Laboratories, where also the reduction of experimental group-size to a singleton had been pioneered by Dr. Dan Ostlind [1, 2].

The liquid that had been added to the diet of that mouse had been fermented by a bacterium that was one of hundreds of microbes that had been sent to Merck & Co. Inc. by Satoshi Ōmura and his team of chemists and microbiologists at the Kitasato Institute in Tokyo. I had the pleasure of visiting Dr. Ōmura in Tokyo many years later; and he shares with me the prize that has brought us here today.

Microbes do not all act alike, or look alike. Both the Kitasato Institute and Merck & Co., Inc. were interested in microbes that stand out from the crowd, and they collaborated in trying to find them. Microbiologists grow weary of finding microbes that have already been found. Professor Ōmura sent us microbes that were unfamiliar to microbiologists. In our new mouse assay, as described above, we found that one of those unfamiliar microbes produced an unfamiliar substance—and that the substance had antiparasitic activity. Furthermore, the antiparasitic activity was of unmatched potency.

Simplicity, in the history of ivermectin, was just a beginning. From then on, there was *complexity*—years of complex basic research and years of complex developmental research. Pharmaceutical development is the epitome, not of simplicity, but of complexity.

The antiparasitic effect seen in the test mouse was an anthelmintic (against parasitic worms) effect. It was quickly confirmed in additional tests, and its potency was so striking that intense interest was aroused. Soon many things were going on at once. The microbiologists described the bacterium as a new species of *Streptomyces* [3]. Fermentation chemists and biologists isolated the mystery substance that killed worms; and they persuaded the bacterium to make it much more abundantly [4]. Analytical chemists removed the main mystery when they used highly sophisticated technology to show that the substance consisted of a complex of eight closely related molecules [5]. It was seen to have structural similarities to the milbemycin pesticides. We named it avermectin. The synthetic chemists made hundreds (eventually thousands) of related compounds, while the parasitologists provided efficacy data and preliminary toxicity data to guide the derivatization program [6, 7]. One of the derivatives (Figure 1) had an efficacy-and-safety profile that was judged to be superior to that of avermectin. The improved structure was made by hydrogenation of the chemical bond of avermectin at the Carbon 22–23 position. It seemed logical that the hydrogenated avermectin should be named "hyvermectin." It was soon learned that in some language "hyver" means "testicle," and so "hyvermectin" became "ivermectin."

Despite being unique in its origin, ivermectin now has many relatives—including doramectin (from a mutant strain of *Streptomyces avermitilis*; selamycin, a derivative of doramectin; nemadectin (from *Streptomyces cyanogriseus*); moxidection a derative of nemadectin; milbemycin oxime (from the macrocyclic lactone milbemycin); eprinomycin (ivermectin derivative with favorable pharmacological distribution in dairy animals).

Meanwhile, the research continued. The parasitologists found out which worms it would kill; [8, 9] the biochemists found how it would kill them—or rather how it would paralyze them [10]. In the case of parasitic worms, paralyzing them is just as good, or from the worm's point of view just as bad, as killing

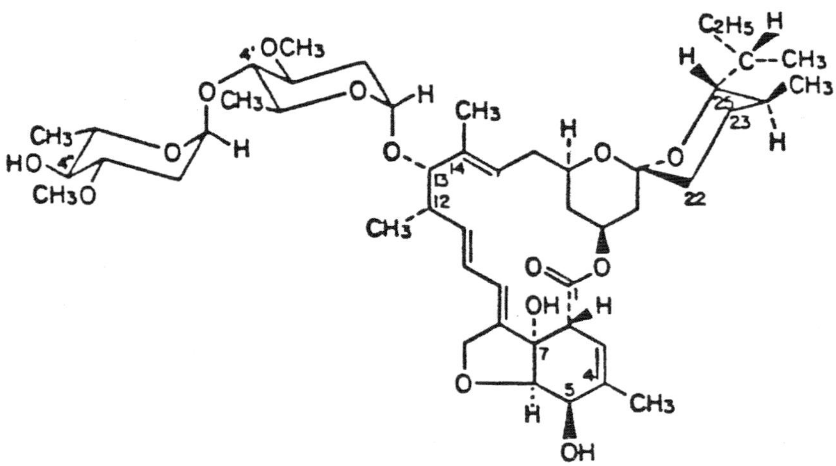

FIGURE 1. The chemical structure of ivermectin (22,23-dihydroavermectin B1a). Its precursor avermectin B1a differs in that the bond at Carbon 22-23 (in the spiroketal group, shown at upper right) has not been hydrogenated.

them. The body will get rid of paralyzed worms. It was discovered that some ecto-parasitic arthropods (including lice and mites) were susceptible to ivermectin, as were endoparasitic insect larvae. The family of macrocyclic lactone antiparasitic agents would become known as "endecticides."

THE MIDDLE

The flood of incoming news was exciting. But those of us who work with new drugs learn to allow ourselves only a subdued form of excitement—for we know that the whole project is likely to collapse with the arrival of tomorrow's bad news. Eventually the project was so promising that it was given 'developmental' status, and even more scientific disciplines were brought into the project. That meant more scientists. In an earlier paper I named 125 Merck scientists and technicians who were listed as authors on some 70 papers published within 10 years of the original discovery [1]. To mention just one discipline: veterinarians with parasitological expertise were recruited. They were graduates of veterinary colleges all over the world, and the breadth and depth of their knowledge was truly astonishing. Under their leadership ivermectin was evaluated against many parasite species in many domestic animal species in many lands. Their expertise was undoubtedly an essential element in the success of ivermectin. The new drug would go on to become the predominant agent in controlling the parasitic diseases that plague the animals on which humans depend for food and fiber—and companionship. Despite the complexity, all the pieces came together to result in the launching of ivermectin as an animal health product in 1981.

Things that are usually bad sometimes turn out to be good. If a broad-spectrum antiparasitic drug turns out to be ineffective against an important parasite, the drug is usually doomed to oblivion. But not always! In dog heartworm disease, caused by the filarial nematode *Dirofilaria immitis*, the adult worm is the most pathogenic stage. Ivermectin is not effective against it—but that is good! Because of their location in the left ventricle and pulmonary artery, injuring and dislodging the worms may result in pulmonary aneurysm. Thus, in the routine de-worming of dogs, killing the adult heartworm can be hazardous to the dog—and to the reputation of the attending veterinarian. Ivermectin, in other words, is ineffective exactly where one would like it to be ineffective.

Nevertheless, ivermectin is commonly used in the prevention of heartworm disease in dogs. Shortly before the discovery of ivermectin, I had instituted a program at Merck to find an agent for the control of heartworm disease. There had been, at the time, few laboratory projects devoted to filarial worms, mainly because of a lack of convenient laboratory models. To establish the life cycle of *D.*

immitis in the laboratory, Lyndia Blair and I proceeded to cultivate large numbers of the mosquito that is the required intermediate host (vector) of the parasite. Initially there was no alternative to using dogs as the definitive host; but then we found that the ferret (*Mustela putorius furo*) is a highly susceptible host for *D. immitis* [11]. It is a suitable host for studying the immature (pre-cardiac) stages of the worm, but the small ferret heart does not readily allow the development of the adult form. Later, in collaboration with Dr. John McCall, we showed that the ferret was also a suitable laboratory host for another filarial parasite, the one that causes lymphatic filariasis (including 'elephantiasis') [12]. Thus, when ivermectin came along, we were immediately able to do the research that led to the first once-a-month treatment for prevention of heartworm in dogs [13]. The product quickly became extremely popular.

The potential value of ivermectin in human medicine was not overlooked. I had always insisted that our written departmental objectives would include the development of new drugs for control of parasites in humans. In the 1960s Nelson in the United Kingdom reported the migration and visualization of onchocercal larvae in the ears of experimentally infected mice, and I had considered the observation as a basis for possible chemotherapeutic assay. When my colleagues found that ivermectin was active against the larvae of *Onchocerca cervicalis* in the skin of horses [14], I knew it was time to take action. My chief, Dr. Jerry Birnbaum, enthusiastically approved my suggestion that Dr. Bruce Copeman in Australia be invited to undertake (with Merck financial support) a trial of ivermectin against a related parasite, *Onchocera gutturosa* in cattle. A trial was arranged through the courtesy of Dr. Ian Hotson, head of Merck animal-health research in Australia, and the ivermectin treatment proved to be effective.

The results of our trials against various parasites in various animals suggested that ivermectin might be effective against several parasitic infections in humans. Being aware of the therapeutic needs in human parasitology, I had no doubt that the greatest potential for filling an unmet need was in River Blindness, which is caused by yet another species of Onchocerca—*Onchocerca volvulus*. The clinical exploration of possible ivermectin usage in humans could not be undertaken lightly; but nor could the prospect of an exceptional clinical benefit be dismissed lightly. Birnbaum and I took that message to the highest levels of Merck research management.

It was an exciting moment for both of us. The head of Merck research at the time was Dr. Roy Vagelos—and he and his top advisers approved a trial of ivermectin in humans. It would be a very cautious test of the efficacy of ivermectin in patients with the beginning stages of River Blindness—before any eye damage had occurred.

In February 1981, the first trials were conducted in Senegal by Dr. Mohammed Aziz of Merck, Dr. Samba Diallo of the University of Dakar, Dr. Michel Larivière of the University of Paris and their colleagues. The initial trials showed that ivermectin was effective against the microscopic worm larvae in the skin of River Blindness patients [15]. That proved to be a landmark in the development of ivermectin for use in humans.

To understand why this was so important, it is necessary to understand that, in River Blindness, unlike the situation in dog heartworm disease, the adult worm is not the primary pathogen. It is the offspring, the microscopic baby worms, that cause the damage to the skin and the eyes. If they can safely be killed, the onset of clinical disease will be blocked. And that is what ivermectin does—as was soon confirmed by many investigators [16].

Onchocerciasis was known to be broadly endemic in francophone Africa. For that reason, results of the clinical trials were compiled and presented, under the leadership of Dr. Philippe Gaxotte of Merck, to the French regulatory

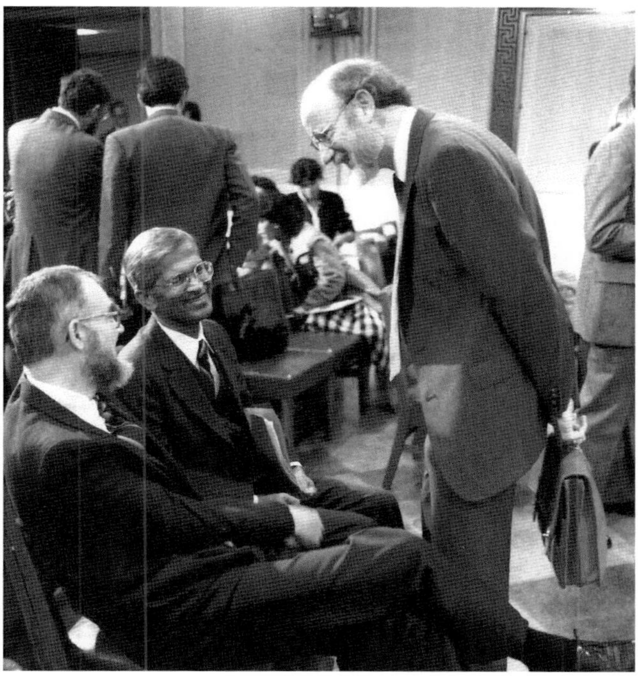

FIGURE 2. The author (right) talks to Dr. Mohammed Aziz (center) and Dr. Kenneth Brown (left) at the 1987 press conference in Washington DC, during which Dr. Roy Vagelos announced that Merck & Co., Inc. would donate ivermectin for the prevention of River Blindness.

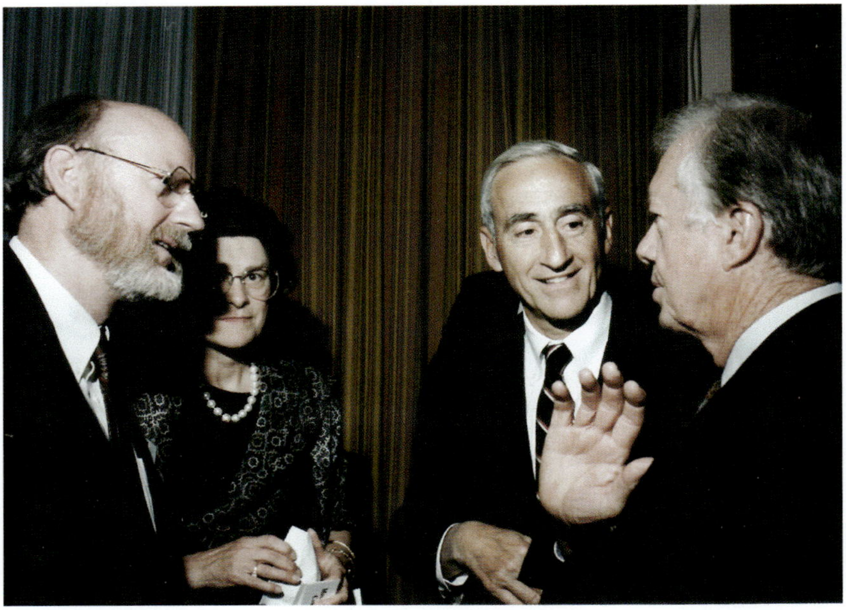

FIGURE 3. Former President Jimmy Carter, head of the Carter Center, discusses River Blindness control with Dr. P. Roy Vagelos, former CEO of Merck & Co., Inc, and the author and his wife. At the United Nations, New York, September 23, 1992.

authorities. Approval of ivermectin for human use was granted in October 1987. The response of Merck leadership came in less than a month.

In 1987 Vagelos, then Merck CEO, announced that Merck & Co. would donate the drug for use against River Blindness (Figure 2). Mohammed Aziz attended that event, but died later in the year. He was succeeded by Dr. Kenneth Brown as director of Merck's development of ivermectin for human use. The extraordinary donation decision has been widely applauded as a historic moment in disease control. It needs no further comment here. The decision led to an unprecedented effort to translate donation of the medicine into distribution of the medicine. The program was undertaken by many groups. I will mention only the World Bank, Merck's Mectizan Donation Program; the World Health Organization; and the Carter Center, but many other agencies participated (Figure 3,4). Over the subsequent 30 years, some 2 billion treatments were distributed. The result was an expanding control of River Blindness, and eventually its certified elimination in several countries [17]. The leaders of that huge program were also numerous—but I will mention one of them here—because he is Swedish! He is Dr. Björn Thylefors [18], and I am honored that he is taking part in some of this week's activities. More recently ivermectin has found a place

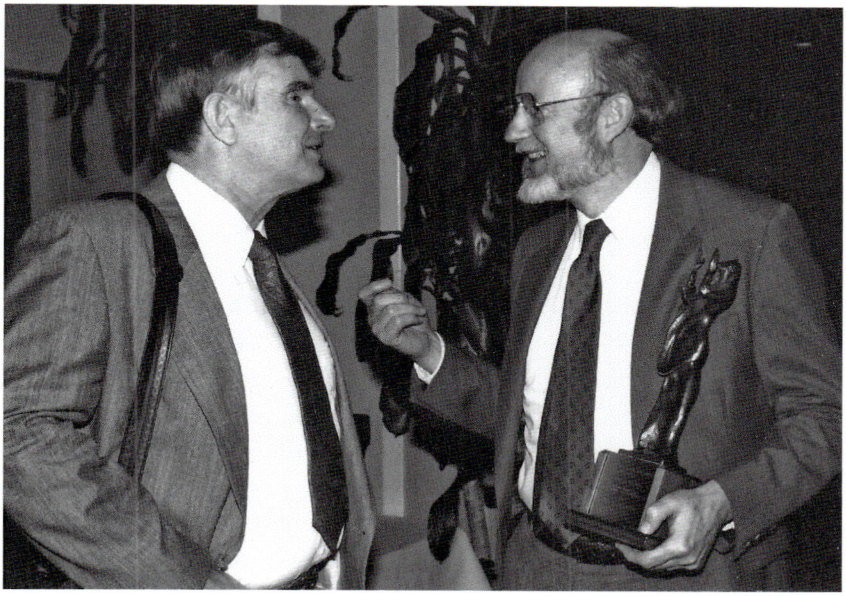

FIGURE 4. Dr. Daniel G. Sissler presenting Helen Keller International Award to Merck & Co., Inc. (accepted by the author for Merck & Co., Inc.). At the United Nations, New York, September 14, 1998.

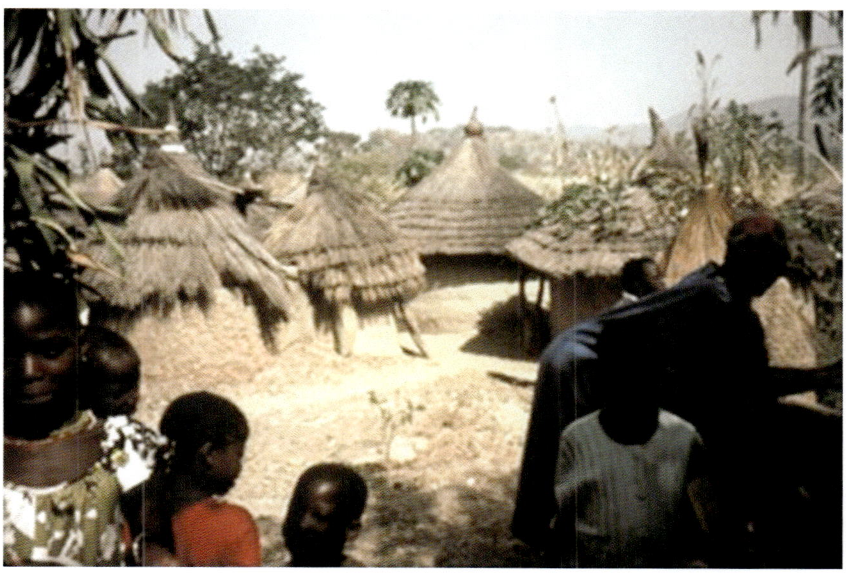

FIGURE 5. One of the remote villages in northern Togo visited by the author. River Blindness was endemic and some of the early community-based trials were being carried out.

in the clinical treatment of several other human diseases, including scabies, and has come to play an important role in the campaign to control lymphatic filariasis (using albendazole in combination with ivermectin or diethylcarbamazine).

THE END

The end of ivermectin is nowhere in sight. This disquisition, however, will end with a glance at the past and a thought for the future.

The accompanying photographs (Figures 5, 6, 7) which I took in West Africa in 1988, are tokens of transition. The bench work had been done; essential field trials in veterinary and human applications had been completed; the feasibility of community-based drug administration for River Blindness control was being explored and the photographs are illustrative of that process. The vast control campaigns directed against River Blindness and lymphatic filariasis were in the offing. They were soon to be carried out by a multitude of care-givers, health workers, administrators and visionary leaders. Their heroic story will be told by others. The photographs shown here are mementoes of a time long gone.

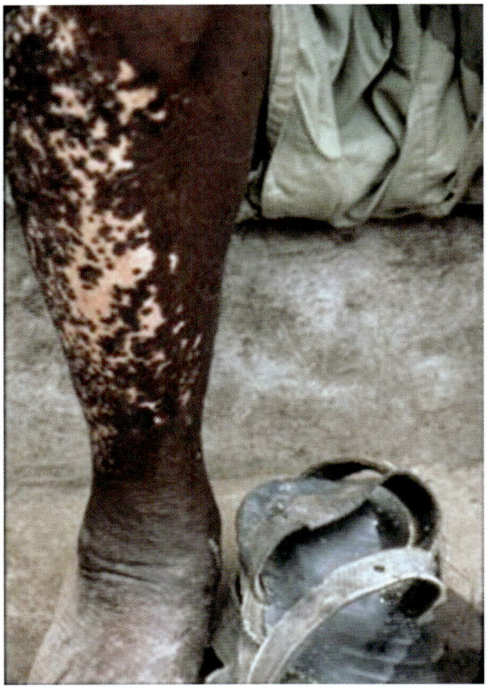

FIGURE 6. One of the many kinds of skin lesion that develop in onchocerciasis over a period of years, following a period of excruciating itching.

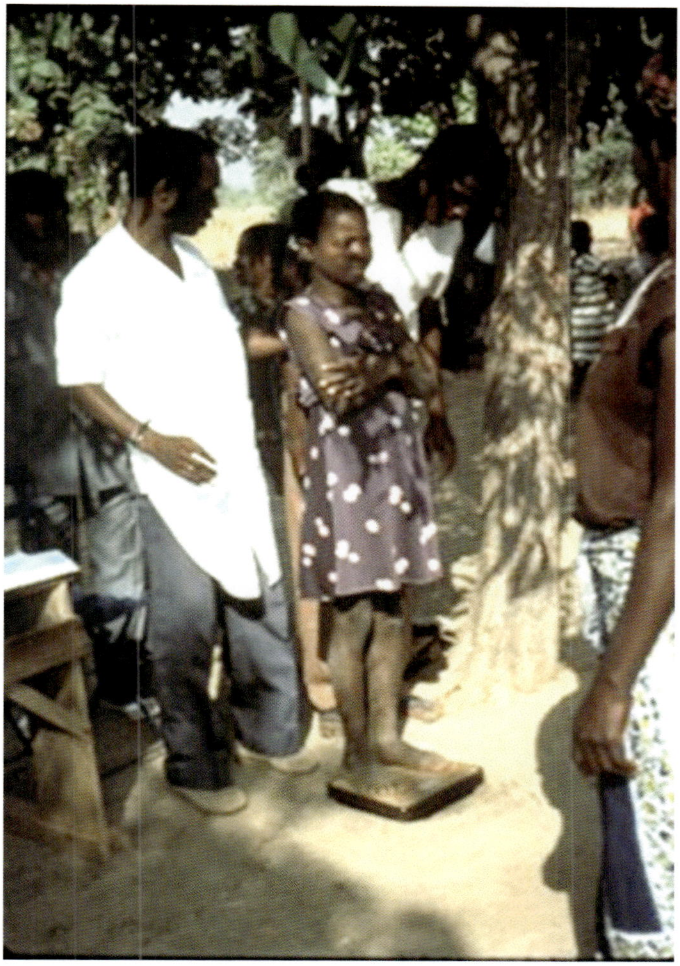

FIGURE 7. An outdoor temporary clinic, where ivermectin was being administered and detailed records were kept.

I now return to that mouse assay with which I began. The operation of that assay was obviously simple. But so was the principle! Thinking it up was a different matter—that was innovative thinking on the part of my colleagues; but the underlying scientific principle was simple. It was bizarre!—but simple. I have described it this way: You line up a series of individual infected mice. You treat each mouse with an unknown amount of an unknown substance that might not be there. Then you check to see if the treatment worked.

It seems to fly in the face of what we are taught about science, with its well-regulated systems and its emphasis on measurement. But we need to understand

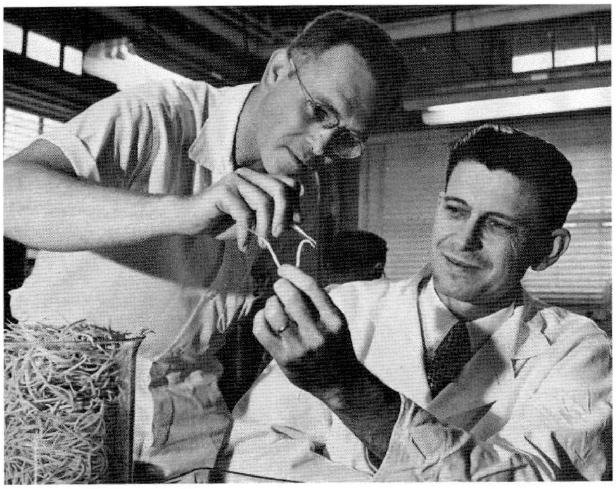

FIGURE 8. Thiabendazole, like other antiparasitic agents, was discovered by simple empirical science. The photo shows two Merck scientists who played key roles in the discovery: parasitologist John R. Egerton (left) and chemist Horace D. Brown (right). Thiabendazole was introduced as a broad-spectrum anthelmintic in 1961.

that this, too, is well-regulated science. Empirical research has been the foundation of the discovery of antiparasitic agents (Figure 8). But "trial and error" research has in recent years been beaten into disrepute and desuetude. And when it is abandoned, we cannot know what price has been paid in "non-discovery."

I have recently made a proposal to search the earth more broadly for new "natural products" as a means of finding novel molecules for chemotherapeutic development [19]. The focus would be primarily on substances produced in microbial fermentation, but could be broadened to include substances made by other forms of life. The target utility of screening new substances would not necessarily be limited to the field of infectious diseases, or even to medicine at all. I have, on occasion, called it my "unpopular proposal"—unpopular because it is destitute of the glamour of "high science;" but though it harkens back, it also looks forward. It would not rely only on science—it would depend crucially on the talent abundantly available in the realms of logistics, finance and management.

The empirical testing of natural products for antiparasitic activity may eventually yield drugs that would be helpful in the multi-agency campaigns that are already underway to control insidious worm diseases such as the soil-transmitted worm infections. Nevertheless, chemotherapeutic disease-control should not be seen as the ultimate objective. Unnatural measures are likely to have unforeseen natural consequences. The broader the activity spectrum of a biodynamic substance, the more we must guard against the hazards of indiscriminate use. Since we cannot count on discriminate use, we should try to control disease without recourse to chemical agents. Despite the current paucity of acceptable vaccines for worm diseases, we may learn how to stimulate or simulate the effective immune responses in a natural yet controllable manner.

In late afternoon I often climb a nearby hill—not a mountain, just a grassy half-mile hill called . . . "Half-mile Hill." From the top I see a marvelous vista of woodland and lake, and a sky often tinted with color as evening falls. It is a moment of uplifting tranquility; and with it comes the realization that many do not live amidst natural beauty and peace. To redress the terrible imbalance, many people around the world are making heroic efforts, and one of their objectives is the improvement of global public health. As we bring science to bear on the problem, I hope we will keep in mind that solutions are sometimes to be found in science that is simple.

ACKNOWLEDGEMENTS

The photographs in Figs 5–7 were taken by the author, and with permission of the subjects. The other photographs are reproduced by permission of Merck & Co., Inc.

LITERATURE

1. Campbell, W.C. 1992. The genesis of the antiparasitic drug ivermectin. In *Inventive Minds: Creativity in Technology*, ed. R.J. Weber, D.N. Perkins, pp. 194–214. New York: Oxford University Press.
2. Campbell, W.C. 2012. History of ivermectin and abamectin: with notes on the history of later macrocyclic lactone antiparasitic agents. *Current Pharmacology and Biotechnology*, **13**: 853–865.
3. Burg, R.W. and E.O. Stapley. 1989. Isolation and characterization of the producing organism. In: Campbell, W.C. 1989 (ed.). *Avermectin and Abamectin*. New York: Springer-Verlag. 363 pp.
4. Omstead, N.M, L. Kaplan, and B.C. Buckland. 1989. Fermentation development and process improvement. In: Campbell, W.C. 1989 (ed.). *Avermectin and Abamectin.* New York: Springer-Verlag. 363 pp.
5. Albers-Schonberg, G., B.H. Arison, J.C. Chabala, A.W. Douglas, P. Eskola, M.H. Fisher, A. Lusi, H. Mrozik, J.L. Smith, and R.L. Tolman. 1981 Avermectins: structure determination. *Journal of the American Chemical Society*, **103**, 4216–4221.
6. Chabala, J.C., H. Mrozik, R.L. Tolman, P. Eskola, A. Lusi, L.H. Peterson, M.F. Woods, and M.H. Fisher. 1980. Ivermectin, a new broad-spectrum antiparasitic agent. *Journal of Medicinal Chemistry*, **23**, 1134–1136.

7. Fisher, M.H. and H. Mrozik. 1989. Chemistry. In: Campbell, W.C. 1989 (ed.). *Avermectin and Abamectin*. New York: Springer-Verlag. 363 pp.
8. Egerton, J.R., D.A. Ostlind, L.S. Blair, C.H. Eary, D. Suhayda, S. Cifelli, R.F. Riek, and W.C. Campbell. 1979. Avermectins, a new family of potent anthelmintic agents: efficacy of the B_1a component. *Antimicrobial Agents and Chemotherapy*. **15:** 372–378.
9. Ostlind, D.A., W.G. Mickle, S. Smith, D.V. Ewanchiw, and S. Cifelli. 2013. Efficacy of ivermectin versus dual infections of *Haemonchus contortus* and *Heligmosomoides polygyrus* in the mouse. *Journal of Parasitology* **99**: 168–169.
10. Turner, M.J. and J.M. Schaeffer. 1989. Mode of action of ivermectin. In: Campbell, W.C. 1989 (ed.). *Avermectin and Abamectin*. New York: Springer-Verlag. 363 pp.
11. Campbell, W.C. and L.S. Blair. 1978. *Dirofilaria immitis*: experimental infections in the ferret (*Mustela putorius furo*). *Journal of Parasitology* **64**: 119–122.
12. Campbell, W.C., L.S. Blair, and J.W. McCall. 1979. *Brugia pahangi* and *Dirofilaria immitis*: experimental infections in the ferret, *Mustela putorius furo*. *Experimental Parasitology* **47**: 327–332.
13. Blair, L.S. and W.C. Campbell. 1978. Trial of avermectin B_{1a}, mebendazole and melarsoprol against pre-cardiac *Dirofilaria immitis* in the ferret (*Mustela putorius furo*). *Journal of Parasitology* **64**(6): 1032–1034.
14. Egerton, J.R., E.S. Brokken, D. Suhayda, C.H. Eary, J.W. Wooden, and R.L. Kilgore. 1981. The antiparasitic activity of ivermectin in horses. *Veterinary Parasitology* **8**: 83–88.
15. Aziz, M.A., B.H. Diallo, I.M. Diop, M. Lariviere, and M. Porta. 1982. Efficacy and tolerance of ivermectin in human *onchocerciasis*. *Lancet* **2**: 171–173.
16. Greene B.M., K.R. Brown, and H.R. Taylor. 1989. Use of ivermectin in humans. In: Campbell, W.C. 1989 (ed.). *Avermectin and Abamectin*. New York: Springer-Verlag. 363 pp.
17. Mectizan Donation Program 2016. Online website: http://www.mectizan.org.
18. Thylefors, B. and M. Alleman. 2006. Towards the elimination of onchocerciasis. *Annals of Tropical Medicine and Parasitology*, **100**:733–746.
19. Campbell, W.C. 2016. Lessons from the history of ivermectin and other antiparasitic agents. Animal.annualreviews.org: doi: 10.1146/annurev-animal-021815-111209. *Annual Review of Animal Biosciences*, in press.

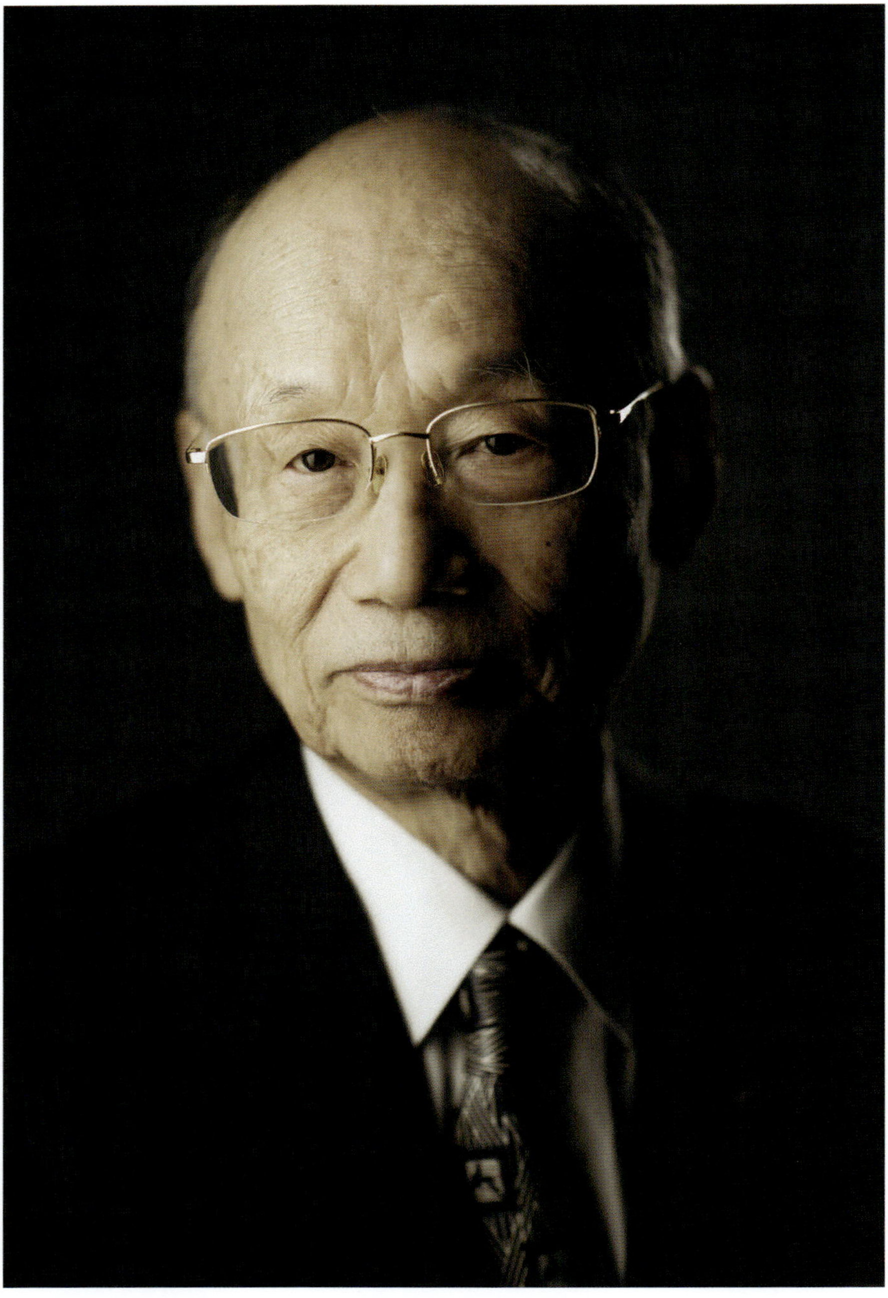

Satoshi Ōmura. © Nobel Media AB. Photo: A. Mahmoud

Satoshi Ōmura

by Andy Crump

In Japan's rural Yamanashi prefecture in the mid-1930s, times were harsh and resources were scarce. The local environment had to provide all the agrarian communities with most of the necessities that they needed for survival. This constituted a valuable and unforgettable lesson for Satoshi Ōmura during his formative years. A oneness with, and profound respect for, Nature was irrevocably instilled in him. Seventy years later, he was to encounter similar conditions to those where he was born and raised when he visited Africa to see first-hand the unmatched beneficial impact of one of the drugs he has discovered—a gift from Japanese soil that has improved the lives and welfare of hundreds of millions of people around the world.

Japan is a predominantly uniform society where the group is held above the individual and familial and social responsibilities remain paramount, as Satoshi's parents taught him from an early age. Those people who understand Japan and the nation's customs and traditions will sympathise with the dilemma that Satoshi faced and struggled to come to terms with throughout his career. A Japanese proverb illustrates the point—"deru kugi wa utareru" (a nail that sticks out will be hammered down). Within such constraints, when one has to adhere to long-standing duties and responsibilities as well as social and cultural norms, it is difficult to think or act differently. To do so, pioneer new paths and develop innovative concepts and techniques, and yet maintain respect and peer acceptance is a singular triumph which requires courage, vision and determination. Fortunately, there is another version of the proverb that is very true in Satoshi's case, "deru kugi wa utareru ga, desugita kugi wa utarenai" (a nail that sticks out will be hammered down, but a nail that sticks out a lot will not).

Satoshi was born into a farming household in Nirasaki in Yamanashi in 1935, the eldest son in a Japanese family, which meant profound traditional family responsibilities. His father was a proactive, leading member of his village and his mother an elementary school teacher and gifted piano player. His parents nurtured in him sensitivity and the deep-seated need to constantly think about others, plus his duty to his parents and siblings, as well as ensuring that he developed excellent life skills to be able to cope with whatever he encountered. With his parents mostly working, Satoshi spent much time with his grandmother, who also repeatedly emphasised that for personal development and satisfaction, it was always best to work for the sake of others—a tenet that has accompanied him throughout his working life.

As is common among many youngsters from a physically active, rural farming background, Satoshi's school years were marked with a perennial struggle between academic and sporting pursuits. He was an adept and successful athlete, excelling in winter sports, such as cross-country skiing, a useful skill in Yamanashi's Southern Alps. His competitive nature, honed by his rise up to national representative levels in skiing, also helped him succeed in his academic endeavours. His sound educational training in Nirasaki led him to qualify for entry to the Faculty of Liberal Arts and Sciences at the University of Yamanashi—perhaps an omen of things to come, as Satoshi has maintained a deep interest in both science and art throughout his life. As many sportsmen will attest, life in university often becomes difficult because of the huge amount of time that needs to be devoted to training and competing. But vital lessons in learning about one's own limits and capabilities in dealing with times in competitions when all seems impossible or beyond one's own limits, can easily be applied to academic challenges, and so Satoshi honed the mental fortitude to succeed in his educational and academic work. Thanks to Professor Senjiro Marut, who would become

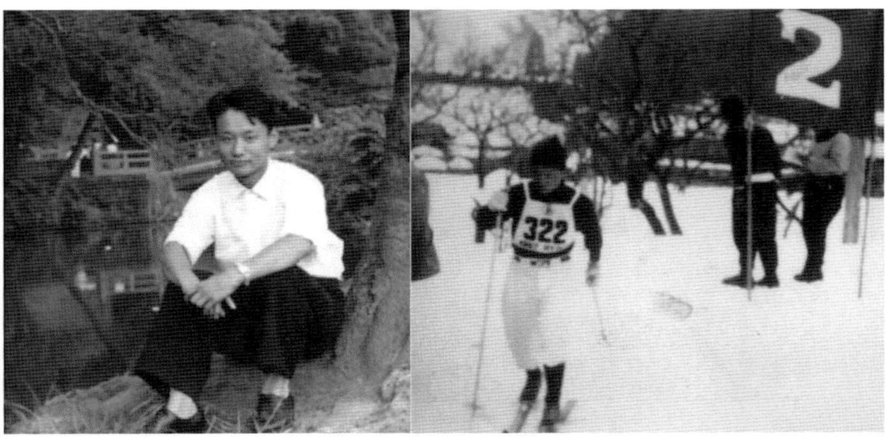

FIGURE 1. Late-1950s: College was a continuous struggle between study and sports.

one of the several key mentors in his life, Satoshi quickly developed an interest in organic chemistry. He also learned about himself, how to try and exceed his limits where possible, to devise his own original approach and methods, based on the evidence of others, but to do things originally, to 'think differently' and, furthermore, to apply those novel thoughts to overcome obstacles, no matter where or when he encountered them.

After graduating, Satoshi began teaching evening classes at a high school in Tokyo. He was deeply impressed by the fact that many of his students attended classes and worked with oil-stained and callous hands, having already been working for a whole day at their predominantly menial jobs, but determined to study and improve their prospects. This stimulated him to also consider how he could best advance his own prospects. However, he quickly became concerned that his sporting efforts may have diminished his scholarly expertise and teaching abilities, so he became determined to recommence his studies to allow himself to teach with greater proficiency for the benefit of his students. He started at

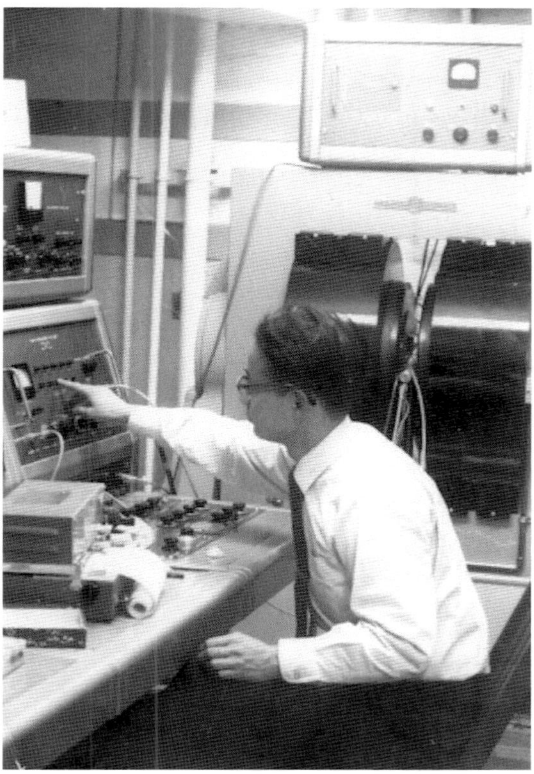

FIGURE 2. 1960s: Satoshi's night-time use of nascent Nuclear Magnetic Resonance (NMR) equipment provided unique insights and skills in molecular structure determination.

the Tokyo University of Education (currently the University of Tsukuba), where he studied chemistry under Professor Koji Nakanishi—a leading expert in the field of natural products organic chemistry and Professor Yojiro Tsuzuki of the Tokyo University of Science, whose laboratory was involved in investigations of the chemical structure of organic compounds using nuclear magnetic resonance (NMR)—a truly cutting-edge technology at the time. While today NMR is commonplace, in those days there was only one such machine nationwide, located at the Tokyo Industrial Laboratory. Although it was used during the daytime by researchers, Satoshi was allowed access to the equipment at night. Working throughout the early morning hours, Satoshi became skilled at analysing the molecular and stereoscopic structures of chemical compounds. His schedule became university study during the day, teaching at night and conducting NMR experiments until dawn.

Despite his exhausting schedule, Satoshi still managed to find time to meet and marry his wife, Fumiko. Throughout those taxing times, Fumiko was a source of great support, often cooking and bringing his evening meal to the laboratory. In addition, Fumiko was a mathematics teacher and an expert with an abacus, to the extent that Satoshi often telephoned her and read out some data which she swiftly computed—without the need of a computer.

It took him 5 long years to obtain his M.S. degree but the extensive knowledge and technical skills acquired during that period became an invaluable foundation for all his later research work. Satoshi eventually received his Masters degree from the Tokyo University of Science in 1963, followed by a Ph.D. in Pharmaceutical Sciences (1968) from the University of Tokyo, and a further doctorate in Chemistry in 1970 from the Tokyo University of Science.

Satoshi began his career as a Research Associate at Yamanashi University in 1963, when he started working in the laboratory of Professor Motoo Kagami in the Department of Fermentation Technology at the University of Yamanashi. The post was arranged by Professor Senjiro Maruta, a mentor from his undergraduate days. Professor Kagami was conducting research on wine and Satoshi recalls being indelibly awed and inspired by yeast microbes that could transform sugar into alcohol overnight, much quicker than even the best of chemists. So began his career-long fascination with, and admiration and respect for, microorganisms.

Two years later, in a quest for a more stimulating environment to facilitate research into microorganisms, Satoshi embarked on his career-long association with the Kitasato Institute. Thus, from 1965 onwards, he has been actively engaged in comprehensive research in the field of bioorganic chemistry, focusing on bioactive substances of microbial origin. Satoshi was a key team member of the Kitasato team due to his expertise in the structural determination of chemicals developed through his NMR work. Under the guidance of Institute Director Toju Hata, the first chemical compound he determined the structure of was the antibiotic Leucomycin. He subsequently accomplished the isolation and structural determination of Cerulenin, a compound with antifungal properties but which, based on the compound's structure which he identified, Satoshi believed should be able to inhibit lipid biosynthesis. He later confirmed this to be the case. Cerulenin, produced by a true fungus, *Acremonium caerulens*, proved to be the first inhibitor of fatty acid (lipid) biosynthesis ever found. It became the lead compound for development of the medically important statins, inhibitors of cholesterol biosynthesis and it remains a pivotal research reagent to this day.

Satoshi quickly realised that this line of work could only be carried out once someone had actually discovered a new compound. He also recognised that finding chemical compounds produced by microbes was a time-consuming and painstaking task. This represented a new challenge that deserved his attention, even though he was, essentially, a chemist. It also meant devising a completely different approach. So began his foray into the development and application of novel screening methods—methods not just to discover antibiotics, but to find any chemical that might be useful to human health and other fields, no matter what they may be. As an example, Satoshi knew that the biosynthesis of alkaloids, which often have specific and pronounced bioactivities, usually follows complex pathways and includes stereospecific steps. Alkaloids (e.g. quinine, atropine, morphine) or alkaloid-containing plants have been used for centuries as remedies, poisons and psychoactive substances. Consequently, he devised a plan to search for alkaloids using Dragendorff's reagent, which simply changed colour in the presence of any alkaloid. Subsequent determination of the structures of any chemical compounds isolated from microbes facilitated identification and understanding of their bioactivity and other properties. Implementing this coordinated approach led him to discover staurosporine, the first indolocarbazole ever identified, which he found had some interesting bioactivity. Indicative of his thinking of working for others, a decade later staurosporine was found by another research group to be the world's first compound capable of preventing the functioning of protein kinases. This revolutionised the search for anticancer agents, staursporine being the lead compound for development of imatinib (Gleevec®) and several other alkaline chemicals that have been developed into the novel anticancer agents currently in widespread and highly successful clinical use. Staurosporine is said to be the most widely used biochemical reagent originating from a naturally-occurring microorganism, with the number of scientific papers based on staurosporine research averaging over 600 annually during the past 20 years.

He also introduced an innovative cell-based screening technique using specific live animal cells. Hymeglusin (1987), a cholesterol biosynthesis inhibitor, and triacsin (1986), an inhibitor of the acyl-CoA synthetase that activates fatty acids, were found using Vero cells and yeast mutants. Diazaquinomycin (1982), an antimetabolite of folic acid, was found using folate-requiring cells. Exploiting a method that used cancerous neuroblast cells from mice, he looked for substances that induced dendrites in such neuroblasts. This approach led to the discovery of Lactacystin, which was found to be an inhibitor of Proteasomes. Lactacystin quickly became a globally renowned research reagent, utilised by a phalanx of researchers, including some past Nobel laureates. Satoshi's success in this field is manifest in the fact that the Nobel laureate chemist, E.J. Corey, named an active derivative of lactacystin (clasto-lactacystinβ-lactone) as omuralide.

In 1971, Satoshi decided to take a sabbatical and work overseas in order to exploit new opportunities to further his work and discoveries. With the help and guidance of Professor Yukimasa Yagisawa, he arranged a lecture tour of universities in Canada and the US and approached them to investigate the possibility of a research position. Receiving a favourable response from all of them, he was attracted by a proposition to work with Professor Max Tishler, ex-Director of Merck, Sharp and Dohme Research Laboratories (MSDRL), who had retired and was setting up a new chemistry department at Wesleyan University in Connecticut. When he arrived to take up his post as Visiting Research Professor, circumstances quickly evolved that would allow him to effectively carry out his research as he pleased as well as meet a continuous flow of leading international chemistry experts who were visiting Professor Tishler, who was so busy that he effectively asked Satoshi to help oversee the running of the laboratory. This led to Satoshi meeting and collaborating with Professor Konrad Bloch of Harvard University, resulting in a joint publication on cerulenin.

Although he was originally scheduled to stay at Wesleyan for three years, the Kitasato Institute recalled Satoshi after a mere 14 months to take over the running of the institute's research programme following the retirement of the existing director. At that point, Satoshi realised that he had to try and secure funding to support the advanced work that he wished to do in Japan and so embarked on a whistle-stop tour of National Institutes of Health (NIH) and several major drug companies in search of funds and to promote the concept of joint research. His idea was to obtain research funding from a corporate sponsor to facilitate and expedite discovery of useful chemical compounds. Development and usage rights would be transferred to the company and, following any commercialisation of a compound, royalties commensurate with the resulting sales income would be paid to Satoshi's research group.

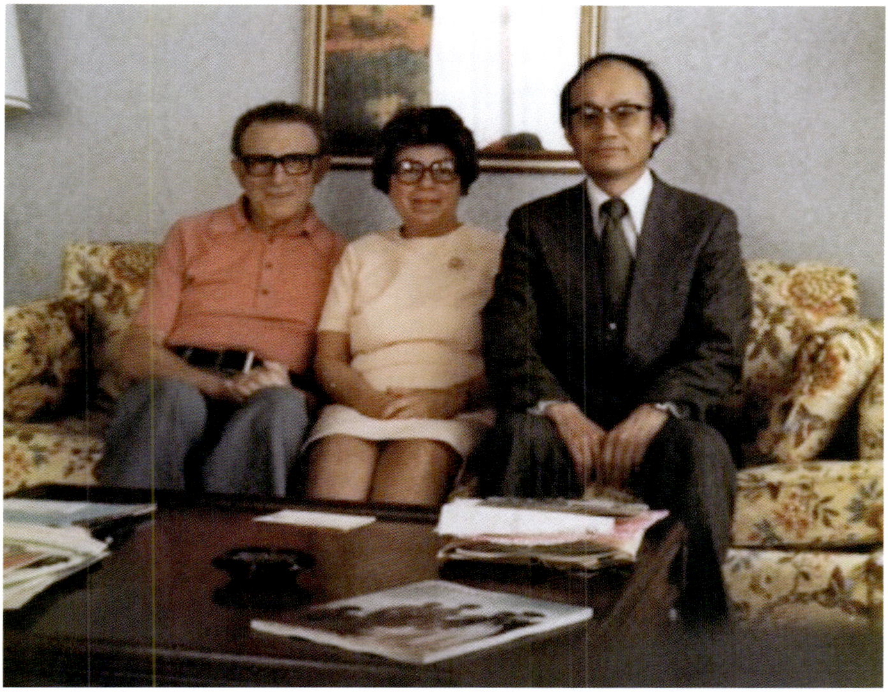

FIGURE 3. Mid-1970s: At Max and Betty Tishler's home. Meeting and being befriended by Max was the critical point in Satoshi's scientific career.

Thanks primarily to his friend and mentor, Max Tishler, Satoshi was able to establish a mutually favourable arrangement with Merck & Company, which allowed optimal exploitation of the comparative advantages of each partner in what would become a pioneering private sector/public sector collaboration. Within the partnership, the Kitasato Institute was responsible for collecting soil samples, identifying unique or promising microbes, isolating and screening chemical compounds and conducting in-vitro evaluations. Merck handled animal testing (in vivo) in innovative animal models, development, production, marketing and distribution. The initial target was to develop drugs for use in livestock and other animals.

The partnership also encompassed a common philosophy—the Kitasato Institute credo, established by Shibasaburo Kitasato, the father of serotherapy, being 'the basis of medicine should be the prevention of disease and that achievements obtained by medical research should be actively applied and widely used to improve public health.' Merck's mission statement was 'to provide society with superior products and services', with George W. Merck's avowed approach being 'we try never to forget that medicine is for the people. It is not for the profits.'

The collaboration produced a variety of new compounds but of greatest significance was avermectin, produced by *Streptomyces avermectinius*, and the dihydro-derivative ivermectin. The producing microorganism was isolated from a soil sample collected on the periphery of a golf course at Kawana in Ito City, Shizuoka Prefecture. The microbe was sent to MSDRL in the US where it was found to display superior antiparasitic activity against the nematode worm, *Nematospiroides dubius*, in MSDRL's unique mouse model. The actinomycete was originally named *Streptomyces avermitilis* (later changed to *avermectinius*) and the active substance was named avermectin. Avermectin represented a completely new class of compound, designated as an 'Endectocide', as it killed a range of different parasites inside as well as outside the body. It was also capable of killing insect vectors.

The safer and more potent ivermectin proved to be a remarkable macrolide anthelmintic antibiotic for veterinary use and was introduced onto the animal health market in 1981. Two years later, it became the world's biggest selling veterinary drug, a position it maintained for over 20 years. In time, and after its unmatched success in animal health, ivermectin was found to be a remarkably effective and safe drug for combating diseases caused by filarial parasitic worms in humans. The world's gravest intractable human filarial diseases were Onchocerciasis (commonly known as River Blindness) and Lymphatic filariasis (commonly known as Elephantiasis). The control—and subsequently, eradication—programmes for these two devastating, disfiguring and stigmatising tropical diseases, which afflict around 1 in 7 of the entire world population, are based primarily on the use of ivermectin, which is being donated free of charge for as long as it is required. Orchestrated by the World Health Organization (WHO), ivermectin, under the brand name Mectizan®, is being administered to almost 300 million people annually in some of the world's poorest and remotest of communities. It is envisaged that Onchocerciasis will be eliminated globally by 2025 (if not sooner) and Lymphatic filariasis by 2020. With respect to Onchocerciasis, disease elimination has virtually been completed in Latin America and is well on the way to success in Africa. The *S. avermectinius* organism discovered by Satoshi in a single sample of Japanese soil remains the only avermectin-producing organism ever found, meaning that single organism has been the sole source of industrial production ever since.

Fortunately, Japan is no longer affected by either of these diseases, Lymphatic filariasis having been eradicated from the country several decades ago.

Merck & Co. Inc. currently supplies enough ivermectin to treat over 250 million people annually free of charge, with both these diseases now in great decline. Ivermectin tablets need to be taken only once a year, which makes it relatively easy to deliver the drug to people in hard-to-reach, poverty-stricken communities. One other key factor is the drug's efficacy at low doses without side effects, the drug is extremely safe and so can be given without the need for medical supervision.

Ivermectin has freed up vast tracts of fertile riverside land for cultivation, creating a secure food supply and work for tens of millions of Africans. With ivermectin preventing blindness and enabling people to continue to farm and work, they are able to experience better living conditions. Thanks to this and other supporting factors, today's African children belong to a generation whose eyesight is comparatively safe, and who will not suffer from disfigurement, lost educational opportunities or social stigma arising from either Onchocerciasis or Lymphatic filariasis. In 2004, Satoshi visited Burkina Faso and Ghana to see in person the immeasurably beneficial impact ivermectin distribution was having on remote rural communities and where, to his surprise, he witnessed conditions similar to those he experienced growing up in rural Yamanashi.

Alongside his discovery work, Satoshi has studied in depth the mechanisms used by microorganisms to produce various kinds of substances, in particular

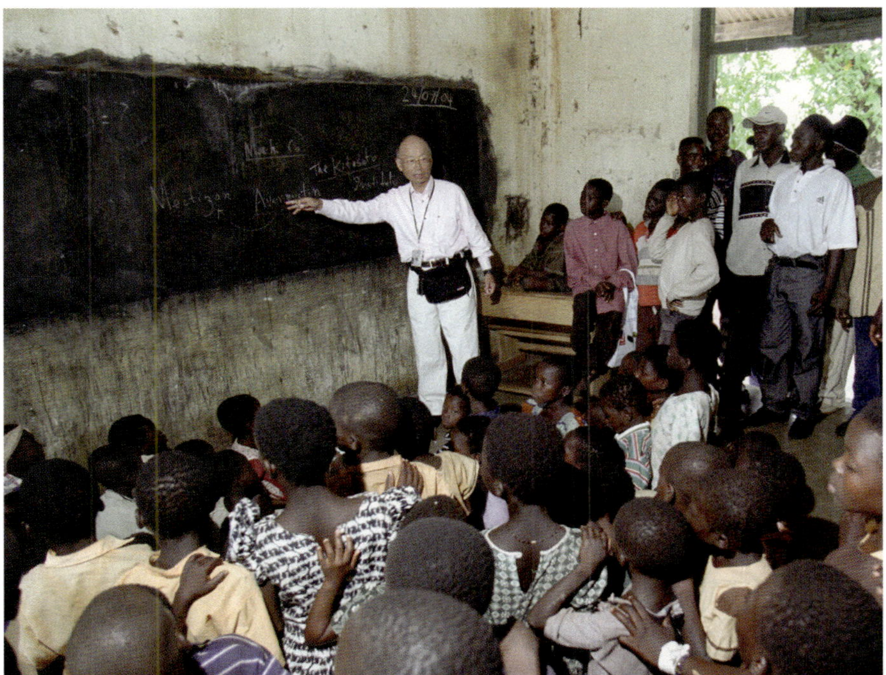

FIGURE 4. Early 2000s in Ghana. Engaging and educating youth in science and social principles—in Japan and internationally—is a deep-rooted passion.

carrying out extensive research at the genetic level. His elucidation and application of the genetic control of chemical compound formation has made it possible to manipulate living microorganisms to produce novel compounds, as well as creating the potential and ability to produce completely synthetic compounds.

As an example of this, Satoshi and his co-workers obtained various mutants of *S. avermectinius* in which part of the biosynthetic pathway of avermectin was blocked. They determined the production pathway by isolating various precursors accumulated in each mutant. Each mutated point on the chromosome was identified, eventually allowing the cloning of all 17 genes concerned with avermectin biosynthesis. Furthermore, the work clarified the function of each gene, providing a complete understanding of the biosynthetic mechanism for producing avermectin. The ground-breaking genetic analysis of *S. avermectinius* was the world's first for a commercially-important actinomycete, and it also demonstrated that the actinomycete has genes which produce 37 kinds of organic compounds (secondary metabolites), besides the immeasurably important avermectin.

Following Satoshi's lead, creation of novel compounds using genetic engineering is now routinely carried out. His original work and continued pioneering research in this area resulted in the appearance of Mederrhodin, created by Satoshi in partnership with England-based Dr David A. Hopwood. This remarkable compound was the first novel synthetic antibiotic created using genetic engineering and is worthy of recognition as being the pioneer compound in a completely new research field with almost limitless potential.

Over the past five decades, Satoshi's drug discovery group at the Kitasato Institute has undertaken advanced and pioneering research based on the profound belief that organic compounds produced by microorganisms have immeasurable promise for use in improving the welfare and health of mankind. His creation and introduction of several highly original methods of isolating useful microorganisms, has led to the discovery of 53 new species of microbes, including 13 novel genera, such as the *Kitasatosporia*, *Longispora* and *Arbophoma*.

Exploiting a broad spectrum of often newly discovered microorganisms isolated predominantly from soil samples, he has discovered around 500 novel organic compounds possessing interesting chemical structures and/or bioactivities, including many now widely-used antibiotics (all indexed and detailed in *Splendid Gifts from Microorganisms, 5th Ed.*, 2015). Among them, 26 compounds and/or their derivatives have entered into widespread common usage as medicines, agents to improve animal health and husbandry, as agrochemicals and as reagents for biochemical research.

Satoshi has also built up an excellent body of research findings on the relationships between chemical structure, bioactivity and mode of action of many macrolide antibiotics, such as leucomycin, tylosin, spiramycin and erythromycin. Among them, rokitamycin, a derivative of leucomycin, together with tilmicosin, a derivative of tylosin, have been used with great effect as human medicines and in animal health.

Overall, the natural organic compounds which have appeared as a result of Satoshi Ōmura's initiatives and endeavours have been used worldwide as medicines, agrochemicals and reagents for biochemical research, and have greatly contributed to progress in the welfare and health of mankind, as well as being essential elements in making major steps forward in biomedical knowledge and understanding possible.

Since 1965, when Satoshi joined the Kitasato Institute as a researcher, he has occupied various posts, culminating in his appointment in 1990 as President, serving as President Emeritus from 2008 to 2012. He has an exemplary record of fundraising and administrative management of the institute, which

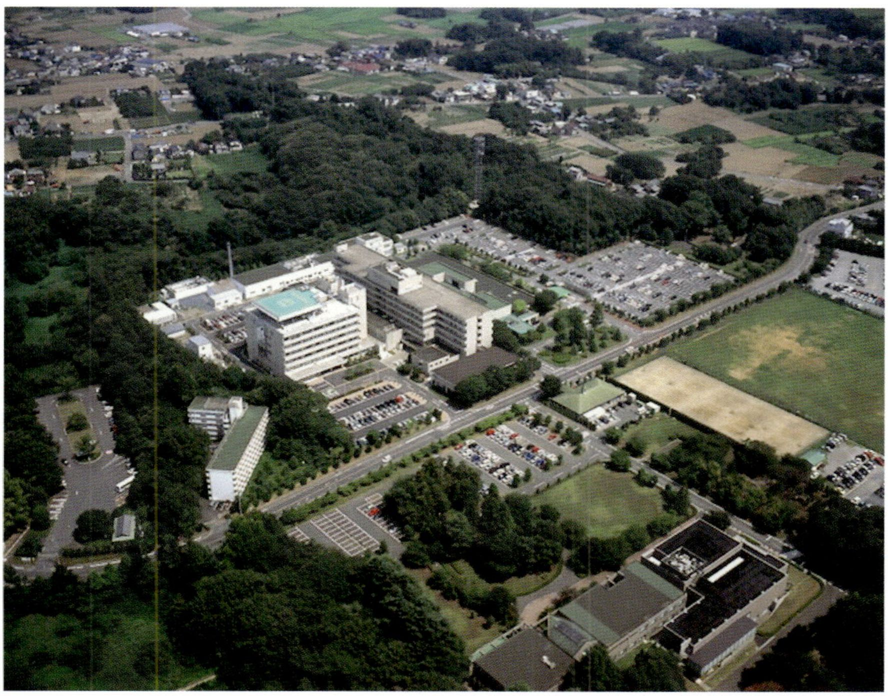

FIGURE 5. The Kitamoto complex in Saitama prefecture, comprising a 440-bed district hospital, residential nursing college and vaccine production plant, was funded by royalties earned from ivermectin sales.

was in an extremely healthy shape when his tenure as President came to an end. He is currently a Distinguished Emeritus Professor and Special Coordinator of the Research Project for Drug Discovery from Natural Products in the Kitasato Institute for Life Sciences, Kitasato University, where he is fully engaged in the continuing search for the treasures that still lie undetected in nature. He was also appointed as inaugural Max Tishler Professor of Chemistry at Wesleyan University (USA) in 2005, a post that he still holds.

Satoshi is being continually recognised internationally in the field of natural products chemistry, and for the application of his discoveries, as evidenced by his numerous awards and honours. Among these are the Hoechst-Roussel Award from the American Society for Microbiology, the Charles Thom Award (Society for Industrial Microbiology, USA), the Robert Koch Gold Medal (Germany), the Prince Mahidol Award (Thailand), the Japan Academy Prize, the Nakanishi Prize of the Japan Chemical Society and American Chemical Society, the Ernest Guenther Award of the American Chemical Society, the Hamao Umezawa Memorial Award of the International Society of Chemotherapy, the Tetrahedron Prize for Creativity in Organic Chemistry, the Arima Award of the International Union of Microbiological Society, the Research Achievement Award of the American Society of Pharmacognosy, the 2014 Canada Gairdner Global Health Award, the Asahi Prize—and now the Nobel Prize in Physiology or Medicine. In 2007 he was decorated with France's Chevalier de L'Ordre National de la Legion d'Honneur award. In 2012 he was designated as a Person of Cultural Merit in Japan, followed by the Order of Cultural Merit in 2015.

He is a member of the Japan Academy, the German Academy of Sciences Leopoldina and the European Academy of Sciences and is a Foreign Associate of the US National Academy of Sciences, the French Academy of Sciences, and the Chinese Academy of Engineering.

His honorary memberships include those of the American Society of Biochemistry and Molecular Biology, the Royal Society of Chemistry, the Chemical Society of Japan, the Japanese Society for Actinomycetes, the Japan Society for Bioscience, Biotechnology and Agrochemistry, as well as his Special Honorary Membership of the Japanese Society of Bacteriology.

Since 1973, he has been a long-standing member of the Editorial Board of the Journal of Antibiotics, serving as an Editor-in-Chief from 2004 to 2013 and now as Editor-in-Chief Emeritus. He has published well over 1,000 scientific articles, and continues to publish extensively. Among his publications, the *Macrolide Antibiotics* (2nd edition) remains a world-leading textbook. He has also published several volumes of personal essays and annually produces his own personalised calligraphy.

Satoshi retains his commitment to engage and groom young researchers in the field of natural product research and to educate them in the correct approach with respect to scientific research, multidisciplinary collaborations and the fundamental importance of good interpersonal associations in working partnerships. As an example of this, 20 years ago, he established the Yamanashi Academy of Sciences in his home prefecture. As part of the academy's operations, 130 high-ranking scientific members regularly visit local schools and colleges to give presentations, meet students and try and encourage them to take up and pursue an interest in the natural sciences.

Although his cross-country skiing days are now behind him, Satoshi is a consummate golfer, when he can find the time. He remains a long-standing and leading patron of Japanese art, remaining very active in this sphere of activity. Having held the post of President of the Joshibi Women's Art University for over 14 years, Satoshi has long championed the concept of Healing Art, it being increasingly accepted that artwork helps create an environment which promotes healing. The extensive collection of original artworks, predominantly by Japanese artists, he has assembled is displayed on the walls of all the hospitals and laboratories with which he is connected. He has also designed and constructed his own art museum, which is open to the public and which he has bequeathed to his hometown of Nirasaki. (see: http://www.nirasakiomura-artmuseum.com/index.html—Japanese only). He also constructed and opened a hot spring facility there because he has always felt the need to repay his hometown for everything that it gave him. He profoundly believes that his life as a scientific researcher is inherently linked to the region where he was born and raised and where his approach to life and wonderment and respect for Nature was instilled in him from a very early age.

(For further information, see: http://www.satoshi-omura.info)

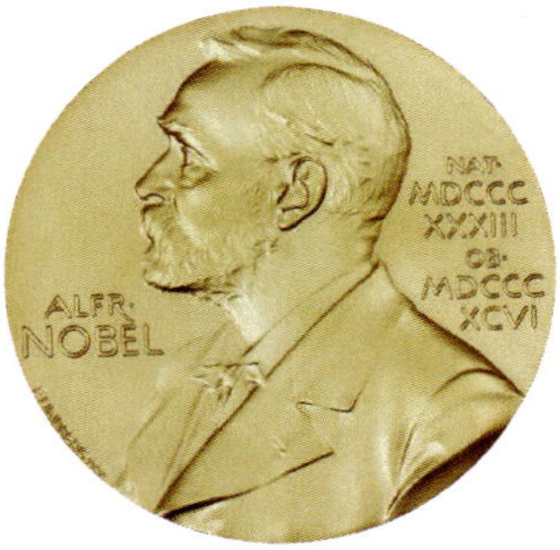

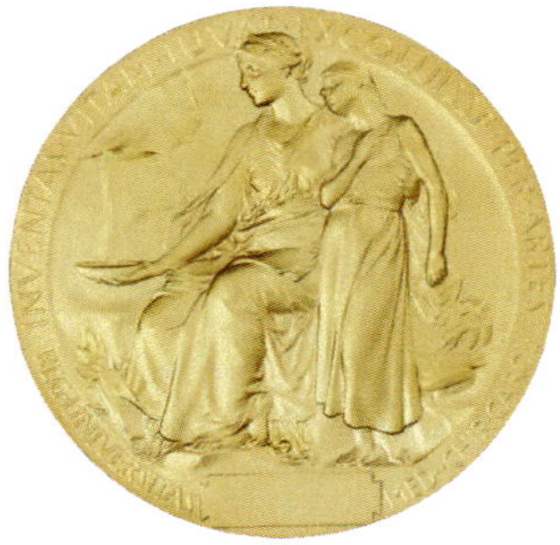

A Splendid Gift from the Earth: The Origins and Impact of the Avermectins

Nobel Lecture, December 7, 2015

by Satoshi Ōmura
Kitasato University, Tokyo, Japan.

The origin of one of the world's foremost, revolutionary, versatile yet relatively unknown drugs lies in Japanese soil—literally and metaphorically. Ivermectin, a multipurpose drug derived from a single microscopic organism discovered in Japanese soil, is being taken free of charge annually by over 250 million people—twice as many people as the entire Japanese population. Its impact on improving the overall health and welfare of hundreds of millions of men, women and children, mostly in poor and impoverished communities, remains unmatched. It continues to defy many preconceived concepts, with no drug resistance developing in humans despite years of extensive monotherapy. This has led to it being included on the World Health Organization's "List of Essential Medicines," a compilation of the most important medications needed in any basic health system. Several international public health experts have also taken the unprecedented step of recommending mass administration of ivermectin to all members of often polyparasitised communities in developing countries as a simple, prophylactic and curative public health intervention [1].

Ivermectin, along with its parent compound, avermectin, are both extremely broad-spectrum antiparasitic agents. Ivermectin is among those few compounds, such as penicillin and aspirin, delineated as 'wonder drugs', all, incidentally, originating from natural products. It is also predominantly a drug for the poor. It is being increasingly used to eliminate intractable tropical diseases, as well to tackle an ever-increasing range of diseases, and is showing promise to provide a solution to hitherto indomitable public health problems. It remains the most potent anti-infective agent in clinical use; the safe single adult dose of around 12 mg once a year comparing favourably with antibiotics like penicillin and tetracycline that require doses of 1000 mg or more per day.

The avermectins, and the derivative ivermectin, were identified in the mid-1970s. The discovery was exceptional, as avermectin represented the world's first 'endectocide', a term specially created to describe the compound which was capable of killing a wide variety of parasitic and health-threatening organisms both inside and outside the body. The avermectins were found to be 2- to 3-fold more potent than compounds in use at the time. Moreover, ivermectin was found to be effective orally, topically or parentally and showed no signs of cross-resistance with commonly used antiparasitic agents [2–4]. Since its discovery, the benefits of ivermectin in terms of global public health and socioeconomic welfare, direct and indirect, have been immeasurable and they continue to accumulate. The discovery occurred at a time when the international community was focussing attention on disregarded and seemingly unconquerable diseases which had been plaguing resource-poor populations throughout the tropics for centuries. The advent of the antiparasitic ivermectin provided a safe, simple and effective solution, now driving several of those seemingly invincible tropical diseases to the brink of eradication.

In science, as elsewhere, it is individuals who are the true agents of change. The discovery of the avermectins was the result of a novel international multidisciplinary research project between a public sector institution (Japan's Kitasato Institute) and a private sector pharmaceutical company (the US-based Merck, Sharp and Dohme). But the successful history of this pioneering public private partnership has been dependent upon the unwavering commitment, ability and quality of scientific and cultural exchanges among the team of exceptional individuals involved, all of whom managed to overcome differences in nationality and working practices and sometimes differing goals.

Likewise, the availability of and access to the drug, its distribution and its enormous and widespread beneficial impact has been dependent upon a combination of an unprecedented drug donation programme plus an exceptional, ground-breaking multifaceted international partnership incorporating, among others, the public and private sectors, multilateral agencies, donor organisations, governments, non-governmental organisations, scientists, health workers and entire disease-affected communities.

IVERMECTIN: PREPARING THE GROUND

In Japan, the Kitasato Institute (KI), founded in 1914 by Shibasaburo Kitasato, known as the father of serotherapy and nominated for the first Nobel Prize in 1901, has long been recognised as a world-leading centre for the discovery of drugs and vaccines, primarily those derived from natural sources. Investigative research and development of chemotherapeutic drugs for practical use is a fundamental core of the work of the institute. Over 100 years ago, in a pioneering breakthrough, Sahachiro Hata, working with Paul Ehrlich, developed salvarsan, a remedy for syphilis, which was a major global health problem at the time. Salvarsan is widely recognised as the world's first chemotherapeutic drug. In the 1930s, Zenjiro Kitasato performed research into plant alkaloids and terpenoids which later led to development of the antitussive compound sapogenin. In the late-1940s, Toju Hata conducted research on antibiotics produced by microbes, leading to discovery of leucomycin in 1953 and the anti-cancer compound mitomycin in 1956.

In the mid-1960s, from a background in studying aspects of fermentation and having garnered significant experience in using the at-the-time novel and nascent Nuclear Magnetic Resonance (NMR) spectroscopy to determine the structure of organic compounds, I was fortunate to join the institute's illustrious alumni, who also include Kiyoshi Shiga and Hideyo Noguchi.

Shortly after joining the KI, having worked on identifying the chemical structure of a handful of compounds, I realised that I could only identify hard-to-find compounds that others had spent a great deal of time, effort and expertise in discovering. Consequently, I decided to challenge myself to actually undertake the discovery process, which was fundamental to identifying new compounds and microbial metabolites, as well as investigate their structure and possible bioactive properties. To that end, coming from a farming family background through which I had developed a profound respect for Nature and its role as a primary source of most of the materials we need for survival, I opted to concentrate on soil microorganisms. Soils often contain 10^9 to 10^{10} microorganisms per gram (dry weight), which possibly represents in excess of 1 million bacterial species [5] and, in my experience, around one third of soil samples tested produce antimicrobial substances. Unfortunately, there is no accepted "Gold Standard" method for isolating and identifying soil bacteria or other microorganisms. A serial dilution and spread-plate method is a reasonably good starting point for isolating bacterial colonies from soil but even at this early stage, the choice of isolation medium is critical and depends on the specific goals. Consequently, devising mechanisms to cope sensibly with this enormous diversity is essential. As a result I refocussed my research on the search for new antibiotics and other biologically interesting microbial metabolites, such as growth factors, enzymes and enzyme inhibitors, based on my conviction that new and innovative screening systems were the key to discovering new compounds—a belief that I have steadfastly maintained to this day.

In science, knowledge and understanding no longer appear quickly. Time, patience, trial and error are all essential ingredients in any screening process. Most screening systems retain their effectiveness but, over the years, I have devised and implemented one or two new screening mechanisms annually, discarding existing systems when resources did not permit them to be kept in operation. Generally, we now routinely have at least 10 customised screening systems operational.

Although many screens prove successful, others do not yield the results envisaged, although this does not mean they are non-functional. In this matter I have always been guided by the words of Louis Pasteur: 'Chance favours the prepared mind'. I believe that this is the key to investigating and unravelling the mysterious world and secrets of microorganisms. This is the mindset that I have always followed and which has allowed Nature to reveal to me almost 500 microbial metabolites that have unique or useful bioactive properties, several of which have proved of incalculable benefit, direct and indirect, to humankind (Fig. 1).

The painstaking work at the KI involves many of the first steps on a long road to creation of a successful drug or useful chemical reagent. We take samples from Nature that contain microoganisms. We then allow the microbes in the sample to grow on agar media plates, slowly cultivating them to produce a pure strain, making sure that we concentrate on novel types. The organism and strain are

- **Microorganisms:**
  - **New genera** **13**
  - **New species & sub-species** **53**
- **New compounds** **483**
- **Useful compounds** **26**
- **Targets for total syntheses** **>100**

FIGURE 1. Discoveries (1965–2014).

then identified, grown in liquid culture and a culture broth is formed. We carry out initial assays on the broth, including an initial metabolite analysis. In the case of the microbe that was the origin of ivermectin, for example, we identified that it also produced a toxic compound, oligomycin, knowledge that proved to be of great value with respect to explaining toxicity problems during later tests in animal models. Once these initial steps have been completed, we can scale up using a jar fermenter which facilitates clearer identification of the organism and its preservation, as well as purification and structural analysis of any promising compound (Fig. 2). We then conserve all microorganisms and compounds in our libraries for future testing and evaluation, either by KI scientists or others.

Generally, during our routine discovery work, we deliberately select unusual microorganisms with the intent to maximise the chances of finding new compounds. In addition, we generally do not have a single, specific objective, preferring to apply initial screens for a variety of bioactive properties. The characteristics of the microbe that we isolated and cultured at the Kitasato Institute and which produced the avermectins were unique and were critical elements in the discovery process [6].

From the outset of my research, I determined that it was highly useful to identify not just a new compound but also the microbe that produced it, usually

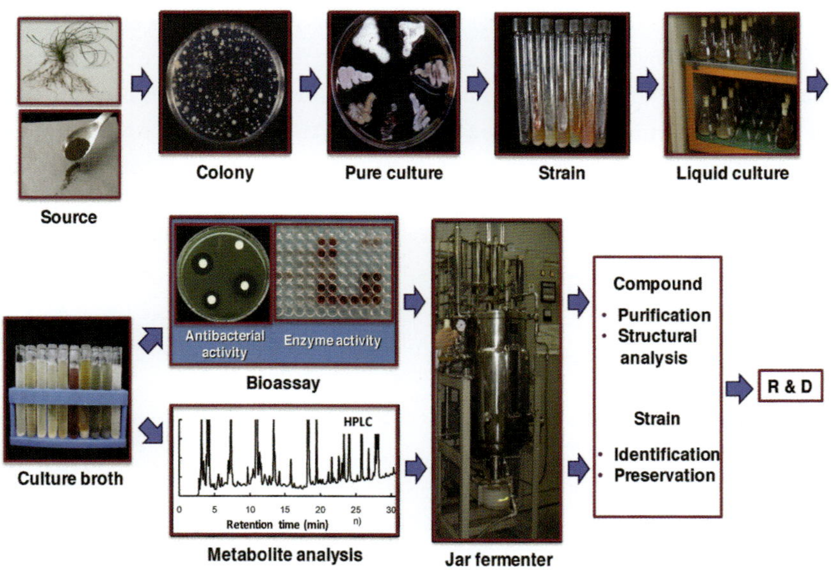

FIGURE 2. Screening for new bioactive compounds.

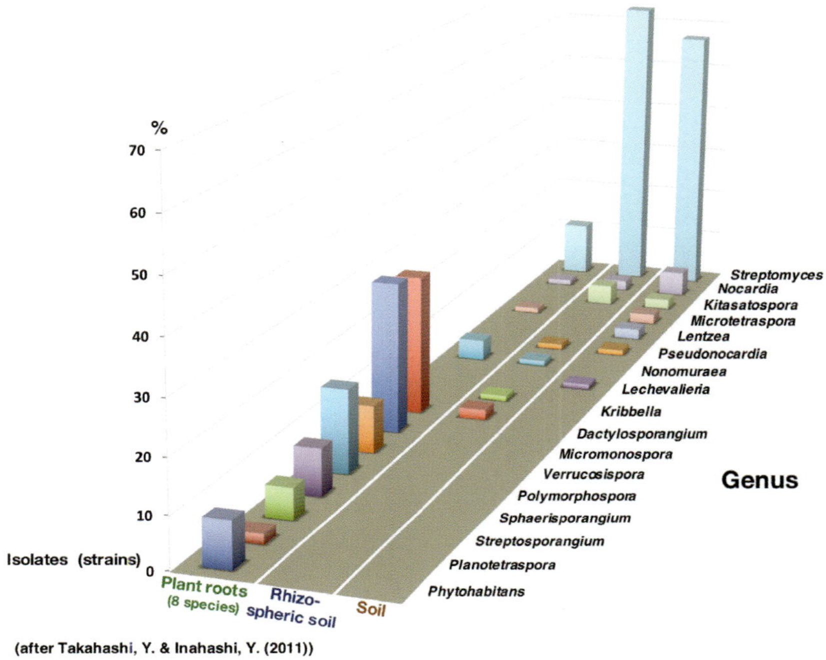

FIGURE 3. Actinomycetes (from plant root and soil samples).

placing both together in a visual presentation, a tradition that I shall maintain in this article. We have attempted to isolate microbes from every kind of natural environment, primarily from soil and latterly from seaweed, plant leaves and plant roots. Figure 3 shows the diversity of microorganisms that have been isolated from plants roots as opposed to soil and provides an indication of how the source can significantly impact the type of microbe found. For example, we have recently identified two new compounds, spoxazomycin (Fig. 4) [7], which displays antitrypanosomal activity, and trehangelin (Fig. 5) [8], a photo-oxidative hemolysis inhibitor from plant root origins.

It goes without saying that all microbes and chemicals are small, well beyond human visual acuity. It therefore seemed sensible to find mechanisms that would clearly signal the presence of something new or potentially useful. Mindful of the fact that, throughout human history, alkaloids, mostly from plant sources, have been the mainstay of traditional medicine, I decided to introduce a new method of 'chemical screening'. This entailed a search and isolation method to identify organic compounds in fermentation broths employing a simple colour-change

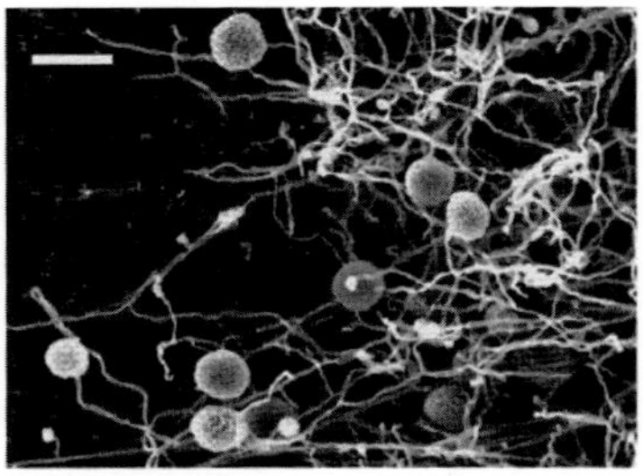

Streptosporangium oxazolinicum K07-0460^{T}
(Bar: 10 μm)

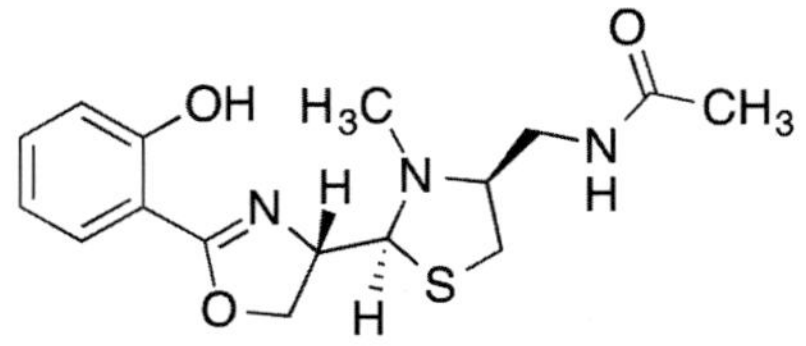

Spoxazomicin A

FIGURE 4.

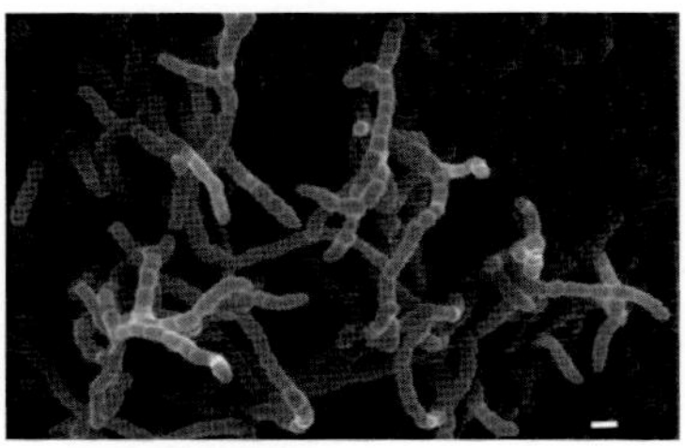

Polymorphospora rubra K07-0510
(Bar: 1 μm)

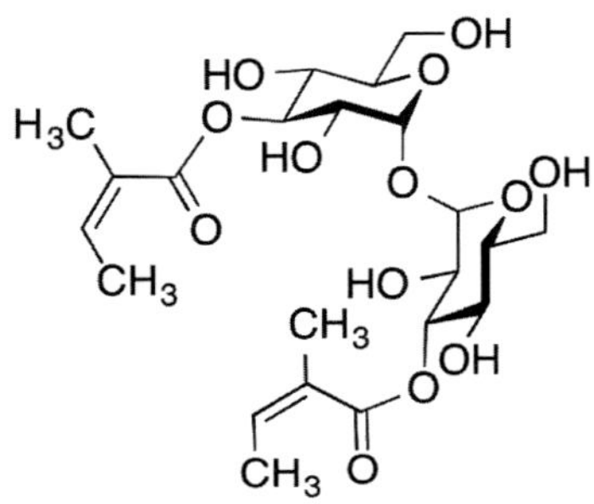

Trehangelin A

FIGURE 5.

reaction. I decided to utilise a simple mechanism using Dragendorff's reagent. Alkaloids, if present, react with the reagent, which contains bismuth nitrate and potassium iodide, to produce an easily visible orange or orange red precipitate.

We implemented this screening system in 1968, based on my profound belief that microorganisms never engage in futility; it is just our lack of knowledge and vision that prevents us from understanding what they produce, how and for what purpose. The first compound isolated through this chemical screening system was the antimicrobial pyrindicin (Fig. 6) [9]. Of far greater significance, in 1977 we isolated the world's first naturally-occurring indolocarbazole compound, staurosporine, produced by *Streptomyces staurosporeus (Lentzea albida)* (Fig.7) [10, 11]. Nine years later, Dr T. Tamaoki found that staurosporine possessed the ability to potently inhibit the functioning of protein kinase C (PKC), the first such compound identified to do so. PKC is a family of enzymes that cause increased expression of oncogenes, thereby promoting cancer progression [12].

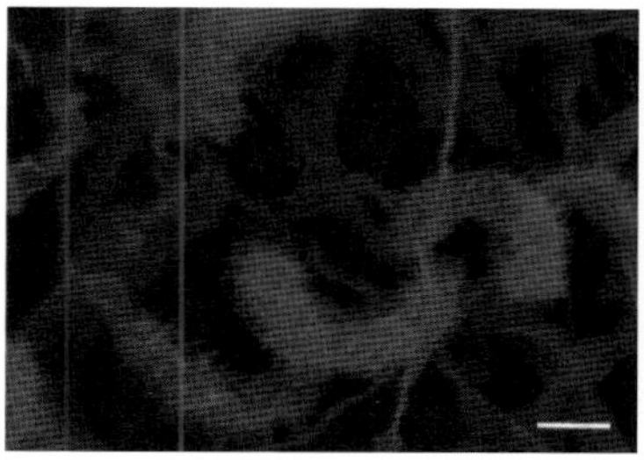

Streptomyces griseoflavus subsp. *pyrindicus* NA-15^{T} (Bar: 1 μm)

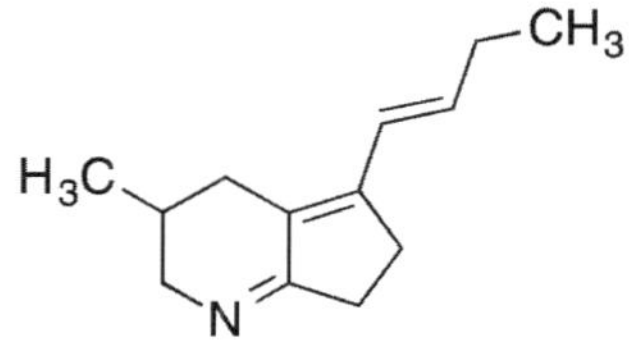

Pyrindicin

FIGURE 6.

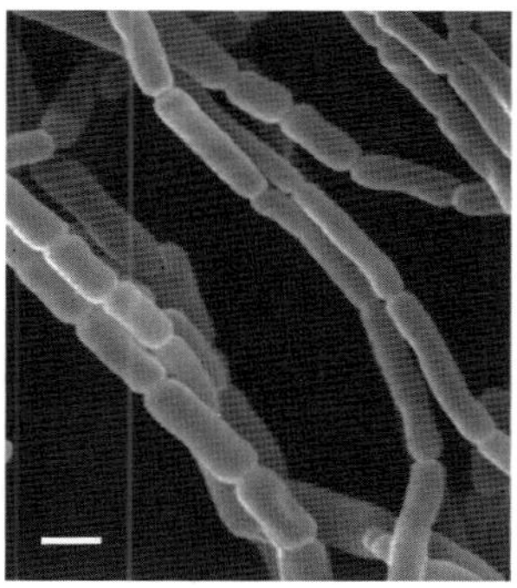

Saccharothrix aerocolonigenes subsp. *staurosporeus* AM-2282^{T} (*Lentzea albida* AM-2282) (Bar: 1 μm)

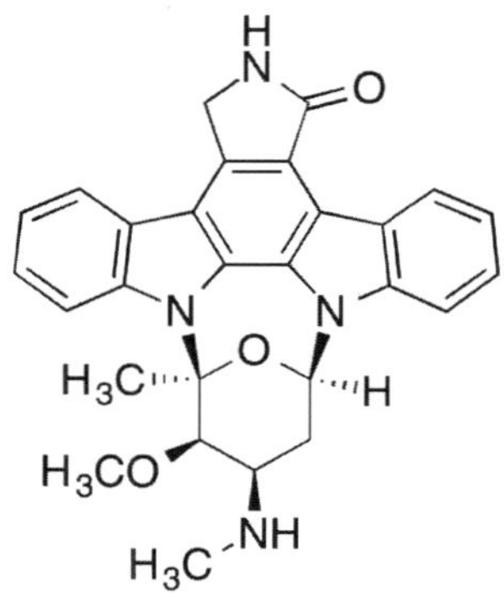

Staurosporine

FIGURE 7.

Almost immediately, staurosporine became one of the world's most prominent research reagents of microbial origin and proved to be the forerunner of many of the recently introduced anti-cancer agents. For example, the development of imatinib (Gleevec®) (Fig. 8) has been directed and influenced by the unique chemical structure and biological activity of staurosporine [13]. For me, the discovery of staurosporine was a significant milestone, not just because of its major impact in science and biomedicine, but because it was a vindication of my beliefs that microorganisms offer a virtually unlimited panoply of beneficial products. It is simply a matter of us finding ways to identify and apply them for the good

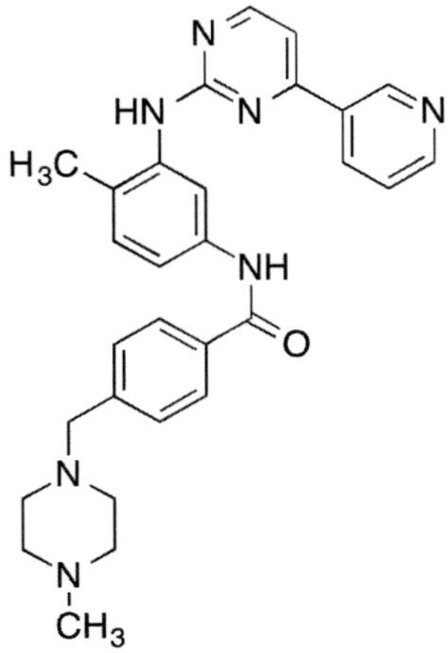

Imatinib (Gleevec®)

FIGURE 8.

of human society. I also firmly believe that the work that I accomplish and the compounds identified and stored can be taken forward or exploited by others for the good of all.

Another novel screening system led to the discovery of lactacystin (Fig. 9), an inhibitor of proteosomes. Lactacystin was found via a method involving induction of neurite outgrowths in Neuro2a, a cell line of murine neuroblastoma cells [14]. This compound proved to be the forerunner for the anticancer agent bortezomib (Fig. 10) (Velcade®).

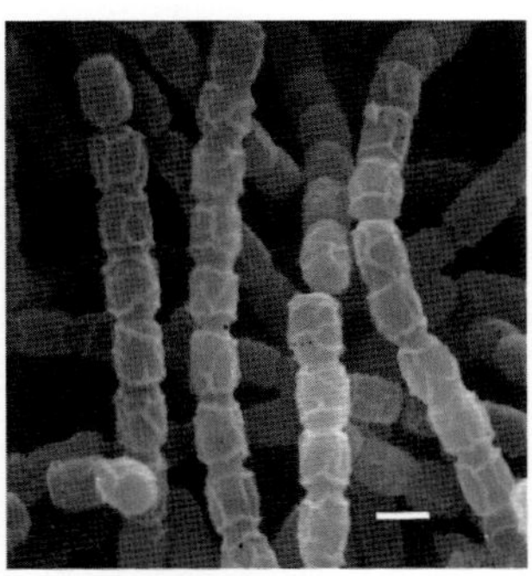

Streptomyces lactacystinicus OM-6519^T
(Bar: 1 μm)

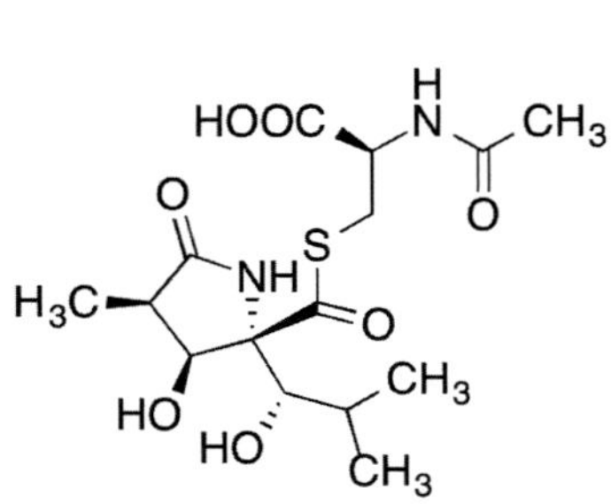

Lactacystin

FIGURE 9.

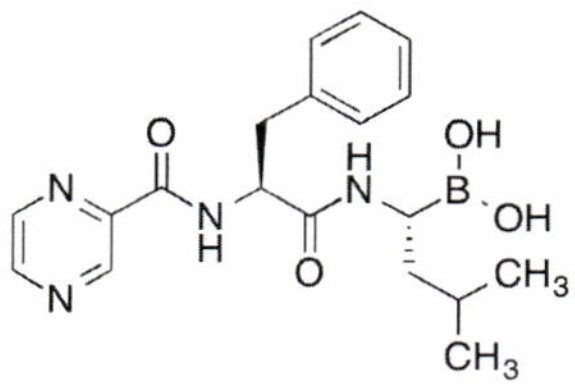

Bortezomib (Velcade®)

FIGURE 10.

The experience, techniques and knowledge gained at the KI in isolating microorganisms, cultivating them, identifying them and then determining the compounds they produce, analysing the chemical structure and elucidating their biological or chemical properties provided an optimal basis for the discovery of ivermectin. However, although we possessed the skill and expertise to discover novel microorganisms and chemicals we had neither the techniques nor the resources to carry out the requisite research and development essential for taking a promising compound though the extremely expensive and often disappointing drug production pipeline. To accomplish that task requires the commitment and extensive resources of a major commercial partner.

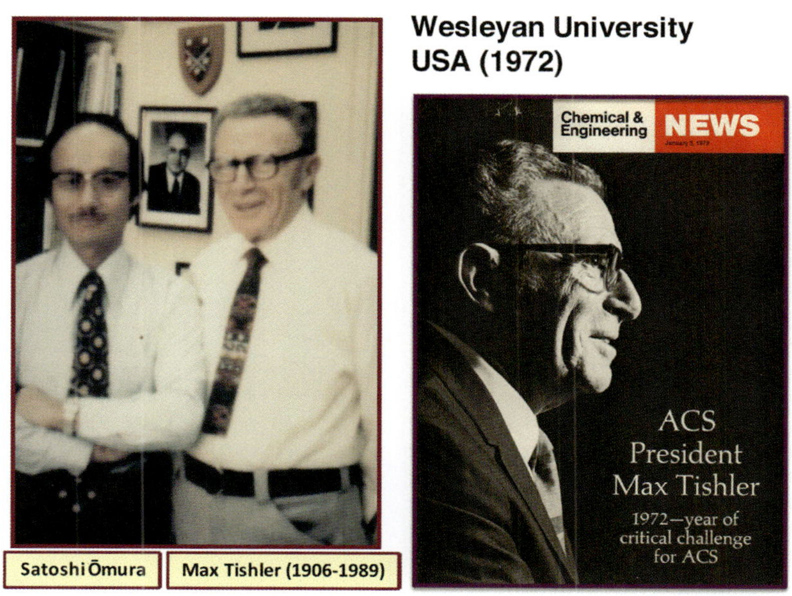

FIGURE 11. Ivermectin: the beginning.

IVERMECTIN: THE BEGINNINGS

In the early 1970s, Professor Yukimasa Yagisawa, General Manager of the Japan Antibiotics Research Association (JARA), encouraged me to exploit the possibilities for research work overseas and the benefits it could provide for both myself and for Japan. He kindly introduced me to key individuals in his network of overseas connections and, as a consequence, in 1971, I was granted a sabbatical that allowed me to take up an invitation from Prof Max Tishler to work as Visiting Research Professor in his newly-formed Chemistry Department at Wesleyan University (Fig. 11.). Max, who almost immediately became President of the American Chemical Society (ACS), had established the department following retirement from his position as President of the Merck Sharp & Dohme Research Laboratory (MDRSL), where he had had a long and distinguished career. My initial work in his laboratory focused on the structural analysis of a new antibiotic, prumycin (Fig. 12)[15] that I had discovered prior to my departure from Japan, as well as on the structure/activity relationships of macrolides [16] and the mode of action of cerulenin (Fig. 13). The contribution that both of these individuals made to my development, as a scientist, educator, and individual, has been inspirational and beyond measure.

My intended stay in the US was curtailed, as I was recalled to head the Research Department at the KI, following the retirement of the then director, and I returned in early 1973. In view of my impending return, and extremely mindful of the critical need to obtain funds to support research work in Tokyo

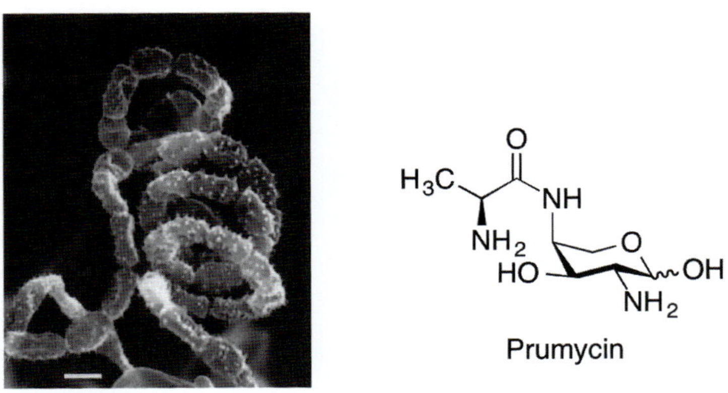

Streptomyces kagawaensis F-1028^{T}
(Bar: 1 μm)

FIGURE 12.

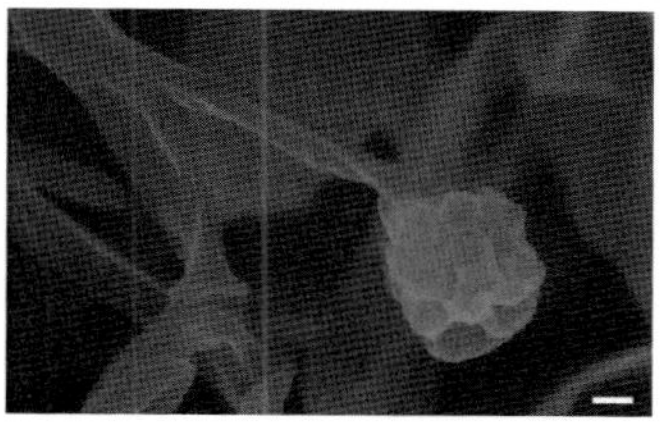

Cephalosporium caerulens KF-140ᵀ
(*Sarocladium oryzae* KF-140)
(Bar: 5 μm)

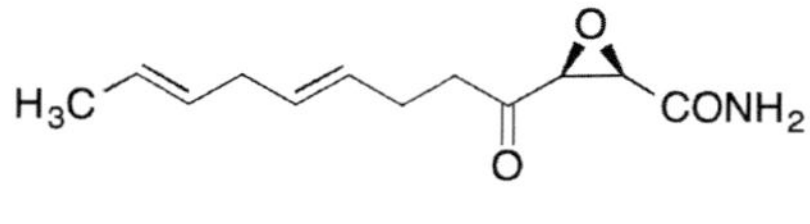

Cerulenin

FIGURE 13.

after I returned, I visited many major US pharmaceutical companies, presenting a proposal for a collaborative research project. I was greatly encouraged because, as I had previously discovered several antibiotics, such as the aforementioned prumycin (an antifungal agent) [17] and cerulenin (an antifungal and inhibitor of fatty acid biosynthesis) [18], as well as leucomycin A_3 (an antimicrobial) (Fig. 14) [19], all of the companies were supportive. At the time, Max, who knew my work and ideas very well, discussed my plan with Dr L.H. Sarett, Max's successor at MSDRL with whom he had worked closely for many years. Max's close connection with Merck and his personal linkage to Dr Lew Sarrett expedited my research collaboration with the MSDRL, which commenced in April 1973. Individuals who played key roles in the alliance are shown in Figure 15. Initially, the goal was to find growth promoting antibiotics suitable for animals, enzyme inhibitors and general purpose antibiotics produced by microorganisms, but the work soon expanded to encompass other targets.

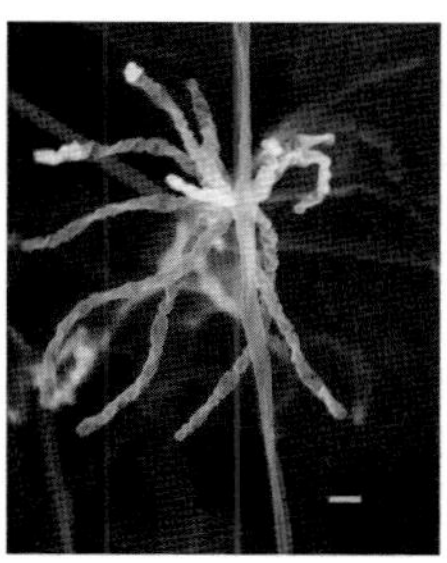

Streptomyces kitasatoensis KA-6ᵀ
(Bar: 1 μm)

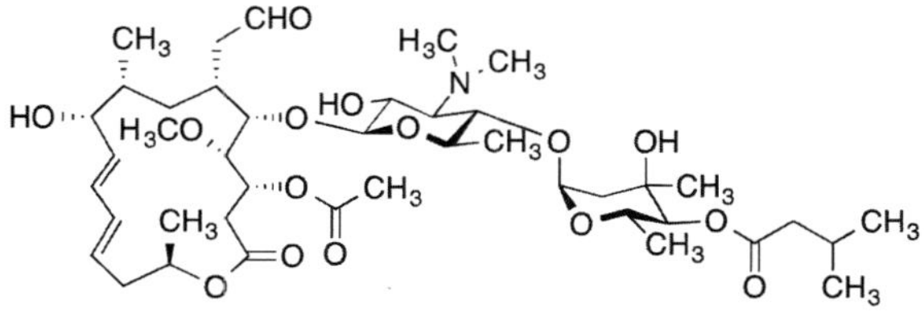

Leucomycin A_3

FIGURE 14.

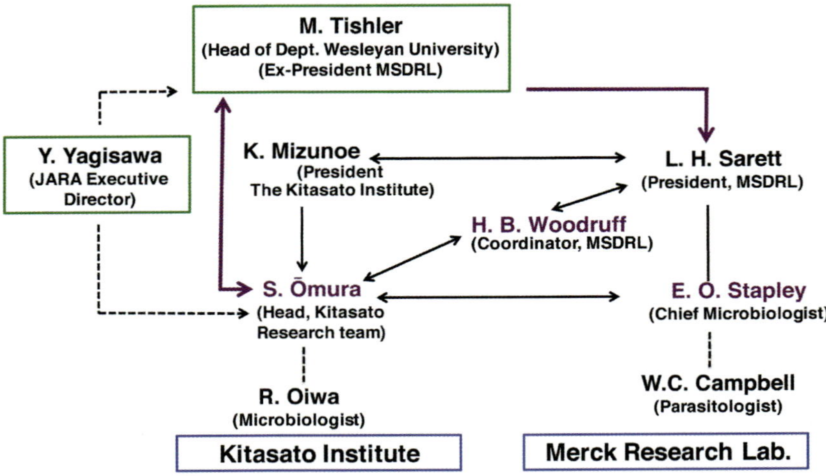

FIGURE 15. Kitasato—MSDRL Collaboration (1973).

IVERMECTIN: THE ADVENT AND USE IN ANIMALS

As the basis of the research initiative, the KI carried out isolation of what we identified as extraordinary microorganisms, culturing them and then undertaking preliminary in vitro evaluation of the bioactivity of any compounds we deemed to be of potential interest, prior to sending the most promising, from our existing library and from newly identified specimens, to MSDRL for in vivo testing.

As a result of the collaboration, a variety of compounds were discovered, the majority exhibiting a range of interesting biological activities and structures. These included luminamycin (Fig. 16) [20], an anti-anaerobic bacterial, vineomycin A_1 (Fig. 17) [21] and setamycin (Fig. 18) [22], both of which have unique structures; elasnin (Fig. 19) [23], the first human elastase inhibitor of microbial origin; and factumycin (Fig. 20), a growth promoting antibiotic for veterinary use [24].

Of far greater importance was avermectin. Simply put, avermectin proved to be one of the world's most remarkable biomedical discoveries, being accompanied by a number of world 'firsts' and having an immeasurably beneficial impact on animal and human health worldwide.

As part of their new in vivo evaluation, and following a suggestion from Max Tishler, the MSDRL introduced a new programme to screen fermentation broths that we identified as being promising [25]. This was done because there was

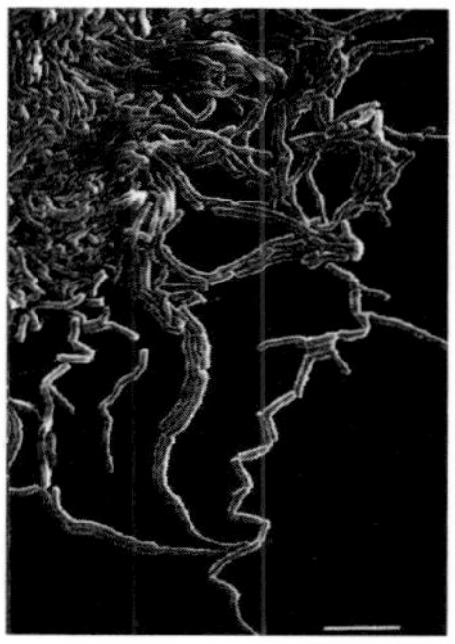

Streptomyces sp. OMR-59
(Bar: 1 μm)

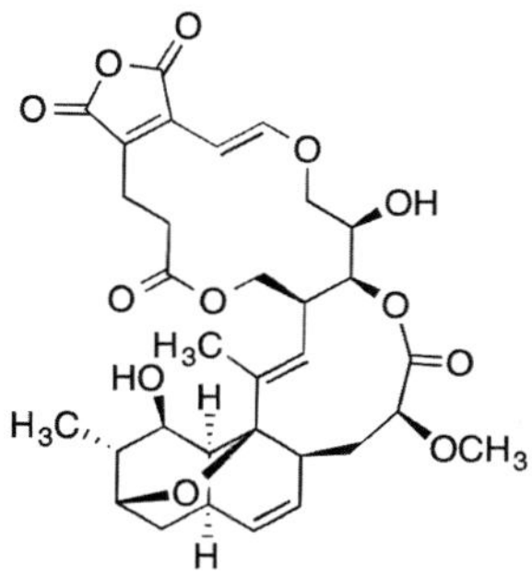

Luminamicin

FIGURE 16.

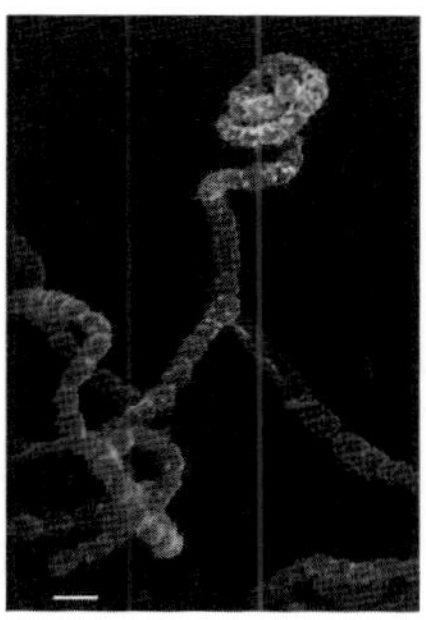

Streptomyces matensis subsp. *vineus* OS-4742^{T} (Bar: 1 μm)

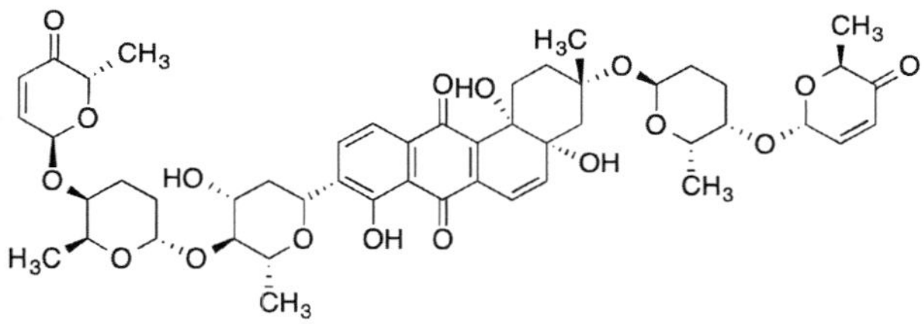

Vineomycin A_1

FIGURE 17.

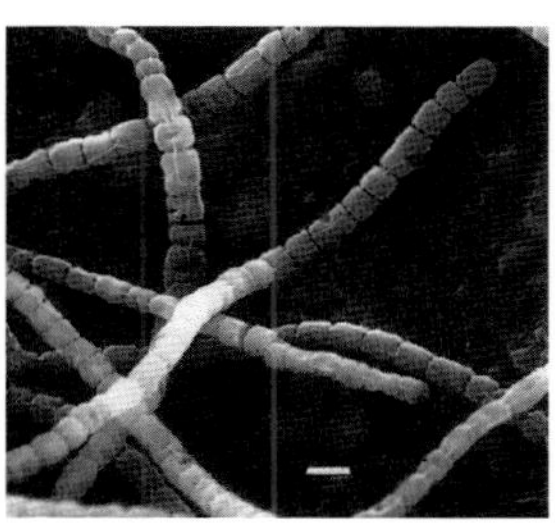

Kitasatospora setae KM-6054^{T}
(Bar: 1 μm)

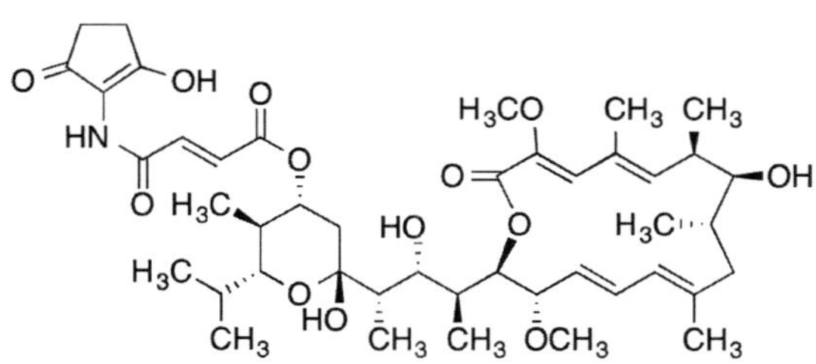

Setamycin

FIGURE 18.

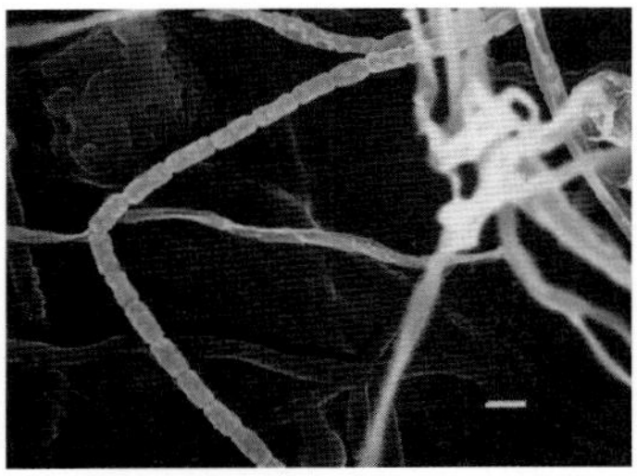

Streptomyces noboritoensis KM-2753
(Bar: 1 μm)

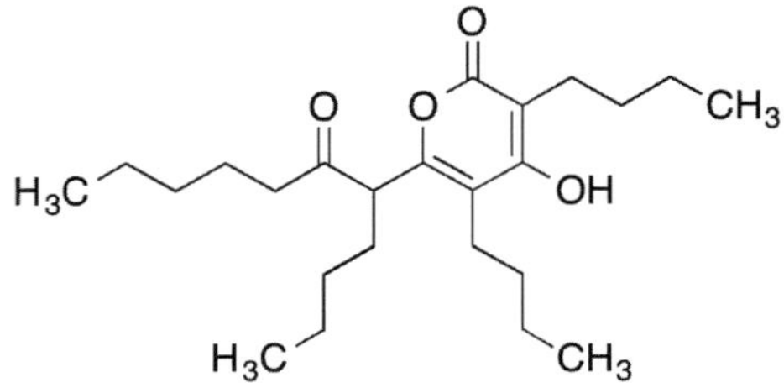

Elasnin

FIGURE 19.

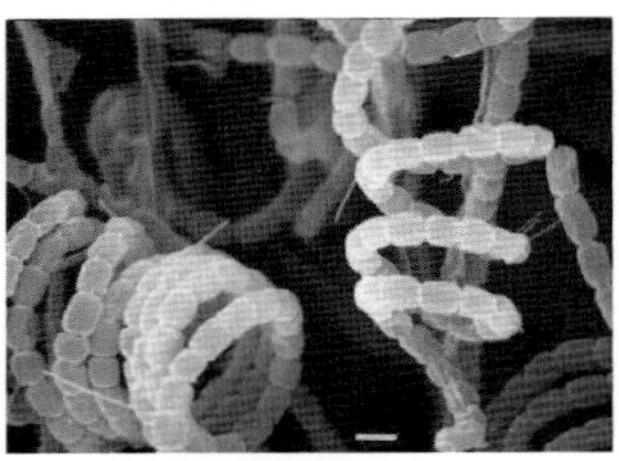

Streptomyces lavendulae OS-4369
(Bar: 1 μm)

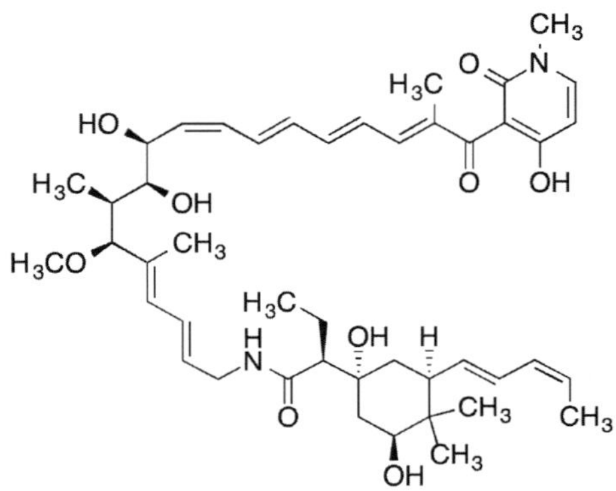

Factumycin

FIGURE 20.

confidence that our broths likely contained interesting compounds. In addition, adding a fermentation broth to the feed of a single animal means it can be tested simultaneously for both efficacy and toxicity, often with results appearing in a week rather than the weeks or months that are usually needed using in vitro tests.

MSDRL researchers screened our microorganisms, which were produced according to our description of the necessary fermentation conditions, the fermentation broths being tested in a novel model of helminth (parasitic worm) infection in which mice were infected with the nematode worm *Nematospiroides dubius (Heligmosomoides polygyrus bukeri)* [26, 27]. In one of the first 50 specially selected microorganisms we sent in 1974, Dr William Campbell and his team found an actinomycete, strain MA-4680, which produced a compound possessing excellent anthelmintic activity with little or no toxicity. The unpurified broth killed all intestinal worms and removed all signs of parasite eggs from the animal's faeces.

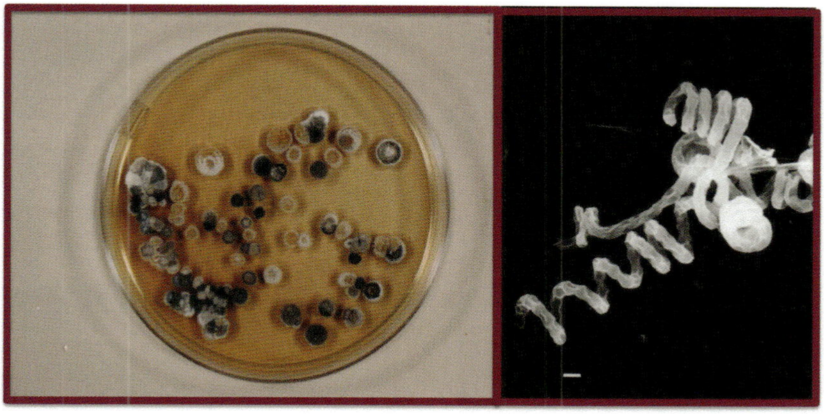

FIGURE 21. The avermectin producing strain.

The producing microorganism (Fig. 21) was originally named *Streptomyces avermitilis* MA-4680 but, in 2002, based on characterization of the original strain and morphological and phylogenetic comparisons, including 16S rDNA sequencing, with closely related members of the genus *Streptomyces*, it was proposed that the organism was in fact a new species and renamed *Streptomyces avermectinius* [28].

After a few trials to confirm the bioactivity findings, isolation chemists were engaged to identify the causal entity. The active ingredient of the broth was identified and named avermectin, which MSDRL chemists found to be a complex mixture of 16-membered macrocyclic lactones, fermentation of *S. avermectinius* producing a mixture of eight avermectin compounds (A1a, A1b, A2a, A2b, B1a, B1b, B2a and B2b) (Fig. 22). Compounds of the B-series containing a 5-hydroxyl group are markedly more active than those of the A-series, which contain a 5-methoxyl group. The four main components, avermectin A1a, A2a, B1a and B2a, constituted 80% of the mixture, with the rest composed of four lower homologs A1b, A2b, B1b and B2b. The structure of the compound was also swiftly elucidated and it was fast-tracked for development [29].

In 1979, the first papers on the avermectins were published, describing the chemicals as a series of macrocyclic lactone derivatives possessing extraordinarily potent anthelmintic properties [30–32]. Up until that time, only a handful of the several thousand microbial fermentation products discovered exhibited

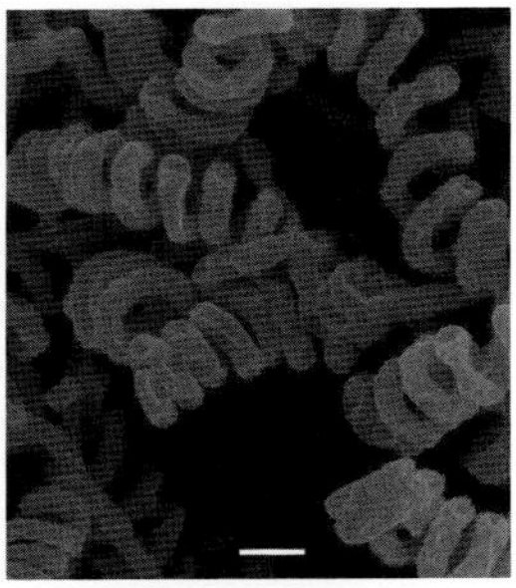

Streptomyces avermectinius (*S. avermitilis*) MA-4680^T (Bar: 2 μm)

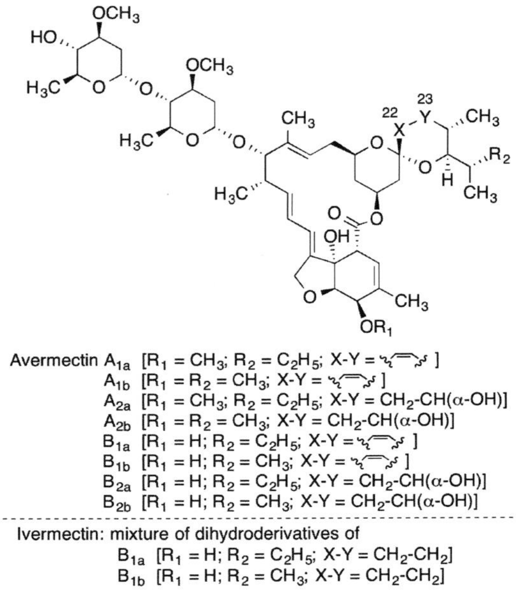

FIGURE 22.

any anthelmintic characteristics. Although structurally similar to macrolide antibiotics and antifungal macrocyclic polyenes, the avermectins did not demonstrate any antibacterial or antifungal activities.

An interdisciplinary team at MSDRL, headed by William Campbell, further investigated the eight active compounds, of which avermectins B1a and B1b were found to have the highest activity. Reduction of the C22–C23 double bond of B1a and B1b compounds with Wilkinson's catalyst improved both the spectrum of activity and safety and the resulting 22,23-dihydro B1 complex (as a mixture of 80% B1a and 20% B1b) was selected for further commercial development under the generic, non-proprietary name ivermectin [33].

The avermectins proved to be effective against roundworms of the intestinal and respiratory tracts as well as filarial parasites [34] and demonstrated biocidal activity against a diverse range of nematodes, insects and arachnids. The mode of action turned out to be both unique and robust, and was 25 times more potent than all currently available anthelmintics. Further analysis revealed that ivermectin was highly efficacious against mite, tick and botfly ectoparasites, organisms that cause massive economic losses in the livestock industry. MSDRL researchers also observed that the compound had remarkable activity against external and internal parasites in horses, cattle, pigs and sheep, effective against, among others, gastrointestinal roundworms, lungworms, mites, lice and hornflies. It was also found to be successful in treating larval heartworms in dogs, but not adult worms, and could be used to treat mange and other conditions in canines. However, no activity was found against flatworms, protozoa, bacteria or fungi [35–38].

The avermectins' broad spectrum of activity, wide therapeutic index, and novel mode of action resulted in them being introduced onto the animal health market in 1981. Two years after their introduction, avermectin-derivative products became the international veterinary sector's biggest seller, accruing annual sales income of around $1 billion, a position maintained for a quarter of a century, the ivermectin-based parasiticide products reportedly becoming MSD's fifth best-selling product group [39].

MSDRL research staff and others around the world have exhaustively searched since the original discovery but no other avermectin-producing organism has ever been found. The strain that we isolated from a single soil sample collected near a golf course bordering the ocean at Kawana in Ito City in the Shizuoka region of Japan remains the only avermectin-producing organism ever found.

Dr Boyd Woodruff of MSDRL was appointed to work alongside our team at the KI in Tokyo, and I am convinced that his personal commitment and expertise were significant factors in making the collaboration such a great success.

IVERMECTIN: MODE OF ACTION

The avermectins potentiate neurotransmission by boosting the effects of glutamate at invertebrate-specific glutamate-gated chloride channels, with minor effects on gamma-aminobutyric acid (GABA) receptors.

In parasites, neurotransmission inhibition occurs via glutamate-gated chloride channels in nerve and muscle cells, preventing their closure [40]. This leads to hyperpolarisation of the neuronal membrane, inducing paralysis of the somatic muscles, particularly the pharyngeal pump, killing the parasite [41, 42]. GABA-related (chloride) channels are commonplace in nematodes, insects and ticks [43–45]. In mammals, GABA receptors and neurons only occur in the central nervous system (CNS) and are thus not accessible [46], ivermectin being safe for vertebrates as it cannot cross the blood-brain barrier. Initial fears that ivermectin was contra-indicated in children under the age of five or who weighed less than 5 kg, where the drug might be able to cross the as yet not fully developed blood/brain barrier, were proven to be unfounded [47].

In humans, ivermectin exerts a peculiar and singular effect that remains poorly understood. The immune response to filarial infection is complex, involving Th2-type systems which counter infective L3 larvae and microfilariae, whereas a combination of Th1 and Th2 pathways are involved in resisting adult worms. It is believed that female adult worms are able to manipulate the immunoregulatory environment to ensure the survival of their microfilarial offspring [48]. Ivermectin treatment of Onchocercal filarial infection causes microfilariae to quickly disappear from the peripheral skin lymphatics. The effect is long lasting, while adult female worms are prevented from releasing microfilariae [49]. Dermal microfilarial loads are reduced by 78% within two days, and by some 98% two weeks after treatment, remaining at extremely low levels for about 12 months. Female worms slowly resume release of microfilaria 3–4 months post-treatment, but at a mere 35% of original production [50]. Regular treatment consequently decreases incidence of infection, interrupts transmission and reduces morbidity and disability. However, the actual mechanism by which ivermectin exerts its effect on microfilariae remains unclear [51].

The half-life of ivermectin in humans is 12–36 hours. The lowest levels of dermal microfilariae occur well after this timeframe, meaning that not all microfilariae are killed in the early days, and microfilariae are known to migrate into deeper dermal layers, sub-cutaneous fat, connective tissue and lymph nodes following ivermectin administration [52]. It is now believed that ivermectin somehow prevents microfilariae from evading the immune system, resulting in the host's own immune response killing the immature worms [53, 54].

Ivermectin does not kill adult worms but suppresses the production of microfilariae by adult female worms, thereby reducing transmission. As the adult worms can continue to produce microfilariae until they die naturally, ivermectin has to be taken once annually for the 16–18 year adult worm lifespan in order to stop transmission.

Th2 responses instil protective immunity against both L3 infective larvae and the microfilaria stage but parasites are able to avoid these responses, which may help explain why drug resistance in parasites in humans has not yet appeared.

IVERMECTIN: DEVELOPMENT FOR HUMAN USE

In the mid-1970s, the global community mobilised itself to address the major problems of neglected tropical diseases. Following the setting up of the Onchocerciasis Control Programme in West Africa (OCP) in 1974, the UN-based Special Programme for Research & Training in Tropical Diseases (TDR) was established in 1975. Onchocerciasis and lymphatic filariasis were two filarial infections among TDR's eight target diseases, with onchocerciasis, at the time, being a major public health problem affecting 20–40 million people in endemic areas, predominantly in Africa (Fig. 23).

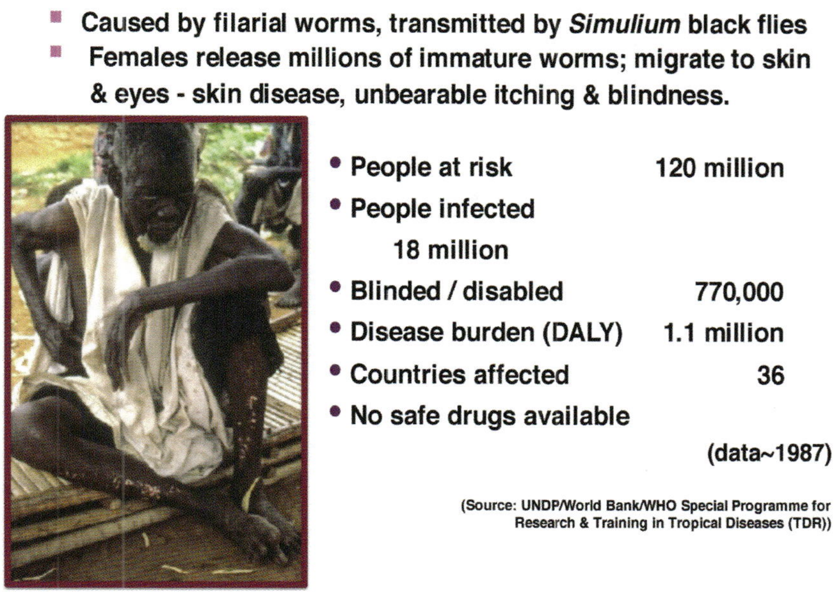

FIGURE 23. Human health goals: Onchocericiasis (River blindness).

Historically found primarily in 30 countries in sub-Saharan tropical Africa, onchocerciasis is caused by a nematode, *Onchocerca volvulus*, which lives for up to 15 years in the human body, female worms continually producing several millions of microfilaria during their lifetime, with the worms being transmitted to humans via the bite of a blood-feeding blackfly.

At the time, there were no safe and acceptable drugs available to treat onchocerciasis, which had plagued Africa for centuries, and nobody was interested in developing anti-*Onchocerca* drugs, as there was no apparent commercial market. Consequently, the OCP based its operations on expensive aerial spraying of insecticides to kill riverine vector fly larvae.

MSDRL scientists soon realised that the anthelmintic potency of ivermectin could help to conquer filarial diseases in humans and joined forces with WHO, nongovernmental organisations, international donors, governments and affected communities to drive forward evaluation of the drug [55].

Meanwhile, with respect to research needs, TDR identified that discovery of effective chemotherapeutic agents was the highest priority, with a macrofilaricide (capable of killing adult worms) substantially preferable to a microfilaricide (which would target immature worms) [56]. Research was hampered by the fact that *Onchocerca* species would not develop to maturity in any rodents, making it impossible to screen compounds against the target organism in a suitable animal model. TDR established a tertiary screen, using cattle, for compounds showing positive results in any secondary screen, the screen being the best predictor of what a compound would do in humans, with well over 10,000 compounds being screened [57, 58].

In reality, ivermectin's role in human medicine began in 1978 inside the MSDRL, with William Campbell being the driving force behind the investigation of the potential for human use. Receiving very positive results after submitting ivermectin to the Australian cattle screen, he subsequently reported to MSDRL management that "an avermectin could become the first means of preventing the blindness associated with onchocerciasis" [59, 60].

In 1981, MSDRL's Mohammed Aziz, previously of the WHO, undertook a small clinical trial of ivermectin in patients with safety paramount. Commencing with a very low dose of 5 μg/kg, he found that a single dose of 30 μ/kg substantially decreased skin microfilariae and confirmed that the effect lasted for at least 6 months, with no serious adverse events. His tests concluded that doses up to 200 μg/kg were safely tolerated [61, 62].

Ivermectin proved to be ideal for combatting Onchocerciasis, which has two main manifestations, dermal damage resulting from microfilariae in the skin and ocular damage arising from microfilariae in the eye. Ivermectin proved to slightly increase microfilariae in the eye upon treatment, followed by a gradual reduction, reaching to near zero within six months. This meant little or no ocular damage. The large ivermectin molecule cannot cross the blood/aqueous humour barrier, stopping it entering the anterior chamber and directly killing or paralysing microfilariae [63]. This made ivermectin a perfect intervention for patients with ocular involvement.

Similarly, evaluation of the impact ivermectin on dermal microfilariae confirmed that it caused almost complete clearance within two days after treatment, reducing the load to virtually zero within eight days. Ivermectin also produces long-term suppression of circulating microfilariae, making it an ideal treatment for patients with dermal involvement [64].

Merck received approval from French authorities in 1987 allowing human use of ivermectin. In a hitherto unprecedented gesture, immediately following registration, ivermectin (branded as Mectizan®) was donated free of charge by Merck & Co. Inc., under the direction of Roy Vagelos (Fig. 24), for the treatment of Onchocerciasis (River Blindness), with KI foregoing all royalties. The donation was for as long as the drug was required, in the amounts that were needed. This represented the first such large-scale drug donation initiative and it has resulted in the world's largest, longest-running and most successful drug donation programme.

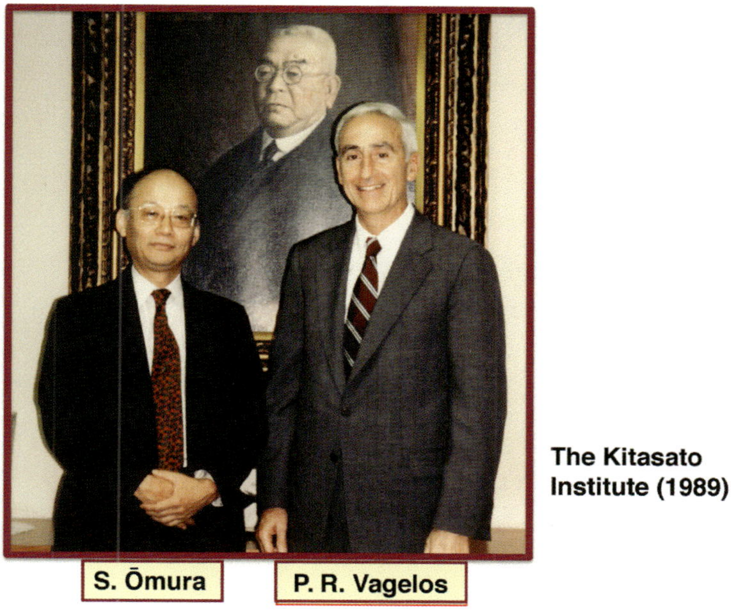

FIGURE 24. Ivermectin—world's most effective drug donation.

Introduced for use in the 11-nation OCP, ivermectin was not a cure. It did not kill adult parasites, a single annual dose simply suppressing symptom-causing onchocercal microfilaria in the skin and eyes and preventing the disease from progressing [65]. To prevent transmission, every eligible member of an affected community needed to take the drug. Ivermectin only kills immature worms, so entire communities in disease endemic areas have to take it for up to 15 years, until the adult female worms die naturally.

Massive clinical trials in Africa proved ivermectin to be a highly effective and safe microfilaricide, which need not be given more frequently than once annually, and showed that it has few side effects, which were dose-dependent, mild and short-lived, with no severe ophthalmological adverse events [66–68]. Ivermectin is very safe and can be given orally in the field by non-medical staff, meaning the drug is ideal for mass treatment programmes.

The African Programme for Onchocerciasis Control (APOC), established in 1995, built on the success of the OCP and extended community-wide mass drug administration (MDA) of ivermectin to 19 other African nations. APOC is recognised as a cost-effective, large-scale public health intervention of enormous significance, preventing an estimated 17.4 million years' worth of healthy

Key partners for Mass Drug Administration (MDA)

- ✓ Merck & Co. Inc. & Mectizan Donation Program
- ✓ Kitasato Institute
- ✓ World Health Organization (WHO)
- ✓ TDR (Special Programme for Research & Training in Tropical Diseases)
- ✓ Onchocerciasis Control Programme - West Africa (OCP)
- ✓ African Programme for Onchocerciasis Control (APOC)
- ✓ World Bank
- ✓ Endemic country governments
- ✓ Non-Governmental Organizations (NGOs)
- ✓ Affected communities & volunteer drug distributors

FIGURE 25. Ivermectin distribution.

life from being lost and freeing all African children taking ivermectin from the dangers of onchocercal blindness and skin disease [69].

In referring to the international efforts to tackle Onchocerciasis in which ivermectin is now the sole control tool, the UNESCO World Science Report concluded, "the progress that has been made in combating the disease represents one of the most triumphant public health campaigns ever waged in the developing world" [70].

The success of the campign to overcome Onchocerciasis is due to the sterling efforts and long-term commitment of a truly international, multidisciplinary coalition, some key partners of which are shown in Figure 25.

EFFECTIVENESS AGAINST OTHER FILARIAL DISEASES

Lymphatic filariasis, also known as elephantiasis, is another devastating, highly debilitating disease that threatens over 1 billion people in more than 80 countries (Fig. 26). An estimated 120 million people in tropical and subtropical regions are infected, 40 million of whom are seriously incapacitated. The disease results from infection with filarial worms, *Wuchereria bancrofti*, *Brugia malayi* or *B. timori*. The parasites are transmitted to humans through the bite of an infected mosquito and develop into adult worms in the lymphatic vessels, causing severe damage and swelling (lymphoedema). Adult worms are responsible for the major disease manifestations, the most outwardly visible forms being painful, disfiguring swelling of the legs and genital organs. Around 25 million men have genital disease (most commonly hydrocoele) and almost 15 million, mostly women, have lymphoedema or elephantiasis of the leg. The psychological and social stigma associated with the disease is immense, as are the economic and productivity losses it causes.

With respect to the use of ivermectin for lymphatic filariasis, again MSDRL took the initial lead. In the mid-1980s, well before ivermectin was approved for human use to treat onchocerciasis, MSDRL scientists were undertaking trials of ivermectin to measure its impact against lymphatic filariasis and to find optimal treatment dosages [71]. Meanwhile, TDR was carrying out multicentre field trials in Brazil, China, Haiti, India, Indonesia, Malaysia, Papua New Guinea, Sri Lanka and Tahiti to evaluate ivermectin, the existing treatment drug, diethylcarbamazine (DEC), and combinations of the two. The results showed that single-dose ivermectin and single-dose DEC worked as well as each other. The combination, even at low dose, proved even more effective, decreasing microfilarial density by 99% after one year and 96% after two years [72–75].

Despite these findings, ivermectin remained unregistered for treatment of lymphatic filariasis until 1998 when approval was granted by French authorities.

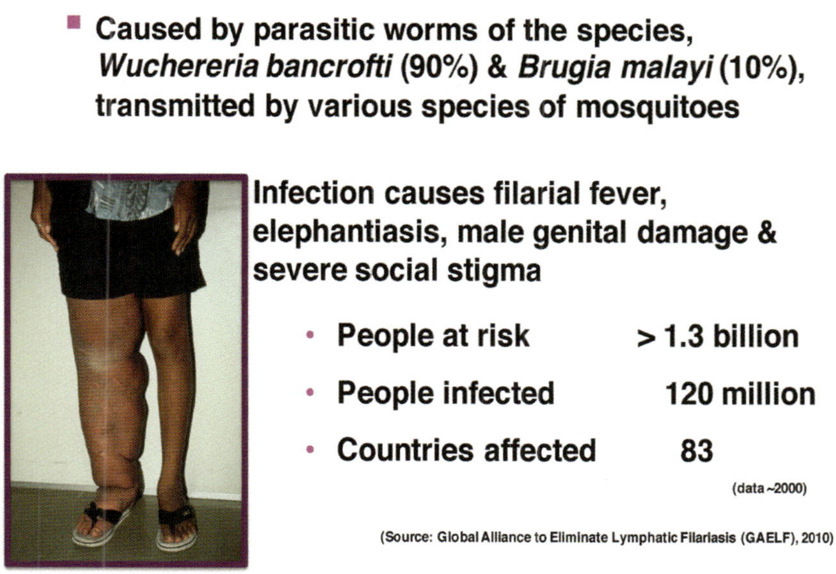

FIGURE 26. Human health goals: Lymphatic filariasis (elephantiasis).

Several years earlier another drug, albendazole, produced by SmithKlineBeecham (now GlaxoSmithKline—GSK) had also been shown to be effective in killing both immature and adult worms. Indeed, field trials had confirmed that once-yearly combinations of albendazole plus DEC or ivermectin were 99% effective in ridding the blood of microfilariae for at least a year after treatment. The primary goal of treating affected communities thus became elimination of microfilariae from the blood of infected individuals so that transmission of infection is interrupted. This opened up the prospect of actually eliminating the disease, something that was made eminently possible thanks to GSK agreeing to donate albendazole. In late-1998, following registration of the drug for lymphatic filariasis, Merck extended its ivermectin donation programme to cover lymphatic filariasis in areas where it co-existed with Onchocerciasis. Subsequently, in 1999/2000, the WHO launched the Global Programme to Eliminate Lymphatic Filariasis (GPELF).

The sheer scale of these disease elimination enterprises is staggering. During the first decade of this century, some 300 million people, roughly the population of the United States, were taking ivermectin tablets annually. In 2014, 328 million ivermectin treatments were requested by disease endemic country governments and approved by the Mectizan Donation Committee. Of this total, 73 million were for combined onchocerciasis/lymphatic filariasis treatments, meaning that around 255 million people were due to receive ivermectin treatment during the year (Fig. 27). In total, 1.4 billion ivermectin treatments have been donated for onchocerciasis (1987–2014) and 1.2 billion for lymphatic filariasis (2000–2014). The goal of elimination of onchocerciasis in Latin America by 2015 has virtually

Ivermectin treatments approved (2014):

Onchocerciasis	**110 million**
Lymphatic filariasis	**218 million**
Sub-total =	328 million
Combined treatments	**73 million**
TOTAL =	**255 million**

Ivermectin treatments administered (2013)

Onchocerciasis	**107 million**
Lymphatic filariasis	**120 million**
TOTAL =	**227 million**

(Source: MDP, WHO(WER), APOC)

FIGURE 27. Ivermectin treatments.

been accomplished, with just one endemic area remaining on the border between Brazil and Venezuela in remote Yanomami Indian communities where some transmission is still occurring [76].

Today, despite enormous advances in the fight to conquer onchocerciasis in Africa, and with the elimination target date fast approaching, an estimated 172 million people are still in need of treatment [77].

COMMERCIAL IVERMECTIN

Besides donated ivermectin being the sole or primary tool in the two global disease elimination programs, commercial for-profit preparations of ivermectin-based drugs are also being put to ever increasing uses. Ivermectin is being used ever more widely as a remedy for strongyloidiasis (an intestinal infection which afflicts 30–100 million people worldwide) and to treat and prevent scabies (a skin infestation of which 300 million cases are reported each year). Each year, more uses for the avermectins, and ivermectin in particular, are being found in human and animal health [78].

Donated Mectizan® is the primary agent for elimination programmes for onchocerciasis and lymphatic filariasis (in combination with albendazole). At-cost ivermectin has also now become:

1. The drug of choice to treat strongyloidiasis, although it is not available in all nations where the disease is endemic [79].
2. Increasingly used to treat scabies (which afflicts around 130 million people worldwide at any one time). Oral ivermectin has been used since 1993 to treat both common scabies and crusted scabies, particularly to control outbreaks in nursing homes where whole-body application of topical agents is impractical [80]. Recently, topical ivermectin lotions were approved and ivermectin is promising to become the future drug of choice for treating scabies [81].
3. The drug of choice for difficult-to-treat *Pediculosis capitis* (head lice infestation), the most common parasitic condition among children worldwide [82]. Oral ivermectin has high efficacy and tolerability and is more effective than topical malathion lotion [83–87]. Topical application is also effective [88].
4. An option for the intestinal infection ascariasis. Although ivermectin is not recommended for human soil transmitted helminth treatment, except for strongyloidiasis, it has activity against ascariasis, hookworm and trichuriasis. Relatively few trials have examined the use of ivermectin

in this respect. A study to compare the three drugs found that ivermectin was as good as albendazole against ascariasis but that combination therapy provided slightly better results [89]. Another study looked at single-dose ivermectin and found it to be as good as 3-day albendazole treatment [90]. Currently, concern is growing about increasing resistance to albendazole and other anthelmintics [91], emphasising the need for new control tools [92].

5. The best option for the food-borne parasitic infection gnathostomiasis. Albendazole and ivermectin are the preferred treatments but ivermectin is more preferable as it can be given in a single dose [93].
6. An option for the parasitic infection mansonellosis. Ivermectin is highly effective against *Mansonella streptocerca*, with a single dose causing long-term suppression of microfilariae [94]. However, it has demonstrated little or no effect against *Mansonella perstans*. Although there is no consensus on the best therapy, the most commonly used drug, DEC, is often ineffective and it is likely that combination therapy will be the best option [95].
7. Used widely 'off-label' (e.g., to kill skin mites in salmon farming). Toxicity in a range of nontarget animals has been reported, including mice, chicken, rhesus monkeys, bats and turtles [96–100].

HOLISTIC HEALTH, WELFARE AND SOCIOECONOMIC IMPACT

Ivermectin is increasingly being viewed as even more of a 'wonder drug' in human health, as it has also been improving the nutrition, general health and wellbeing of billions of people worldwide ever since it was first used to treat onchocerciasis in humans in 1988. It is ideal in many ways, being multipurpose, highly effective and broad-spectrum, safe, well tolerated and can be easily administered (a single, annual oral dose).

Over the 25-year period that communities in Africa and Latin America have been taking ivermectin to combat river blindness and elephantiasis, anectdotal reports of secondary and non-target benefits have been burgeoning. The benefits described range from an increase in the libido of men to the ability of the tablets to kill termites. Research is accelerating to explore the veracity of these perceived additional benefits and to try and quantify the true overall impact that ivermectin may provide in communities undergoing MDA.

From a purely medical standpoint, ivermectin is known to kill a range of intestinal parasitic worms. The outcome is a visible and tangible sign, people observing worms in their stools. Consequently, owing to this outward manifestation, villagers feel better and are simultaneously encouraged to continue complying with the drug regime.

Work in Brazil investigating the overall health impact of ivermectin in MDA communities indicates that after two standard doses of ivermectin given 10 days apart, intestinal worm burdens are decimated. Infestations with Strongyloides, Enterobius, and Ascaris were completely cured, whereas other worm burdens were cut to 50–85% of original levels. With regard to external parasites, 99% of pediculosis was cured, compared with scabies (88%) and tungiasis (64%) [101, 102]. Another analysis showed that children in a community that underwent 17 years of ivermectin treatment showed markedly reduced prevalence and intensities of *Trichuris trichiuria* infections and that even children not eligible for treatment displayed reductions, indicating that ivermectin benefitted all members of the community by helping to reduce transmission [103].

In a survey of 3,125 community members in Nigeria who had been receiving ivermectin MDA, the results were also diverse and impressive. Among those treated, with regard to onchocerciasis, there was an 18.5% reduction in body itching, along with reduced skin rash (17.3%), reports of 11.7% better vision, and a 6.6% darkening of 'leopard skin'. Moreover, in addition to the targeted improvements, 24.6% of individuals reported being dewormed, 22.3% said their appetite had increased, 7.9% felt that they had experienced a noticeable reduction in arthritic or other musculoskeletal pain, 6.6% of men declared their libido had improved, 4.5% of community members said their head lice had disappeared, and 4.5% of women described a reversal of secondary amenorrhea [104].

Health:

- **55.7% improved vision**
- **54% dewormed**
- **50.3% better skin**
- **44.4% reduced itching**
- **31.4% less head lice**
- **Less ill health, less high blood pressure, less epilepsy**
- **Better fertility & improved libido**

Social:

- **75.6% reported improved ability to work**
- **28.3% improved self respect/esteem**
- **26.4% better peer acceptance**
- **15.6% improved school attendance**
- **9.1% better home relationships**

(Source: Okeibunor, J.C. *et. al.* (2011))

FIGURE 28. Ivermectin mass drug administration secondary benefits: Africa (4-country study).

In a subsequent comprehensive four-country study of MDA patients in Africa, diverse health and social impacts and perceptions were quantified (Fig. 28). Overall, 84.7% felt ivermectin had provided multiple and substantial health and social welfare benefits. All patients reported being better able to sleep at night and were of the opinion that the MDA had improved their social, psychological, and economic wellbeing, with both food productivity and food security being improved [105].

BENEFITS IN JAPAN

The discovery of avermectin has contributed greatly towards improving the lives and living standards of billions of people around the world, as well as to improving the health of livestock and pets. Development, donation and distribution of the drug have been associated with many highly beneficial precedents. The substantial royalties earned by the Kitasato Institute on sales of ivermectin in animal health have also been used wisely and beneficently. They have funded a great deal of highly-focused research, have been used to obtain 27 hectares of land at Kitamoto City in Saitama Prefecture and to construct a vaccine production facility as well as a 440-bed district general hospital and a nursing college. At present, over 1,000 patients per day visit the hospital, which covers a catchment area that was previously grossly underserved with medical facilities. We placed a ceramic plate of a scanning electron micrograph of *S. avermectinius* at the entrance hall of the Kitamoto hospital to illustrate the true foundations on which the building has been constructed and to remind us all of the bounty that still lies hidden in soil, in Japan and elsewhere, awaiting discovery.

GENETICS OF *S. AVERMECTINIUS* AND AVERMECTIN BIOSYNTHESIS

Soon after its use became widespread in animal health, ivermectin resistance began to appear, at first in small ruminants but also more significantly in cattle parasites, especially *Cooperia* spp. [106]. It is well known that high-level resistance to ivermectin appears in free-living *Caenorhabditis elegans* [107]. Thankfully, despite over 30 years of constant worldwide use, there have been no reports of resistance in canine heartworms or among equine *Strongyloides* parasites. More importantly, despite some 25 years of constant monotherapy in humans, no convincing evidence of resistance in *Onchocerca volvulus* has yet been found, although there are indications that resistance may be starting to develop and that resistant parasites are being selected [108, 109].

Chemists have achieved the total synthesis of the avermectins. However to fully understand the biosynthesis of the avermectins, and to allow us to manipulate *S. avermectinius* into producing modified analogues, we mapped the entire genome of the microorganism.

Our work in terms of mapping of biosynthetic genes, elucidation of biosynthetic pathways and overall genome analysis of the avermectin-producing microorganism, *S. avermectinius* MA-4680^{T} allowed us to create mutant organisms in which avermectin biosynthesis was blocked. Thorough stepwise analysis allowed identification of single-point mutations, elucidating the structures of biosynthetic intermediates produced by each mutant and determination of their locations in the biosynthetic pathways. Moreover, the information taken from these blocked mutants became the basis for the cloning of gene clusters for avermectin biosynthesis.

In 1999, we reported that 17 genes of *S. avermectinius* encode enzymes that are involved in avermectin biosynthesis (Fig. 29) [110–113]. Of these, those encoding four type-I polyketide synthases are concerned with lactone formation, via 12 cycles and 53 steps. The remainder act on pathway-specific regulation,

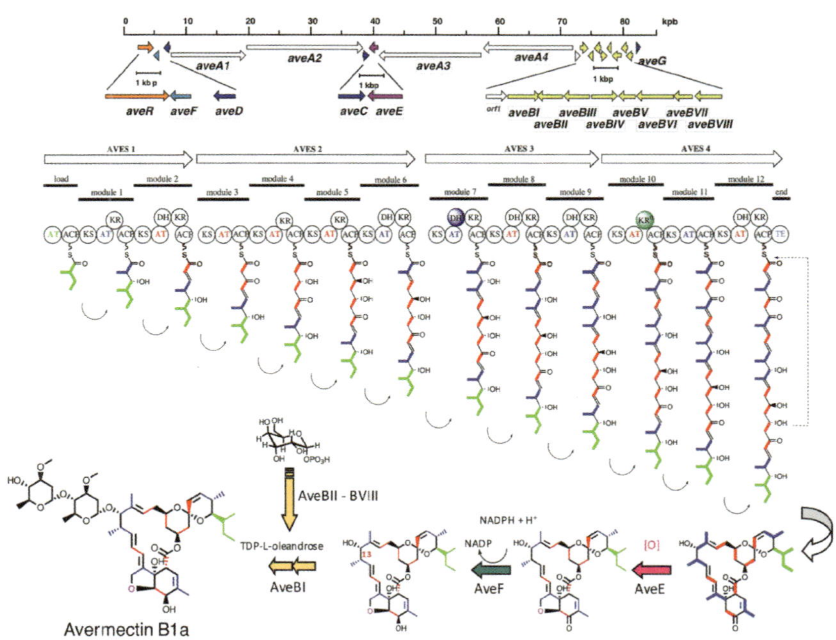

FIGURE 29. *S. avermectinius*: avermectin biosynthesis.

with 12 genes being involved in modification of the lactone ring, biosynthesis of oleandrose and its glycosylation.

The functions of the 17 genes were analysed by cloning. As shown in Figure 29, four genes, *aveA1*, *aveA2*, *aveA3*, and *aveA4*, are involved in the biosynthesis of the basic skeleton of the aglycone moiety. AVES1/AVES4, whose synthesis is governed by these four genes, are multifunctional proteins composed of 3973, 6239, 5532, and 4681 amino acids, respectively.

There are a total of 12 modules in these four large, multifunctional proteins. The AT (acyltransferase) domain transports acyl groups necessary for acyl-chain elongation, one after another, to the ACP (acylcarrier protein) domain present in each module. The acyl groups are then condensed by the catalytic action of the KS (β-oxoacyl-ACP synthase) domain. The resultant β-oxoactyl-ACP is reduced by the KR (β-oxoacyl-ACP reductase) domain and β-hydroxyacyl-ACP is further dehydrated by the DH (dehydratase) domain. The chain elongation reactions and lactonisation at the final step by TE (thioesterase) domain form the basic skeleton of lactone and the nascent lactone is further modified by cytochrome P450 (AveE: CYP171A1) and C5- ketoreductase (AveF) to form avermectin aglycones. Through reaction of the *aveB1-aveBVII* gene's products, namely AveBIIwAveBIII, L-oleandrose is synthesised from glucose-1-phosphate as TDP-L-oleandrose and linked to the aglycone-lactone, completing avermectin biosynthesis. The presence of the hydroxyl group at position 13, which allows the binding of L-oleandrose, is extremely important, as the presence of two L-oleandroses produces the potent antinematode activity of avermectin. The DH domain in module 7 at AVES3 is originally involved in the C13-OH dehydration reaction, but when histidine is substituted for tyrosine in its catalytic active center (consensus motif: HxxxGxxxxP/S), the domain becomes dysfunctional. Subsequently, biosynthesis progresses, while the hydroxyl group at position 13 remains, forming lactone. This single-point mutation, which has resulted in huge health benefits for humankind, allows the sugar (L-oleandrose) binding and subsequent biosynthesis of avermectin, which has superior anthelmintic activity compared to metabolites without the sugar moiety, such as milbemycin and nemadectin (FIg. 29) [114].

Our group completed analysis of the entire genome (9,025,608 bases) of *S. avermectinius* MA-4680^{T}) in 2003 [115, 116]. The information obtained, which represented the first genome analysis of an industrially important actinomycete, provided a major boost for research of secondary metabolites of microorganisms. We initially estimated that there were 32 such clusters, finally determining that there are 37 clusters involved (Fig. 30) [117]. The production of oligomycin,

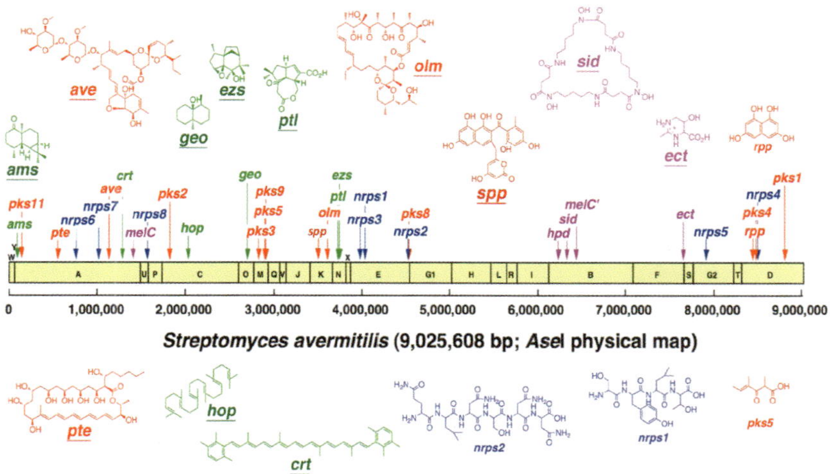

FIGURE 30. Distribution of gene clusters for secondary metabolite biosyntheses in *Streptomyces avermectinius* (*avermitilis*).

along with avermectin, was already known but production of 10 secondary metabolites, including the polyene macrolide, filipine III (*pte*), carotene (*crt*), pentalenolactone (*ptl*), geosmin (*geo*), and nocardamin (*sid*) were all predicted by the genetic analysis, and later confirmed by isolating each metabolite from a fermentation broth of *S. avermectinius*. This created a new research mechanism, whereby production of compounds with specific structures can be predicted by gene analysis and later confirmed through actual production and isolation. The mechanism by which secondary metabolites are produced in *S. avermectinius* has now been fully clarified and work is progressing to engineer the producer microorganism to manufacture yet more potent 'designer' compounds.

We have created an improved strain of *S. avermectinius*, which contains only 80% of the original genome, by removing sequences unnecessary for compound

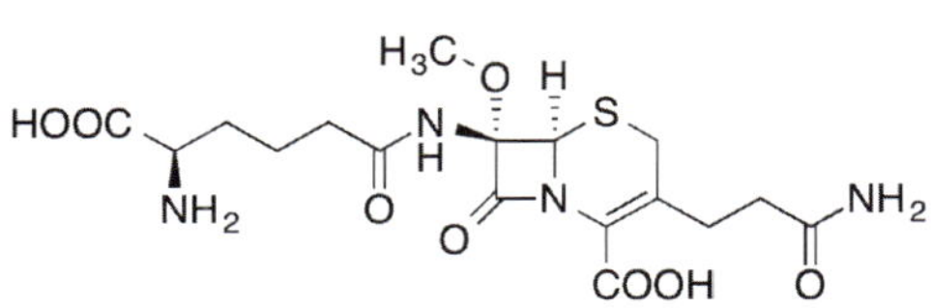

Cephamycin C

FIGURE 31.

production by the site-specific and homologous recombination technique. Using the genome-minimised strain, the heterologous expression of gene cluster for cephamycin C (Fig. 31) biosynthesis from a *S. clavuligerus* genomic library, was attempted, resulting in astonishing production of bioactive compounds [118]. This is a highly innovative foray in biotechnology, which should provide clues to guide applied research on genetic manipulation and customised culturing systems to facilitate productivity of a range of useful compounds.

IVERMECTIN: THE FUTURE

In addition to the gradual appreciation of the diverse health and socioeconomic benefits that ivermectin does provide, research is beginning to shed light on the promise of ivermectin and the prospects of it combatting a range of diseases and for killing vectors of disease-causing parasites. Box 1 provides an indicator of the potential that has been identified thus far, particularly against diseases of the poor, and provides an insight into the wide spectrum of benefits of ivermectin that may yet lie undiscovered and unexploited.

CONCLUDING REMARKS

Ivermectin has continually proved to be astonishingly safe for human use. Indeed, it is such a safe drug, with minimal side effects, that it can be administered by non-medical staff and even illiterate individuals in remote rural communities, provided that they have had some very basic, appropriate training. This fact has helped contribute to the unsurpassed beneficial impact that the drug has had on human health and welfare around the globe, especially with regard to the campaign to fight onchocerciasis.

In reality, the renewed interest in fighting tropical diseases, including the involvement of the pharmaceutical industry, which has become increasingly evident over the past four decades, and which has saved lives and improved the welfare of billions of people, notably the poor and disadvantaged in the topics, can be traced back to the 1987 introduction of ivermectin for use in humans. The remarkable and unparalleled donation of ivermectin can rightly be seen to be the origin of this philanthropic largesse.

Today, ivermectin is being increasingly used worldwide to combat other diseases in humans, and new and promising properties and uses for ivermectin and other avermectin derivatives are continuing to be found. Of perhaps even greater significance is the evidence that the use of ivermectin has both direct and indirect beneficial impact on improving community health. Above all, ivermectin has proved to be a medicine of choice for the world's rural poor.

According to many experts, a post-antibiotic era—in which common infections and minor injuries can kill—is a very real possibility, with WHO Director General Dr Margaret Chan declaring "the rise of antibiotic resistance is a global health crisis, and governments now recognise it as one of the greatest challenges for public health today."

My work has always been guided by five fundamental creeds: the almost unlimited abilities of microorganisms to produce novel compounds; the crucial need to establish 'gold-standard' screening systems; recognition that screening is not just a routine exercise; the major contribution of basic research; and the need to assign the highest value to maintaining human relationships and partnerships.

As science advances and our knowledge improves, it is clear to me that the elucidation of suitable targets for medicines, and our expectations for finding remedies to treat both known and as-yet unknown diseases and conditions, will not only improve but also accelerate. Genomic mapping and identification of lead compounds have progressed significantly since the turn of the century, as evidenced by the mapping of the human genome. As mentioned above, research is also expected to develop substantially based on the findings of biosynthetic studies and from the investigation of naturally-occurring substances that boast hitherto unseen structures. I firmly believe that Nature's microbes produce metabolites offering unmatched promise toward meeting our needs, although the introduction of novel screening methods will be key to achieving optimal results. Thus, success will only be restricted by our vision and our innovation—or lack of it. Fortunately, we have access to some of the innovation we need through genetic engineering and the number of non-natural compounds obtained is increasing rapidly to supplement the never-ending stream of novel compounds that Nature can supply.

For 50 years, I have worked alongside specialised researchers in fields such as Biochemistry, Microbiology, and Clinical medicine. My approach has always been influenced by the tenet "One encounter, one chance." This encompasses the deep reverence that is an essential part of the Tea Ceremony (or Chanoyu), which is held in the highest esteem in Japanese culture. As well as the certain fact that exact circumstances at any point in time will never happen again, I believe it is important to seize opportunities as and when they arise. And to maintain profound respect and consideration for all my colleagues—as well as for Nature and the microorganisms I work with. Such sentiments form the fundamental basis for all good scientific research and discovery.

BOX 1. POTENTIAL USES OF IVERMECTIN

- **Streptocerciasis:** occurs in Central Africa due to infection with the nematode *Dipetalonema streptocerca* transmitted by the bite of insects of the genus *Culicoides*. Ivermectin kills the disease-causing microfilaria [B1].
- **Trichinosis:** globally, 11 million individuals are infected with Trichinella roundworms, which can be killed by ivermectin [B2].
- **Myiasis:** infestation by fly larvae that grow inside the host. It is a relatively common affliction of people in poor, rural tropical communities. Surgical removal of the parasites is often the only remedy. Oral myiasis has been successfully treated with ivermectin [B3].
- **Vector control:** The avermectins are toxic to almost all insects, causing water balance difficulties, as well as disruption of moulting and metamorphosis, death occurring from between 1 and 30 days [B4]. Ivermectin kills a wide variety of insects [B5, B6] and is highly effective against bedbugs, capable of eradicating or preventing bedbug infestations [B7].
- **Malaria:** Mosquitos (*Anopheles gambiae*) that transmit *Plasmodium falciparum*, the most dangerous malaria-causing parasite in Africa, can be killed by the ivermectin present in the human bloodstream after a standard oral dose [B8–B10]. At sub-micromolecular levels, ivermectin inhibits the nuclear import of polypeptides of the signal recognition particle of *P. falciparum* (PfSRP), killing the parasites. This raises the possibility that ivermectin could become a useful, novel malaria transmission control tool [B11, B12].
- **Leishmaniasis:** Ivermectin kills sandflies (*Phlebotomus papatasi*) that transmit the parasites that cause leishmaniasis and has been suggested as a means to help control them [B13, B14]. Ivermectin also kills various stages of the disease-causing parasite, *Leishmania major* [B15, B16].
- **Trypanosomiasis:** Ivermectin has promise as a systemic drug against the tsetse fly vectors of African trypanosomiasis (Sleeping Sickness) [B17, B18]. There is scope for investigating the use of ivermectin in the treatment of trypanosomiasis from several aspects [B19].
- **Schistosomiasis:** A research collaboration was established between the Kitasato Institute and the Oswaldo Cruz Institute (Fiocruz) in Brazil in 2008 to test ivermectin analogues and compounds from the chemical libraries of each institute in screening systems being operated in the two institutions. Promising results were immediately found with regard to the impact of ivermectin on the intermediate host snails responsible

for maintaining the schistosomiasis re-infection cycle, offering the prospect of using ivermectin to help control one of the world's major neglected diseases [in press].

- **Antiviral:** Ivermectin is a broad-spectrum inhibitor of importin a/b nuclear import, demonstrating potent antiviral activity towards HIV-1 and dengue viruses [B20].

  Ivermectin also strongly inhibits replication of several flaviviruses (yellow fever dengue, Japanese encephalitis, and tick-borne encephalitis) [B21, B22].
- **Antibacterial:** Ivermectin prevents *Chlamydia trachomatis* infection [B23]. It is also reported to be bactericidal against a range of mycobacterial species, including *Mycobacterium tuberculosis* [B24] and *M. ulcerans* [B25].
- **Anticancer:** Ivermectin promotes cell death in leukaemia cells and ME-180 cervical cancer cells [B26–B28]

ACKNOWLEDGEMENTS

I would like to convey my sincerest gratitude to all those concerned in my being chosen as a recipient of the 2015 Nobel Prize in Physiology or Medicine, which I humbly receive on behalf of everyone who has helped me on every step of a wonderful journey of discovery.

I would also like to express my particular and profound thanks to all the people who have supported me and my research on the discovery, development and deployment of the avermectins/ivermectin, to Professor Andy Crump for his invaluable cooperation in the preparation of this account and, of course, to my family for their unwavering and paramount support.

REFERENCES

1. Speare, R. & Durrheim, D. (2004) Mass treatment with ivermectin: an underutilized public health strategy. *Bull. World Health Organ.*, 82 (8); 559–636.
2. Campbell, WC. (1981) An introduction to the avermectins. *N. Z. Vet. J.* 29; 174–178.
3. Ostlind, DA., Cifelli, S. & Lang, R. (1979) Insecticidal activity of the parasitic avermectins. *Vet. Rec.* 105; 168.
4. Putter, I., MacConnell, JG., Preiser, FA., Haidri, AA., Ristich, SS. & Dybas, RA. (1981) Avermectins: novel insecticides, acaricides and nematicides from a soil microorganism. *Experientia* 37; 963–964.
5. Gans, J., Wolinsky, M. & Dunbar, J. (2005) Computational improvements reveal great bacterial diversity and high metal toxicity in soil. *Science* 309; 1387–1390.

6. Stapley, EO. & Woodruff, HB. (1982) Avermectins, antiparasitic lactones produced by *Streptomyces avermitilis* isolated from a soil in Japan. 154–170 In: *Trends in Antibiotic research: Genetics, biosyntheses, actions & new substances* (Eds; Umezawa, H., Demain, AL., Hata, T., & Hutchinson, CR.) JARA.
7. Inahashi, Y., Iwatsuki, M., Ishiyama, A., Namatame, M., Nishihara-Tsukashima, A., Matsumoto, A., Hirose, T., Sunazuka, T., Yamada, H., Otoguro, K., Takahashi, Y., Ōmura, S. & Shiomi, K. (2011) Spoxazomicins A-C, novel antitrypanosomal alkaloids produced by an endophytic actinomycete, *Streptosporangium oxazolinicum* K07-0460T. *J. Antibiot.* 64; 303–307.
8. Nakashima, T., Okuyama, R., Kamiya, Y., Matsumoto, A., Iwatsuki, M., Inahashi, Y., Yamaji, K., Takahashi, Y. & Ōmura, S. (2013) Trehangelins A, B and C, novel photo-oxidative hemolysis inhibitors produced by an endophytic actinomycete, *Polymorphospora rubra* K07-0510. *J. Antibiot.* 66; 311–317.
9. Ōmura, S., Tanaka, H., Awaya, J., Narimatsu, Y., Konda, Y. & Hata, T. (1974) Pyrindicin, a new alkaloid from a *Streptomyces* strain. Taxonomy, fermentation, isolation and biological activity. *Agric. Biol. Chem.* 38; 899–906.
10. Ōmura, S., Iwai, Y., Hirano, A., Nakagawa, A., Awaya, J., Tsuchiya, H., Takahashi, Y. & Masuma, R. (1977). A new alkaloid AM-2282 of *Streptomyces* origin. Taxonomy, fermentation, isolation and preliminary characterization. *J. Antibiot.* 30; 275–282.
11. Nakano, H. & Ōmura, S. (2009) Chemical biology of natural indolocarbazole products: 30 years since the discovery of staurosporine. *J. Antibiot.* 62; 17–26.
12. Yamasaki, T., Takahashi, A., Pan, J., Yamaguchi, N. & Yokoyama, KK. (2009). Phosphorylation of Activation Transcription Factor-2 at serine 121 by protein kinase C controls c-Jun-mediated activation of transcription. *J. Biol. Chem.* 284; 8567–8581.
13. Atwell, S., Adams, JM., Badger, J., Buchanan, MD., Feil, IK., Froning, KJ., Gao, X., Hendle, J., Keegan, K., Leon, BC., Müller-Dieckmann, HJ., Nienaber, VL., Noland, BW., Post, K., Rajashankar, KR., Ramos, A., Russell, M., Burley, SK. & Buchanan, SG. (2004) A novel mode of Gleevec binding is revealed by the structure of spleen tyrosine kinase. *J. Biol. Chem.* 279; 55827–55832.
14. Ōmura, S., Fujimoto, T., Otoguro, K., Matsuzaki, K., Moriguchi, R., Tanaka, H., & Sasaki Y. (1991) Lactacystin, a novel microbial metabolite, induces neuritogenesis of neuroblastoma cells. *J. Antibiot.* 44; 113–116.
15. Ōmura, S., Katagiri, M., Atsumi, K., Hata, T., Jakubowski, AA., Bleecker-Springs, E. & Tishler, M. (1974) Structure of prumycin. *J. Chem. Soc., Perkin Trans.* 1; 1627–1631.
16. Ōmura, S., Tishler, M., Nakagawa, A., Hironaka, Y. & Hata, T. (1972) Relationships of structure and microbiological activities of the 16-membered macrolides. *J. Med. Chem.* 15; 1011–1015.
17. Hata, T., Ōmura, S., Katagiri, M., Atsumi, K. & Awaya, J. (1971) A new antifungal antibiotic, prumycin. *J. Antibiot.* 24; 900–901.
18. Sano, Y., Nomura, S., Kamio, Y., Ōmura, S. & Hata, T. (1967) Studies on cerulenin. III. Isolation and physico-chemical properties of cerulenin. *J. Antibiot.* 20; 344–348.
19. Ōmura, S., Katagiri, M., Umezawa, I., Komiyama, K., Maekawa, T., Sekikawa, K., Matsumae, A. & Hata, T. (1968) Structure-biological activities relationships among leucomycins and their derivatives. *J. Antibiot.* 21; 532–538.

20. Ōmura, S., Iwata, R., Iwai, Y., Taga, S., Tanaka, Y. & Tomoda, H. (1985) Luminamicin, a new antibiotic. Production, isolation and physico-chemical and biological properties. *J. Antibiot.* 38; 1322–1326.
21. Ōmura, S., Tanaka, H., Oiwa, R., Awaya, J., Masuma, R. & Tanaka, K. (1977) New antitumor antibiotics, OS-4742 A1, A2, B1 and B2 produced by a strain of *Streptomyces. J. Antibiot.* 30; 908–916.
22. Ōmura, S., Otoguro, K., Nishikiori, T., Oiwa, R. & Iwai, Y. (1981) Setamycin, a new antibiotic. *J. Antibiot.* 34; 1253–1256.
23. Ōmura, S., Nakagawa, A. & Ohno, H. (1979) Structure of elasnin, a novel elastase inhibitor. *J. Am. Chem. Soc.* 101; 4386–4388.
24. Gullo, VP., Zimmerman, SB., Dewey, RS., Hensens, O., Cassidy, PJ., Oiwa, R. & Ōmura S. (1982) Factumycin, a new antibiotic (A40A): fermentation, isolation and antibacterial spectrum. *J. Antibiot.* 35; 1705–1707.
25. Sarrett, LH. & Roche, C. (1995) Max Tishler. In *Biographical memoirs* 66, 352–369 National Academies Press.
26. Miller, TW. & Gullo, VP. (1989) Avermectins and related compounds: In *Natural Products Isolation: Separation Methods for Antimicrobials* (Eds. Wagman, GH and Cooper, R.) Journal of Chromatography Library, Volume 43. Elsevier, Amsterdam. pp. 347–376
27. Campbell, WC., Fisher, MH., Stapley, EO., Albers-Schonberg, G. & Jacob, TA. (1983) Ivermectin: a potent new antiparasitic agent. *Science* 221; 823–828.
28. Takahashi, Y. Matsumoto, A., Seino, A., Ueno, J., Iwai, Y. & Ōmura, S. (2002) *Streptomyces avermectinius* sp. nov., an avermectin-producing strain. *Int. J. Syst. Evol. Microbiol.* 52; 2163–2168.
29. Albers-Schönberg, G., Arison, BH., Chabala, JC., Douglas, AW., Eskola, P., Fisher, MH., Lusi, A., Mrozik, H., Smith, JL. & Tolman, RL. (1981) Avermectins: Structure determination. *J. Am. Chem. Soc.* 103; 4216–4221.
30. Burg, RW., Miller. BM., Baker, EE., Birnbaum, J., Currie, SA., Hartman, R., Kong, YL., Monaghan, RL., Olson, G., Putter, I., Tunac, JB., Wallick, H., Stapley, EO., Oiwa, R. & Ōmura, S. (1979) Avermectins, new family of potent anthelmintic agents: producing organisms and fermentation. *Antimicrob. Agents Chemother.* 15; 361–367.
31. Miller, TW., Chaiet, L., Cole, DJ., Cole, LJ., Flor, JE., Goegleman, RT., Gullo, VP., Joshua, H., Kempf, AJ., Krellwitz, WR., Monaghan, RL., Ormond, RE., Wilson, KE., Albers-Schönberg, G. & Putter, I. (1979) Avermectins, new family of potent anthelmintic agents: isolation and chromatographic properties. *Antimicrob. Agents Chemother.* 15; 368–371.
32. Egerton, JR., Ostlind, DA., Blair, LS., Eary, CH., Suhayda, D., Cifelli, S., Riek, RF., & Campbell, W. (1979) Avermectins, new family of potent anthelmintic agents: efficacy of the B1A component. *Antimicrob. Agents Chemother.* 15; 372–378.
33. Chabala, JC., Mrozik, H., Tolman, RL., Eskola, P., Lusi, A., Peterson, LH., Woods, MF., Fisher, MH. & Campbell, WC. (1980) Ivermectin, a new broad-spectrum antiparasitic agent. *J. Med. Chem.* 23; 1134–1136.
34. Campbell, WC. (1981) Efficacy of the avermectins against filarial parasites: a short review. *Vet. Res. Commun.* 5; 251–262.
35. Hotson, IK. (1982). The avermectins: A new family of antiparasitic agents. *J. South African Vet. Assoc.* 53; 87–90.

36. Barth, D. & Sutherland, IH. (1980) Investigations of the efficacy of ivermectin against ectoparasites in cattle. *Zentral. Bakt. Parasit. Infect. Hyg.* 57; 319.
37. Centurier, C. & Barth, D. (1980) On the efficacy of ivermectin versus ticks (*O. moubata*, *R. appendiculatus* and *A. variegatum*) in cattle. *Zentral. Bakt. Parasit. Infect. Hyg.* 58; 319–320.
38. Campbell, WC. (Ed.) (1989) *Ivermectin and abamectin*. Springer-Verlag, New York. 363pp.
39. Frost, L. Reich, MR. & Fujisaki, T. (2002) A partnership for ivermectin: Social worlds and boundary objects. In *Public-Private: Partnerships for Global Health* (Ed. Reich MR). Harvard University Press. pp. 87–114.
40. Ōmura, S. (2002) In *Macrolide Antibiotics—Chemistry, Biology and Practice* 2nd edn (Ed. Ōmura, S.) 571–576 Academic Press, San Diego.
41. Duce, R. & Scott, RH. (1985) Actions of dihydroavermectin B1a on insect muscle. *Br. J. Pharmacol.* 85; 395–401.
42. Geary, TG., Sims, SM., Thomas, EM., Vanover, L., Davis JP., Winterrowd, CA., Klein, RD., Ho, NF. & Thompson, DP. (1993) *Haemonchus contortus*: ivermectin induced paralysis of the pharynx. *Exp. Parasitol.* 77; 88–96.
43. Fritz, LC., Wang, CC. & Gorio, A. (1979) Avermectin B1a irreversibly blocks postsynaptic potentials at the lobster neuromuscular junction by reducing muscle membrane resistance. *Proc. Natl Acad. Sci.* (USA) 76; 2062–2066.
44. Mellin, TN., Busch, RD. & Wang, CC. (1983) Post-synaptic inhibition of invertebrate neuromuscular transmission by avermectin B1a. *Neuropharmacology* 22; 89–96.
45. Turner, M. & Schaeffer JM. (1989) In *Ivermectin and Abamectin* (ed. Campbell, WC.) pp. 73–88 (Springer-Verlag, New York).
46. Campbell, WC. (1985) Ivermectin: an update. *Parasitol. Today* 1; 10–16.
47. del Mar Saez-De-Ocariz, M., McKinster, CD., Orozco-Covarrubias, L., Tamayo-Sánchez, L. & Ruiz-Maldonaldo, R. (2002) Treatment of 18 children with scabies or cutaneous larva migrans using ivermectin. *Clin. Exp. Dermatol.* 27; 264–267.
48. Maizels, RM. & Lawrence, RA. (1991) Immunological tolerance: the key feature in human filariasis? *Parasitol. Today* 7; 271–276.
49. Taylor, HR. & Greene, BM. (1989) The status of ivermectin in the treatment of human onchocerciasis. *Am. J. Trop. Med. Hyg.* 41; 460–466.
50. Plaisier, AP., Alley, ES., Boatin, BA., Van Oortmarssen, GJ, Remme, H., De Vlas, SJ., Bonneux, L. & Habbema, JD. (1995) Irreversible effects of ivermectin on adult parasites in onchocerciasis patients in the Onchocerciasis Control Programme in West Africa. *J. Infect. Dis.* 172; 204–210.
51. Basáñez, M-G., Pion, SD., Boakes, E., Filipe, JA., Churcher, TS. & Boussinesq, M. (2008) Effect of single-dose ivermectin on *Onchocerca volvulus*: a systematic review and meta-analysis. *Lancet Infect. Dis.* 8; 310–322.
52. Duke, BO., Soula, G., Zea-Flores, G., Bratthauer, GL & Doumbo, O. (1991) Migration and death of skin-dwelling *Onchocerca volvulus* microfilariae after treatment with ivermectin. *Trop. Med. Parasitol.* 42; 25–30.
53. Mackenzie, CD., Geary, TG. & Gerlach, JA. (2003) Possible pathogenic pathways in the adverse clinical events seen following ivermectin administrations in onchocerciasis patients. *Filaria J.* 2 (Suppl. 1); S5.
54. Moreno, Y., Nabhan, JF., Solomon, J., MacKenzie, CD, & Geary, TG. (2010)

Ivermectin disrupts the function of the excretory-secretory appartus in microfilariae of *Brugia malayi*. *Proc. Nat. Acad. Sci USA*. 107; 20120–20125.

55. Crump, A. & Ōmura, S. (2011) Ivermectin, "Wonder drug" from Japan: the human use perspective. *Proc. Jpn. Acad. Ser. B: Phys. Biol. Sci.* 87; 13–28.
56. Fujisaki, T & Reich, M. (1998) TDR's contribution to the development of ivermectin for onchocerciasis. TDR, Geneva. (TDR/ER/RD/98.3)
57. WHO/TDR (1976) Participation of the Pharmaceutical sector. (TDR/WP/76.30)
58. Lucas, AO. (2002) Public-Private Partnerships: Illustrative examples. In *Public-Private Partnerships for Public Health* (Ed. Reich M). Harvard University Press, Cambridge, Mass. USA. pp 19–39.
59. Campbell WC. (2012) History of avermectin and ivermectin, with notes on the history of other macrocyclic lactone antiparasitic agents. *Curr. Pharm. Biotech.* 13; 853–865.
60. Sturchio, JL. (1992) The Decision to Donate Mectizan: Historical Background. Merck & Co., Inc. Rahway, New Jersey, USA (unpublished document).
61. Aziz, MA., Diallo, S., Diop, IM., Larivière, M. & Porta, M. (1982) Efficacy and tolerance of ivermectin in human onchocerciasis. *Lancet* 2; 171–173.
62. Coulaud, JP., Larivière, M., Gervais, MC., Gaxotte, P., Aziz, A., Deluol, AM & Cenac, J. (1983) Treatment of human onchocerciasis with ivermectin. *Bull. Soc. Pathol. Exot. Filiales.* 76; 681–688.
63. Dadzie, KY., Bird, AC., Awadzi, K., Schulz-Key, H., Gilles, HM. & Aziz, MA. (1987) Ocular findings in a double-blind study of ivermectin versus diethylcarbamazine versus placebo in the treatment of onchocerciasis. *Brit. J. Opthalmol.* 71; 78–85.
64. Larivière, M., Aziz, M., Weimann, D., Ginoux, J., Gaxotte, P., Vingtain, P., Beauvais, B., Derouin, F., Schultz-Key, H., Basset, D. & Sarfati, C. (1985) Double-blind study of ivermectin and diethylcarbamazine in African onchocerciasis patients with ocular involvement. *Lancet* 326; 174–177.
65. Taylor, HR. & Greene, BM. (1989) The status of ivermectin in the treatment of human onchocerciasis. *Am. J. Trop. Med. Hyg.* 41; 460–466.
66. Awadzi, K. (1980) The chemotherapy of onchocerciasis II: Quantification of the clinical reaction to microfilaricides. *Ann. Trop. Med. Parasitol.* 74; 189–197.
67. Awadzi, K., Dadzie, KY., Shulz-Key, H., Haddock, DR., Gilles, HM., & Aziz, MA. (1985) The chemotherapy of onchocerciasis X. An assessment of four single dose treatment regimes of MK-933 (ivermectin) in human onchocerciasis. *Ann. Trop. Med. Parasitol.* 79; 63–78.
68. Campbell, W.C. (1991) Ivermectin as an antiparasitic agent for use in humans. *Annu. Rev. Microbiol.* 45; 445–474.
69. Coffeng, LE., Stolk, WA., Zouré, HG., Veerman, JL., Agblewonu, KB., Murdoch, ME., Noma, M., Fobi, G., Richardus, JH., Bundy, DA., Habbema, D., de Vlas, SJ. & Amazigo, UV. (2013) African Programme for Onchocerciasis Control 1995–2015: model-estimated health impact and cost. *PLoS Negl. Trop. Dis.* 7; e2032.
70. *UNESCO World Science Report 2005*. p.198. UNESCO, 2005, Paris.
71. Diallo, S., Aziz, MA., Ndir, O., Badiane, S, Bah, IB. & Gaye, O. (1987) Dose-ranging study of ivermectin in the treatment of Filariasis due to *Wuchereria bancrofti*. *Lancet* 329; 1030.

72. WHO/TDR (1995) *Tropical Disease Research: Progress 1975–94*. p. 95. WHO, Geneva.
73. Kumaraswami, V., Ottesen, EA. & Vijayasekran, V (1988) Ivermectin for treatment of *Wuchereria bancrofti* filariasis: efficacy and adverse reactions. *J. Am. Med. Assoc.* 259; 3150–3153.
74. Ottesen, EA., Kumaraswami, V. & Vijayasekran, V. (1990) A controlled trial of ivermectin and diethylcarbamazine in lymphatic filariasis. *N. Eng. J. Med.* 322; 1113–1117.
75. Richards Jr, FO., Eberhard, ML., Bryan, RT., Mcneeley, DF., Lammie, PJ., Mcneeley, MB., Bernard, Y. Hightower, AW. & Spencer, HC. (1991) Comparison of high-dose ivermectin and diethylcarbamazine for activity against Bancroftian filariasis in Haiti. *Am. J. Trop. Med. Hyg.* 44; 3–10.
76. Mectizan Donation Program (2015) *Annual Highlights* (2104) MDP, Atlanta.
77. WHO (2015) *Weekly Epidemiological Report* 90, 49; 661–680.
78. Ōmura, S. & Crump, A. (2014) Ivermectin: panacea for resource-poor communities? *Trends Parasitol.* 30; 445–455.
79. World Health Organization (2014) Strongyloidiasis: Key Facts, World Health Organization, Geneva.
80. Ohtaki, N., Taniguchi, H. & Ohtomo, H. (2003) Oral ivermectin treatment in two cases of scabies: effective in crusted scabies induced by corticosteroid but ineffective in nail scabies. *J. Dermatol.* 30; 411–416.
81. Karthikeyan, K. (2005) Treatment of scabies: newer perspectives. *Postgrad. Med. J.* 81; 7–11.
82. Pilger, D., Heukelbach, J., Khakban, A., Oliveira, FA., Fengler, G. & Feldmeier H. (2010) Household-wide ivermectin treatment for head lice in an impoverished community: randomized observer-blinded trial. *Bull. World Health Organ.* 88; 90–96.
83. Heukelbach, J., Wilcke,T., Winter, B. & Feldmeier H. (2005) Epidemiology and morbidity of scabies and *Pediculosis capitis* in resource-poor communities in Brazil. *Br. J. Dermatol.* 153; 150–156.
84. Chosidow, O., Giraudeau, B., Cottrell, J., Izri, A., Hofmann, R., Mann, SG. & Burgess I. (2010) Oral ivermectin versus malathion lotion for difficult-to-treat head lice. *N. Engl. J. Med.* 362; 896–905.
85. Nofal, A. (2010) Oral ivermectin for head lice: a comparison with 0.5% topical malathion lotion. *J. Ger. Soc. Dermatol.* 8; 985–988.
86. Currie, MJ., Reynolds, GJ. & Glasgow, N. (2010) A pilot study of the use of oral ivermectin to treat head lice in primary school students in Australia. *Pediatr. Dermatol.* 27; 595–599.
87. Ameen, M., Arenas, R., Villanueva-Reyes, J., Ruiz-Esmenjaud, J., Millar, D., Domínguez-Dueñas, F., Haddad-Angulo, A. & Rodríguez-Alvarez M. (2010) Oral ivermectin for treatment of *Pediculosis capitis*. *Pediatr. Infect. Dis. J.* 29; 991–993.
88. Pariser, DM., Meinking, TL., Bell, M., & Ryan, WG. (2012) Topical 0.5% ivermectin lotion for treatment of head lice. *N. Engl. J. Med.* 367; 1687–1693.
89. Belizario, VY., Amarillo, ME., de Leon, WU., de los Reyes, AE., Bugayong, MG. & Macatangay, BJ. (2003) A comparison of the efficacy of single doses of albendazole, ivermectin, and diethylcarbamazine alone or in combinations against *Ascaris* and *Trichuris* spp. *Bull. World Health Organ.* 81; 35–42.

90. Marti, H., Haji, HJ., Savioli, L., Chwaya, HM., Mgeni, AF., Ameir, JS. & Hatz C. (1996) A comparative trial of a single-dose ivermectin versus three days of albendazole for treatment of *Strongyloides stercoralis* and other soil-transmitted helminth infections in children. *Am. J. Trop. Med. Hyg.* 55; 477–481.
91. Bieri, FA., Li. YS., Yuan, LP., He, YK., Gray, DJ., Williams, GM. & McManus DP. (2014) School-based health education targeting intestinal worms—further support for integrated control. *PLoS Negl. Trop. Dis.* 8, e2621.
92. Bethony, J., Brooker, S., Albonico, M., Geiger, SM., Loukas, A., Diemert, D. & Hotez PJ. (2006) Soil-transmitted helminth infections: ascariasis, trichuriasis, and hookworm. *Lancet* 367; 1521–1532.
93. Nontasut, P., Bussaratid, V., Chullawichit, S., Charoensook, N. & Visetsuk, K. (2000) Comparison of ivermectin and albendazole treatment for gnathostomiasis. *Southeast Asian J. Trop. Med. Public Health* 31; 374–377.
94. Fischer, P., Tukesiga, E. & Büttner, DW. (1999) Long-term suppression of *Mansonella streptocerca* microfilariae after treatment with ivermectin. *J. Infect. Dis.* 180; 1403–1405.
95. Bregani, ER., Rovellini, A., Mbaidoum, N. & Magnini MG. (2006) Comparison of different anthelminthic drug regimens against *Mansonella perstans* filariasis. *Trans. R. Soc. Trop. Med. Hyg.* 100; 458–463.
96. Skopets, B., Wilson, RP., Griffith, JW. & Lang, CM. (1996) Ivermectin toxicity in young mice. *Lab. Anim. Sci.* 46; 111–112.
97. Kim, JS. & Crichlow, EC. (1995) Clinical signs of ivermectin toxicity and efficacy of antigabaergic convulsants as antidotes for ivermectin poisoning in epileptic chickens. *Vet. Hum. Toxicol.* 37; 122–126.
98. Iliff-Sizemore, SA., Partlow, MR. & Kelley ST. (1990) Ivermectin toxicology in a rhesus macaque. *Vet. Hum. Toxicol.* 32; 530–532.
99. DeMarco, JH., Heard, DJ., Fleming, GJ., Lock, BA. & Scase, TJ. (2002) Ivermectin toxicosis after topical administration in dog-faced fruit bats (*Cynopterus brachyotis*). *J. Zoo Wildl. Med.* 33; 147–150.
100. Teare, JA. & Bush, M. (1983) Toxicity and efficacy of ivermectin in chelonians. *J. Am. Vet. Med. Assoc.* 183; 1195–1197.
101. Heukelbach, J., Winter, B., Wilcke, T., Muehlen, M., Albrecht, S., de Oliveira, FA., Kerr-Pontes, LR., Liesenfeld, O. & Feldmeier, H. (2004) Selective mass treatment with ivermectin to control intestinal helminthiasis and parasitic skin diseases in a severely affected population. *Bull. World Health Organ.* 82; 563–571.
102. Heukelbach, J., Wilcke, T., Winter, B., Sales de Oliveira, FA., Sabóia Moura, RC., Harms, G., Liesenfeld, O. & Feldmeier, H. (2004) Efficacy of ivermectin in a patient population concomitantly infected with intestinal helminths and ectoparasites. *Arzneimittelforschung* 54; 416–421.
103. Moncayo, AL., Vaca, M., Amorim, L., Rodriguez, A., Erazo, S., Oviedo, G., Quinzo, I., Padilla, M., Chico, M., Lovato, R., Gomez, E., Barreto, ML. & Cooper, PJ. (2008) Impact of long-term treatment with ivermectin on the prevalence and intensity of soil-transmitted helminth infections. *PLoS Negl. Trop. Dis.* 2, e293.
104. Anosike, JC., Dozie, IN., Ameh, GI., Ukaga, CN., Nwoke, BE., Nzechukwu,

CT., Udujih, OS. & Nwosu, DC. (2007) The varied beneficial effects of ivermectin (Mectizan) treatment, as observed within onchocerciasis foci in southeastern Nigeria. *Ann. Trop. Med. Parasitol.* 101; 593–600.

105. Okeibunor, JC., Amuyunzu-Nyamongo, M., Onyeneho, NG., Tchounkeu, YF., Manianga, C., Kabali, AT. & Leak, S. (2011) Where would I be without ivermectin? Capturing the benefits of community-directed treatment with ivermectin in Africa. *Trop. Med. Int. Health* 16; 608–621.

106. Kaplan, RM. (2004) Drug resistance in nematodes of veterinary importance: a status report. *Trends Parasitol.* 20; 477–481.

107. Dent, JA. (2000) The genetics of ivermectin resistance in *C. elegans*. *Proc. Nat. Acad. Sci. (USA)* 97; 2674–2679.

108. Wolstenholme, AJ. (2004) Drug resistance in veterinary helminths. *Trends Parasitol.* 20; 469–476.

109. Lustigman, S. & McCarter, JP. (2007) Ivermectin resistance in *Onchocerca volvulus*: Toward a genetic basis. *PLoS Negl Trop Dis.* 1; e76.

110. Ikeda, H., Wang, L.-R., Ohta, T., Inokoshi, J. & Ōmura, S. (1998) Cloning of the gene encoding avermectin B 5-O-methyltransferase in avermectin-producing *Streptomyces avermitilis*. *Gene* 206; 175–180.

111. Ikeda, H. & Ōmura, S. (1997) Avermectin biosynthesis. *S. Chem. Rev.* 97; 2591–2609.

112. Ikeda, H., Nonomiya, T., Usami, M., Ohta, T. & Ōmura, S. (1999) Organization of the biosynthetic gene cluster for the polyketide anthelmintic macrolide avermectin in *Streptomyces avermitilis*. *Proc. Natl. Acad. Sci. (USA)* 96; 9509–9514.

113. Ikeda, H., Nonomiya, T. & Ōmura, S. (2001) Organization of biosynthetic gene cluster for avermectin in *Streptomyces avermitilis*: analysis of enzymatic domains in four polyketide synthases. *J. Ind. Microbiol. & Biotechnol.* 27; 170–176.

114. Carter, GT, Nietsche, JA., Hertz, MR., Williams, DR., Siegel, MM., Morton, GO., James, JC. & Borders, DB. (1988) LL-F28249 antibiotic complex: a new family of antiparasitic macrocyclic lactones. Isolation, characterization and structures of LL-F28249 alpha, beta, gamma, lambda. *J. Antibiot.* 41; 519–529.

115. Ōmura, S., Ikeda, H., Ishikawa, J., Hanamoto, A., Takahashi, C., Shinose, M., Takahashi, Y., Horikawa, H., Nakazawa, H., Osonoe, T., Kikuchi, H., Shiba, T., Sakaki, Y. & Hattori, M. (2001) Genome sequence of an industrial microorganism *Streptomyces avermitilis*: deducing the ability of producing secondary metabolites. *Proc. Natl. Acad. Sci. (USA)* 98; 12215–12220.

116. Ikeda, H., Ishikawa, J., Hanamoto, A., Shinose, M., Kikuchi, H., Shiba, T., Sakaki, Y., Hattori, M. & Ōmura. S. (2003) Complete genome sequence and comparative analysis of the industrial microorganism *Streptomyces avermitilis*. *Nat Biotechnol.* 21; 526–531.

117. Nett, M., Ikeda, H., Moore, BS. (2009) Genomic basis for natural product biosynthetic diversity in the actinomycetes. *Nat. Prod. Rep.* 26; 1362–1384.

118. Komatsu, M., Uchiyama, T., Ōmura, S., Cane, D. E. & Ikeda, H. (2010) Genome-minimized *Streptomyces* host for the heterologous expression of secondary metabolism. *Proc. Natl. Acad. Sci. (USA)* 107; 2646–2651.

BOX REFERENCES

B1. Fischer, P., Bamuhiiga, J. & Büttner, DW. (1997) Treatment of human *Mansonella streptocerca* infection with ivermectin. *Trop. Med. Int. Health* 2; 191–199.

B2. Basyoni, MM. & El-Sabaa, AA. (2013) Therapeutic potential of myrrh and ivermectin against experimental *Trichinella spiralis* infection in mice. *Korean J. Parasitol.* 51; 297–304.

B3. Shinohara, EH., Martini, MZ., de Oliveira Neto, HG. & Takahashi, A. (2004) Oral myiasis treated with ivermectin: case report. *Braz. Dent. J.* 15; 79–81.

B4. Strong, L. & Brown, TA. (1987) Avermectins in insect control and biology: a review. *Bull. Entomol. Res.* 77; 357–389.

B5. Jackson, HC. (1989) Ivermectin as a systemic insecticide. *Parasitol. Today* 5; 146–156.

B6. Tesh, RB. & Guzman, H. (1990) Mortality and infertility in adult mosquitoes after the ingestion of blood containing ivermectin. *Am. J. Trop. Med. Hyg.* 43; 229–233.

B7. Sheele, JM., Anderson, JF., Tran, TD., Teng, YA., Byers, PA., Ravi, BS. & Sonenshine DE. (2013) Ivermectin causes *Cimex lectularius* (Bedbug) morbidity and mortality. *J. Emerg. Med.* 45; 433–440.

B8. Chacour, C., Lines, J. & Whitty, CJM. (2010) Effect of ivermectin on *Anopheles gambiae* mosquitoes fed on humans; the potential of oral insecticides in malaria control. *J. Infect. Dis.* 202; 113–116.

B9. Kobylinski, KC., Deus, KM., Butters, MP., Hongyu, T., Gray, M., da Silva, IM., Sylla, M. & Foy BD. (2010) The effect of oral anthelmintics on the survivorship and re-feeding frequency of anthropophilic mosquito disease vectors. *Acta Trop.* 116; 119–126.

B10. Kobylinski, KC., Sylla, M., Chapman, PL., Sarr, MD. & Foy BD. (2011) Ivermectin mass drug administration for humans disrupts malaria parasite transmission in Senegalese villages. *Am. J. Trop. Med. Hyg.* 85; 3–5.

B11. Panchal, M., Rawat, K., Kumar, G., Kibria, KM., Singh, S., Kalamuddin, M., Mohmmed, A., Malhotra, P. & Tuteja R. (2014) *Plasmodium falciparum* signal recognition particle components and anti-parasitic effect of ivermectin in blocking nucleo-cytoplasmic shuttling of SRP. *Cell Death Dis.* 5, e994.

B12. Foy, BD., Kobylinski, KC., da Silva, IM., Rasgon, JL. & Sylla, M. (2011) Endectocides for malaria control. *Trends Parasitol.* 27; 423–428.

B13. Mascari, TM., Mitchell, MA., Rowton, ED. & Foil, LD. (2008) Ivermectin as a rodent feed-through insecticide for control of immature sand flies (Diptera: Psychodidae). *J. Am. Mosq. Control Assoc.* 24; 323–326.

B14. Kadir, MA., Aswad, HS., Al-Samarai, AM. & Al-Mula, GA. (2009) Comparison between the efficacy of ivermectin and other drugs in treatment of cutaneous leishmaniasis. *Iraqi J. Vet. Sci.* 23 (Suppl. II); 175–180.

B15. Hanafi, HA., Szumlas, DE., Fryauff, DJ., El-Hossary, SS., Singer, GA., Osman, SG., Watany, N., Furman, BD. & Hoel, DF. (2011) Effects of ivermectin on blood-feeding *Phlebotomus papatasi* and the promastigote stage of *Leishmania major*. *Vector Borne Zoonotic Dis.* 11; 43–52.

B16. Rasheid, KA. & Morsy, TA. (1998) Efficacy of ivermectin on the infectivity of *Leishmania major* promastigotes. *J. Egypt Soc. Parasitol.* 28; 207–212

B17. Distelmans, W., D'Haeseleer, F. & Mortelmans J. (1983) Efficacy of systemic administration of ivermectin against tsetse flies. *Ann. Soc. Belg. Med. Trop.* 83, 119–125.

B18. Pooda, SH., Mouline, K., De Meeûs, T, Bengaly, Z. & Solano, P. (2013) Decrease in survival and fecundity of *Glossina palpalis gambiensis vanderplank 1949* (Diptera; Glossinidae) fed on cattle treated with single doses of ivermectin. *Parasit. Vectors* 6; 165

B19. Udensi, UK. & Fagbenro-Beyioku, AF. (2012) Effect of ivermectin on *Trypanosoma brucei brucei* in experimentally infected mice. *J. Vector Borne Dis.* 49; 143–150.

B20. Wagstaff, KM., Sivakumaran, H., Heaton, SM., Harrich, D. & Jans, DA. (2012) Ivermectin is a specific inhibitor of importin a/b-mediated nuclear import able to inhibit replication of HIV-1 and dengue viruses. *Biochem. J.* 443; 851–856.

B21. Mastrangelo, E., Pezzullo, M., De Burghgraeve, T., Kaptein, S., Pastorino, B., Dallmeier, K., de Lamballerie, X., Neyts, J., Hanson, AM., Frick, DN., Bolognesi, M. & Milani M. (2012) Ivermectin is a potent inhibitor of flavivirus replication specifically targeting NS3 helicase activity: new prospects for an old drug. *J. Antimcrob. Chemother.* 67; 1884–1894.

B22. Tay, MY., Fraser, JE., Chan, WK., Moreland, NJ., Rathore, AP., Wang, C., Vasudevan, SG. & Jans, DA. (2013) Nuclear localization of dengue virus (DENV) 1-4 nonstructural protein 5: protection against all 4 DENV serotypes by the inhibitor ivermectin. *Antiviral Res.* 99; 301–306.

B23. Pettengil, MA., Lam, VW., Ollawa, I., Marques-da-Silva, C. & Ojcius, DM. (2012) Ivermectin inhibits growth of *Chlamydia trachomatis* in epithelial cells. *PLoS ONE* 7; e48456

B24. Lim, LE., Vilchèze, C., Ng, C., Jacobs, WR. Jr, Ramón-García, S. & Thompson, CJ. (2013) Anthelmintic avermectins kill *Mycobacterium tuberculosis*, including multidrug-resistant clinical strains. *Antimicrob. Agents Chemother.* 57; 1040–1046.

B25. Omansen, TF., Porter, JL., Johnson, PD., van der Werf, TS., Stienstra, Y. & Stinear, TP. (2015) In-vitro activity of avermectins against *Mycobacterium ulcerans. PLoS Negl Trop Dis.* Mar 5;9(3); e0003549. doi: 10.1371/journal.pntd.0003549.

B26. Sharmeen, S., Skrtic, M., Sukhai, MA., Hurren, R., Gronda, M., Wang, X., Fonseca, SB., Sun, H., Wood, TE., Ward, R., Minden, MD., Batey, RA., Datti, A., Wrana, J., Kelley, SO. & Schimmer AD. (2010) The antiparasitic agent ivermectin induces chloride-dependent membrane hyperpolarization and cell death in leukemia cells. *Blood* 116; 3593–3603.

B27. Shen, M., Zhang, Y., Saba, N., Austin, CP., Wiestner, A. & Auld, DS. (2013) Identification of therapeutic candidates for chronic lymphocytic leukemia from a library of approved drugs. *PLoS ONE* 8; e75252

B28. Furusawa, S., Shibata, H., Nishimura, H., Nemoto, S., Takayanagi, M., Takayanagi, Y. & Sasaki, K-I. (2010) Potentiation of doxorubicin-induced apoptosis of resistant mouse leukaemia cells by ivermectin. *Pharm. Pharmacol. Commun.* 6; 129–134.

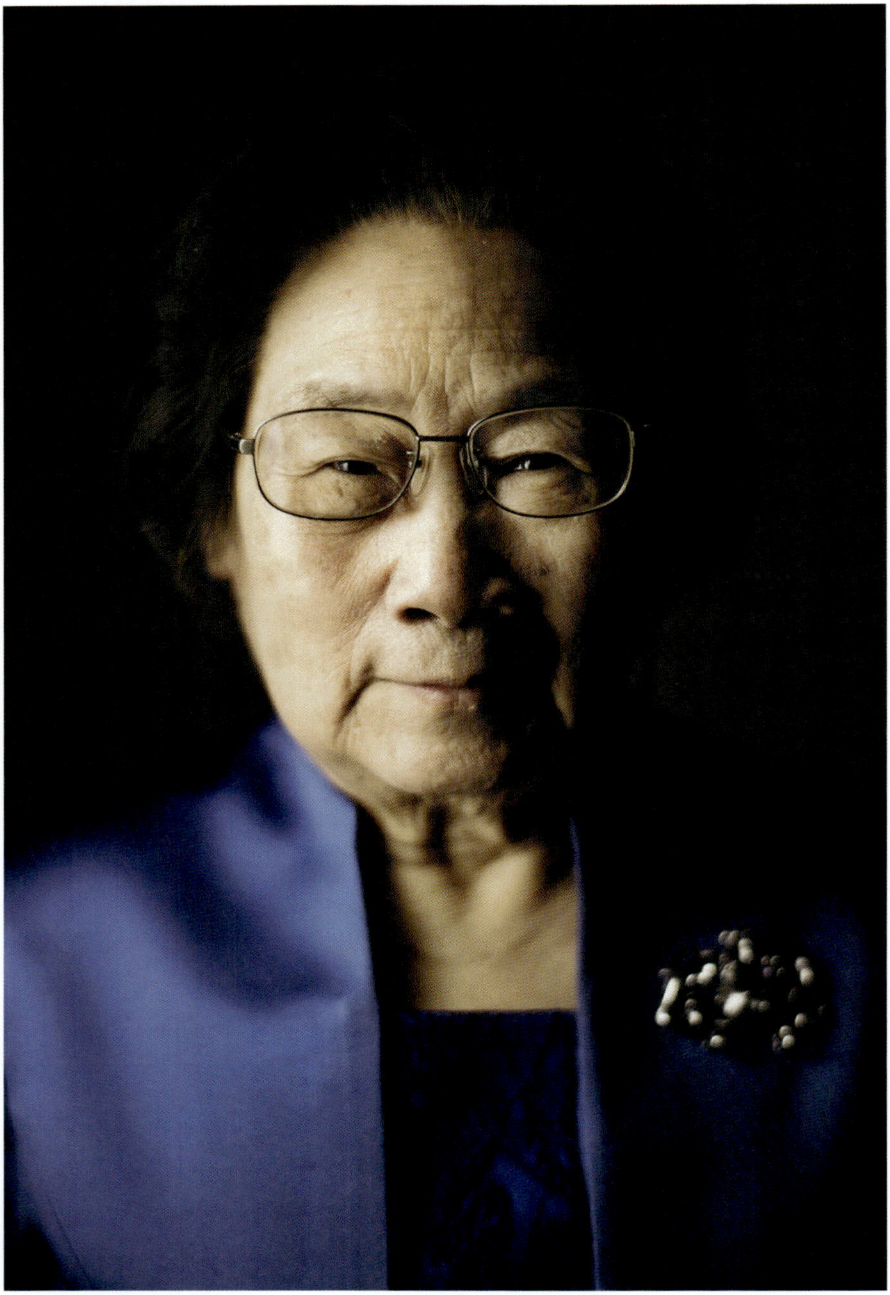

Tu Youyou. © Nobel Media AB. Photo: A. Mahmoud

Tu Youyou

MY CHILDHOOD

I was born on December 30, 1930 in Ningbo, a city on the east coast of China with a rich culture and over seven thousand years of history. Although it was a tumultuous age in China when I was a child, I was lucky enough to have completed a good education from primary to middle school.

My father worked in a bank while my mother looked after my four brothers and me, the only girl in our family. According to a recently discovered family tree, my ancestors lived in Ningbo for many generations. Our family's long history of highly valuing children's education and always considering this as the family's top priority allowed me to have good opportunities for attending the best schools in the region—from the private Ningbo Chongde Primary School (1936–1941) and later the private Ningbo Maoxi Primary School (1941–1943) to the private Ningbo Qizheng Middle School (1943–1945) and the private Ningbo Yongjiang Girls' School (1945–1946).

I unfortunately contracted tuberculosis at the age of sixteen and had to take a two-year break and receive treatment at home before I resumed my study at the private Ningbo Xiaoshi High School (1948–1950) and Ningbo High School (1950–1951). This experience led me to make a decision to choose medical research for my advanced education and career—if I could learn and have (medical) skills, I could not only keep myself healthy but also cure many other patients. After graduation from high school, I attended the university entrance examination and fortunately I was accepted by the Department of Pharmacy and became a student at the Medical School of Peking University.

MY UNIVERSITY LIFE

My choice of learning pharmacy was driven by my interests, curiosity, and a desire to seek new medicines for patients. In 1941, an Institute of Chinese

Materia Medica was found at Peking University. The institute late developed into the Department of Pharmacy in the Medical School in 1943. In 1952, the second year of my university training, the Medical School was divided from Peking University and became the independent Beijing Medical College. By that time, significant efforts and investment were made in building the university's infrastructure and curriculum. Most pharmacy courses such as pharmacognosy, medicinal chemistry and phytochemistry were designed and taught by returnees such as Professors Lin Qishou (林启寿) and Lou Zhicen (楼之岑) who had received educations and advanced degrees in Western countries. Although pharmacognostical study or called "crude drugs" was my major, my training was not limited to that field and I had great chances to attend all basic training in the pharmaceutical sciences. In the pharmacognosy course, Professor Lou Zhicen conveyed knowledge on the origins of medicinal plants and trained us how to classify, distinguish and identify these plants based on their botanical descriptions etc. In the phytochemistry course, Professor Lin Qishou gave a comprehensive introduction and hands-on training on how to extract active ingredients from the plants, how to select proper extraction solvents, how to carry out chemistry studies and determine the structures of the chemicals isolated from the plants etc. These courses provided scientific insights into the herbs and plants and more importantly, explained how these herbal medicines work, in a way different from traditional Chinese medicine.

MY FIRST JOB AND A LIFE-LONG COMMITMENT

This December, we celebrated the 60th anniversary of the China Academy of Chinese Medical Sciences (CACMS). This was also the 60th anniversary of my career. After graduation from the university in 1955, I was assigned to work in the Institute of Chinese Materia Medica of the newly established Academy of Traditional Chinese Medicine under the China Ministry of Health. The academy has been growing and expanding rapidly over last sixty years along with change of its name from the Academy of Traditional Chinese Medicine to the China Academy of Traditional Chinese Medicine and now the China Academy of Chinese Medical Sciences. However, its mission of focusing on professional training, research and continuous exploring and development of Chinese medicines for human healthcare through utilization of evolving sciences and technologies has never changed. It is the academy's mission and establishment that have provided me with good opportunities to utilize my knowledge, skills and experience while being exposed to new areas of research.

My first research project was on *Lobelia chinensis* (半边莲), an herb commonly prescribed in the traditional Chinese medicine for the treatment of *Schistosomiasis*, a disease caused by *Schistosoma* type parasitic flat worms. In fact, my first publication was on the pharmacognostical study of *Lobelia chinensis*, co-authored with my mentor, Professor Lou Zhicen, in 1958. I completed another study on pharmacognostical evaluation of *Radix Stellariae* (银柴胡) before I went for a full-time training program on Chinese medical theory and practice organized by the Ministry of Health for professionals with a Western (modern) medical background between 1959 and 1962. This training further added in-depth knowledge on traditional Chinese medicines to my Western medical background.

Over the last sixty years, I have held different responsibilities at the academy, from head of the Chemistry Department (1973–1990) to head of the Artemisinin Research Center of the China Academy of Chinese Medical Sciences (1997–) and various academic assignments from associate professor (1979–1985), professor (1985–), and now chief professor of the China Academy of Chinese Medical Sciences.

WESTERN AND TRADITIONAL CHINESE MEDICINE—A UNIQUE COMBINATION

China lacked medical resources in the early 1950s. There were only around twenty thousand physicians and several tens of thousands of traditional Chinese medical practitioners in the country. To fully utilize these limited resources and explore Chinese medicines, the national leadership launched programs in an effort to promote the ideas of enhancing the healthcare services through a "combination of Western and traditional Chinese medicines." Medical school graduates or young doctors were encouraged to learn traditional Chinese medicines, while experienced traditional Chinese medical practitioners were asked to enrich their knowledge by attending training courses on Western medicine. This unique combination not only proved beneficial to patients but also enabled further exploration and development of Chinese medicine and its application through modern scientific approaches.

The Ministry of Health of China organized a number of full-time training courses in the late 1950s in which scientists with Western medical backgrounds were given opportunities for systemic training on the traditional Chinese medicine. In my two and a half year training program, I learned traditional Chinese medical theory and gained experience from clinical practice. Another training program I attended was on the processing (炮制) of Chinese Materia Medica.

This processing skill is a unique and exclusive pharmaceutical technology and has been widely used for the preparation of Chinese materia medica. The traditional way of processing was developed and summarized from thousands of years of experience in the traditional Chinese medical practices, with a belief that processing could alter the properties and functions of remedies, increase medical potency and reduce toxicity and side effects. In fact, differences in chemical compositions have been detected between herbs treated with different processes. Knowledge of such processing, in combination with the scientific explanation, benefited my work enormously.

ASSIGNMENT OF THE ANTIMALARIAL DRUG RESEARCH TASK

Malaria is a life-threatening epidemic disease. It was, however, effectively treated and controlled by chloroquine and quinolines for a long period of time until the development of drug-resistant malaria *plasmodium* parasites, namely *plasmodium falciparum*, in the late 1960s following the catastrophic failure of a global attempt to eradicate malaria. Resurgence of malaria and rapidly increased mortality posed a significant global challenge, especially in the South East Asian countries. In the 1960s, the Division of Experimental Therapeutics at the Walter Reed Army Institute of Research (WRAIR) in Washington, DC launched programs to search for novel therapies to support the US military presence in South East Asia. US military force involved in the Vietnam War suffered massive casualties due to disability caused by malaria infection. Up to 1972, over 214,000 compounds were screened with no positive outcomes.

In China, the military institutes started confidential antimalarial research in 1964. In 1967, the Chinese leadership set up a group office for malaria control (abbreviated as the National 523 Office) to coordinate nationwide research. Several thousand compounds were screened between 1967 and 1969 but no useful medicines were found.

In 1969, two directors and another member from the National 523 Office visited the Academy of Traditional Chinese Medicine and the Institute of Chinese Materia Medica, seeking help in searching for novel remedies among Chinese medicines.

It was in the middle of the great cultural revolution in China. Almost every institute was impacted and all research projects were stalled. A lot of experienced experts were sidelined. After thoughtful consideration, the academy's leadership team appointed me to head and build a Project 523 research group at the Institute of Chinese Materia Medica. My task was to search for antimalarial drugs among traditional Chinese medicines.

As a young scientist, I was so overwhelmed and motivated by this trust and responsibility. I also felt huge pressure from the high visibility, priority, challenges as well as the tight schedule of the task. The other challenge was the impact on my family life. By the time I accepted the task, my elder daughter was four years old and my younger daughter was only one. My husband had to be away from home attending a training campus. To focus on research, I left my younger daughter with my parents in Ningbo and sent my elder daughter to a full-time nursery where she had to live with her teacher's family while I was away from home for the project. This continued for several years. My younger daughter couldn't recognize me when I visited my parents three years later, and my elder daughter hid behind her teacher when I picked her up upon returning to Beijing after a clinical investigation.

TRADITIONAL CHINESE MEDICINE AND ITS RELEVANCE TO MALARIA

Our long journey searching for antimalarial drugs began with collection of relevant information and recipes from traditional Chinese medicine.

Malaria was one of the epidemic diseases with the most comprehensive records in traditional Chinese medical literature, such as *Zhou Li* (周礼), a classical book in ancient China published in the Zhou Dynasty (1046–256 B.C.). Other literature includes the *Inner Canon of the Yellow Emperor* (黄帝内经) published around the time of the Chun Qiu and Qin Dynasties (770–207 B.C.), the *Synopsis of Prescriptions of the Golden Chamber* (金匮要略) published in the Han Dynasty (206 B.C–220 A.D.), the *General Treatise on the Causes and Symptoms of Diseases* (诸病源候论) published in the Sui Dynasty (581–618 A.D.), the Qian Jin Fang or *Prescriptions Worth a Thousand Pieces of Gold* (千金方) and the Wai Tai Mi Yao or *Secret Medical Essentials of a Provincial Governor* (外台密要) published in the Tang Dynasty (618–907 A.D.), a book on malaria (痎疟论疏) published in the Ming Dynasty (1368–1644 A.D.) and the *Malignant Malaria Guide* (瘴疟指南) published in the Qing Dynasty (1644–1911 A.D.), the *Prescription for Universal Relief* (普济方) published in the Ming Dynasty, 1368–1644 A.D.), *etc.*

After thoroughly reviewing the traditional Chinese medical literature and folk recipes and interviewing experienced Chinese medical practitioners, I collected over two thousand herbal, animal and mineral prescriptions within three months after initiation of the project. From these two thousand recipes, I summarized 640 prescriptions in a brochure entitled "Antimalarial Collections of Recipes and Prescriptions" (抗疟单秘验方集). I circulated copies of the brochure to other research groups outside the institute for reference through the national project 523 office in April 1969.

A HANDFUL OF QINGHAO IMMERSED IN TWO LITERS OF WATER, WRING OUT THE JUICE AND DRINK IT ALL (青蒿一握, 以水二升渍, 绞取汁, 尽服之)

We started our experiments on dichroine using animal models. The study was soon stopped due to its severe side effects. From May 1969, extracts of over hundred herbs were prepared and tested in rodent malaria, with few promising results found up to June 1971.

After multiple experiments and failures, I re-focused on reviewing the traditional Chinese medical literature. One of the herbs, Qinghao (青蒿) (the Chinese name for the herbs in the *Artemisia* family), showed some effects in inhibiting malaria parasites during initial screening, but the result was inconsistent and not reproducible. I repeatedly read relevant paragraphs in the literature where the use of Qinghao was recorded as relieving malaria symptoms.

In Ge Hong's *A Handbook of Prescriptions for Emergencies* (肘后备急方), I noticed one sentence "A handful of Qinghao immersed in two liters of water, wring out the juice and drink it all" (青蒿一握, 以水二升渍, 绞取汁, 尽服之) when Qinghao was mentioned for alleviating malaria fevers. Most herbs were typically boiled in water and made into a decoction before taken by the patients.

This unique way of using Qinghao gave me the idea that heating during extraction might have destroyed the active components and the high temperature might need to be avoided in order to preserve the herb's activity. Ge Hong's handbook also mentioned "wring out the juice." This reminded me that the leaf of Qinghao might be one of the main components prescribed. I redesigned experiments in which the stems and leaves of Qinghao were extracted separately at a reduced temperature using water, ethanol and ethyl ether.

SAMPLE NO. 191, A SYMBOLIC BREAKTHROUGH IN ARTEMISININ DISCOVERY

We produced extracts from different herbs including Qinghao using the modified process and subsequently tested those ethyl ether, ethanol and aqueous extracts on rodent malaria. On October 4, 1971, we observed that sample number 191 of the Qinghao ethyl ether extract showed 100% effectiveness in inhibiting malaria parasites in rodent malaria. In subsequent experiments, we separated the extracts into a neutral portion and a toxic acidic portion. The neutral portion showed the same effect when tested in malaria-infected monkeys between December 1971 and January 1972.

On March 8, 1972, I reported these findings at the National Project 523 meeting held in Nanjing. This encouraging news evoked overwhelming interest from antimalarial drug research teams across the country.

"SHENG NONG TASTED HUNDRED HERBS," WHY COULDN'T WE?

Starting in March 1972, the team started to produce large quantities of Qinghao extract in preparation for clinical studies. Most pharmaceutical workshops were shut down during the great cultural revolution. Without manufacturing support, we had to extract herbs ourselves using household vats etc. The team worked very long hours every day including the weekends. Due to lack of proper equipment and ventilation, and long-term exposure to the organic solvents, some of my team members included myself started to show unhealthy symptoms. This, however, did not stop our efforts.

Some conflicting information was seen from the animal toxicological studies. It was already in the middle of the summer and very limited time was available to us before the malaria epidemic season would end. We would have to delay the study for at least a year if we continued our debate on toxicity. To expedite the safety evaluation, I asked to take the extracts voluntarily. The leaders at the institute approved my request. In July 1972, two other team members and myself took the extracts under close monitoring in the hospital. No side effect was observed in the one-week test window. Following the trial, another five members volunteered in the dose escalation study. This safety evaluation won us precious time and allowed us to start and complete the clinical trial in time.

Traditional Chinese medicine started with a story: "Sheng Nong tasted a hundred herbs." Sheng Nong was an ancient Chinese medical practitioner. To understand the efficacy and toxicity of the herbs, he tasted over a hundred herbs himself and recorded all the details, which left us with a lot of precious information. Although Qinghao was prescribed as an herbal medicine for thousands of years, the dose of the active ingredients in these prescriptions was much lower than that in the Qinghao extract we tested. Our desire to get the clinical trial completed and have the medicine for our patients as soon as possible was the real driving force behind our action.

SUCCESS IN THE FIRST CLINICAL TRIAL

The first clinical trial on the Qinghao extract was carried out in Hainan province between August and October 1972. We treated a total of twenty-one local and migrant malaria patients, nine infected by *Plasmodium falciparum*, eleven infected by *Plasmodium vivax* and one with mixed malaria infections.

The patients were divided into three groups with different dose regimens. We closely monitored the patients' body temperature and the changes in the numbers of parasites in their blood specimens. The trial was successful: all patients recovered from the fevers and no malaria parasites were detected after treatment. Nine malaria patients were also successfully treated with the Qinghao extract in Beijing No. 302 hospital.

The results from the first clinical trial in Hainan and Beijing No. 302 hospital were reported in the National Project 523 meeting held in Beijing in November 1972. The success of the first clinical trial and previous evidence observed in rodent malaria and monkey studies steered nationwide antimalarial drug research toward Qinghao.

ARTEMISININ AND DIHYDROARTEMISININ

We started isolation and purification of neutral Qinghao ethyl ether extract parallel with the clinical trial in 1972. Between April and June of 1972, a few crystals were isolated from the extract. The team finally isolated several crystals using silica gel column chromatography in November 1972, of which one showed effectiveness against malaria. The compound was later named artemisinin, or Qinghaosu (青蒿素) in Chinese.

We carried out a clinical trial of artemisinin between August and October 1973 using artemisinin tablets, which however did not yield the desired results. We examined the tablets returned from the clinical center and found that the tablets were too hard to disintegrate. We resumed the study using artemisinin capsules at the end of September 1973. Since it was already toward the end of the epidemic season, we only treated three patients and all of them recovered after administration of artemisinin capsules.

Dihydroartemisinin was found in September 1973 in an experiment where I tried to derivatize artemisinin for a structural activity relationship evaluation. The carboxyl group related peak disappeared and was replaced by the hydroxyl group related peak in the IR spectrum after a reduction reaction using sodium borohydride. This experimental result was verified in a repeat experiment carried out by team members. In a subsequent test in rodent malaria, we noticed that a significantly reduced dose was sufficient to achieve the same efficacy as artemisinin when dihydroartemisinin was administered.

We completed a series of development activities on the chemistry, pharmacology, pharmacokinetics, stability, and clinical trials on artemisinin and dihydroartemisinin according to regulatory requirements. The China Ministry of Health granted an Artemisinin New Drug Certificate to the Institute of Chinese Materia Medica in 1986 and a Dihydroartemisinin New Drug Certificate in 1992, respectively. Dihydroartemisinin is ten times more potent than artemisinin clinically, again demonstrating the "high efficacy, rapid action and low toxicity" of the drugs in the artemisinin category.

"BENCH TO BEDSIDE"—COLLABORATION EXPEDITED TRANSLATION FROM A DISCOVERY TO A MEDICINE

We started to determine the chemical structure of artemisinin in December 1972. The first thing we verified was that the compound did not contain nitrogen. This gave us a hint that the compound we found could be a new chemical different from quinolines. The team late confirmed that the compound was a new sesquiterpene lactone containing a peroxy group with a formula of $C_{15}H_{22}O_5$ and a molecular weight of 282.

In the 1970s, instruments and capabilities were very limited at each individual institute. The team at the Institute of Chinese Materia Medica collaborated with the Institute of Materia Medica, China Academy of Medical Sciences, who confirmed the formula of the artemisinin molecule. We started collaboration with the Shanghai Institute of Organic Chemistry and the Institute of Biophysics of the Chinese Academy of Sciences on artemisinin chemical structure analysis in 1974. The stereo structure was finally determined using X-ray crystallography at the Institute of Biophysics. This was one of the first applications reported in China in determining an absolute molecular configuration utilizing the scattering effects of oxygen atoms by X-ray diffraction technique.

No doubt, collaboration and collective efforts expedited the translation from discovery to new medicine. Colleagues from the Academy of Traditional Chinese Medicine, the Shangdong Provincial Institute of Chinese Medicine, the Yunnan Provincial Institute of Materia Medica, the Institute of Biophysics of the Chinese Academy of Sciences, the Shanghai Institute of Organic Chemistry of the Chinese Academy of Sciences, the Guangzhou University of Chinese Medicine, the Academy of Military Medical Sciences and many other institutes made significant contributions in their respective areas of responsibility during the development process. The leadership team from the National 523 Office played an important role in ensuring logistic support and coordinating nationwide collaboration.

QINGHAO AND ARTEMISIA ANNUA L.

The herb Qinghao was frequently mentioned in the traditional Chinese medical literature for various clinical applications besides alleviating malaria symptoms. These applications include relieving itches caused by scabies and scabs, treating malignant sores, killing lice, retaining warmth in joints, improving visual acuity, etc. However, little explanation was given on either the species or effective parts of the plant in the traditional Chinese medical literature.

According to plant taxonomy, there are at least six species in the *Artemisia* family: *Artemisia annua* L., *Artemisia apiacea* Hance, *Artemisia scoparia* Waldst. et kit., *Artemisia capillaries* Thunb., *Artemisia japonica* Thunb., and *Artemisia eriopoda* Bunge. The traditional Chinese medical literature only mentioned Qinghao (the general name of *Artemisia* in Chinese). By the time that our research on artemisinin was being carried out, two Qinghao (*Artemisia*) species were listed in the Chinese Pharmacopoeia and four others were also being prescribed.

We carried out a thorough investigation and confirmed that only *Artemisia annua* L. (sweet wormwood) contains artemisinin. In addition to identification of the right species, we also verified the best regions for growing Qinghao, the best collection season and the officinal part of the plant.

OUR DISCOVERY SAVES PATIENTS' LIVES WHILE SCIENTIFIC COMMUNITIES RECOGNIZE OUR CONTRIBUTIONS

I always feel that nothing can be more rewarding than the fact that artemisinin, since its discovery, has saved many malaria patients' lives. Over the past several decades, more than two hundred million malaria patients have received artemisinin or artemisinin combination therapies.

The scientific community never forgets any significant contribution to healthcare. I appreciate the numerous awards granted by the government and organizations in China. This includes the Award for Progress in Antimalarial Research Achieved by the Project 523 Scientific Team by the China National Science Conference in 1978, the National Scientific Discovery Award for the Antimalarial Drug Qinghaosu by the China Ministry of Science and Technology in 1979, the Invention Award (as the first inventor) by the China National Congress for Science and Technology in 1982, the Award for Young and Middle-aged Experts with Outstanding Contributions by the China State Council in 1984, the Highest Honorary Award of the China Academy of Traditional Chinese Medicine in 1992, the Top Ten National Achievements for Progress in Science and Technology award from the China State Scientific and Technological Commission in 1992, the First-rate Award of National Achievements in Science and Technology by the National Award Committee for Advances in Science and Technology in 1992, the National Model Worker award from the China State Council in 1995, the Award for Outstanding Achievement in Traditional Chinese Medicine by the Guangzhou Zhongjing Award Foundation for Traditional

Chinese Medicine in 1995, the Outstanding Scientific Achievement Award by the Hong Kong Qiu Shi Science and Technologies Foundation in 1996, the Top Ten Healthcare Achievements in New China by the China Ministry of Health in 1997, the Woman Inventor of the New Century award by the China National Bureau of Intellectual Property in 2002, the Golden Medal of the 14th National Invention Exhibition by the China National Bureau of Intellectual Property in 2003, the Award for Development of Chinese Materia Medica by the Cyrus Chung Ying Tang Foundation in 2009 and the China GlaxoSmithKline Award for Outstanding Achievements in Life Science in 2011.

I sincerely thank the Prince Mahidol Award Foundation (Thailand) for presenting me with the 2003 Prince Mahidol Award, the Albert and Mary Lasker Foundation (USA) for presenting me with the 2011 Lasker-DeBakey Clinical Medical Research Award and the Warren Alpert Foundation and Harvard Medical School (USA) for awarding me the 2015 Warren Alpert Foundation Prize (co-recipient). I am, once again, sincerely grateful to the Nobel Foundation (Sweden) for awarding me the 2015 Nobel Prize in Physiology or Medicine as a co-recipient.

RESEARCH EFFORTS CONTINUE

The discovery of artemisinin inspires us to approach research through the integration of diversified disciplines. Exploring the treasury of traditional Chinese medicine has provided us with a unique path leading to success, while utilizing modern scientific techniques and approaches are no doubt an effective and efficient way of realizing and expediting discoveries.

We are continuing our research efforts on artemisinin to understand its action mechanisms and to prevent or delay the development of artemisinin-tolerant or -resistant malaria. Expanding the clinical applications of artimisinin is also of interest to public health. We know what it can do, but we need to know why and how it does this, what else it can do and how it can do better . . .

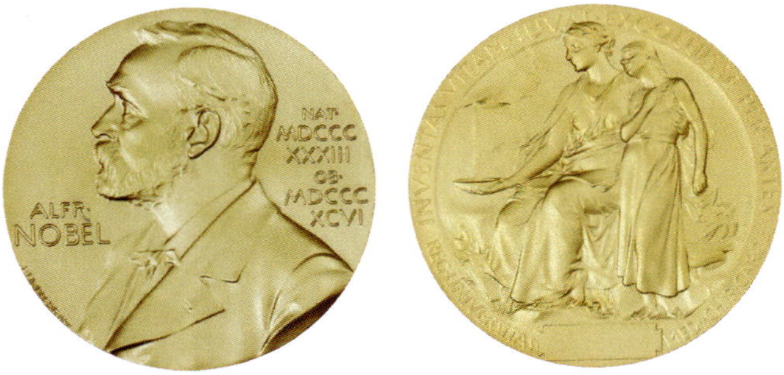

Artemisinin—A Gift from Traditional Chinese Medicine to the World

Nobel Lecture, December 7, 2015

by Tu Youyou
Institute of Chinese Materia Medica, China Academy of Chinese Medical Sciences, Beijing, China.

Dear respected Chairman, General Secretary, Esteemed Nobel Laureates, Ladies and Gentlemen,

It is my great honor to give this lecture today at Karolinska Institute. The title of my presentation is: Artemisinin—A Gift from Traditional Chinese Medicine to the World.

I would like to thank the Nobel Assembly and the Nobel Foundation for awarding me the 2015 Nobel Prize in Physiology or Medicine. This is not only an honor for myself, but also a recognition and motivation for all scientists in China. I would also like to express my sincere appreciation for the great hospitality of the Swedish people which I have received during my short stay over the last few days.

Thanks to Dr. William C. Campbell and Dr. Satoshi Omura for their excellent and inspiring presentations. The story I will tell today is about the diligence and dedication of Chinese scientists during the search for antimalarial drugs from traditional Chinese medicine forty years ago under considerably under-resourced research conditions.

INTRODUCTION

Malaria

Malaria has long been a devastating and life-threatening global epidemic disease in human history. Hippocrates, a Greek physician, described the disease as "marsh fevers," "agues," "tertian fevers," "quartan fevers," and "intermitten fevers" in his treatise "On Airs, Waters, and Places" in 400 B.C. [1]. A detailed description of malaria symptoms can also be found in 黄帝内经 (Huangdi Neijing, the *Inner Canon of the Yellow Emperor*, written around the time of the Chun Qiu and Qin Dynasties, 770–207 B.C.), the earliest traditional Chinese medical literature source [2].

Since malaria commonly originated and spread in humid areas surrounding marshes and swamps, the disease was considered associated with "bad air" hovering around the region, which is how the word "malaria," a combination of Medieval Italian "mal" (bad) and "aria" (air), was derived [3].

It was not known that the disease was caused by parasites until the French scientist Charles Louis Alphonse Laveran discovered the single-celled *Plasmodium* parasite in blood smears from malaria patients in 1880 [4]. In 1897, Ronald Ross, a British military doctor, found *Plasmodium* "eggs," oocysts, in the guts of female mosquitoes and late verified that *Anopheles* mosquitoes were responsible for transmission of malaria parasites between subjects [5]. These findings explained how the disease was transferred from malaria patients to the healthy population through a vector—female *Antopheles* mosquitoes. Both Laveran and Ross received the Nobel Prize in Physiology or Medicine in recognition of their exceptional contribution in understanding the origins of malaria.

There are over a hundred species of *Plasmodium*. Five of them infect humans, among which *Plasmodium malariae*, *Plasmodium ovale*, *Plasmodium vivax*, and deadly *Plasmodium falciparum* cause malaria whereas *Plasmodium knowlesi* hardly poses any threat to humans. Camillo Golgi, an Italian scientist and Nobel Laureate, raised an idea for differentiation of the *Plasmodium* species in 1886 when he demonstrated the correlation between the periodicity of paroxysms (the chill and fever pattern in the patient) with the 72-hour life cycle of development of *Plasmodium malariae*. In observing 48-hour cycles of development from other patients, he came to the conclusion that there must be more than one species of malaria parasite responsible for these different patterns of cyclical infection [6].

Human malaria symptoms are closely associated with the complex life cycle of malaria parasites. Malaria parasites present as sporozoites, merozoites, gametocytes, gametes and oocysts through their life cycle either in the vector (the definitive host) or in the infected subjects, *e.g.* humans (the secondary host). Healthy individuals are infected by an invasion of the thread-like sporozoites following a mosquito bite. The sporozoites then, through blood circulation, enter the liver cells where each sporozoite develops into a schizont containing thousands of tiny rounded merozoites over a period of one or two weeks. The schizont releases the merozoites into the bloodstream when it matures and bursts. For some malaria species, for example, *Plasmodium vivax* and *Plasmodium ovale*, some sporozoites will develop into hypnozoites, which can reside in the liver for months or years before developing into schizonts. This causes relapses in infected people. The merozoites, once they have escaped from the liver cells to the blood stream, are taken up by the red blood cells where they asexually produce new infective merozoites until the red cells burst, which initiates another round of asexual multiplication. Some of the merozoites develop into gametocytes that, once taken by female *Anopheles* mosquitoes through blood meal, mature to form sperm-like male gametes or large, egg-like female gametes. Fertilization of gametes produces an oocyst filled with infectious sporozoites in the mosquitoes' guts. The oocyst then bursts and releases sporozoites, which migrate to mosquitoes' salivary glands, ready to attack their next victim. Since all forms of *Plasmodium* parasites are hidden in either the liver or red blood cells during most of their life cycles, they are well camouflaged from the immune system. This makes it more challenging to trigger a defense through either a natural immune response or vaccination [7].

Treatment of malaria relies on chemotherapy, using medicines that act on various phases of *Plasmodium* parasite life cycles. These medicines include quinoline compounds, sulfadoxine/pyrimethamine, mefloquine (Lariam), lumefantrine, doxycycline, artemisinin and artemisinin-based combination therapies (ACTs). The most commonly used ACTs consist of an artemisinin component plus other antimalarial drugs such as mefloquine (ASMQ), lumefantrine (Coartem), amodiaquine (ASAQ), piperaquine (Duo-Cotecxin), and pyronaridine (Pyramax).

Vector control such as use of insect repellants, insecticide-treated mosquitoes nets (INTs), indoor residual spraying as well as elimination of stagnant water etc. is still the main approach for malaria prevention, although some malaria vaccines are under development. Some preventative medicines, for example, chloroquine, doxycycline, mefloquine (Lariam), primaquine, and a combination of atovaquone and proguanil (Malarone) may be used should prophylaxis be deemed necessary [8].

To promote early diagnosis and effective treatment of malaria, the World Health Organization (WHO) published the third edition of its *Guidelines for the treatment of malaria* in April 2015. The organization recommends that "All cases of suspected malaria be confirmed using parasite-based diagnostic testing (either microscopy or rapid diagnostic test) before administering treatment. Results of parasitological confirmation can be available in 30 minutes or less. Treatment solely on the basis of symptoms should only be considered when a parasitological diagnosis is not possible" [9].

In addition, in order to address the increasing incidences of artemisinin-tolerant or -resistant malaria, the WHO issued its *Global Plan for Artemisinin Resistance Containment* (*GPARC*) and *Emergency Response to Artemisinin Resistance in the Greater Mekong Subregion* in which a systematical tier approach is recommended via situational management in controlling, containing and eliminating occurrence and spread of artemisinin-resistant malaria [10–11].

"Expanding access to artemisinin-based combination therapies (ACTs) in malaria-endemic countries has been integral to the remarkable recent success in reducing the global malaria burden. No alternative antimalarial medicine is currently available offering the same level of efficacy and tolerability as ACTs. The emergence of artemisinin resistance in the Greater Mekong subregion (GMS) is therefore a matter of great concern. Resistance to other antimalarial medicine was also detected first in GMS, eventually appearing elsewhere. In Africa there is evidence that the spread of resistance coincided with increases in child mortality and morbidity" [9].

Traditional Chinese medicine's views on malaria

Malaria was known as a disease by our Chinese ancestors long time ago. A Chinese character inscription 疟 (malaria in Chinese) was found in the oracle ruins from between 1401 and 1122 B.C. Comprehensive descriptions on malaria symptoms, epidemics and relief of its unique periodic fevers and chills were provided in subsequent ancient medical literature, such as 周礼 (*Zhou Li*, a classical book in ancient China, the Zhou Dynasty, 1046–256 B.C.), 黄帝内经 (*The Inner Canon of the Yellow Emperor*, from around the time of the Chun Qiu and Qin Dynasties, 770–207 B.C.), 金匮要略 (*The Synopsis of Prescriptions of the Golden Chamber*, the Han Dynasty, 206 B.C–220 A.D.), 诸病源候论 (*On Causes and Symptoms of Diseases*, the Sui Dynasty, 581–618 A.D.), 千金方 (Qian Jin Fang) and 外台密要 (Wai Tai Mi Yao) (the Tang Dynasty, 618–907 A.D.), 痎疟论疏 (a book on malaria, the Ming Dynasty, 1368–1644 A.D.) and 瘴疟指南 (*Malignant Malaria Guide*, the Qing Dynasty, 1644–1911 A.D.). Several ancient texts from the central Asian countries, Assyria and India also described some basic features of malaria.

In fact, traditional Western and Chinese medicine agreed on their basic understanding of malaria. Our Chinese ancestors believed that malaria was caused by an invasion of 外邪 (exogenous evil) into the human body. The term "exogenous evil" was further explained as 疟气 (malaria gas), 疟邪 (pathogen of malaria disease), 瘴毒 and 瘴气 (miasm, miasma). This consensus remained in traditional Chinese medicine for more than two thousand years since it was first described in 黄帝内经 (in the *Inner Canon of the Yellow Emperor*, from around the time of the Chun Qiu and Qin Dynasties, 770–207 B.C.). Similarly, in the medieval period, Western medical practitioners believed that inhaling rotten gases from marshes and swamps was the cause of malaria.

Malaria was one of the epidemic diseases with the most comprehensive records in traditional Chinese medical literature. For example, 普济方 (Pu Ji Fang, *Prescription for Universal Relief*, the Ming Dynasty, 1368–1644 A.D.), one of the most comprehensive Chinese medicine prescription texts, contained at least four chapters entitled 诸疟门 (Chu Nue Men) on malaria.

The herb Qinghao

The term "Qinghao" is a general synonym in Chinese for the herbs in the *Artemisia* family.

Qinghao is one of the most common herbs that have been prescribed in traditional Chinese medical practice for over two thousand years. In Chinese medical terms, it offers the functions of clearing deficient heat, cooling and detoxifying blood, eliminating osteopyrexia and fever, freeing from summer heat, ceasing the recurrence of malaria fevers, removing jaundice, etc.

In 神农本草经 (*Sheng Nong's Herbal Classic*, the Qin and Han Dynasty, around 221 B.C. to 220 A.D.), the oldest herbal classic in China, Qinghao was listed in an inferior category under the name of 草蒿 with a description of having an inherent nature of "bitterness and cold" and its main clinical application was in relieving itches caused by scabies and scabs, treating malignant sores, killing lice, retaining warmth in joints, and improving visual acuity [12].

Although the herb Qinghao was documented in the traditional Chinese medical literature, however, few details were given on either the species or the effective parts of the plant when clinical application was mentioned.

According to plant taxonomy, there are at least six species in the *Artemisia* family: *Artemisia annua* L., *Artemisia apiacea* Hance, *Artemisia scoparia* Waldst. et kit., *Artemisia capillaries* Thunb., *Artemisia japonica* Thunb., and *Artemisia eriopoda* Bunge. Our studies confirmed that only *Artemisia annua* L. contains meaningful quantities of artemisinin [13].

Relief of malaria symptoms, *i.e.* periodic fevers using Qinghao was first recorded by 葛洪 (Ge Hong) in 肘后备急方 (*A Handbook of Prescriptions for Emergencies*, the East Jin Dynasty, around 317–420 A.D.). The application was subsequently mentioned in other literature such as 圣济总录 (Sheng Ji Zonglu, *General Records of Holy Universal Relief*, the Song Dynasty, 960–1279 A.D.), 丹溪心法 (Danxi Xinfa, Danxi, Mastery of Medicine, the Yuan Dynasty, 1271–1368

A.D.), 普济方 (Pu Ji Fang, *Prescription for Universal Relief*, the Ming Dynasty, 1368–1644 A.D.) in which Qinghao soup, Qinghao pills for malaria relief, and Qinghao powders were described for relieving malaria symptoms. In addition to a summary of experience from earlier practitioners, 李时珍 (Li Shi Zhen) recorded his own practice in treating periodic "fevers and colds" in 本草纲目 (*Compendium of Materia Medica*, the Ming Dynasty, 1368–1644). Malaria-related information could also be found in 本草备要 (*Essentials of Materia Medica*, the Qing Dynasty, 1644–1911 A.D.) and 温病条辨 (*Detailed Analysis of Epidemic Warm Diseases*, the Qing Dynasty, 1644–1911 A.D.).

In addition to the documentation in the traditional Chinese medical literature, some empirical formulas was also very popular in some regions, for example, a recipe from Jiangsu province mentioned collecting Qinghao leaves on the day of 端午 (The Dragon Boat Festival) and drying them in the shade, mixing with equal amount of cortex cinnamomi powders, taking 一钱 (a weight unit, equal to approximately 3.72 grams) together with warm wine when having colds and with cold wine when having fevers in 五更 (time traditionally used in China, 3 to 5 a.m.) on the day of a malaria episode, avoiding stimulating foods while taking medicines " to reduce malaria symptoms."

No doubt, clinical practice in alleviating malaria symptoms utilizing Qinghao—inherited from traditional Chinese medical literature—provided some useful information leading to the discovery of artemisinin.

DISCOVERY OF ARTEMISININ

Background

Malaria was effectively treated and controlled by chloroquine and quinolines for a long period of time until development of drug resistant malaria in the late 1960s following the catastrophic failure of a global attempt to eradicate malaria. Resurgence of malaria and rapidly increased mortality due to loss of effective treatment presented a serious global challenge, in particular, in the regions with prevalence of malaria associated with the drug resistant *Plasmodium* parasites, especially *Plasmodium falciparum*.

South East Asia was one of the most severe endemic areas in the late 1960s. As reported, during the Vietnam War, casualties in the US military force caused by medical disability due to the full seasonal prevalence of malaria reached four to five times higher than casualties from actual direct combat in 1964. Malaria infected nearly half of total military individuals or around five hundred thousand US soldiers in 1965. Fighting malaria became one of the top medical priorities and challenges for the US Army in Vietnam. A program coordinated through the Division of Experimental Therapeutics at the Walter Reed Army Institute of Research (WRAIR) in Washington, DC was launched to search for new antimalarial drugs. The program involved numerous research institutes and a vast investment. Up to 1972, over 214,000 compounds were screened by the Walter Reed Army Institute of Research which, however, ended up with no breakthrough findings or discoveries of novel antimalarial medicines.

Confidential antimalarial research was initiated within the Chinese military in 1964. Research on novel antimalarial medicines became an important political assignment for the medical researchers in the Chinese army.

A national office for malaria control, known as the 523 Office (for purposes of confidentiality, the project was named for May 23, the date when it was initiated; the Office was terminated in March 1980) was established in 1967 with a mission of organizing and coordinating antimalarial drug research activities in seven provinces and cities across the country. Several thousand compounds were screened between 1967 and 1969. However, no effective antimalarial drugs were identified [15].

Initial screening

In 1969, two directors and one member from the National Project 523 Office visited the Institute of Chinese Materia Medica of the Academy of Traditional Chinese Medicine, seeking help in searching for novel antimalarial drugs from Chinese medicines. I was appointed by the leadership team at the Academy of Traditional Chinese Medicine to build and head the Project 523 research group at the institute.

I started by collecting information on the relevant traditional Chinese medicines. Within three months, I gathered over two thousand herbal, animal and mineral prescriptions for either internal or external uses by reviewing ancient traditional Chinese medical literatures and folk recipes, and interviewing experienced Chinese medical practitioners for potential prescriptions and herbal recipes. I then narrowed down the prescriptions from two thousand to 640 and summarized the recipes in a brochure entitled **抗疟单秘验方集** ("Antimalarial Collections of Recipes and Prescriptions"). I circulated copies of the brochure to other research groups outside the institute for reference through the National Project 523 Office in April 1969.

We started with experiments on dichroine using animal models. The study was soon abandoned due to its severe side effects. From May 1969, aqueous and ethanol extracts of over hundred herbs were prepared and tested in rodent

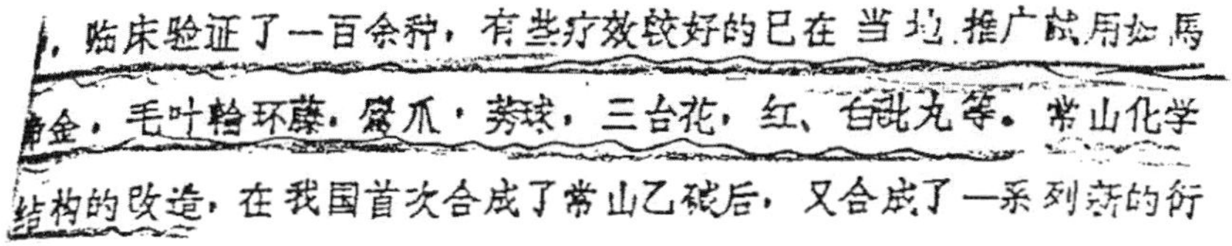
，临床验证了一百余种，有些疗效较好的已在当地推广试用如馬
鞭金，毛叶轮环藤，鹰爪，萝球，三台花，红、白砒丸等。常山化学
结构的改造，在我国首次合成了常山乙碱后，又合成了一系列新的衍

FIGURE 1. Copy of a paragraph from the summary of the National Malaria Control Research Meeting, issued by the National Leading Group Office for Malaria Control on June 1, 1971.

malaria with few promising results found up to June 1971. The paragraph in the summary of national malaria control research meeting shown on Figure 1 updated the antimalarial drug research, saying that "over a hundred clinical verifications were conducted; some of the (herbal medicines) showing some clinical relevance has been further tested locally, including herbal *dichodrae, ktze cycleanine, talon, ball atrazine, clerodendron serratum*, red and white arsenic pills etc" [16].

Extract Sample No 191 and Focus on Qinghao Research

We started to focus on the herb Qinghao in 1971 but achieved no promising results after multiple experiments. In September 1971, a modified procedure was designed to reduce the extraction temperature by immersing or distilling Qinghao using ethyl ether. The extracts we obtained were then treated with an alkaline solution to retain the neutral portion by removing acidic impurities.

In the experiments carried out on October 4, 1971, sample No. 191, *i.e.* the neutral portion of the Qinghao ethyl ether extract, was found 100% effective on rodent malaria when administered orally at a dose of 1.0 g/kg for three consecutive days (Figure 2). The same results were observed when tested in malaria-infected monkeys between December 1971 and January 1972. This breakthrough finding became a critical step in the discovery of artemisinin.

In the same studies, extracts from *air potato yam, pomegranate, rhizoma smilacis glabrae*, and extract of Qinghao using other solvents were also tested with negative or no comparable results.

I reported our findings at the nationwide Project 523 meeting held in Nanjing on March 8, 1972, saying that "We have screened over a hundred types of single and combination herbal recipes since July 1971 and found that Qinghao ether extract showed 95–100% inhibition of rodent malaria. We performed further purification to retain the effective neutral portion by removing the non-effective toxic acidic portion. We observed the same efficacy when we tested the

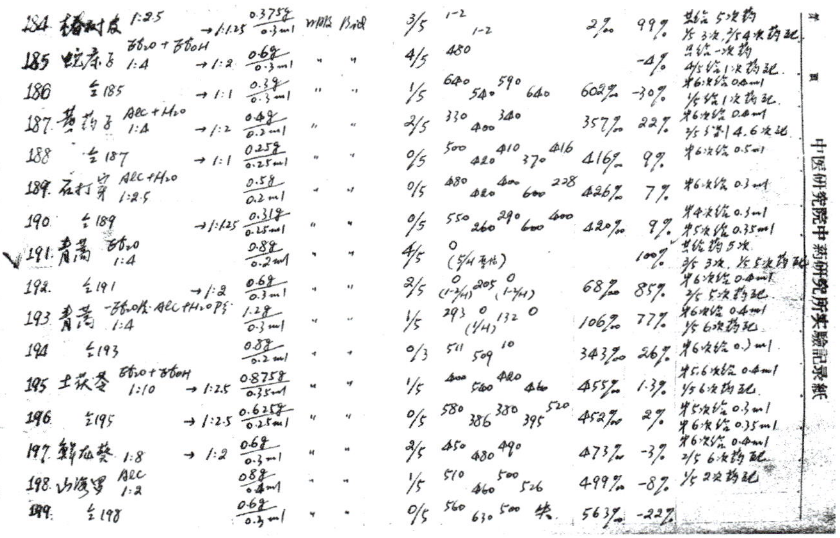

FIGURE 2. Copy of the original laboratory notebook record showing 100% inhibition of the malaria parasite by Qinghao neutral extract when testing on a rodent malaria model.

Qinghao ether extract and the neutral portion on the monkey malaria model in late December." (Figure 3)

This report attracted overwhelming interests and triggered nationwide collaboration in research on Qinghao and Qinghao extracts. We received multiple letters from other institutes requesting that we share information on our findings and experience [17], to which we responded with thorough explanations (Figure 4).

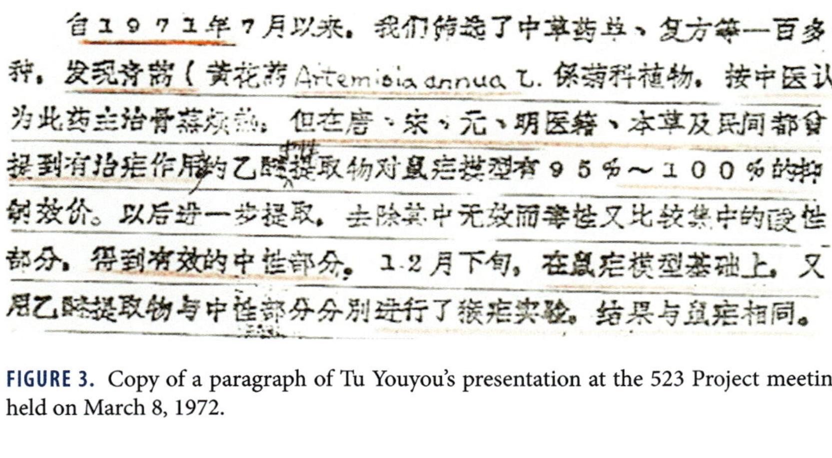

自1971年7月以来，我们筛选了中草药单、复方等一百多种，发现青蒿（黄花蒿 Artemisia annua L. 係菊科植物，按中医认为此药主治骨蒸烦热，但在唐、宋、元、明医籍、本草及民间都曾提到有治疟作用）的乙醚提取物对鼠疟模型有95%～100%的抑制效价。以后进一步提取，去除其中无效而毒性又比较集中的酸性部分，得到有效的中性部分。12月下旬，在鼠疟模型基础上，又用乙醚提取物与中性部分分别进行了猴疟实验，结果与鼠疟相同。

FIGURE 3. Copy of a paragraph of Tu Youyou's presentation at the 523 Project meeting held on March 8, 1972.

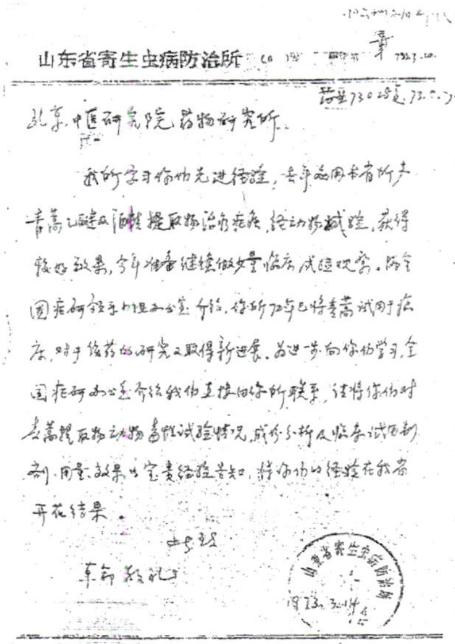
山东省寄生虫病防治所

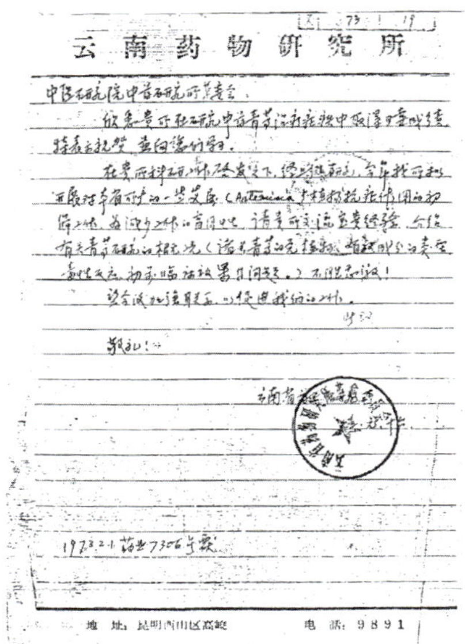
云南药物研究所

地址：昆明西山区高峣 电话：9891

FIGURE 4. Copy of the letters from the Shandong Institute of Parasitic Diseases (left) and Yunnan Provincial Institute of Materia Medica (right) requesting sharing of information on the findings made by the team at the Institute of Chinese Materia Medica, Academy of Traditional Chinese Medicine.

First clinical trial on Qinghao extract and nationwide collaboration in subsequent development

We subsequently carried out a clinical trial between August and October 1972 in Hainan province (twenty-one cases) and simultaneously at Beijing 302 hospital (nine cases). This was the first time the neutral Qinghao ethyl ether extract was tested in humans. In the trial carried out in Hainan province, a total of twenty-one local and migrant malaria patients, nine infected by *Plasmodium falciparum* and eleven infected by *Plasmodium vivax*, were treated in three dose groups and all of them recovered from the fevers with full clearance of malaria parasites. All nine patients were successfully treated at Beijing 302 hospital. The results from the first clinical trial in Hainan and Beijing 302 hospital were reported in the nationwide project 523 meeting held in Beijing in November 1972. The national office for malaria control issued a communication on malaria control research on November 5, 1972 to record the clinical findings (Figure 5).

> "In the expedited clinical trial on the twenty-one cases of local and migrant malaria patients in August, the Qinghao extract from the Beijing (research) district showed relatively good efficacy (over

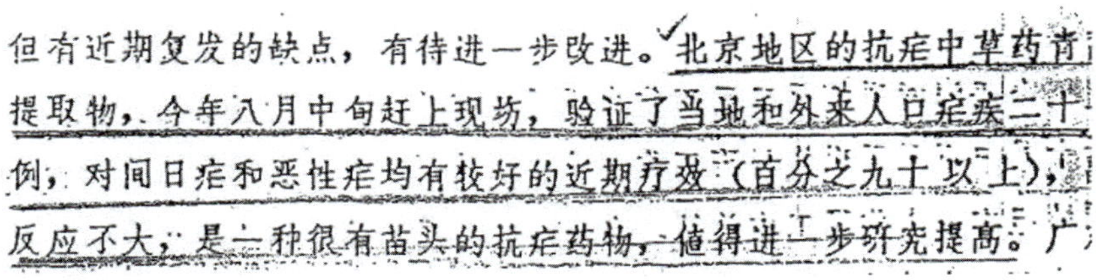
但有近期复发的缺点，有待进一步改进。北京地区的抗疟中草药青
提取物，今年八月中旬赶上现场，验证了当地和外来人口疟疾二十
例，对间日疟和恶性疟均有较好的近期疗效（百分之九十以上），
反应不大，是一种很有苗头的抗疟药物，值得进一步研究提高。广

FIGURE 5. Copy of a paragraph from the communication on malaria control research issued by the National Leading Group Office for Malaria Control on November 5, 1972.

90%) against *Plasmodium vivax* and *Plasmodium falciparum*. This is a promising antimalarial drug with potential for further improvement" [18].

Proving the efficacy of neutral Qinghao ethyl ether extract in the experiments on rodent and monkey malaria models in October 1971 and the subsequent clinical trial between August and October 1972 steered nationwide antimalarial research towards Qinghao.

Figure 6 summarizes the antimalarial research program carried out by the team at the Institute of Chinese Materia Medica, Academy of Traditional Chinese

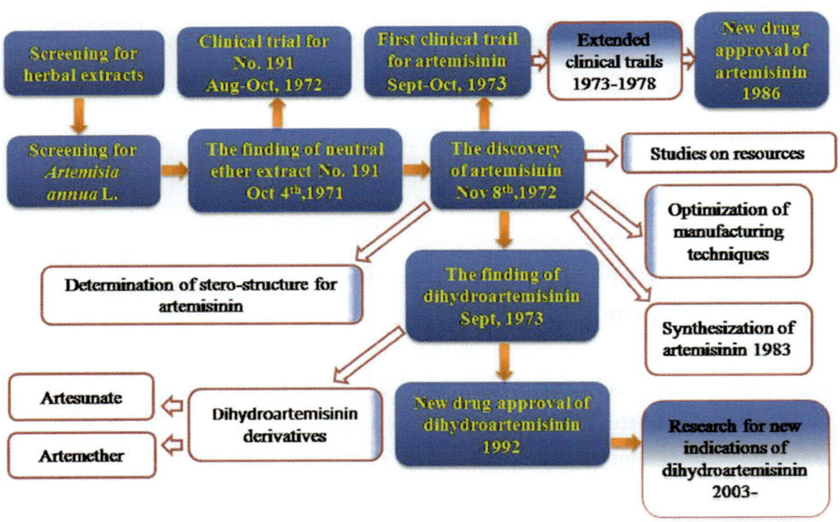

FIGURE 6. Summary of the work completed by the research team at the Institute of Chinese Materia Medica, Academy of Traditional Chinese Medicine (boxes with blue background). Work completed through collaboration between the Institute of Chinese Materia Medica and other institutes (Boxes transitioning from blue to white), and work completed through collaboration between other research teams across the nation (boxes in white).

Medicine in which the programs highlighted in blue were accomplished by the team at the Institute of Chinese Materia Medica while the programs highlighted in blue and white were completed through the joint efforts by the teams at the Institute of Chinese Materia Medica and other institutes. Other research teams across the nation collaboratively completed the non-highlighted programs.

The team at the Institute of Chinese Materia Medica independently completed screening on Qinghao herbal extracts, and herb Qinghao (*Artemisia annua* L. more specifically), proved the efficacy of neutral Qinghao ethyl ether extract (Sample No 191) in animal models in October 1971, completed the first clinical trial and proved the clinical efficacy of neutral Qinghao ethyl ether extract between August and October 1972, isolated and discovered artemisinin in November 1972, completed the first clinical trial on artimisinin between September and October 1973, discovered dihydroartemisinin, completed development activities, applied for and received artemisinin new drug approval in 1986 and dihydroartemisinin new drug approval in 1992. We collaborated with other institutes nationwide on extended clinical trials between 1973 and 1978, determination of the stereo structure of artemisinin, research on dihydroartemisinin derivatives, searches for Qinghao resources, optimization of manufacturing techniques, and research on new indications for dihydroartemisinin after 2003. Other institutes across the country synthesized and developed a number of artemisinin derivatives, *i.e.* artemeter, artesunate and arteether into new drugs.

Purification of artemisinin and chemistry studies

We started further isolation and purification of neutral Qinghao ethyl ether extract parallel with the clinical trial and verification. In August 1972, we observed a good separation of the purified neutral extract by silica gel thin-layer chromatography. In November 1972, an effective antimalarial compound was isolated from the neutral Qinghao ethyl ether extract by the team at the Institute of Chinese Materia Medica. The compound was later named artemisinin or Qinghaosu in Chinese.

We started to determine the chemical structure of artemisinin in December 1972 through elemental analysis, spectrophotometry, mass spectrum, polarimetric analysis and other techniques.

The compound was further purified with different re-crystallization processes and tested at the department of analytical chemistry of the Institute of Materia Medica, China Academy of Medical Sciences. Based on the elemental analysis and results from other studies, colleagues at the Institute of Material Medica verified that the compound contained no nitrogen and had a potential formula of $C_{15}H_{22}O_5$ on April 27, 1973 (Figure 7). We started collaboration with the Shanghai Institute of Organic Chemistry and the Institute of Biophysics of Chinese Academy of Sciences on artemisinin chemical structure analysis in 1974. The stereo-structure was finally determined by X-ray crystallography, which verified that artemisinin was a new sesquiterpene lactone containing a peroxy group (Figures 8 and 9). This was one of the first applications reported in China in determining an absolute molecular configuration utilizing the scattering effects of oxygen atoms by X-ray diffraction technique [19, 20]. Table 1 presents some of the physical and chemical test results for artemisinin chemical and stereo structure determination. The stereo structure of artemisinin was pub-lished in 1977 and cited by *Chemical Abstracts* [20, 21].

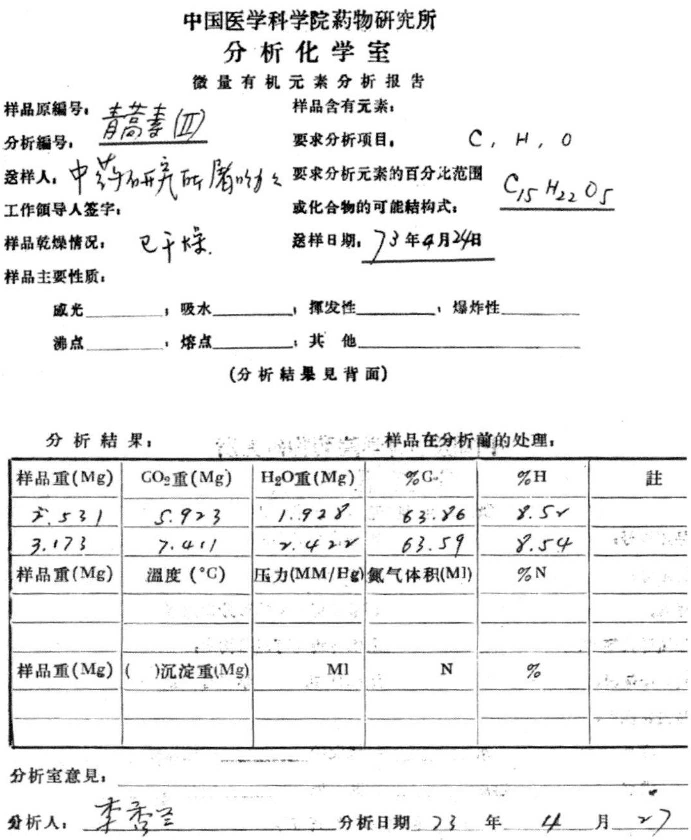
中国医学科学院药物研究所

分析化学室

微量有机元素分析报告

样品原编号：青蒿素(II)　　样品含有元素：

分析编号：　　要求分析项目：C，H，O

送样人：中药研究所屠呦呦　　要求分析元素的百分比范围或化合物的可能結构式：$C_{15}H_{22}O_5$

工作領导人签字：

样品乾燥情况：已干燥　　送样日期：73年4月24日

样品主要性质：

感光____，吸水____，揮发性____，爆炸性____

沸点____，熔点____，其他____

(分析結果見背面)

分析結果：　　样品在分析前的处理：

样品重(Mg)	CO_2重(Mg)	H_2O重(Mg)	%C	%H	註
2.531	5.923	1.928	63.86	8.52	
3.173	7.411	2.422	63.59	8.54	
样品重(Mg)	溫度 (°C)	压力(MM/Hg)	氮气体积(Ml)	%N	
样品重(Mg)	( )沉淀重(Mg)	Ml	N	%	

分析室意見：

分析人：李秀兰　　分析日期 73 年 4 月 27

FIGURE 7. The elements analysis report by the collaborative institution, the Institute of Matria Medica, Chinese Academy of Medical Sciences, on April 27, 1973.

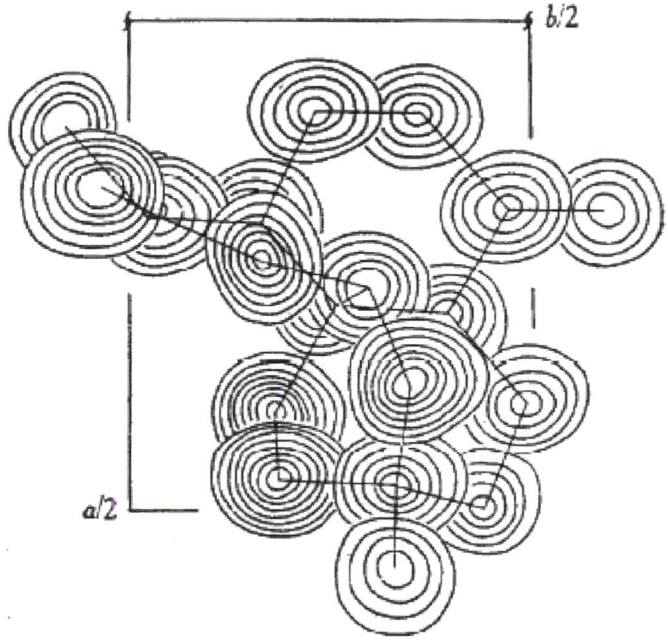

FIGURE 8. Three-dimensional electron density of the artemisinin crystal [20].

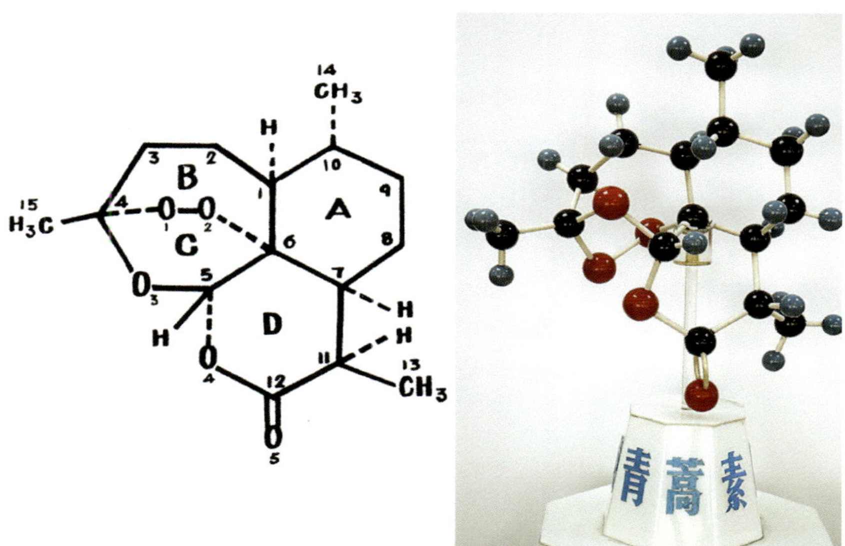

FIGURE 9. Chemical and stereo structures of artemisinin.

TABLE 1. Determination of chemical and stereo structure of artemisinin

Test	Result
Appearance	White, needle shape crystaslline
Melting point	156–157 °C
Optical rotation	$[\alpha]^{17}{}_{D}$: +66.3 °
High resolution mass spectrum	m/z 282.1472 $[M]^+$
Elemental analysis	C: 63.72%, H: 7.86%
UV absorption	–
Solubility	Readily soluble in chloroform, acetone, ethyl acetate, benzene Soluble in ethanol, ethyl ether Slightly soluble in cold petroleum ether Insoluble in water
IR (KBr)	1745cm^{-1}, 831cm^{-1}, 881cm^{-1}, 1115cm^{-1}
^{1}H-NMR	(CCl_4, 100M Hz, Hexamethyl disiloxane) δ: 0.93 (doublet, J=*6Hz), 1.06 (doublet,J=6Hz),1.36 (singlet),3.08–3.44 (multiplet)
^{13}C-NMR	(Chloroform, 22.63M Hz) δ: 12,19,23 (quartlet), 25,25.1,37,35.5 (triplet), 32.5,33,45,50,93.5 (doublet), 79.5,105,172 (singlet)
X-ray crystallography	Crystallographic parameters: D_2^4—P_{212121} Lattice constant: a = 24.098 Å, b = 9.468 Å, c = 6.399 Å, Measured density: d_o = 1.30 g/cm^3 Calculated density: d_c = 1.294 g/cm^3 Number of molecules in an asymmetric unit: 4

Artemisinin structure—efficacy correlation and artemisinin derivatives

In order to determine the functional groups in the artemisinin molecule, we chemically modified the peroxyl and carboxyl groups of the molecule.

We produced deoxyartemisinin through reduction of the peroxyl group to an epoxy group by subjecting the artemisinin in the palladium and calcium carbonate methanol solution under room temperature and pressure, and then treating it using an acetone and n-hexane mixture.

We also produced dihydroartemisinin by reducing the carboxyl group to a hydroxyl group using sodium borohydride. Dihydroartemisinin was further reduced to dihydro-deoxyartemisinin by reacting in a palladium and calcium carbonate methanol solution.

Compound	Graph of chemical structures	Dose mg/kg/day × 3	Clearance of parasites
Artemisinin	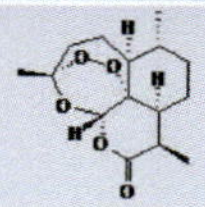	**50-100**	**Yes**
Dihydroartemisinin	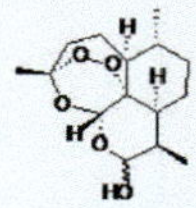	**12.5**	**Yes**
Acetate of dihydroartemisinin	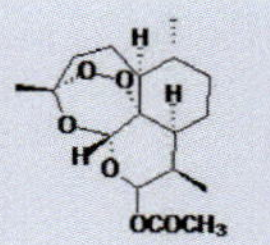	**6**	**Yes**
Deoxyartemisinin	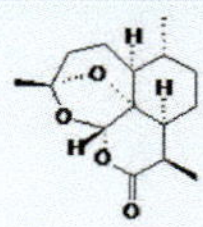	**100**	**No**

FIGURE 10. Structure—Activity relationship of compounds derived from artemisinin.

Some new compounds were obtained by derivatizing through the hydroxyl group of dihydroartemisinin.

Figure 10 shows the effective doses and observation in clearance of malaria parasites when the structure-modified compounds were administered. The results showed that the dose was reduced from 50–100 mg/kg/day for artemisinin to 12.5 mg/kg/day and 6 mg/kg/day for dihydroartemisinin and acetate of dihydroartemisinin. The dose was similar between deoxyartemisinin and artemisinin. However, deoxyartemisinin was unable to clear malaria parasites. This study verified that the peroxyl group in the artemisnin molecule was critical for its antimalarial function while reducing the carboxyl group to hydroxyl group improved the efficacy as well as allowed derivatization of artemisinin to form new compounds. This led to the development of dihydroartemisinin and other compounds such as artemether, artesunate, and arteether into new antimalarial drugs (Figure 11). Up to now, no clinical application has been reported with other artemisinin derivatives except for the four presented here.

New antimalaria medicines—artemisinin and dihydroartemisinin

The team at the Institute of Chinese Materia Medica carried out a series of development activities on the chemistry, pharmacology, pharmacokinetics and stability of artemisinin and dihydroartemisinin and performed clinical trials

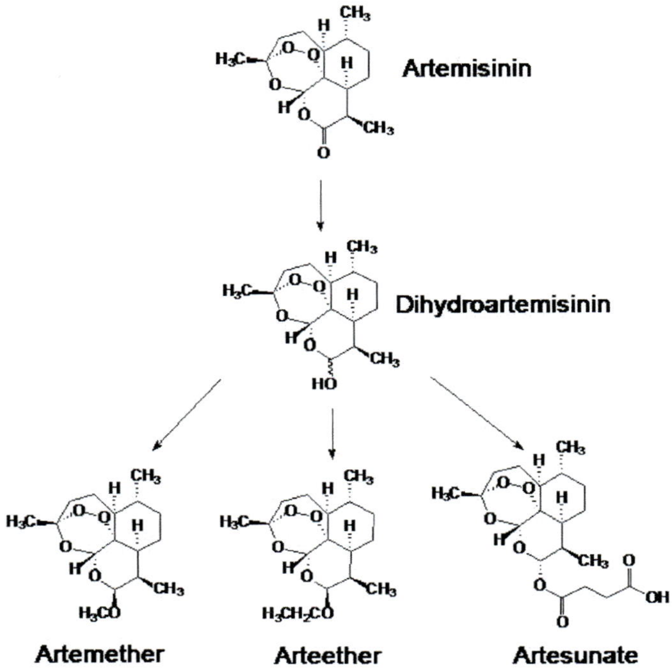

FIGURE 11. Artemisinin and artemisinin derivatives.

according to regulatory requirements. The China Ministry of Health granted an Artemisinin New Drug Certificate (Figure 12, left) to the Institute of Chinese Materia Medica in 1986 and a Dihydroartemisinin New Drug Certificate (Figure 12, right) in 1992, respectively. Dihydroartemisinin is ten times more potent than artemisinin clinically, again demonstrating the "high efficacy, rapid action and low toxicity" of the drugs in the artemisinin category.

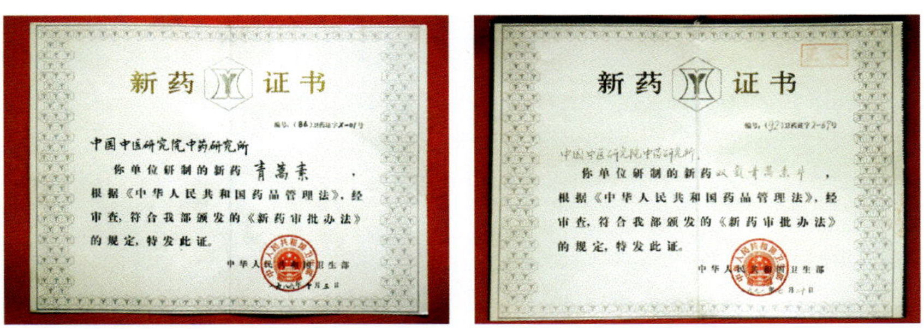

FIGURE 12. The Artemisinin New Drug Certificate granted in 1986 (left) and the Dihydroartemisinin New Drug Certificate granted in 1992 (right).

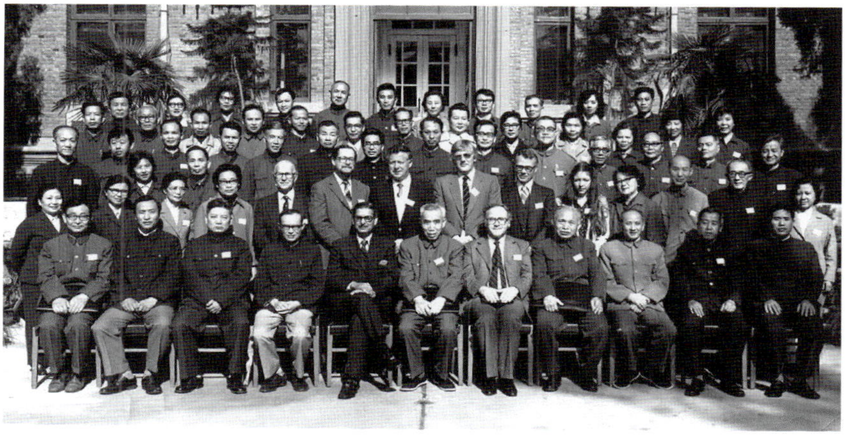

FIGURE 13. Delegates to the 4th Meeting of The SWG-Chemal "Qinghaosu" held by the World Health Organization (WHO), the World Bank and United Nations Development Program (UNDP) in Beijing in 1981.

Worldwide attention to artemisinin

The World Health Organization (WHO), the World Bank and United Nations Development Program (UNDP) held the 4th joint Malaria Chemotherapy Science Working Group meeting in Beijing in 1981 (Figure 13). A series of presentations on artemisinin and its clinical application, including my report "Studies on the Chemistry of Qinghaosu," received positive and enthusiastic responses. In the 1980s, several thousand malaria patients were successfully treated with artemisinin and its derivatives in China.

DISCOVERY OF ARTEMISININ WAS NOT AN EASY WIN

After this brief review, you may comment that this is no more than an ordinary drug discovery process. However, it was not a simple and easy journey in the discovery of the artemisinin from Qinghao, a Chinese herbal medicine with over two thousand years of clinical application, especially in the 1970s when research was significantly under-resourced in China.

Commitment to a clearly defined goal assures success in discovery

The Institute of Chinese Materia Medica of the Academy of Traditional Chinese Medicine joined the antimalarial drug research Project 523 in 1969. I was appointed the head to build the Project 523 research group at the institute by the

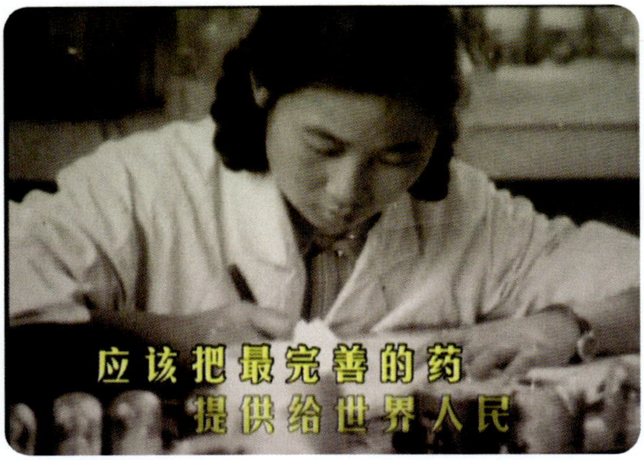

FIGURE 14. Screen shot from the TV program "To Develop and Provide the Best Drugs for People around the World."

academy's leadership team and was in charge of searching for novel antimalarial drugs from Chinese medicines. It was a confidential military program with a high priority. As a young scientist in her early career life, I felt overwhelmed by the trust and responsibility received for such a challenging and critically important task. I had no choice but to fully devote myself to accomplishing my duties (Figure 14).

Knowledge is prologue in discovery

Figure 15 shows a photo taken soon after I joined the Institute of Chinese Materia Medica. Professor Lou Zhicen (left), a famous pharmacognosist, was mentoring me on how to differentiate herbs. I graduated from Beijing Medical College in 1955 after four years of training on modern pharmaceutical sciences and later attended a training course on theories and practices of traditional Chinese medicine designed for professionals with a modern (Western) medicine training background between 1959 and 1962. "Fortune favors the prepared mind" and "What's past is prologue." My prologue of integrated training in both modern and Chinese medicine prepared me for the challenges when the opportunities to search for antimalarial Chinese medicines became available.

Information collating and accurate deciphering are the foundation for success in research

After accepting the tasks, I collected over two thousand herbal, animal and mineral prescriptions for either internal or external use by reviewing ancient

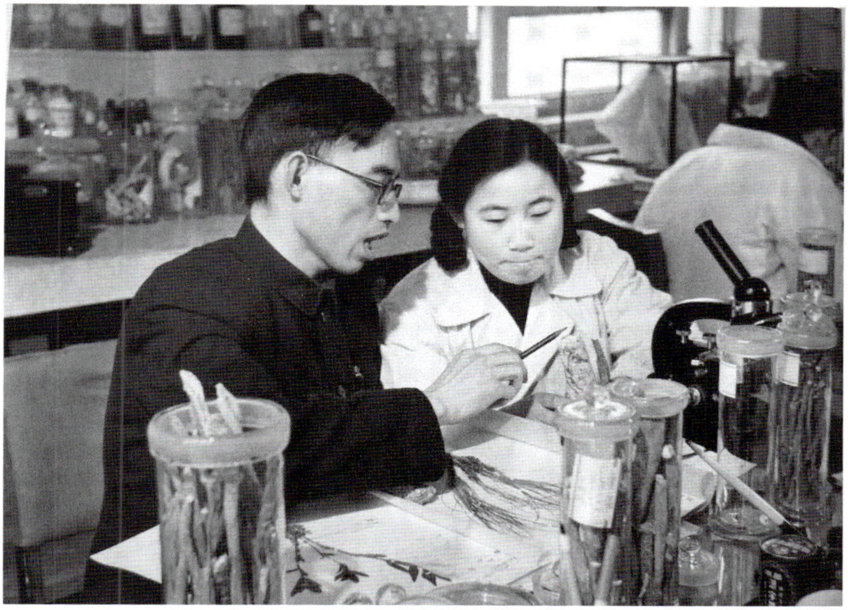

FIGURE 15. Professor Lou Zhicen (left), a famous pharmacognosist, mentoring the author on how to differentiate herbs.

traditional Chinese medical literature and folk recipes, interviewing well-known and experienced Chinese medical doctors who provided me prescriptions and herbal recipes. I summarized six hundred forty prescriptions in a brochure 抗疟单秘验方集 ("Antimalarial Collections of Recipes and Prescriptions") (Figure 16). It was this information collection and deciphering that laid a sound foundation for the discovery of artemisinin. This also differentiates the approaches taken by Chinese medicine and general phytochemistry in searching for novel drugs.

Thorough literature reviewing inspires an idea leading to success

I reviewed the traditional Chinese literature again when our research stalled, following numerous failures. In reading 肘后备急方 written by 葛洪 (Ge Hong's *A Handbook of Prescriptions for Emergencies*, the East Jin Dynasty, around 317–420 A.D.) (Figure 17), I further pondered the sentence 青蒿一握, 以水二升渍, 绞取汁, 尽服之 (A handful of Qinghao immersed in two liters of water, wring out the juice and drink it all) which recommended cold Qinghao for alleviating malaria symptoms. Most herbs were typically boiled in water and made into decoction before taken by the patients.

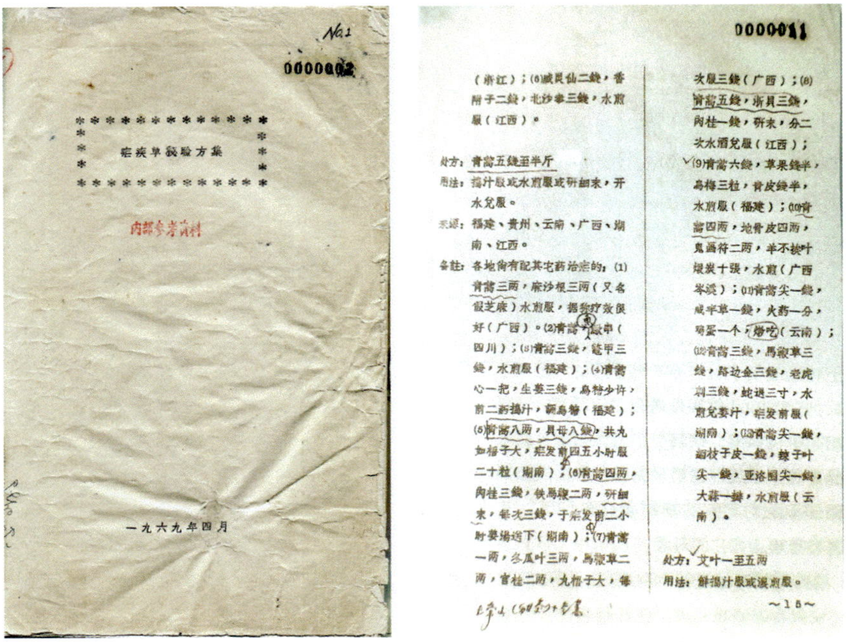

FIGURE 16. Antimalarial collections of recipes and prescriptions.

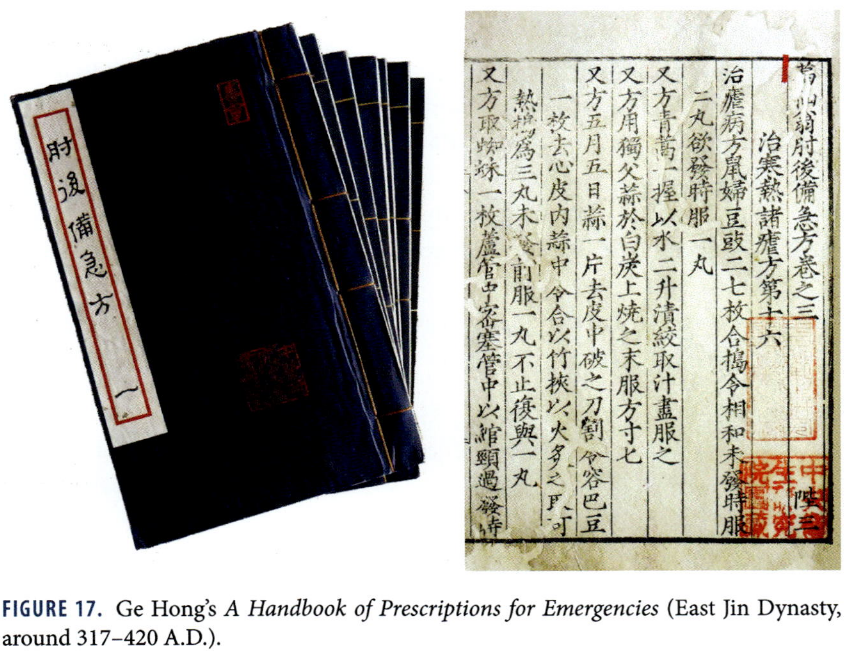

FIGURE 17. Ge Hong's *A Handbook of Prescriptions for Emergencies* (East Jin Dynasty, around 317–420 A.D.).

This unique way of using Qinghao suddenly gave me the idea that heating might need to be avoided during extraction, in order to preserve the herb's activity. I subsequently redesigned the experiments by extracting the leaves and stems of Qinghao separately at a low temperature using water, ethanol and ethyl ether [22].

The earliest mentioning of Qinghao's application as an herbal medicine was found on the silk manuscripts entitled 五十二病方 (*Prescriptions for Fifty-two Kinds of Disease*) unearthed from the third Han Tomb at Mawangdui. Its medical application was also recorded in 神农本草经 (*Sheng Nong's Herbal Classic*), 补遗雷公炮制便览 (Bu Yi Lei Gong Pao Zhi) and 本草纲目 (*Compendium of Materia Medica*) (Figure 18) etc.

Although the herb Qinghao was widely documented in the traditional Chinese medical literature, however, few details were given on either the species or effective parts of the plant when clinical application was mentioned.

According to plant taxonomy, there are at least six species in the *Artemisia* family; *Artemisia annua* L., *Artemisia apiacea* Hance, *Artemisia scoparia* Waldst. et kit., *Artemisia capillaries* Thunb., *Artemisia japonica* Thunb., and *Artemisia eriopoda* Bunge. However, no clear classification was given for the Qinghao (the

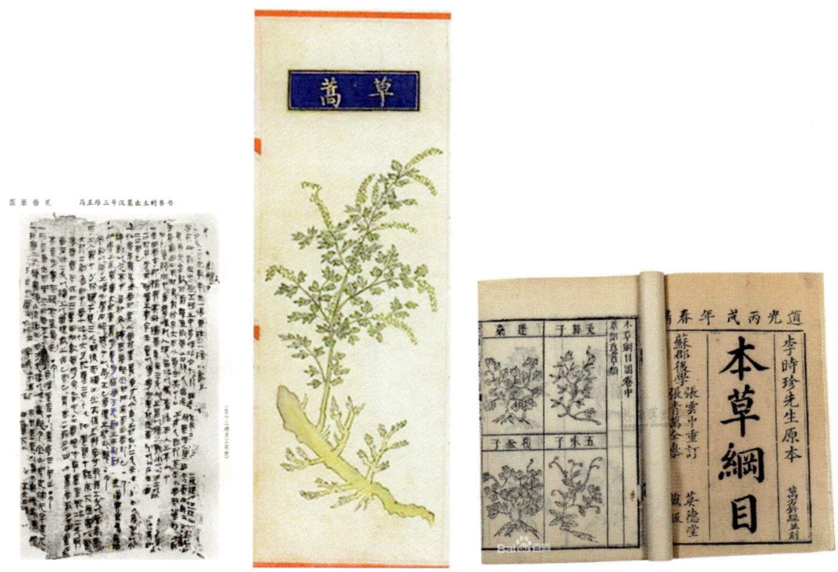

FIGURE 18. *Prescriptions for Fifty-Two Kinds of Disease*, unearthed from the Third Han Tomb at Mawangdui (left), *Bu Yi Lei Gong Pao Zhi* (middle), and *Compendium of Materia Medica* (right).

general name of the *Artemisia* family) regardless of numerous mentions of the name Qinghao in the literature, nor did the texts specify the effective parts of the plant. All the species in Qinghao (*Artemisia*) family were used. By the time that research on artemisinin was carried out, two Qinghao (*Artemisia*) species were listed in the Chinese Pharmacopoeia and four others were also being prescribed.

Our studies confirmed that only *Artemisia annua* L. (sweet wormwood) contains meaningful quantity of artemisinin. We subsequently carried out a thorough study on the herb Qinghao.

Figures 19 and 20 show illustrative descriptions of plants and epidermis structures of leaves from different species in the *Artemisia* family [23]. Figure 21 shows the thin-layer chromatographic spectrums of extracts from *Artemisia annua* L., *Artemisia scoparia* Waldst. et kit., *Artemisia eriopoda* Bunge, *Artemisia capillaris* Thunb., *Artemisia japonica* Thunb., and *Artemisia apiacea* Hance [23].

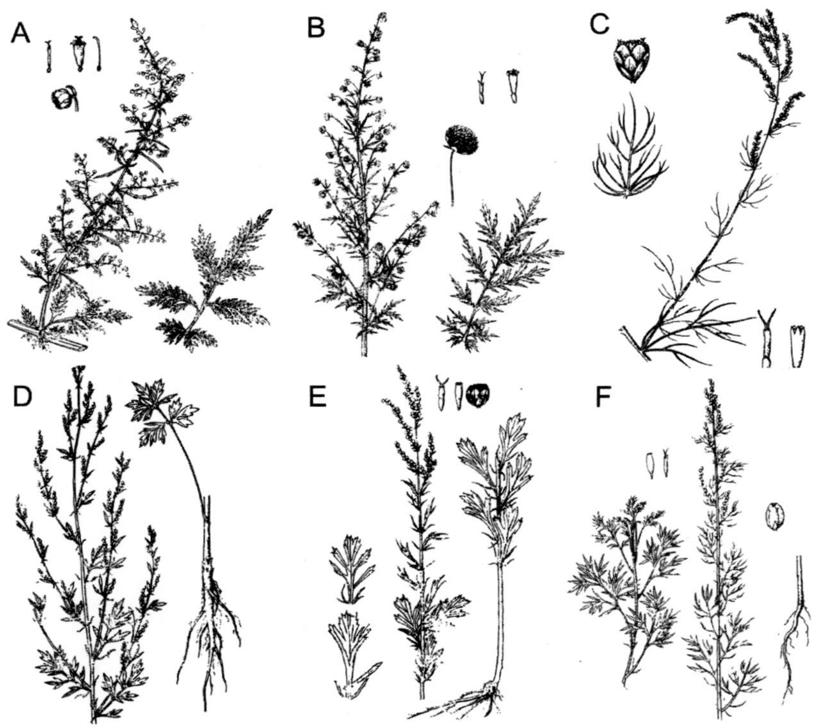

FIGURE 19. Illustrative description of six species in the artemisia family A. *Artemisia annua* L., B. *Artemisia apiacea* Hance C. *Artemisia capillaris* Thunb., D. *Artemisia eriopoda* Bunge, E. *Artemisia japonica* Thunb., F. *Artemisia scoparia* Waldst. et kit.

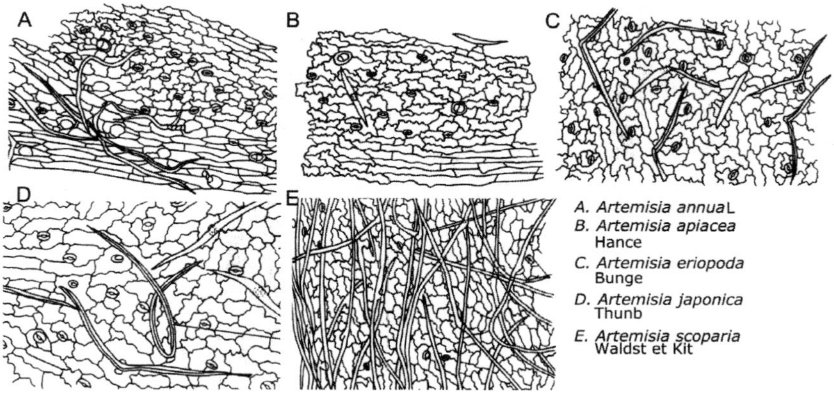

FIGURE 20. Illustrative epidermis structures of leaves from different species in the *Artemisia* family (*Artemisia capillaries* Thunb. has the epidermis structure similar to *Artemisia scoparia* Waldst. et Kit.).

Samples No 2 (*Artemisia annua* L. from Hainan province) and No 3 (*Artemisia annua* L. from Beijing) have peaks eluted at the same retention time as the artemisinin reference standard (sample No. 1) while No. 4 (*Artemisia scoparia* Waldst. et kit.), No. 5 (*Artemisia eriopoda* Bunge), No. 6 (*Artemisia capillaris* Thunb.), No. 7 (*Artemisia japonica* Thunb.) and No. 8 (*Artemisia apiacea* Hance)

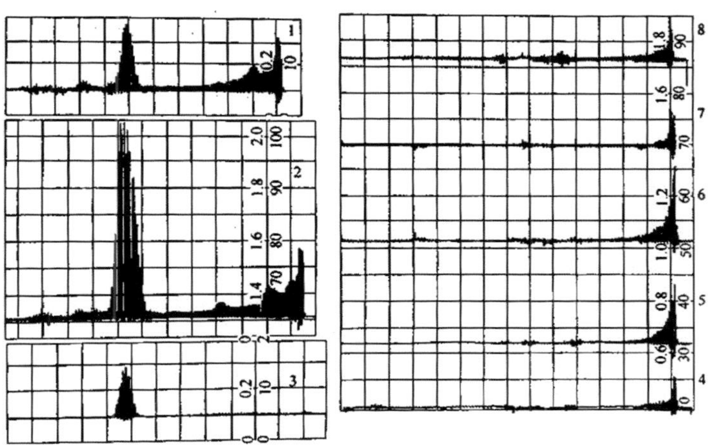

FIGURE 21. Thin-layer chromatographic spectrums of the extracts (Kieselgel 60 F254, mobile phase: Petroleum ether/ethyl acetate = 85/15) from 1. Artemisinin reference standard 2. *Artemisia annua* L. from Hainan province, 3. *Artemisia annua* L. from Beijing, 4. *Artemisia scoparia* Waldst. et kit., 5. *Artemisia eriopoda* Bunge, 6. *Artemisia capillaris* Thunb., 7. *Artemisia japonica* Thunb., 8. *Artemisia apiacea* Hance.

do not have any peaks or do not contain artemisinin. The peak from the sample No. 2 (*Artemisia annua* L. from Hainan province) was much higher than that from the sample No. 3 (*Artemisia annua* L. from Beijing) suggesting that *Artemisia annua* L. growing in Hainan province contained more artemisinin compared to the *Artemisia annua* L. collected from Beijing.

In addition to the confusion in finding the right plant, variables such as the part and origin of the plant, its harvest season, low artemisinin content in the plant, extraction and purification process etc. added extra difficulties in the discovery of artemisinin. Success in identifying effectiveness of neutral Qinghao ethyl ether extract was not a simple and easy win.

No doubt, traditional Chinese medicine provides a rich resource. Nevertheless, it requires our thoughtful consideration to explore and improve.

Persistence in the face of challenges

Research conditions were relatively poor in China in the 1970s. In order to produce sufficient quantities of Qinghao extract for clinical trials, our team carried out extraction using several household water vats (Figure 22). Some team members' health deteriorated due to long-term exposure to large quantities of organic

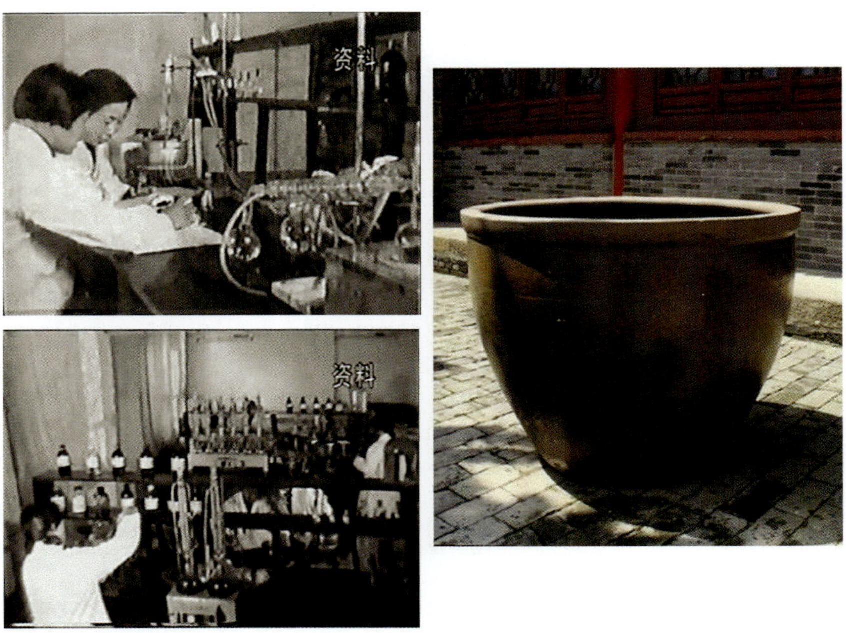

FIGURE 22. Under-resourced research conditions in 1970s China.

solvents and insufficient ventilation equipment. In order to launch clinical trials sooner while not compromising patient safety, based on the limited safety data from the animal study, the team members and myself volunteered to take Qinghao extract ourselves to assure its safety. In 1973, unsatisfactory results were observed in the clinical trial using artemisinin tablets, the team carried out a thorough investigation and verified poor disintegration of the tablets as the root cause, which allowed us to quickly resume the trial using capsules and confirmed artemisinin's clinical efficacy in time.

Collaborative team efforts expedited translation from scientific discovery to effective medicine

An antimalarial drug research symposium was held by the national project 523 office in Nanjing on March 8, 1972. At this meeting, on behalf of the Institute of Chinese Materia Medica, I reported the positive readouts of Qinghao extract No. 191 observed in animal studies performed on rodent malaria and monkeys. The presentation evoked significant interest. On November 17, 1972, I reported the results of the successful treatment of thirty clinical cases at the national conference held in Beijing. This triggered nationwide collaboration in research on Qinghao for malaria treatment.

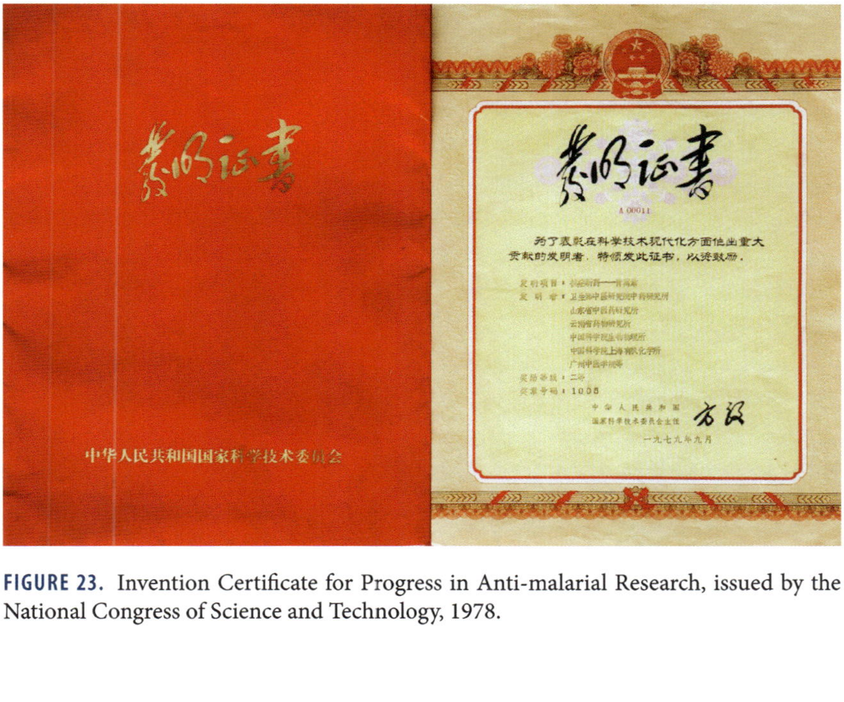
中华人民共和国国家科学技术委员会
A 00011
为了表彰在科学技术现代化方面作出重大贡献的发明者，特颁发此证书，以资鼓励。
中华人民共和国
国家科学技术委员会主任
一九七九年九月

FIGURE 23. Invention Certificate for Progress in Anti-malarial Research, issued by the National Congress of Science and Technology, 1978.

Today, I would like to express my sincere appreciation again to my fellow Project 523 colleagues at the Academy of Traditional Chinese Medicine for their devotion and exceptional contributions during the discovery and subsequent application of artemisinin. I would like to, once again, thank and congratulate our colleagues from the Shandong Provincial Institute of Chinese Medicine, the Yunnan Provincial Institute of Materia Medica, the Institute of Biophysics of Chinese Academy of Sciences, the Shanghai Institute of Organic Chemistry of the Chinese Academy of Sciences, the Guangzhou University of Chinese Medicine, the Academy of Military Medical Sciences and many other institutes for their invaluable contributions in their respective areas of responsibility during our collaboration and their help in caring for malaria patients (Figure 23).

I would also like to express my sincere respect to the national 523 office leadership team for their continuous efforts in organizing and coordinating the antimalarial research programs.

Without collective efforts, we would not have been able to present artemisinin—our gift to the world—in such a short period of time.

MALARIA CONTROL AND RESISTANCE OR TOLERANCE TO ARTEMISININ DRUGS

Malaria remains a severe challenge to global public health

"The findings in this year's World Malaria Report demonstrate that the world is continuing to make impressive progress in reducing malaria cases and deaths," Dr. Margaret Chan, Director-General of World Health Organization, commented in the recent *World Malaria Report* [24].

The report indicated positive progress in malaria control as a result of continuous intervention: "Since the year 2000, average malaria infection prevalence declined 46% in children aged 2–10, from 26% to 14% in 2013. The number of malaria infections at any one time dropped 26%, from 173 million to 128 million in 2013. Malaria mortality rates have decreased by 47% worldwide and by 54% in the WHO Africa Region . . . . By 2015, if the annual rate of decrease over the past 13 years is maintained, malaria mortality rates are projected to decrease by 55% globally and by 62% in the WHO Africa Region. Malaria mortality rates in children aged under 5 years are projected to decrease by 61% globally and 67% in the WHO Africa Region."

Nevertheless, statistically, approximately 3.3 billion people across 97 countries or regions are still at risk of contracting malaria and around 1.2 billion people live in high-risk regions where the annual infection rate is at or above one per 1000 [24].

According to the latest statistical estimate, approximately 198 million cases of malaria occurred globally in 2013, causing 584,000 deaths, with 90% of these in severely affected African countries and 78% being children below age five. Only 70% of malaria patients receive artemisinin combination therapies (ACTs) in Africa and as high as 56 millions to 69 millions of child malaria patients do not have ACTs available for them [24].

A severe warning about parasites resistant to artemisinin

Plasmodium falciparum resistance to artemisinin has been detected in five countries of the Greater Mekong subregion: Cambodia, the Lao People's Democratic Republic, Myanmar, Thailand and Vietnam. In many areas along the Cambodia–Thailand border, *Plasmodium falciparum* has become resistant to most available antimalarial medicines.

Tolerance of the *Plasmodium falciparum* to mono artemisinin therapy has increased significantly. Although artemisinin-based combination therapies are still highly efficacious, increases in the rates of treatment failure with artesunate–mefloquine in Thailand and with dihydroartemisinin-piperaquine in Cambodia have been reported. There was evidence of genetic changes in the parasites, *i.e.* mutations in the Kelch 13 (K13) propeller domain associated with their reduced susceptibility and slow clearance [25].

It is an even more serious concern—or a severe warning—that resistance to artemisnin is not only detected in the Greater Mekong sub-region but has also appeared in some African regions [25].

Global plan for artemisinin-resistant containment

WHO launched the Global Plan for Artemisinin Resistant Containment (GPARC) in January 2011 with a goal to maximize protection to artemisinin combination therapies as an effective treatment for *Plasmodium falciparum* malaria. Artemisinin resistance has been confirmed within the Greater Mekong sub-region, and potential epidemic risk is undergoing a critical review. Over a hundred experts involved in the program reached unanimous agreement that the chance of containing and eradicating artemisinin-resistant malaria is very limited and there is an urgent need to constrain artemisinin resistance.

A proactive matrix approach by stopping the spread of resistant parasites, increasing monitoring and surveillance to evaluate the artemisinin resistance threat; improving access to diagnostics and rational treatment with artemisinin combination therapies, investing in artemsinin resistance-related research, and motivating action and mobilizing resources is encouraged by WHO to contain or eliminate artemisinin resistance where it already exists and prevent artemisinin resistance where it has not yet appeared [8].

To protect the efficacy of artemisinin combination therapies, I strongly urge global compliance with WHO's Global Plan for Artemisinin Resistant Containment. This is our responsibility as scientists and medical doctors in the field.

CHINESE MEDICINE, A GREAT TREASURE

Before concluding, I would like to briefly discuss Chinese medicine. "Chinese medicine and pharmacology are a great treasure-house. We should explore them and raise them to a higher level." (Figure 24). Artemisinin was explored using this resource. From our research experience in discovering artemisinin, we learned the strengths of both Chinese and Western medicine. There is great potential for future advances if these strengths can be fully integrated. We have a substantial amount of natural resources from which our fellow medical researchers can develop novel medicines.

Since "Tasting a hundred herbs by Sheng Nong," we have accumulated substantial experience in clinical practice, integrated and summarized the medical application of most nature resources over the past several thousand years through Chinese medicine. Adopting, exploring, developing and advancing these practices would allow us to discover more novel medicines beneficial to global healthcare.

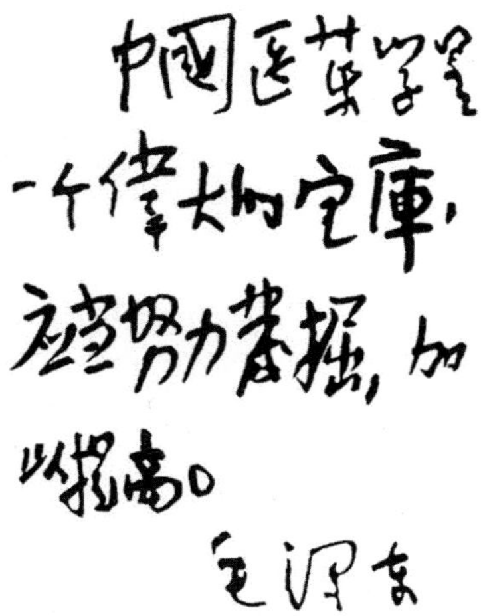

FIGURE 24. Handwriting of Mao Zedong: "Chinese medicine and pharmacology are a great treasure-house. We should explore them and raise them to a higher level."

To end my lecture, I would like to share with you a well-known poem, "On the stork tower," written during the Tang Dynasty by Wang Zhihuan (688–742 AD).

> "The sun along the mountain bows; The Yellow River seawards flows;
> You will enjoy a grander sight; By climbing to a greater height."

Let us reach to a greater height to appreciate Chinese culture and find the beauty and treasure in the territory of traditional Chinese medicine!

ACKNOWLEDGEMENTS

I would like to thank all my colleagues in China and overseas for their contributions to the discovery, research and clinical applications of artemisinin!

I am deeply grateful to all my family members for their continuous understanding and support!

I sincerely appreciate your kind attention!

Thank you all!

REFERENCES

1. Hippocrates, *On Airs, Waters, and Places*. 400 B.C. London: Sydenham Society; 1849:179–222.
2. 黄帝内经 疟论篇 第三十五 (Section Thirty Five, Chapter on Malaria of Inner Canon of Yellow Emperor).
3. Ernst Hempelmann and Kristine Krafts, Bad air, amulets and mosquitoes: 2,000 years of changing perspectives on malaria, *Malaria Journal* 2013, **12**:232. (http://www.malariajournal.com/content/12/1/232).
4. Alphonse Laveran—Nobel Lecture: Protozoa as Causes of Diseases. December 11, 1907. "Alphonse Laveran—Nobel Lecture: Protozoa as Causes of Diseases." Nobelprize.org. Nobel Media AB 2014. Web. Jan 1, 2016. http://www.nobelprize.org/nobel_prizes/medicine/laureates/1907/laveran-lecture.html.
5. Ronald Ross—Nobel Lecture, Researches on Malaria, December, 12, 1902. "Ronald Ross—Nobel Lecture: Researches on Malaria." Nobelprize.org. Nobel Media AB 2014. Web. Jan 1, 2016. http://www.nobelprize.org/nobel_prizes/medicine/laureates/1902/ross-lecture.html.
6. William E. Collins and Geoffrey M. Jeffery, Plasmodium malariae: Parasite and Disease, *Clin Microbiol Rev.* 2007 Oct; **20**(4): 579–592.
7. National Institutes of Health National Institute of Allergy and Infectious Diseases (NIAID) Science Education, *Understanding Malaria, Fighting an Ancient Scourge.*
8. Centers for Disease Control and Prevention, *Choosing a Drug to Prevent Malaria* (http://www.cdc.gov/malaria/travelers/drugs.html).
9. WHO, *Guidelines for the treatment of malaria*, Third edition, April 2015.

10. WHO, *Global Plan for Artemisinin Resistance Containment* (GPARC).
11. WHO, *Emergency Response to Artemisinin Resistance in the Greater Mekong Subregion.*
12. 神农本草经 卷三 下经 草 下品 草蒿 (*Sheng Nong's Herbal Classic*, Volume 3).
13. 屠呦呦等, 青蒿及青蒿素类药物, 第9页, 化工出版社 (Tu Youyou *et al. Artemisia and Artemisinin Drugs*, page 9, Chemical Industry Press ISBN 978-7-122-00857-2).
14. COL Christian F. Ockenhouse, History of U.S. Military Contributions to the Study of Malaria, *Military Medicine*, 170, 4:12, 2005.
15. 钱伟长, 刘德培, 20世纪中国知名科学家学术成就概览 · 医学卷 · 药学分册, 333页 (Qian Wei-Chang, Liu De-Pei, Chinese Famous Scientist of the 20th Century Academic Overview, Volume Medicine, Pharmacy, Page 333, Science Press ISBN 978-7-03-041517-2)
16. 疟疾防治研究工作领导小组, 全国疟疾防治研究工作座谈会议的总结, 1971年6月1日 (The National Leading Group Office for Malaria Control, Summary of National Malaria Control Research Meeting, 1st Jun 1971).
17. 屠呦呦等, 青蒿及青蒿素类药物, 第40页,化工出版社 (Tu Youyou *et al.* Artemisia and Artemisinin Drugs, page 40, Chemical Industry Press ISBN 978-7-122-00857-2).
18. 全国疟疾防治研究工作领导小组, 疟疾防治研究工作情况交流 (14), 1972年11月5日 (The National Leading Group Office for Malaria Control, Communication on Malaria Control Research, 5th November 1972).
19. 屠呦呦等, 青蒿及青蒿素类药物, 第45–56页, 化工出版社 (Tu Youyou *et al.* Artemisia and Artemisinin Drugs, pages 45–56, Chemical Industry Press ISBN 978-7-122-00857-2).
20. 青蒿素结构研究协作组, 一种新型的倍半萜内酯-青蒿素 科学通报1911, 3: 142 (Research Group for Artemisinin: A New Sesquiterpene Lactone—Artemisinin, *Chinese Science Bulletin*, 1977, 3:142).
21. C.A. 1977, 87, 98788g.
22. 葛洪, 肘后备急方, 卷三, 治寒热诸疟方第十六 (Ge Hong, *A Handbook of Prescriptions for Emergencies*, the 3rd Volume, Recipe No. Sixteen for Treating Cold and Fevers of Malaria, East Jin Dynasty, 300–400 A.D.).
23. 屠呦呦等, 青蒿及青蒿素类药物, 第13–30页,化工出版社 (Tu Youyou *et al. Artemisia and Artemisinin Drugs*, pages 13–26, Chemical Industry Press ISBN 978-7-122-00857-2).
24. WHO, World Malaria Report 2014, ISBN 978 92 4 156483 0.
25. Elizabeth A. Ashley *et al*, Spread of Artemisinin Resistance in *Plasmodium falciparum* Malaria, *New England Journal of Medicine*, 2014; **371**:411–423 July 31, 2014.